General Epidemiology for Health Professionals

General Epidemiology for Health Professionals

Editor

Ram Chandra Goyal MBBS MD (Community Medicine)

FIAPSM (Fellowship of Indian Association of PSM) FIPHA (Fellowship of Indian Public Health Association)

Head, Community Health Services
Trichy SRM Medical College, Hospital and Research Center
Irungalur, Trichy, Tamil Nadu, India

Ex-Dean, Rural Medical College, Ahmednagar, Maharashtra, India

CBS

CBS Publishers & Distributors Pvt Ltd

New Delhi • Bengaluru • Chennai • Kochi • Kolkata • Mumbai

Hyderabad • Jharkhand • Nagpur • Patna • Pune • Uttarakhand

General Epidemiology
for Health Professionals

ISBN: 978-93-88902-97-7

First Edition: 2021

Published by Satish Kumar Jain and Produced by Varun Jain for

CBS Publishers & Distributors Pvt Ltd
4819/XI, Prahlad Street, 24 Ansari Road, Daryaganj, New Delhi 110 002, India
Ph: 011-23289259, 23266861, 23266867 Fax: 011-23243014 Website: www.cbspd.com
e-mail: delhi@cbspd.com; cbspubs@airtelmail.in

Corporate Office: 204 FIE, Industrial Area, Patparganj, Delhi 110 092
Ph: 011-4934 4934 Fax: 011-4934 4935 e-mail: publishing@cbspd.com; publicity@cbspd.com

Branches

- **Bengaluru:** Seema House 2975, 17th Cross, K.R. Road, Banasankari 2nd Stage, Bengaluru 560 070, Karnataka
  Ph: +91-80-26771678/79 Fax: +91-80-26771680 e-mail: bangalore@cbspd.com
- **Chennai:** 7, Subbaraya Street, Shenoy Nagar, Chennai 600 030, Tamil Nadu
  Ph: +91-44-26680620, 26681266 Fax: +91-44-42032115 e-mail: chennai@cbspd.com
- **Kochi:** 42/1325, 1326, Power House Road, Opp. KSEB, Power House, Ernakulam 682 018, Kochi, Kerala
  Ph: +91-484-4059061-67 Fax: +91-484-4059065 e-mail: kochi@cbspd.com
- **Kolkata:** 6/B, Ground Floor, Rameswar Shaw Road, Kolkata-700 014, West Bengal
  Ph: +91-33-22891126, 22891127, 22891128 e-mail: kolkata@cbspd.com
- **Mumbai:** 83-C, Dr E Moses Road, Worli, Mumbai-400018, Maharashtra
  Ph: +91-22-24902340/41 Fax: +91-22-24902342 e-mail: mumbai@cbspd.com

Representatives

• **Hyderabad**	0-9885175004	• **Jharkhand**	0-9811541605	• **Nagpur**	0-9421945513
• **Patna**	0-9334159340	• **Pune**	0-9623451994	• **Uttarakhand**	0-9716462459

Printed at: Rashtriya Printers, Dilshad Garden, Delhi, India

to

health professionals
who strive for the
globally healthy communities

List of Contributors

Badrinarayan Mishra MBBS MD (Community Medicine) DSA DSM
Professor
Department of Community Medicine
RD Gardi Medical College
Ujjain, Madhya Pradesh, India

Himanshu Negandhi MD (Community Medicine) Master of Medicine (Clin Epi)
Additional Professor
Department of Community Medicine
Indian Institute of Public Health, Delhi
Public Health Foundation of India

Mabashshera Firdos Khan
Tutor
Department of Community Medicine
All India Institute of Medical Sciences
Nagpur, Maharashtra, India

Mohan K Doibale MBBS MD (PSM) DTT DHA CIT FIAPSM FIPHA
Professor and Head
Department of Community Medicine (PSM)
Government Medical College
Aurangabad, Maharashtra, India

Paramita Sengupta MBBS MD (Community Medicine) MPH (UK)
Dean, Professor and Head
Department of Community and Family Medicine
All India Institute of Medical Sciences
Kalyani, West Bengal, India

Pradeep Deshmukh MBBS MD (Community Medicine)
Professor and Head
Department of Community Medicine
All India Institute of Medical Sciences
Nagpur (MS), India

Pradeep Kumar MBBS MD (Community Medicine)
Professor
Department of Community Medicine
Dr M K Shah Medical College
Ahmadabad, Gujarat, India

Purushottam Giri MBBS, MD (PSM)
Professor
Department of Community Medicine
IIMSR Medical College
Badnapur, District Jalna (MS), India

Ram Chandra Goyal MBBS MD (Community Medicine) FIAPSM (Fellowship of Indian Association of PSM) FIPHA (Fellowship of Indian Public Health Association)
Head
Community Health Services
Trichy SRM Medical College, Hospital and Research Center
Irungalur, Trichy (TN) India
Ex-Dean, Rural Medical College
Ahmednagar (MS), India

Sanjay P Zodpey MBBS, MD (PSM)
Professor and Vice President (Academics)
Public Health Foundation of India, New Delhi, India
Director, Indian Institute of Public Health
New Delhi, India

Vinay Rao MBBS MD (Community Medicine)
Associate Professor
Department of Community Medicine
Father Muller Medical College
Mangalore, Karnataka, India

Preface

Epidemiology is the cornerstone in health sciences, be it be human or animal. Epidemiology has paved the way in all clinical disciplines apart from promotive and preventive health. The practice of epidemiology has forced us to study social, political, genetic, macro- and micro-environment, legal, economic, GIS, management and other issues to understand dynamics of health. This help us to develop effective and efficient public health policies and programs applicable local to global level.

An idea of writing this book came to my mind when I saw my students struggling to understand and comprehend societal dynamics to implement principles of epidemiology while practicing public health. I also realized while working in developed countries that every health professional, clinical/non-clinical, must know the basics of epidemiology to undertake clinical/public health practice. Therefore, I felt the need to bring out this book *General Epidemiology for Health Professionals*.

We, the contributors, have tried hard to create an 'aura of conscience' among clinical practitioners regarding analytical and holistic approach to their practice for their health seekers through this book penned by eminent public health professionals.

The contributors have helped write an extremely integrated, illustrative comprehensive book comprising 20 chapters. Apart from basic principles of epidemiology, it also includes an introduction to spatial epidemiology, applied epidemiology, field epidemiology, epidemiological statistics, and basics of infectious disease modelling, surveillance system, ethical issues and practical tools.

This book has the following strengths:

1. The contributors are eminent mentors, facilitators and practitioners of public health epidemiology.
2. It is based on local to global examples.
3. Comprehensive with inclusion of chapters like spatial epidemiology, applied epidemiology, field epidemiology, basics of infectious disease modelling, and international health regulations.
4. Liberal use of graphical depiction for better comprehension.
5. Easier ways of understanding concepts and calculations.
6. Simple language without complex technical jargons for better understanding, even by a primary healthcare professional.
7. Based on more than four decades of cumulative experience.

This book is crafted in such a way that all health professionals (national and international) will be able to decipher concepts and practice epidemiology for the larger good. The book will be especially beneficial to graduates and postgraduates, medical/health teachers and practitioners and to some extent, advanced learners. I am sure all policy makers, managers and their colleagues will be immensely benefitted.

The readers will appreciate the constraints of length and breath, scope, facts and interpretation of each topic mentioned in this book. We have worked hard to include all basics with some advanced elements to fulfil the quest of the readers.

I look forward to all my readers to help enrich this book and the topics therein by sharing their valuable suggestions, so we can incorporate them for the betterment of the next edition.

Ram Chandra Goyal
Email: drgoyal45@gmail.com

Acknowledgements

My journey into the medical profession started from my village, where I was the witness, sufferer and survivor of the ravages of the disease known as smallpox.

The next milestone in my life and education was solely due to my alma mater, Mahatma Gandhi Institute of Medical Sciences (MGIMS). This internationally acclaimed institution is located in Sewagram, Wardha which is also home to the Sewagram Ashram, home to Mahatma Gandhi for a brief period of time. I too stayed in Sewagram Ashram as a part of my initiation and later in another remote village during the first year of my medical education. It was during this time that we were unknowingly exposed to a world class system that taught us societal dynamics and application of epidemiology.

My sincere gratitude towards the innumerable pure souls that I interacted and learned from. These include but are definitely not limited to teachers, guides, colleagues, students, policy makers and implementers with whom I interacted during the various classes, field work, discussions, workshops, conferences, etc.

I am extremely indebted to my colleagues at Al-Arab University, Benghazi, Libya, who encouraged me pen down this book. I started planning the chapters and writing the topics of the books along with my Indian colleagues but was not able to pursue our goal to fruition due to an abrupt departure as a result of the 2011 Civil War.

It is around this time that I started work on what is now my first book, *Research Methodology for Health Professionals*' published by Jaypee Brothers, New Delhi to whom I am so very thankful. Upon the successful completion and launch of this book, the dormant wish and zeal to complete my earlier work took seed. Fuelled by the motivation and encouragement of my beloved wife, Baby Goyal, I took up the task of reframing and redesigning the proposed book and invited eminent professionals of repute in the field of public health and epidemiology. I am indeed grateful to all my learned contributors who gladly accepted my invitation and contributed their experienced writings with full enthusiasm.

I would like to extend my warm and heartfelt thanks to Prof (Dr) Sanjay P Zodpey, Prof (Dr) Pradeep Kumar, Dr Mohan K Doibale, Prof (Dr) BN Mishra, Prof (Dr) Paramita Sengupta, Prof (Dr) Pradeep Deshmukh, Prof (Dr) Purushottam Giri, Prof (Dr) Vinay Rao, Himanshu Negandhi and Mabashshera Firdos Khan for their valuable contributions to this book.

I sincerely thank to CBS Publishers & Distributors Pvt Ltd, New Delhi, for accepting this manuscript for publication and promotion.

I also wish to thank all persons who are unnamed here for their direct and indirect support in helping me to complete this book.

Last but not the least, my unconditional love and affection to my wife Baby and my family: Abhishek, Abhilasha, Dhiraj and Pranonita. Thank you all for your support at all times during the completion of this book.

Ram Chandra Goyal

Contents

Chapter

1

Introduction to Epidemiology

Ram Chandra Goyal

HISTORICAL AND DEVELOPMENTAL BACKGROUND OF EPIDEMIOLOGY

INTRODUCTION

The understanding of epidemiology should help to achieve health for all and this concept probably exists since the existence of human being. The development of epidemiology to its present form has its roots even before the primary documented descriptions written by Hippocrates, the 'Father of Medicine'.

The intension of author is to briefly review the development of modern epidemiology so that one can understand how keen observation, self-acquired knowledge and a critical but positive attitude help in understanding of health and disease.

To review of past, present and future of epidemiology may be classified under following headings.

A. Early epidemiology, extending from the fifth century BC to around 1830;
B. Classical epidemiology, from around 1830 to the 1940s;
C. Modern epidemiology, from the 1940s to the present.

Early Epidemiology

Numerous keen epidemiological observations were made in the past and have been handed down in surviving documents, based at best on simple or crude methods of investigation.

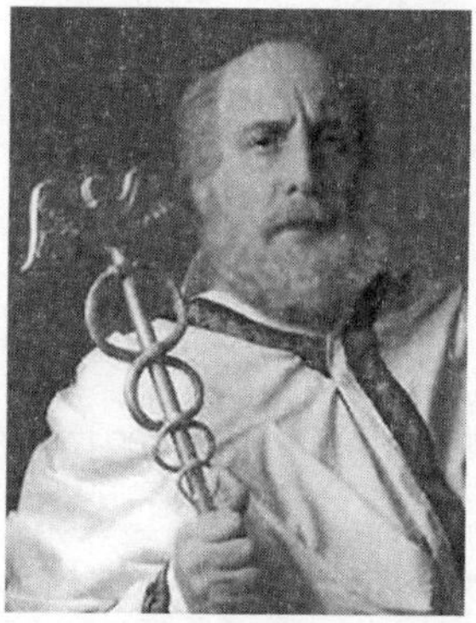

Hippocrates (ca 460–ca 375 BC)
'The Father of Medicine'

Hippocrates (ca 460–ca 375 BC) attempted to explain disease occurrence from a rational rather than a supernatural viewpoint. He suggested that environmental and host factors such as behaviour might influence the development of disease.

Epidemiological theories were also elaborated to explain the spreading of diseases, mainly the 'epidemics'. Hippocrates developed the medical approach by providing concise, accurate, and complete descriptions of actual clinical cases, including diseases such as tetanus, typhus, and phthisis. This remained 'without parallel until the late seventeenth century'. However, in his book on *Airs, Waters and Places*, he clearly identified as a seminal environmental scientist—the general dependence of health not on magical influences but on an identifiable array of natural external factors (Box 1.1 and Fig. 1.1).[1]

Hippocrates states in his writings on *De Affectionibus*, "When you face a sick person you should ask him from what he is suffering, for what reason, for how many days, what he eats and what are his bowel movements". To all these questions one should add "What work does he do?"

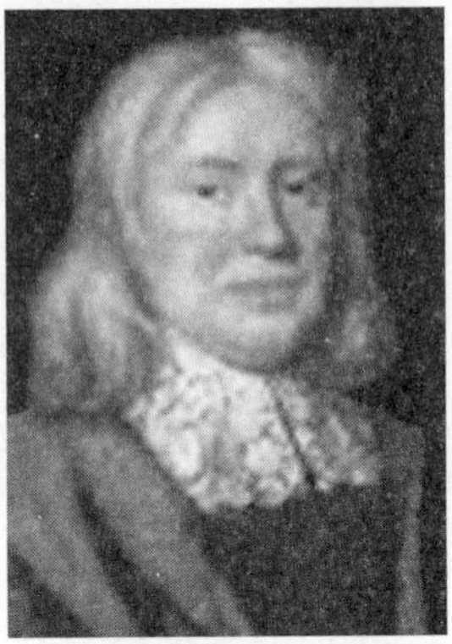

Thomas Sydenham (1624–1689)

Box 1.1

Whoever wishes to investigate medicine properly should proceed, thus—in the first place to consider the seasons of the year, and what effects each of them produces. Then the winds, the hot and the cold, especially such as are common to all countries, and then such as are peculiar to each locality. In the same manner, when one comes into a city to which he is a stranger, he should consider its situation, how it lies as to the winds and the rising of the sun; for its influence is not the same whether it lies to the north or the south, to the rising or to the setting sun. One should consider most attentively the waters which the inhabitants use, whether they be marshy and soft, or hard and running from elevated and rocky situations, and then if saltish and unfit for cooking; and the ground, whether it be naked and deficient in water, or wooded and well watered, and whether it lies in a hollow, confined situation, or it elevated and cold; and the mode in which the inhabitants live, and what are their pursuits, whether they are fond of drinking and eating to excess, and given to indolence, or are fond of exercise and labor.

Hippocrates

On Airs, Waters and Places

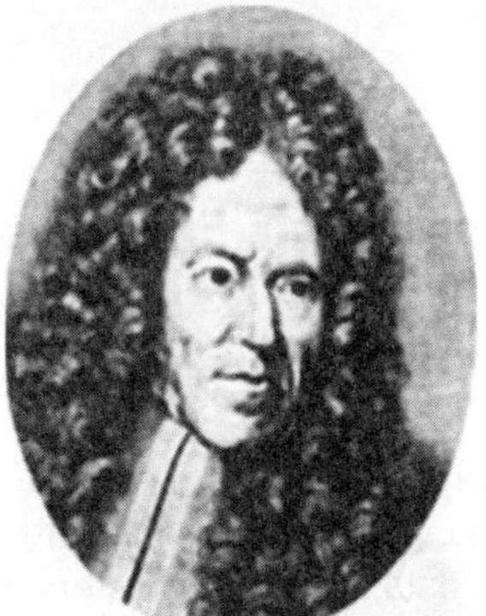

Bernardino Ramazzini (1633–1714)
'The founder of occupational medicine'

Thomas Sydenham (1624–1689), revived the clinical observation and brought attention back to the circumstances surrounding the occurrence of clinical cases.

In the year 1700, **Bernardino Ramazzini (1633–1714)**, the founder of occupational medicine, in his book on occupational diseases, *De Morbis Artificum Diatriba* (*Diseases of Workers*) outlined the health hazards of chemicals, dust, metals, repetitive or violent motions, odd postures, and other disease-causative agents encountered by workers in 52 occupations. He conjectured that the relatively high incidence of breast cancer among nuns was due to celibacy.[2]

Sixty-two years later, **Percival Pott (1775)**, was among the first ones to do a comparative observation in quantitative terms. He reported that scrotal cancer was very frequent among London chimney workers, and that their death rate due to this disease was more than 200 times higher than that of other workers.

Giovanni Maria Lancisi (1654–1720), anatomist and clinician, 'personal physician to Pope' in his book on *De Subitaneis Mortibus* (1707), reported a detailed pathological

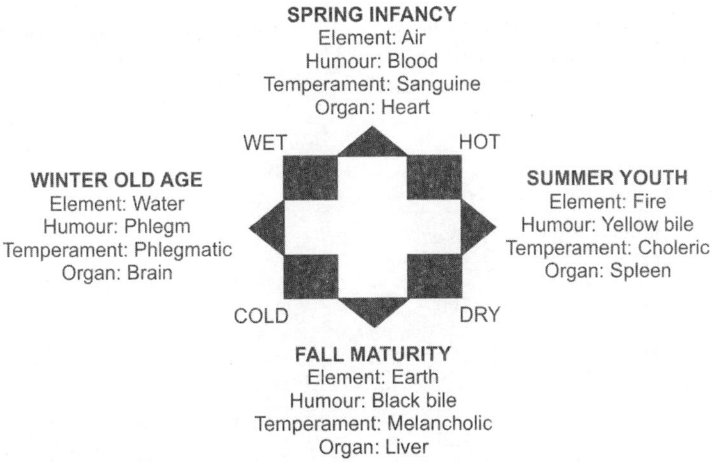

Fig. 1.1: Natural external factors of health

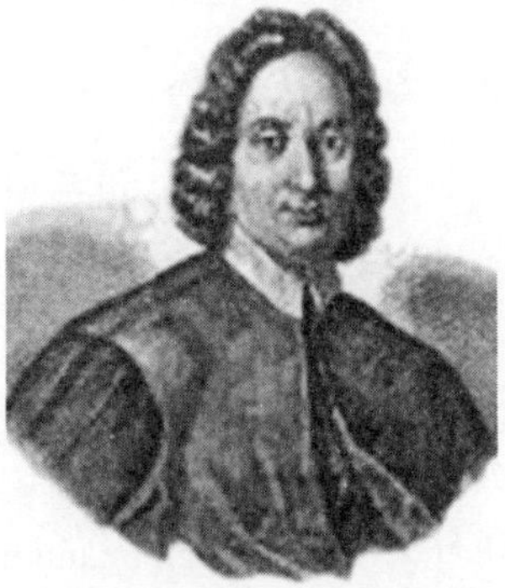

Giovanni Maria Lancisi (1654–1720)

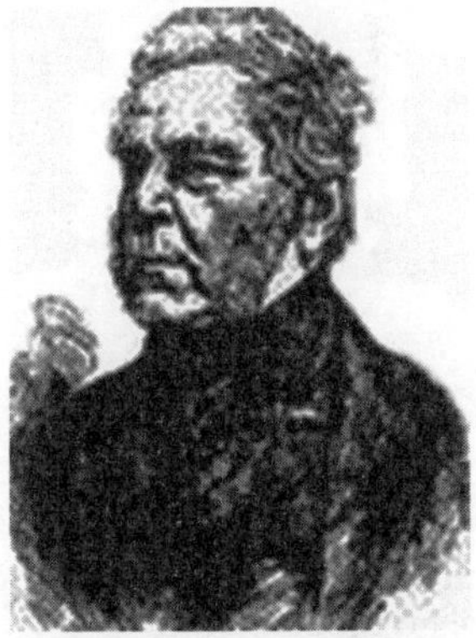

John Graunt (1620–1674)
'The founder of demography'

investigation of a series of sudden deaths in Rome, is probably the first epidemiological study of a non-communicable condition (Lebowitz, 1970).

Demographic approach was already developing in the latter part of the fourteenth and in the fifteenth centuries, e.g. in Florence and Venice the counting of deaths and some early form of death certification specifying the cause in broad terms (e.g. 'plague' or 'not plague' during such epidemics) were current and established practices.[3]

The major step forward from recording, counting, and accounting to a quantitative analysis of the data was the later accomplishment of **John Graunt (1620–1674)** in London, who can be regarded as the founder of demography. His *Natural and Political Observations Upon the Bills of Mortality* (1662) was based on a series of weekly bills covering individual deaths and their causes in the London area back to 1603 (Tables 1.1–1.3).[4]

John Graunt's most original creation was 'life tables'—a new way to present population and mortality statistics by calculating survivorship on a chart. Using this method John Graunt was able to predict the number of persons who would survive to each successive age on his chart and the life expectancy of the groups from year to year. Development of the life tables has been hailed as marking the beginning of the science of demography. The types of charts John Graunt originated remain in use even today.[5]

Such charts made an impact on the pioneer demographic work of other noted astronomers and scientists, including Edmund Halley, England's astronomer royal.

Table 1.1: First life table

Age (years)	*Number dying*	*Number surviving*
Birth	0	100
6	36	64
16	24	40
26	15	25
36	9	16
46	6	10
56	4	6
66	3	3
76	2	1
86	1	0

Table 1.2: Counting the dead: The bills of mortality

Disease	*Number*	*Disease*	*Number*
Abortive and stilborn	445	Quinsie	7
Affrighted	1	Rising of the lights	98
Aged	628	Scurvey	9
Ague	43	Suddenly	62
Apoplex, and Meagrom	17	Surfeit	86
Bloody flux	348	Teeth	470
Bruised and ulcers	28	Thursh and sore mouth	40
Burst and rupture	9	Tympany	13
Cancer and wolf	10	Tissick	34
Canker	1	Vomiting	1
Childbed	171	Worms	27

Table. 1.3: Some of the observations of John Graunt are as under which show some early theories and concept in epidemiology

"That about one-third of all that were quick die under 5 years old, and about thirty six per centum under six"	High infant mortality
"That some diseases, and casualties keep a constant proportion, whereas some others are very irregular"	Differential mortality rates
"That a fourth part more die of the plague than are set down"	Underreporting
"There hath been in London within this age four times of great mortality—1592, 1603, 1625, and 1638, whereof that of 1603 was the greatest"	Cyclic (periodic) occurrence of disease
"That plagues always come in with king's reigns is most false"	Testable hypotheses
"That in London there has been twelve burials for eleven Christenings. That in the country there has been contrary-wise, sixty-three Christenings for fifty-two burials."	Urban-rural differences
"There come yearly to dwell at London about 6000 strangers out of the country, which swells the burials about 200 per annum"	Migration
"That there are about 6 millions, and a half of people in England, and Wales"	Census taking
"That every wedding one with another produces four children"	Fertility rates
"There being 14 males to 13 females, and males being prolifique 40 years, and females but 25, it follows that in effect there be 560 males to 325 females"	Sex ratio Death of women in child-birth

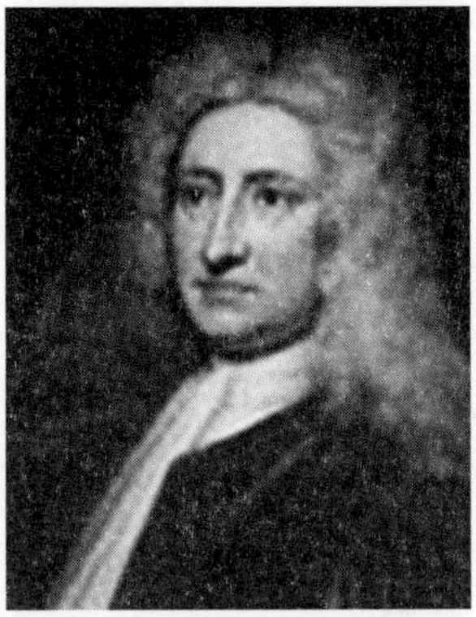

Edmund Halley (1656–1742)
'Inventor of first empirical life tables'

Edmund Halley (1656–1742), invented the first empirical life tables (after John Graunt, demographic studies), particularly in France, mathematical tools were being developed for dealing with chance events and probabilities, which were equally applicable to the study of such collective phenomena as births, deaths, etc.

One of the earlier theories regarding the fact that the most frequent and fatal diseases appeared obviously 'communicable', either from person to person or from fomites, has a forerunner in the Latin poet Lucretius (first–second century BC). In his poem *De Rerum Natura* hints that 'seeds' of disease can pass from a sick to a healthy individual.

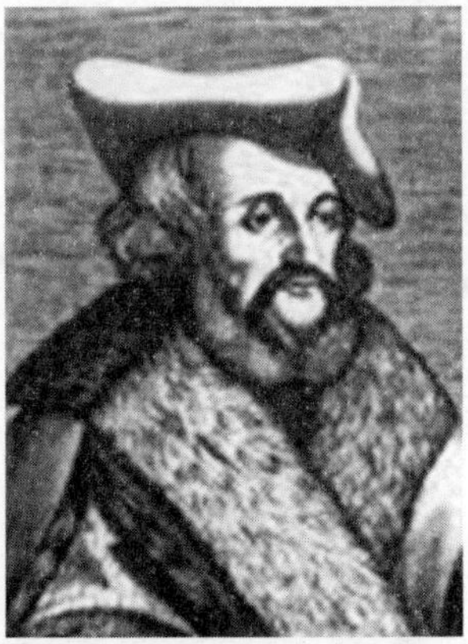

Gerolamo Fracastoro (1478–1553)

Later on **Gerolamo Fracastoro (1478–1553),** in his book *De Contagione et Contagiosis Morbis* (1546), presented the first clear and coherent germ theory of disease. Fracastoro theorized that a variety of diseases are caused by transmissible, self-propagating entities (germs) which, however, were conceived more as substances akin to present day viruses than to bacteria.

He thought that these agents were specific to each disease and could spread from person to person or through infected articles (fomites) or at a distance. He went as far as arguing that treatment should consist of the destruction of the germs by either heat or cold, or of their evacuation from the body, or by checking the putrefaction processes caused by these germs, or by neutralizing them by antagonistic substances. He studied new disease making ravages in his time and named as syphilis (1530).

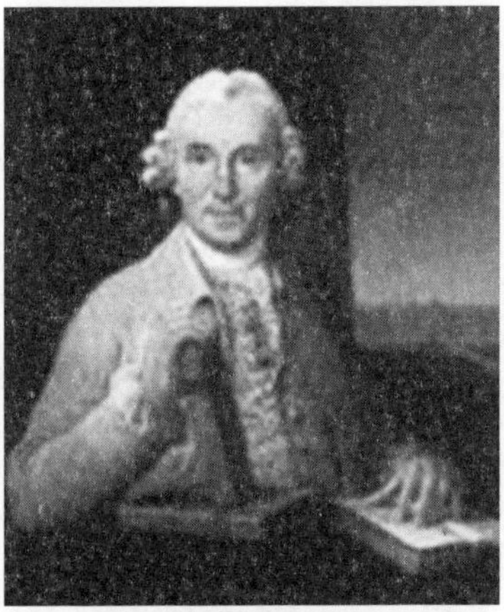

James Lind (1716–1794)
'The first one to conduct clinical trial'

James Lind (1716–1794), is being considered as the first one to do a clinical trial—a planned, comparative, and quantitative experiment on humans in order to learn something about the efficacy of a curative or preventive treatment in a clinical setting. In 1747, he tried out six different supplements to the basic diet of 12 sailors suffering from scurvy, and found that citrus fruits, and only these cured the patients. Later in 1771, he also compared quinine to treat malaria with less well-defined control therapies (Lind, 1771).[6]

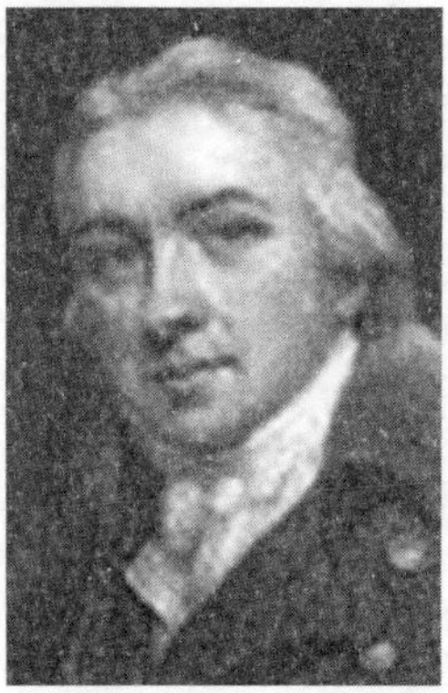

Edward Jenner (1749–1823)
'Inventor of smallpox vaccine and the first one to conduct preventive trialí

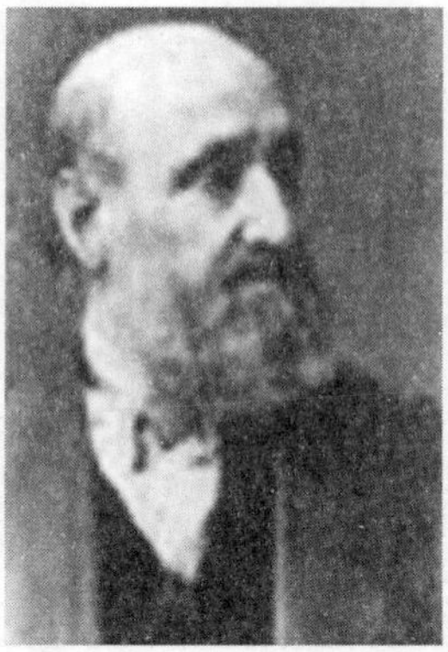

William Farr (1807–1883)
'The Father of Modern Vital Statistics and Surveillance'

Edward Jenner (1749–1823)—the first more or less rigorous trial of a preventive measure was performed by Jenner with 23 vaccinated people, but he still used what is now being called 'historical controls', i.e. he compared these vaccinated people with unvaccinated ones of the past who had not been specially selected beforehand for the purpose of the trial (Jenner, 1798).

The three streams in early epidemiology—medical, demographic and theoretical, coalesced in an effective way only towards the end of the eighteenth and beginning of the nineteenth centuries, giving rise to epidemiology as we recognize it today, an investigation of diseases and their aetiology at the population level.[7]

Classical Epidemiology

With the beginning of the industrial transformation of western Europe, starting in Great Britain and propagating from the mid-eighteenth century to the continent in the next decades, 'crowd diseases' emerged which struck the populations amassed in the slums of the fast-growing centers of industrial development (London, Glasgow, Manchester, Paris, Lyon, Berlin, etc.). This provided the decisive stimulus and observational field for epidemiology, which developed as the investigation facet of a vast public health movement.

In Great Britain medical registration of deaths had been introduced in 1801 and in 1838, **William Farr (1807–1883)** introduced a national system of recording causes of death. Once the mechanism started to work it provided a wealth of data which Farr himself first analyzed with great skill, making full use of life table techniques and of procedures for standardizing rates. He was also instrumental in building up a classification of diseases for statistical purposes, both national and international. His analyses, published from the Registrar General's Office at regular intervals, gave a picture of the evolving health condition of the population of Great Britain and drew the attention of all social investigators during the Victorian period, including Marx and Engels.

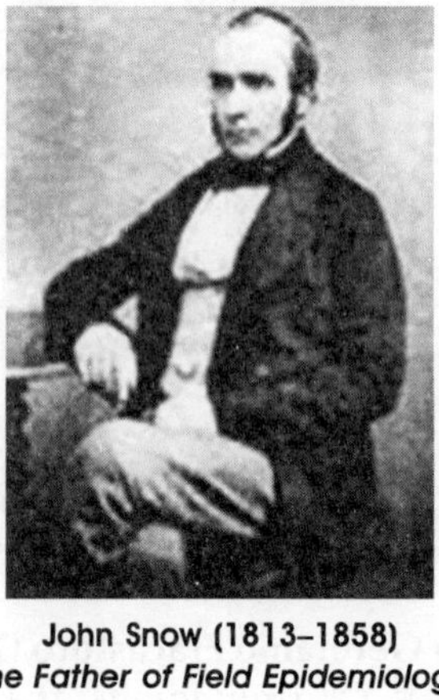

John Snow (1813–1858)
'The Father of Field Epidemiology'

The most celebrated early observational epidemiological study is that of **John Snow (1813–1858)** on cholera in London in 1853. Cholera (Asiatic cholera) had started to rage in India and then moved westwards, the first epidemic hitting Great Britain in 1831–32, causing at least 60,000 deaths. Snow directly investigated the subsequent major epidemic episodes in London in 1849 and 1854, focusing attention on the role that polluted water in the spread of the disease.

Among a number of other observations he noted (Table 1.4) that, while in 1849 and 1854 roughly the same number of deaths had occurred in the London districts supplied by the water company of Southwark and Vauxhall, a marked reduction in deaths had occurred in those districts supplied by the Lambeth company. No major change in population had occurred between 1849 and 1854 but, unlike Southwark and Vauxhall, the Lambeth company had changed its sources of water supply, moving higher up the Thames, probably above, as Snow conjectured, the greatest source of contamination by city sewage.[8]

Table 1.4: Mortality from cholera in the areas of London supplied by the Southwark and Vauxhall, and Lambeth Water Companies in 1849 and 1854 (From Snow, 1853)

Districts with water supplied by	*Number of deaths attributed to cholera*	
	1849	*1854*
Southwark and Vauxhall Company	2261	2458
Lambeth Company	162	37
Both companies	3905	2547

Indeed, when he computed death rates from cholera (Table 1.5), they were more than 20 times lower for the districts supplied by the Lambeth company in respect to those supplied by Southwark and Vauxhall. Strong corroboration of these findings came from a more refined investigation: In some areas the water supplies for the two companies happened to be closely intermixed, some houses receiving their water from the Lambeth company and others from Southwark and Vauxhall.

Table 1.5: Mortality from cholera in the districts of London supplied by the Southwark and Vauxhall, and the Lambeth companies, July 8 to August 26, 1854 (From Snow, 1853)

Districts with water supplied by	*Population 1851 census*	*Deaths from cholera population*	*Cholera death rate per 1000*
Southwark and Vauxhall company	167,654	844	5.0
Lambeth company	19,133	18	0.9
Both companies	300,149	652	2.2

The number of houses and the size of the pertinent populations belonging to each company were known, but a door-to-door inquiry was needed, and indeed carried out by Snow, on all cholera cases to ascertain to which company the water supply of their homes belonged. This allowed the correct calculation of valid rates of cholera occurrence. The results are shown in (Table 1.6), which clearly demonstrates that even within the same physical area the origin of the water supply separates in a clear cut way those populations with high and low rates of disease occurrence.[9]

In France, the influence of great mathematicians such as D'Alembert, Condorcet, the Swiss Euler and Bernoulli family, Lagrange and Laplace who worked on probability and statistics during the eighteenth and early nineteenth century was strongly felt in the medical field.

Pierre Louis (1787–1872), who introduced the 'numerical method' in medicine and produced statistical evidence. At the first Congress of Italian Scientists, in Pisa in 1838 (*Atti della prima riumione degli scienziati italiani 1939*), it was proposed that to compare

Table 1.6: Mortality from cholera in London, July 8 to August 26, 1854, related to source of individual water supply in three groups of districts (from Snow, 1855)

Group of districts with water supplied by	*Water supply of individual houses*	*Population, 1851 census*	*Deaths from cholera*	*Cholera death rate per 1000 population*
Southwark and Vauxhall company	Southwark and Vauxhall company	167,654**	738	4.4
Lambeth company	Lambeth company	19,133**	4	0.2
Both companies	Southwark and Vauxhall company	98,862	419	4.2
	Lambeth company	154,615	80	0.5
Rest of London		1,921,972	1,422	0.7

** Overestimated by a small amount, since this figure includes population with no water supply.

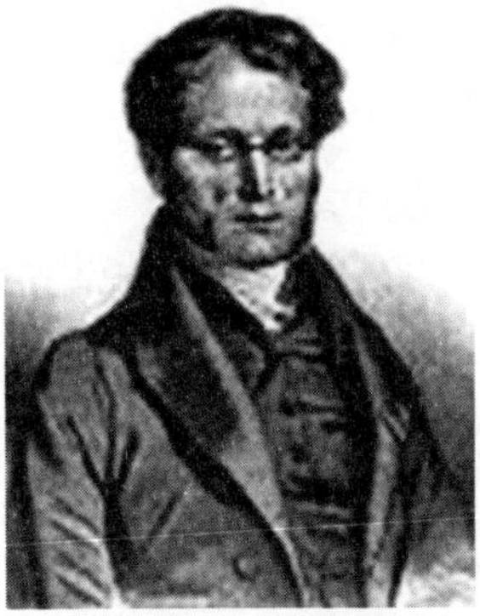

Pierre Louis (1787–1872)
Introduced the 'numerical method' in medicine

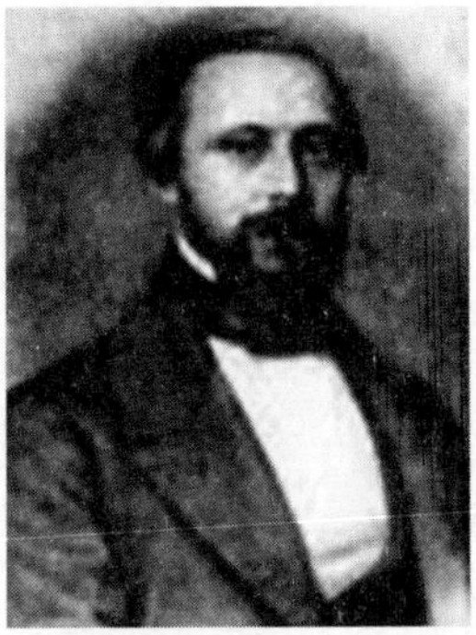

Rudolf Virchow (1821–1902)
'The founder of (microscopic) cellular pathology'
'A believer in role of social science in medicine'

different treatments, the best method would be to administer them in different wards of large hospitals to which access of patients would be on a strict rotation basis without any possibility of choice on the part of the physicians. The outcome of each treatment would then be carefully recorded and counted and the whole process, as well as the interpretation of the results identifying the superior treatment (if any), would be strictly monitored and reported by a steering committee.[10]

German scientist **Rudolf Virchow (1821–1902)** work in pathology is regarded as a cornerstone of modern medicine. He believed that 'medicine is a social science'. At the International Congress of Statistics in 1855, Rudolf Virchow stated the form of the bulletin indicated by Mr Farr can be recommended from the practical and medical point of view, because it contains one column for the disease, and another for the consequences of the diseases that have been the immediate cause of death; for it is one of the most important aims of statistics to know not only the direct causes of death but also the indirect ones, i.e. the pathological state which produces the truly lethal alterations. The mechanism itself of death is of interest for practical statistics only in the case of crime, or of a lesion due to violence, or of accident.[11]

One can clearly recognize here the basic concept and structure of current death certification, separating underlying causes from proximate causes, as well as the separate classification of accidents and traumatic events even now present in the International Classification of Diseases (ICD).

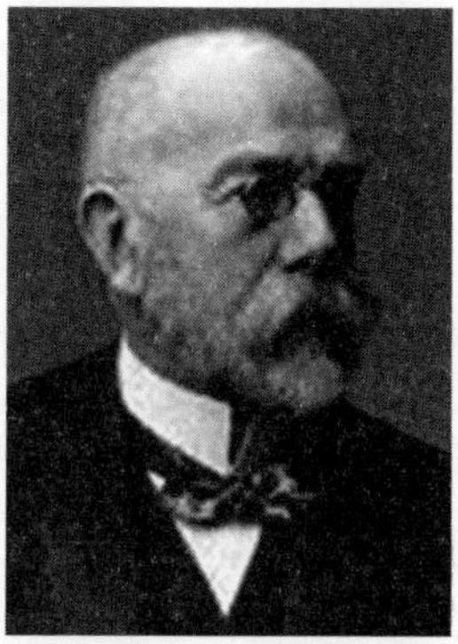

Robert Koch (1843–1910)
'Discovered the anthrax disease cycle (1876); and the bacteria responsible for tuberculosis (1882) and cholera (1883)'

Robert Koch (1843–1910), in the wake of the fundamental discovery of microorganisms by Louis Pasteur (1822–1895), not only to contribute to the discovery of the agents of several diseases (anthrax, tuberculosis, etc.), but also to formulate a set of criteria for establishing causality in epidemiological studies. Robert Koch in his postulates stated that a microorganism to be regarded as a causative agent of a disease should fulfill the following criteria.

Microorganism should be:

i. Found in all subjects with the disease;
ii. Grown *in vitro* (in a suitable medium);
iii. Capable of reproducing the disease in some animal species.
iv. Recovered from the infected animals

Perhaps it is the third criterion which more sharply differs from those nowadays quoted in the literature, following the guidelines put forward by A B Hill, which include as one element supporting causality 'the biological plausibility'. This is much weaker and less strict than the ability to reproduce the disease in some animal species, which reflects an attitude of giving full weight to the result of experiments in animals, a feature which became somewhat blurred with the advent of the 'new epidemiology' in the 1940s.

Modern Epidemiology

Individual studies on cancer, non-rheumatic cardiovascular diseases, and psychiatric diseases, can be traced well back in time, but one can take as a convenient turning point for the rise of the modern epidemiology the period around 1940s.

One of the milestones in the development of modern epidemiology is the 'tobacco and health story'. Among the first one, Pearl (1938) reported using insurance data that the expectation of life for smokers was substantially reduced in respect to non-smokers. The second, one might single out the observation by Ochsner and De Bakey (1939) of high frequency of smokers among the lung cancer patients coming to their hospital in those early days of thoracic surgery.

These were followed by other statistical findings of a general nature pointing to a dramatic increase of lung cancer rates in men throughout the 1940s, in particular in the US and the UK.

In 1950, three hospital-based case control studies were published (Doll and Hill, Levin *et al.*, and Wynder and Graham), which clearly showed causal association between tobacco smoking and lung cancer.

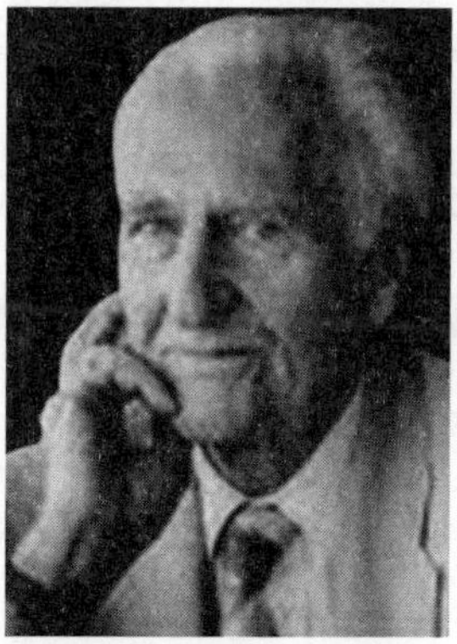

Sir Richard Doll (1912–2005)
An eminent epidemiologist 'Through case-control studies they (along with Sir A B Hill) established a link between cigarette smoking and lung cancer'

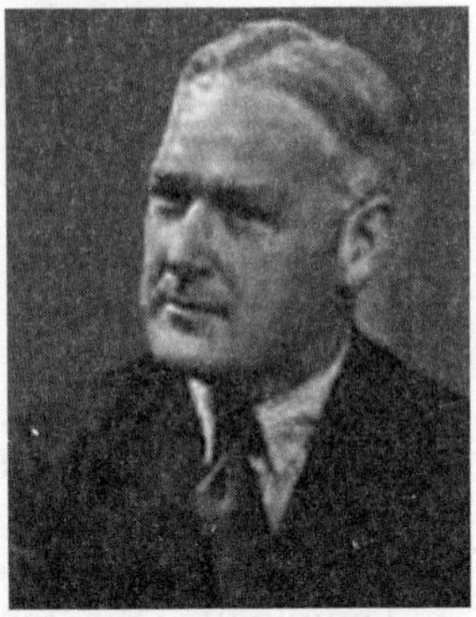

Sir Austin Bradford Hill (1897–1991)
A brilliant statistician 'Through case-control studies they (along with Sir Richard Doll) established a link between cigarette smoking and lung cancer'

The case-control study by **Doll and Hill** was much more sophisticated in methodological terms. Over the whole period of investigation from 1948 to 1952, they recruited 1357 male and 108 female patients with lung cancer from several hospitals in London and matched them with respect to age and sex to the same number of patients hospitalized for non-malignant conditions. The study showed strong indication for a positive association between smoking and lung cancer. Despite the methodological concerns regarding case-control studies, Doll and Hill themselves believed that smoking was responsible for the development of lung cancer. The study became a landmark that inspired future generations of epidemiologists to use this methodology.[12,13]

It remains to this day a model for the design and conduct of case-control studies, with excellent suggestions on how to reduce or eliminate selection, interview, and recall bias. Because of the strong evidence, they started a cohort study of 20,000 male British physicians in 1951, known as the 'British Doctors' Study. These were followed to further investigate the association between smoking and lung cancer. The authors compared mortality from lung cancer among those who never smoked with that among all smokers and with those who smoked various numbers of cigarettes per day (Doll and Hill, 1964).

The term 'cohort study' was introduced by Frost in 1935 to describe a study that compared the disease experience of people born at different periods, in particular the sex- and age-specific incidence of tuberculosis, and the method was extended to the study of non-communicable disease by Korteweg who used it 20 years later to analyze the epidemic of lung cancer in the Netherlands.

The famous cohort study was the 'Framingham Heart Study' that was based on the population of Framingham, a small community in Massachusetts. The study was initiated in 1948 to yield insights into causes of cardiovascular diseases (CVD). For this purpose, 5209 participants free from coronary heart disease (CHD), 30 to 62 years of age, were examined and then followed for nearly 50 years to determine the rate of occurrence of new cases among persons free of disease at first observation.[14]

The intensive biennial examination schedule, long-term continuity of follow-up and investigator involvement, and incorporation of new design components over its decades-long history have made this a uniquely rich source of data on individual risks of CVD events. The study served as a reference and good example for many subsequent cohort studies in this field adopting its methodology. In particular, analysis of these data led to the development of the perhaps most important modelling technique in epidemiology, the multiple logistic regression.[14]

Two other leading examples of cohort studies conducted within a single population or for comparison of multiple populations to assess risk factors for cardiovascular events are the Whitehall Study of British civil servants (Rose and Shipley, 1986) and the Seven Countries Study of factors accounting for differences in CHD rates between populations of Europe, Japan, and North America (Keys 1980; Kromhout *et al.*, 1995).[15]

In contrast to the above cohort studies that focused on cardiovascular diseases, the US Nurses' Health Study is an impressive example of a multipurpose cohort study. It recruited over 120,000 married female nurses, 30 to 55 years of age, in a mail survey in 1976. In this survey, information on demographic, reproductive, medical and lifestyle factors was obtained. Nurses were contacted every 2 years to assess outcomes that occurred during that interval and to update and to supplement the exposure information collected at baseline. Various exposure factors like use of oral contraceptives, post-menopausal hormone therapy, and fat consumption were related to different outcomes such as cancer and cardiovascular disease (Lipnick *et al.*, 1986). The most recent results have had an essential impact on the risk-benefit assessment of post-menopausal hormone therapy speaking against its use over extended periods (Chen *et al.*, 2002).[16]

This phase of the development of epidemiology received new input from the two-way exchange between epidemiology and clinical medicine, which has been a constant feature in the history of the subject. As previously exemplified Ramazzini, a clinician, and Snow, a physician (pioneering anesthesia), had enlarged clinical observations by looking for causes of disease at the population level; conversely, Louis had brought the methods of population studies into the clinical domain to evaluate the effects of medical acts in patient populations. The 'new epidemiology' clearly highlights this dual exchange.

A yardstick in this development was the publication in 1972 by Archie Cochrane (1909–1988); (Cochrane, 1972) of a brilliant essay advocating a systematic use of the randomized trial method to evaluate procedures in the areas of clinical and health services.

Today's epidemiology: Today, as yesterday, epidemiology as a population approach to health and disease embraces two bodies of knowledge—first, epidemiological methods of investigation and, second, epidemiological substantive notions developed by application of such methods (biological and social facets). Both bodies of knowledge have undergone substantial expansion since World War II with the development of the 'new epidemiology'.

These developments have taken place concurrently within an accelerated evolution in the whole field of biology and health, and one can single out four traits, particularly salient in Europe and other economically developed areas of the world.

1. The unprecedented advances of research in some domains like immunology, the neurosciences, and, most prominently, molecular genetics and cell and developmental biology.
2. The advances in clinical medicine at the diagnostic and therapeutic levels. Till recently the only approach to disease control was curative and preventive approach but nowadays, treatments capable of effectively influencing length and quality of survival are available for a number of serious conditions, both infectious and non-infectious.
3. The escalating costs of all healthcare delivery systems, whether private, public or mixed, have brought to the forefront issues of effective and efficient use of available resources which were of negligible importance, or almost unknown, three or four decades ago.
4. The renewed awareness among professionals and the general public of the dependence of health on the environment, material and social, personal, local or general. In parallel with this goes the realization that tangible deterioration of the environment does take place because of shortsighted human activities.

These developments and their interrelationship change the pattern of the factors capable of promoting, damaging or restoring health, and impose a virtually continuous reappraisal and adaptation of the healthcare system and, more generally, of all plans of action aimed at influencing health.[17]

Tomorrow's epidemiology: Following are three major challenges in future development of epidemiology and epidemiologists.[18]

THE CHALLENGE OF RAPIDLY GROWING BIOLOGY

The accelerated developments in molecular biology were taken up by epidemiologists to measure markers of exposure, early biological effects, and host characteristics that influence response (susceptibility) in human cells, blood, tissue and other material. These techniques augment the standard tools of epidemiology in the investigation of low-level risks, risks imposed by complex exposures, and the modification of risks by genetic factors. The use of such biomarkers of exposure and effect has led to a boom of the so-called molecular epidemiology, a methodological approach with early origins. These developments were accompanied by the sequencing of the human genome and the advances in high-throughput genetic technologies that led to the rapid progress of genetic epidemiology.

THE CHALLENGE OF DEVELOPING SOCIETY

The composition and behaviour of society is changing world-over with increasing ageing population, changing reproduction, persistent inequalities in health conditions between different sections of society, in particular gender, occupation, and socio-economic categories. Monitoring trends and identifying causal factors in this area, which could be labelled 'social epidemiology', characterizing in a major way of their involvement in public health.

THE CHALLENGE OF DIVERSIFICATION VERSUS INTEGRATION

As in all other scientific and technical branches of activity, epidemiology has been recently, and continues to, specialize along different axes.

A first axis is methodology versus substantive studies; areas of current and future development in methodology are, for example, the treatment of exposure measurements and errors of measurement to reduce misclassification and improve study power, methods in genetic epidemiology, modelling of the exposure–response relationship with multiple longitudinal measurements.

A second axis is diversification of different fields of substantive interest, e.g. cancer epidemiology, epidemiology of ageing, etc. A whole area of specialization is 'clinical epidemiology', the application of epidemiological methods within the clinical domain, both for studies evaluating diagnostic, prognostic, therapeutic, and rehabilitative procedures and for evolving formal methods of optimal clinical decision-making. Another rapidly growing branch is 'evidence-based medicine' (EBM), which employs formal methods to assemble and evaluate the existing evidence on the effects of medical interventions.

A final axis of diversification tends to separate those who specialize in investigative aspects for routine or research purposes from those who plan and implement interventions. In clinical medicine this has produced a variety of specialists in purely diagnostic activities (clinical chemists, clinical pathologists, diagnostic radiologists, imaging specialists), different from the therapist who decides and acts on the basis of the diagnosis; similarly, in the public health area, the epidemiologist may become more and more a pure specialist in aetiological and evaluative investigations, leaving others to decide what to do.

The successes in epidemiology have largely derived from its working as the investigative component of health, studying the distribution and determinants of health and diseases in populations. This essence should continue to be preserved in the foreseeable future by incorporating into epidemiological research. The new opportunities are currently arising in particular from the fields of genetics, environmental sciences, clinical medicine, and healthcare. The well-designed epidemiological studies can provide strong and reliable evidences for formulation of health policies to provide highest level of health to the population to lead a quality of life.

TIMELINE HISTORY OF EPIDEMIOLOGY AND PUBLIC HEALTH

Antiquity:	Concepts of health closely tied to religion, superstitions, magic, ..., etc.
460–375 BC:	Hippocrates—role of environmental factors in disease
129–216 D:	Galen—re-emphasized the role of environmental factors in disease
1334:	Petrarch—introduced the concept of comparison
1346–1350:	Bubonic plague epidemics in Europe
1439–1541:	Paracelus—toxicology founder
1546:	Gerolamo Fracastoro published book *"De Contagione et Contagiosis Morbis"*, presented the first clear and coherent germ theory of disease
1654–1720:	Giovanni Maria Lancisi—probably the first epidemiological study of a non-communicable condition
1662:	John Graunt—bills of mortality and the 'law of mortality'. The first life table giving the probability of dying at each age.
1700:	Bernadino Ramazzini—'Father of Occupational Epidemiology'; published diseases of workers: Also breast cancer in nuns
1706–1777:	Francois Bossier de Lacroix (known as Sauvages)—systematic classification of diseases (*Nosologia Methodica*)
1747:	James Lind — scurvy experiment
1775:	Percival Pott—scrotum cancer findings among chimney workers
1798:	Edward Jenner—cowpox vaccination against smallpox
1787–1872:	Pierre Charles Alexandre Louis (1787–1872)—introduced the 'numerical method' in medicine
1819–1901:	Pettenkofer—first one to put up concept of multifactorial causation of diseases
1834:	William Farr—the Father of Modern Vital Statistics and Surveillance
1847:	Ignaz Semmelweiss (Vienna)—discovered transmission and prevention of puerperal fever
1848:	Rudolf Virchow—"medicine is a social science"
1849:	John Snow—waterborne transmission of cholera
1851:	John Grove—*on the nature of epidemics* (presented the germ theory)
1882:	Robert Koch—discovered causative agent for anthrax and tuberculosis and proposes Koch's postulates
1914–1918:	Joseph Goldberger studies pellagra
1918:	First pandemic of influenza
1928:	Alexander Flaming—discovery of penicillin
1930:	Frost W H—first professor of epidemiology
1938:	John Paul—introduced the term clinical epidemiology
1948:	World Health Organization (WHO)
1948:	Framingham study
1950:	Sir Richard Doll and Sir Austin Bradford Hill—case control study on tobacco smoking and lung cancer
1951:	Cornfield *et al.*—founded an era of risk relativism
1951:	CCI conference—defined screening
1966:	Sachett DL—established first clinical epidemiological research unit
1977:	Global eradication of smallpox.
1978:	Alma Ata—developed primary healthcare
1988:	Last John M—defined epidemiology (widely accepted)
1994:	Cairo conference—defined reproductive health

References

1. Francis Adams (translator). On Airs, Waters, and Places by Hippocrates, Written 400 BC. Available at http://classics.mit.edu/Hippocrates/airwatp l.8.8.html
2. Rodolfo Saracci. Introducing the history of Epidemiology in book Teaching Epidemiology. Oxford Scholarship Online Monographs April 2010.Downloaded on 15th Dec. 2010. Available at http://fds.oup.com/www.oup.com/pdf/13/9780192630667.pdf pp 3–25.
3. Lilienfield, AM (ed.). Times, places and persons. Aspects of the history of epidemiology. The Johns Hopkins University Press, Baltimore. 1980.
4. Graunt, John. Natural and Political Observations—made upon the Bills of Mortality, 1662... echo.mpiwg-berlin.mpg.de/content/demo
5. Graunt, John. Natural and Political Observations mentioned in a following Index, and made upon the Bills of Mortality, 1665... echo.mpiwg-berlin.mpg.de/content/demo
6. Lind J. A treatise of the scurvy. In three parts. Containing an inquiry into the nature, causes and cure, of that disease. Together with a critical and

chronological view of what has been published on the subject. Edinburgh: Printed by Sands, Murray and Cochran for A Kincaid and A Donaldson,1753: http://www.jameslindlibrary.org/illustrating/records/a-treatise-of-the-scurvy-in-three-parts-containing-an-inquiry

7. Edward Jenner. Jenner's quest for a Smallpox Vaccine (1798); An Inquiry into the Causes and Effects of the Variolae Vaccinae, Known by the Name of the Cow-Pox http://www.ourcivilisation.com/smartboard/shop/jennere/index.htm
8. Snow John. Snow on Cholera: Being a Reprint of Two Papers. New York: The Common wealth Fund; London: H. Milford, Oxford University Press; 1936. Down loaded from http://nrs.harvard.edu/urn
9. Snow John.On the Mode of Communication of Cholera, 8 volumes, London, 1849;2nd ed. 1855.
10. Centers for Disease Control and Prevention (CDC). Introduction to epidemiology (lesson 1) from Principles of Epidemiology in Public Health Practice, 3rd Edition (SS-1000). Published by US Department of Health and Human Services, Centers for Disease Control and Prevention, Office of Workforce and Career Development Atlanta, available at http://www.cdc.gov/pp 1–7.
11. Virchow R. Collected essays on public health and epidemiology. Vol. 1. Science History Publications, Canton, MA.; 1985.
12. Doll R, Hill AB. Smoking and carcinoma of the lung: Preliminary report. BMJ, 1950;(ii):739–48.
13. Doll R, Hill AB. Mortality in relation to smoking: ten years' observation of British doctors. BMJ, 1964; (i):1399–1410 and 1460–7.
14. Framingham heart study foundation. Available on http://www.framinghamheartstudy.org/about/index.
15. Lipnick RJ, Buring JE, Hennekens CH, Rosner B, Willett W, Bain C, Stampfer MJ, Colditz GA, Peto R, Speizer FE. Oral contraceptives and breast cancer: a prospective cohort study. JAMA, 1986; 255:58–61.
16. Chen WY, Colditz GA, Rosner B, Hankinson SE, Hunter DJ, Manson JE, Stampfer MJ, Willett WC, Speizer FE. Use of postmenopausal hormones, alcohol, and risk for invasive breast cancer. Ann Intern Med 2002;137(10):798–804.
17. Alfredo Morabia (editor). A history of epidemiologic methods and concepts. Publisher: Birkhäuser, Basel; 2004.
18. Victor JS, Wayne DR. Evolving historical perspective (Ch. 2), from Understanding the Fundamentals of Epidemiology an evolving text Fall Ed. Published by University of North Carolina at Chapel Hill; 2000:17–30.

DEFINITION, OBJECTIVES, AND APPROACH IN EPIDEMIOLOGY

DEFINITION

The word epidemiology comes from the Greek words ***epi***, meaning on or upon, ***demos***, meaning people, and ***logos***, meaning the study of. In other words, the word epidemiology has its roots in the study of a population(s).

The various dictionaries define the epidemiology as follows:

1. The branch of medicine that investigates the causes and control of epidemics (Webster's New World College Dictionary, 2010)
2. All the elements contributing to the occurrence or non-occurrence of a disease in a population; ecology of a disease (Webster's New World College Dictionary, 2010)
3. The branch of medicine that deals with the study of the causes, distribution, and control of disease in populations (the American Heritage, Dictionary of English Language, 4th ed., 2010.).

Some of the authors who have written on the subject, ranging from Hippocrates to those of the present day are given below.[1]

1. That branch of medical science which treats of epidemics (Parkin, 1873)
2. The science of the mass phenomena of infectious diseases (Frost, 1927)
3. The study of disease, any disease, as a mass phenomenon (Greenwood, 1934)
4. Epidemiology is the study of the distribution and determinants of disease frequency in man. (Mac Mahon, 1960)

Many definitions have been proposed, but the following definition captures the underlying principles and public health spirit of epidemiology:

Last J M (1988) defined epidemiology is "the **study** of the **distribution** and **determinants** of **health-related states or events** in

specified populations, and the **application** of this study to the **control** of health problems"[2,3]

Key terms in this definition reflect some of the important principles of epidemiology.[2,3]

- **Study** includes: surveillance, observation, hypothesis testing, analytic research and experiments.
- **Distribution** refers to analysis of—times, persons, places and classes of people affected.
- **Determinants** include factors that influence health—biological, chemical, physical, social, cultural, economic, genetic, behavioural, etc.
- **Health-related states and events** refer to—diseases, causes of death, behaviours such as use of tobacco, positive health states, reactions to preventive regimes and provision and use of health services.
- **Specified populations** include those with identifiable characteristics, such as occupational groups.
- **Application** to prevention and control the aims of public health—to promote, protect, and restore health.

Details of Each Components

Study

Epidemiology is data-driven and relies on a systematic and unbiased approach to the collection, analysis, and interpretation of data. Basic epidemiologic methods tend to rely on careful inquiry, observation and use of valid comparison groups to assess whether what was observed differs from what might be expected, e.g. number of cases of tuberculosis in a particular area during a particular time period or the frequency of an exposure among persons with disease. In fact, epidemiology is often described as the basic science of public health because:

- It is a quantitative discipline that relies on a working knowledge of probability, statistics, and sound research methods.
- It is a method of causal reasoning based on developing and testing hypotheses grounded in such scientific fields as biology, behavioural sciences, physics, and ergonomics to explain health-related behaviours, states, and events.
- It provides the direction for practical and appropriate public health action based on scientific and causal reasoning.

Distribution

It can be discussed under two sub-headings: i. pattern, and ii. frequency

i. **Pattern** refers to the occurrence of disease or health-related events by time, place, and person. Time patterns may be annual, seasonal, weekly, daily, hourly, weekday versus weekend, or any other breakdown of time that may influence disease or injury occurrence. Place patterns include geographic variation, urban/rural differences, and location of work sites or schools. Personal characteristics include demographic factors which may be related to risk of illness, injury, or disability such as age, sex, marital status, and socio-economic status, as well as behaviours (lifestyle) and environmental factors.

ii. **Frequency** refers not only to the number of health events such as the number of cases of tuberculosis/diarrhea/AIDS/diabetes in a population, but also to the relationship of that number to the size of the population. The frequencies help to compare disease occurrence across different populations, time and places.

Determinants

Determinants include factors that influence health, the occurrence of disease and health-related events. There are many determinants but these may be divided in two broad categories—(1) Host factors, e.g. age, sex, occupation, education, immunity, nutritional status, health status, etc. (which determines the susceptibility of the individual) and (2) Environmental factors—living and non-living, e.g. air, water and pollution, housing condition, heat, cold, etc. (determines host exposure to the specific agent).

They assess whether groups with different rates of disease differ in their demographic characteristics, genetic or immunologic make-up, behaviours (lifestyle), environmental factors including past or present exposure, and/or other so-called potential risk factors.

Health-related States or Events

In fact, the term health-related states or events may be seen as anything that affects the well-being of a population. However, epidemiology was originally focused exclusively on epidemics of communicable diseases subsequently it expanded to endemic communicable diseases and non-communicable infectious diseases. By the middle of the 20th century, additional epidemiologic methods had been developed and applied to chronic diseases, injuries, birth defects, maternal-child health, occupational health, and environmental health. Then epidemiologists began to look at behaviours related to health and well-being, such as physical exercise, use of personal protective devices, and seat belt. Health-related events like natural or man-made disasters, lifestyle (smoking, irresponsible sexual behaviour, etc.) terrorism and other social problems, etc. are also studied. Epidemiologists now can make use of genetic markers to assess the risk of disease.

Specified Populations

The epidemiologist's main concern is the health of the group of people in a family, community or population but the clinician is only concerned about the health of an individual. Therefore, the clinician and the epidemiologist have different responsibilities when faced with a person with illness, e.g. when a patient with tuberculosis disease presents, both is interested in establishing the correct diagnosis. However, while the clinician usually focuses on treating and caring for the individual, the epidemiologist focuses on identifying the exposure or source that caused the illness; the number of other persons who may have been similarly exposed; the potential for further spread in the community; and interventions to prevent additional cases or recurrences.

The pattern of various health problems/diseases among different populations, e.g. rural, urban, migratory, nomadic, tribal, vulnerable, marginalized, remote, unreachable, etc. are different.

Application

Any discovery or inventions related to human and their environment should always be targeted toward the benefits to the human population without which the discovery is useless; so is true for epidemiology. The practice of epidemiology is both a science and an art. It is not only the study of health in a population; it also involves applying the knowledge gained by the studies to prevent and control diseases or adverse health related events through community-based practices.

APPROACHES IN EPIDEMIOLOGY

The practice of epidemiology relies on a systematic approach. The epidemiologist, ask and or observe, counts cases or health events, and describes them in terms of time, place, and person; divides the number of cases by an appropriate denominator to calculate rates, ratios or proportions; analyzes, compares these over time or groups of population or places, draw inferences, decide and act to improve the situation.

The following are the approaches in epidemiology.

A. Asking questions
B. Making comparisons
C. Making decisions
D. Application (implementation of interventions)

Asking Questions

Epidemiology is a way to explore the facts which are usually carried out by number of methods like interviewing and discussions (asking questions), observations and experimentations. The first step is crucial as it may lead to some aetiological clue (observational study—descriptive) and motivate explorer for further study (analytical and experimental) the disease or health event in question.

Any kind of study will be incomplete if it does not describe the what, who, where, when, and why/how of a situation/disease or health event, e.g.

i. What is the event?	(The problem)
ii. Where did it happen?	(Place distribution)
iii. When did it happen?	(Time distribution)
iv. Who are affected?	(Person distribution)
v. Why did it happen?	(Causes and risk factors)
vi. How did it happen?	(Mode of transmission)

Making Comparisons

Epidemiology is basically focusing its perspective on groups or populations rather than individuals. Various tools are needed to compare different characteristics relating to disease occurrence between populations in relation to different time periods, different places or different groups of persons. The comparison of groups may be done in terms of morbidity, mortality, disability, fertility, etc. the comparison of morbidity or mortality in populations with and without a certain exposure or the comparison of exposure between diseased subjects and a control group. Inclusion of an appropriate reference group (non-exposed or non-diseased) for comparison with the group of interest is a condition for causal inference.

One of the first considerations before making comparisons is to ensure what is known as 'comparability' between the study and control groups. In other words, both the groups should be similar so that "like can be compared with like". For facts to be comparable, they must be accurate, and they must be gathered in a uniform way. The comparability can be best achieved by randomization or matching. Another alternative is standardization which usually has a limited application to a few characteristics such as age, sex and parity.

Making Decisions

Epidemiological reasoning and decision making consists of three major steps. First, a statistical association between an explanatory characteristic (exposure) and the outcome of interest (disease) is established.

Then, from the pattern of the association a hypothetical (biological) inference about the disease mechanism is formulated that can be refuted or confirmed by subsequent studies. Finally, when a plausible conjecture about the causal factor(s) leading to the outcome has been established then decisions are taken.

In practice, these three major steps are interwoven in an iterative process of hypothesis generation by descriptive and exploratory studies, statistical confirmation of the presumed association by analytical studies and, if feasible, implementation and evaluation of intervention activities, i.e. experimental studies. Based on results/finding, actions/programs are designed and decided to implement (if beneficial) to population.

Application (implementation of interventions)

It is necessary to uses the scientific methods of descriptive, analytic, experimental epidemiology as well as experiences, epidemiologic judgments, and understanding of local conditions in 'diagnosing' the health of a community and proposing appropriate, practical, affordable and acceptable public health interventions to control and prevent disease in the community. The inferences of epidemiological studies can be applied to a whole population or sub-group in defined geographical areas or a family or an individual depending of the situation, e.g. prevention of genetic diseases.

Warren Winkelstein (2000) described the need for a 'more **expansionist approach**' in order to address disease problems arising from pollution, global warming, population growth, poverty, social inequality, civil unrest, and violence. Even without taking the further step of proposing that epidemiology should attempt to reduce these conditions themselves, the challenges for epidemiology are daunting.[3]

AIM AND OBJECTIVES OF EPIDEMIOLOGY (MILTON TERRIS)[4]

Epidemiology is multidisciplinary, problem-oriented applied research. The ultimate **aim** of epidemiology is to lead to effective action to eliminate or reduce the health problem or its consequences; and promote the health and well-being of society as a whole.

Broad objectives

1. To discover the agent, host, and environmental factors that affect health, in order to provide the scientific basis for the prevention of disease and injury and the promotion of health.
2. To determine the relative importance of causes of illness, disability, and death, in order to establish priorities for research and action.
3. To identify those sections of the population which have the greatest risk from specific causes of ill health (and benefit from specific interventions), in order that the indicated action may be directed appropriately (targeting).
4. To evaluate the effectiveness of preventive and therapeutic health programs and services in improving the health of the population.
5. To study the natural history of disease from its precursor states through its manifestations and clinical course.
6. To conduct surveillance of disease and injury occurrence in populations and of the levels of risk factors—passive (receive reports), active (poll practitioners, conduct surveys)
7. To investigate outbreaks (e.g. hospital-acquired infections, disease clusters, food-borne and waterborne infections) to identify their source and controlling epidemics (e.g. measles, rubella, coronary heart disease, overweight).

VARIETIES OF EPIDEMIOLOGY

Classical epidemiology is population-oriented and addresses the community origin of health problems, e.g. nutrition, behaviour, psycho-social state of the population, etc.

Clinical epidemiology is patient-orientated to health settings and aimed at improving diagnosis, treatment and prognosis of patients who already suffer a medical condition.

In clinical epidemiology, the patient comes to the doctor; in classical epidemiology, the investigator goes out into the community to find persons who have the disease or experience of the suspected causal factor in question. Clinical epidemiology is based on biomedical concepts with an ever-increasing concern for refining the technique of diagnosis and treatment at the individual level. The subject matter of clinical medicine is easily 'perceived' by such techniques as clinical and laboratory examinations including post-mortem reports.[4]

Sackett defined clinical epidemiology as 'the application, by a physician who provides direct patient care, of epidemiologic and biostatistical methods to the study of diagnostic and therapeutic processes in order to effect an improvement of health' (Sackett 1969).[5]

As epidemiology continues to develop and to expand into new areas, the field has diversified into many forms and discipline; some of them are mentioned as under.[6]

1. Surveillance, 'shoe-leather' epidemiology (outbreak investigations, and epidemic control)
2. Microbial epidemiology—biology and ecology of pathogenic microorganisms, their lifecycles, and their interactions with their human and non-human hosts
3. 'Risk factor' epidemiology—searching for exposure–disease associations that may provide insights into etiology and avenues for prevention
4. Healthcare epidemiology—assess accuracy, efficacy, effectiveness, and unintended consequences of methods of

prevention, early detection, diagnosis, treatment, and management of health conditions

5. Molecular epidemiology—investigate disease at the molecular level to precisely characterize pathological processes and exposures, to elucidate mechanisms of pathogenesis, and to identify precursor conditions
6. Genetic epidemiology—the confluence of molecular biology, population studies, and statistical models with an emphasis on heritable influences on disease susceptibility and expression.
7. Social epidemiology—the branch of epidemiology that studies the social distribution and social determinants of health at the population level
8. Pharmaco-epidemiology—defined as the application of epidemiologic knowledge, methods, and reasoning to the study of the effects and uses of drugs in human populations
9. Occupational epidemiology—it is the broad field of epidemiology to identify the causes of disease in a population in order to intervene to remove them. Occupational epidemiology is an exposure-oriented discipline; it is thus the systematic study of illnesses and injuries related to the workplace environment.
10. Environmental epidemiology—"the study of the effect on human health of physical, biological, and chemical factors in the external environment. By examining specific populations or communities exposed to different ambient environments, environmental epidemiology seeks to clarify the relation between physical, biological, and chemical factors and human health".
11. Reproductive epidemiology—the studies of distribution and determinants of diseases directly related to reproduction.
12. Nutritional epidemiology—to describe the distribution and variation in the nutritional behaviour of individuals and groups and, primarily but not exclusively, to relate that behaviour to some health outcome, to explore the causal relationship between exposure and outcome.
13. Big epidemiology (defined as upwards of $100 million for a study)—multisite collaborative trials, such as the hypertension detection and follow-up program (HDFP), Coronary Primary Prevention Trial (CPPT), Multiple Risk Factor Intervention Trial (MRFIT), women's health initiative (WHI).
14. Entrepreneurial epidemiology—building institutions and careers by winning research funding and facilities.
15. Testimonial epidemiology—giving depositions and testifying in court or in legislative hearings on the state of epidemiologic evidence on a matter of dispute.
16. Global epidemiology—assessing the effects of human activity on the ecosystem that supports life on Earth.

CHARACTERISTICS OF EPIDEMIOLOGY

Those studies which fulfill the following criteria should ideally be considered as epidemiologic studies.

- Studies basically observational, rather than experimental;
- Studies focuses on free-living human populations defined by geography, worksite, institutional affiliation, occupation, migration status, health conditions, exposure history, or other characteristics rather than a group of highly-selected individuals studied in a clinic or laboratory;
- Studies deals with aetiology and control of disease, rather than with phenomena that are not closely tied to health status;
- Those with multidisciplinary, empirical approach directed at understanding or solving a problem rather than on advancing theory within a discipline.

However, not all epidemiologic studies have these characteristics. One can find out the scoring system using following formula to conclude weather the study is epidemiological or not.

$$\text{Score} = 1n\ (n^{y})k^{s}d^{2}/pc$$

where:

n = number of subjects

y = number of years of follow-up

k = total direct costs (in $1,000,000)

s = sponsor (international organizations = 4, Ministry of health = 3, other public organizations = 2, corporate = 1)

d = principal investigator's degree (PhD – Epid = 5, MD plus MPH-epid = 4, MD = 3, MPH = 2, other health doctorate = 1)

p = number of first-authored publications that the PI will author

c = % of the principal investigator's and co-investigator's salary that will be covered

The higher the score, the more likely that the study is epidemiology.

References

1. Victor JS, Wayne DR. Epidemiology- definition, functions and characteristics (Ch.1), from Understanding the Fundamentals of Epidemiology an evolving text Fall Ed. Published by University of North Carolina at Chapel Hill; 2000;3–16.
2. Centers for Disease Control and Prevention (CDC). Introduction to epidemiology (lesson 1) from Principles of Epidemiology in Public Health Practice, 3rd Edition (SS-1000). Published by US Department of Health and Human Services, Centers for Disease Control and Prevention, Office of Workforce and Career Development Atlanta, available at http://www.cdc.gov/pp 1–21.
3. Bonita R, Beaglehole R, Kjellström T. Basic epidemiology, 2nd edition Published by World Health Organization, Geneva, Switzerland, 2006.
4. Milton Terris. The Society for Epidemiologic Research (SER) and the future of Epidemiology. Am J Epidemiol 1992;136(8):909–15, p 912).
5. Sackett D. Clinical epidemiology. Am J Epidemiol 1969;89:125–8.
6. Wolfgang Ahrens, Klaus Krickeberg, Iris Pigeot. An Introduction to Epidemiology (Ch.1) from Wolfgang Ahrens and Iris Pigeot (Ed). Handbook of Epidemiology. Springer-Verlag Berlin Heidelberg, Germany, 2005.

EPIDEMIOLOGY AND PUBLIC HEALTH

The primary quest is to achieve healthy population in healthy nation. It requires a focused vision, mission, goals, objectives and targets.

Public health has been defined by the institute of medicine committee as a mission, i.e."the fulfillment of society's interest in assuring the conditions in which people can be healthy". The substance of public health was defined as: "Organized community efforts aimed at the prevention of disease and the promotion of health. It links many disciplines and rests upon the scientific core of epidemiology."[1]

The 'basic science of public health work' is not only depends on epidemiology but other basic public health sciences subjects like clinical medicine, sociology, toxicology, molecular biology, anthropology, nutrition, sanitary engineering, policy analysis, risk assessment, industrial hygiene, economics, and political science are also contribute to health of the population.[2,3]

Epidemiology is a philosophy and methodology that can be applied to learning about and resolving a very broad range of health problems. The 'art' of epidemiology is knowing when and how to apply the various epidemiological strategies creatively to answer specific health questions; it is not enough to know what the various study designs and statistical methodologies. Hence, it is considered as 'art and science'.[4]

The full value of epidemiological research is only realized when it is translated into health policy and the subsequent planning and implementation of disease or injury prevention and control programs.

Epidemiology is the branch of public health which attempts to discover the causes of disease in order to make disease prevention possible.

There are many definitions of epidemiology (described previously); some of the epidemiologists agree to definition, "the study of the distribution and determinants of disease frequency in human populations"[1–4] and other with Last JM as mentioned in dictionary of epidemiology but all epidemiologists, however, will agree that epidemiology concerns itself with populations rather than individuals.

Epidemiology has been described as the 'art of the possible', because epidemiologists work with human populations, they are rarely able to manipulate events or the environment as can the laboratory scientist. They must, therefore, exploit situations as they exist naturally to advance knowledge. They must be both pragmatic and realistic.[5,6]

They must realize both the capabilities and limitations of the discipline. Morris has said that the "epidemiologic method is the only way to ask some questions..., one way of asking others and no way at all to ask many" (Morris, 1975). The art of epidemiology is to know both when epidemiology is the method of choice and when it is not, and how to use it to answer the question.

EPIDEMIOLOGICAL INQUIRY FRAMEWORK LEADING TO PUBLIC HEALTH ACTION

Accurate epidemiologic information/knowledge will help in the process of public health planning, implementation and evaluation. The following table will help to understand how information/knowledge is generated and use to the end point for proving the healthcare.

1. **Acquisition and validation of knowledge:** This phase relates to the actual invention or discovery and its validation by other researchers before it is accepted as evidence. This can be achieved through various epidemiological methods experimental studies, e.g. Hippocrates's, John Snow's, John Graunt's, Virchow's, etc. contribution were made by keen observations.
2. **Acceptability of knowledge:** Second phase starts when the knowledge is put to practical use in clinical/epidemiological settings. While the initiation is by individual clinicians, professional bodies constitute expert groups to develop or modify the guidelines by using the techniques of meta-analysis and consensus development.
3. **Application of knowledge:** Third phase starts when an accepted epidemiological practice finds its way into a national level policy, plan or programme. It has to enter into the public health research agenda since health service or operational research would be needed for further research.

Interfaces mentioned above are critical for the transfer of evidence from one phase to the other, finally resulting into a successful translation of epidemiological research (Table 1.7) to public health policy/programme.

EPIDEMIOLOGIC EVIDENCE AND PUBLIC HEALTH ACTION

The epidemiologic information needs to be provided clearly and objectively to public health policymakers, planners and decision makers for preparing health policies, planning, implementation and evaluation of various strategies. However, public health workers should not wait for full proof scientific evidence to make decisions/judgements to resolve the problem for those who must make public health policy decisions, because inaction may worsen the situation. The ideal public health policymaker would fully incorporate the relevant scientific evidence from epidemiology and other sources, ambiguous and incomplete though it may be, and integrate that evidence with other relevant considerations to reach a wise decision.

In recent years, biomedical research has led to remarkable discoveries and capabilities but in many instances it was possible to decisions for prevention without the full knowledge of the pathogenic agent/causative factor. Sir Austin Bradford Hill (1968: 300), wrote that the incomplete and tentative nature of scientific knowledge "... does not confer upon us a freedom to ignore the knowledge we

Table. 1.7: Epidemiological inquiry framework leading to public health action

Steps	*Level of knowledge*	*Conceptual end-point*	*Type of activity required*
Acquisition and validation of knowledge	Knowledge acquisition	First documented/ reported study	Basic innovative epidemiological research
	Knowledge validation	Other studies confirming the finding	Basic epidemiological research
Acceptability of of knowledge	Knowledge transfer	Epidemiological/public health/clinical practice	Epidemiological/clinical/ health research including trials
	Knowledge dissemination	Good epidemiological practices and public health policies and guidelines	Meta-analysis and consensus development
Application of knowledge	Knowledge application	Development of national/ international public health policies/protocols/guidelines/standards	Operational research and consensus development
	Knowledge translation	Implementation of health policies	Technical, economical, managerial, etc. Evaluation and advocacy

already have, or to postpone the action that it appears to demand at a given time." But the judgement of what action is demanded by existing knowledge is often complex and controversial.

The following examples are given in Tables 1.8 and 1.9.[7]

Many population-based epidemiological studies, done in a country, is being applied to other countries for the benefit of population in cost effective manner. All these studies have shown definite causation and association.

EPIDEMIOLOGY, PUBLIC HEALTH AND POLITICS

The quantitative character of epidemiology and its strong emphasis on methods does not make this science immune to the influence of politics and ideology. Even descriptive epidemiological assessments or epidemiological profiles are imbued with theoretical assumptions shaped by the institutional setting under which epidemiological investigations are conducted.[8]

The term political epidemiology expresses the importance of political and bureaucratic processes in coping with epidemiological information. Political assimilability might well be the overriding consideration when the epidemiological picture of a particular health problem is confused, inadequate, and contradictory or a matter of considerable economic import.[9]

Politics can affect population health through various social processes such as, grassroots organizing, social movements, wars, strikes, protests and non-government organizations.

Public policies, and their relation to health, are still not the part of mainstream in epidemiology, which continues to consider health as apolitical, and applies a definition of health that is centered on the individual illness

Table 1.8: Discoveries of dieseases and their prevention

Disease	*Discoverer of preventive measure*	*Year of discovery preventive measure*	*Year of discovery of agent*	*Discoverer of agent*	*Causative or preventive agents*
Scurvy	J Lind	1753	1928	A Szent-Györgyi	Ascorbic acid
Pellagra	J Goldberger	1755	1924	G Casal *et al.*	Niacin
Scrotal cancer	P Pott	1775	1933	JW Cook *et al.*	Benzo(a)pyrene
Smallpox	E Jenner	1798	1958	F Fenner	Orthopoxvirus
Puerperal fever	I Semmelweis	1847	1879	L Pasteur	*Streptococcus*
Cholera	J Snow	1849	1893	R Koch	*Vibrio cholerae*
Bladder cancer	L Rehn	1895	1938	WC Hueper *et al.*	2-Naphthylamine
Yellow fever	W Reed *et al.*	1901	1928	A Stokes *et al.*	Flavivirus
Oral cancer	R Abbe	1915	1974	D Hoffmann *et al.*	N-nitrosonomicotine

Source: Wynder EL. Invited commentary: Studies of mechanism and prevention. Am J Epidemiol 1994: 547–549.

Table 1.9: Population-based risk factors studies

Type of study	*Risk factors*
Framingham study	Risk factors of coronary heart disease
Doll and Hill study	Cigarette smoking and lung cancer
US Nurses' Health Study	Multipurpose cohort study
Oslo heart study	Diet–smoking trial
The Multiple Risk Factor Intervention Trial (MRFIT) study	Effect of smoking, high blood pressure and elevated cholesterol levels on mortality due to CHD
Role of folic acid during pregnancy	Prevention of neural tube defect

rather than on society health problems. As a result, health policies are equated to healthcare services policies, and inequalities in health distribution are considered to be the result of individual problems or of how healthcare is implemented. This perspective has the effect of directing political attention towards the most manageable variable, the healthcare services. However, health inequalities have a political basis. Information on health inequality is not sufficient in order to decide what is inevitable and what is unjust, and such a decision does not depend solely on logic and empirical research, but also on an assessment of politics and ideology.

The scientist, the epidemiologist must communicate freely their research findings for making public process, including policy within a societal and political context. Many a times, there is economization and trading of epidemiological studies by the large players for their benefits which may increase the social inequalities in health.

Let us consider achievements of "The Millennium Development Goals (MDG, in spite of initial political support, we are at halfway through the proposed timescale, the expected progress has not been achieved. One has to identify those factors that are hindering MDG achievement and develop future policies and proposals with greater coherence and supported by a broader, empirical knowledge base including the politics. An interdisciplinary approach, medical humanities or otherwise, is a promising avenue for addressing health and health inequities.[10]

PARTNERSHIP BETWEEN EPIDEMIOLOGY AND PUBLIC HEALTH IN SOUTH-EAST ASIA REGION

Recently (March 2010), WHO regional office for South-east Asia reiterated that epidemiology is the core for development of public health. The Delhi Declaration on Epidemiology advocated by South-east Asia Regional Conference on Epidemiology in March 2010 on various issues related to epidemiology and public health, some of them are as follows (Delhi Declaration on Epidemiology, March 2010):

1. **Promote** epidemiology as a core discipline of public health, and as an essential tool for rational evidence-based health action and for addressing, with socio-cultural sensitivity, issues related to equity in health with social justice;
2. **Recognize** the essential role of epidemiology, together with suitable laboratory back-up, in providing evidence-based information, in partnership with health and health-related sectors and the community, for advocacy, planning interventions, monitoring and evaluation in health;
3. **Strengthen** epidemiology and public health by creating an enabling environment and establishing career structures at national, state, provincial and district levels. In addition augment capacity by mandating competent background and level of expertise for persons responsible for health of populations;
4. **Emphasize** the use of epidemiology for strengthening health system and primary healthcare;
5. **Strengthen and reform** epidemiology and public health education, training and research in the region by all possible means, including establishing regional networks to enable sharing of expertise and information, particularly through the use of modern information technology.

Finally with the rapid development in all discipline in health sciences, there is a need for innovative, transdisciplinary approaches in newer field of epidemiology.

To conclude, epidemiology and public health should go hand-in-hand to develop good policies based on evidence-based knowledge to achieve health for all globally.

References

1. Institute of Medicine, Committee for the Study of the Future of Public Health, Division of Healthcare Services. The Future of Public Health. Washington, DC: National Academy Press. 1988;pp 40–41.
2. Russell LB. The knowledge base for public health strategies. Am J Public Health 1997;87:1597–98.
3. David A Savitz, Charles Poole, William C Miller. Reassessing the Role of Epidemiology in Public Health. American Journal of Public Health. 1999; 89(8):1158–61.
4. Roger Detels. Epidemiology: The foundation of public health (Ch 6.1.) in Detels R, McEwen J, Beaglehole R, Tanaka H (Eds). Oxford Textbook of Public Health (4th edn). Oxford University Press, USA, 2002.
5. Bonita R, Beaglehole R, Kjellström T. Basic epidemiology, 2nd edn. Published by World Health Organization, Geneva, Switzerland; 2006;165–67.
6. Neil Pearce. A Short Introduction to Epidemiology. Second Edition, Occasional Report Series No. 2, Centre for Public Health Research, Massey University Wellington Campus, Private Box 756, Wellington, New Zealand. 2005;9–11.
7. Wynder EL. Invited commentary: Studies of mechanism and prevention. Am J Epidemiol 1994;547–49.
8. Avilés LA. Epidemiology as discourse: The politics of development institutions in the Epidemiological Profile of El Salvador. J Epidemiol Community Health 2001;55:164–71.
9. Arthur Brownlea. Social Science and Medicine. Part D: Medical Geography. 1981;15(1):57–67. doi:10.1016/0160-8002(81)90016-2.
10. Gil-González D, Ruiz-Cantero MT, Álvarez-Dardet C. How political epidemiology research can address why the millennium development goals have not been achieved: Developing a research agenda. Journal of Epidemiology and Community Health 2009,63(4): 278–80.

SPATIAL EPIDEMIOLOGY: AN OVERVIEW

"From now on, space by itself and time by itself are doomed to fade away into mere shadows, and only a kind of union of the two will preserve an independent reality."

—Hermann Minkowski, 1908

INTRODUCTION

The word spatial (also **spacial**) originated from Latin word **'spatium'** meaning **'space'** in mid 19th century.

As we know that there are three types of epidemiology (descriptive epidemiology, analytical and experimental), the descriptive epidemiology deals with time, place and person. However, much attention is not given to descriptive epidemiology specially place distribution.

Spatial epidemiology is the description and analysis of geographically indexed health data with respect to demographic, environmental, behavioural, socio-economic, genetic, and infectious risk factors. It is part of a long tradition of geographic analyses dating back to the 1800s when maps of disease rates in different countries began to emerge to characterize the spread and possible causes of outbreaks of infectious diseases such as yellow fever and cholera (Walter 2000).[1] Over the ensuing decades, it grew in complexity, sophistication, and utility. Spatial epidemiology extends the rich tradition of ecologic studies that use explanations of the distribution of diseases in different places to better understand the etiology of disease (Doll 1980; Keys 1980).[2,3]

Although epidemiologic research focusing on place or location historically received considerably less attention, modern epidemiology increasingly incorporates the spatial perspective into research designsand models.

Spatial factors have also become prominent features in etiologic research, especially concerning host-vector-agent interactions, but also in guiding social and environmental epidemiologic investigations. Spatial methods are also progressively incorporated into health services research focused on specificdiseases, health conditions, or risk factors.

DEFINING SPATIAL EPIDEMIOLOGY

The geographical epidemiology is defined as "the description of spatial patterns of disease incidence and mortality." According to Lawson spatial epidemiology is "concerned with the analysis of the spatial/geographical distribution of the incidence of disease." It incorporates the spatial perspective into the research design and analysis of the distribution, determinants, and outcomes of all aspects of health and well-being across the continuum from diseases prevention to recovery.[4–6]

Spatial epidemiology is not synonymous with health and/or medical geography. Health geography is the primarily focused on spatial patterns and context, whereas spatial epidemiology is inherently focused on populations.

Concepts of Place and Vicinity[7–11]

Health is an outcome of different factors, such as personal characteristics (age, gender, social class), the physical and social environments, an individual interacts with, cultural norms, and both the provision and utilization of health services. Person's residential area and workplace are also important in determining the health status.

For example, in India, the pregnant women living in remote rural/tribal areas may have to travel longer distances to reach primary health centers, usually get delayed in accessing the emergency facilities for delivery. Various diseases are also typically distributed from one place to another, e.g. kala azar is more common in Bihar and Odisha than Maharashtra.

A neighborhood is typically defined as the geographic area relevant to the specific health outcome being studied. However, neighborhoods can be delineated by the extent of the individual's spatial interaction or administratively delimited at the scale at which policies are implemented (country, state, district, villages, houses).

Graphical information systems (GIS) have really been around for as long as there have been maps (Fig. 1.2).

At the heart of the matter is the emphasis on 'where'? — 1. Where do disease's spread? 2. Where are the persons or communities most at risk? 3. Where are resources located that best supply their demand or potential demand? 4. And, of course, once we know 'where', we are in a much better position to ask 'why'.

GIS has a language all its own. The World Geodetic System (WGS84) is a graphical representation of the world, that transforms a 3D sphere to 2D map made of points, lines, polygons, (vectors), grids (raster), and their associated data attributes.

In general, you can represent topography with a series points (each with its own value), in a grid (a tessellated plane of pixel-like data, e.g. digital camera images and computer screens), or with contour lines (polygons).

Computing just makes them more comprehensive, accurate and available to non-cartographic folks. There are a number of open source and free tools available to epidemiologists to help incorporate GIS into their armamentarium. The two most important are GRASS 1 and R. There has also been some movement away from toolbox programs (like ArcGIS) to more service-oriented tools, like Google Earth (to which R and GRASS can also interface).

Need for Spatial Methods

All epidemiological studies are spatial! When do we need to 'worry', i.e. acknowledge the spatial component? "Are we explicitly interested in the spatial pattern of disease incidence?" For example, disease mapping, cluster detection. Is the clustering a nuisance quantity that we wish to acknowledge, but are not explicitly interested in? For example, spatial regression. If we are interested in the spatial pattern then, if the data are not a complete enumeration, we clearly need the data to be randomly collected in space.[12]

Elliott *et al.* identified four types of spatial analyses in epidemiology:

1. Disease mapping,
2. Geographical correlation studies,
3. Risk assessment in relation to point or line sources, and
4. Cluster detection and disease clustering.

Types of Data

An important distinction is whether the data arise as: Point data in which exact residential location exist for cases and non-cases, or count data in which aggregation (typically over-administrative units), has been carried out.

GIS can answer the following questions.

Condition: What is .... ?

Location: Where .... ?

Trend: What is the change since.......?

Pattern: What spatial pattern........... ?

Modelling: What if ....?

GIS applications in public health/epidemiology:

- Simple visualization
- Mapping risk
- Location allocation
- Mapping disease spread
- Neighborhoods and health

Functions of GIS

1. Prepare thematic maps
2. Overlaying the pieces of information
3. Creation of buffer areas nearby selected points
4. To do specific calculations, e.g. proportions, distances, etc.
5. Create link between database and maps
6. Process aerial and satellite images
7. To provide extrapolation techniques

Fig. 1.2: Graphical information system

These data are ecological in nature, in that they are collected across groups, in spatial studies the groups are geographical areas.

Type of Studies for Collection of Data

All descriptive studies can be used for spatial epidemiology; however, ecological and cross-sectional studies are more suitable. Cross-sectional studies typically examine the distribution of exposures and outcomes simultaneously, frequently through use of population-based administrative health data or representative sample surveys. Studies using cross-sectional designs rarely integrate the spatial perspective directly because spatial referents for each observation are not collected or are at a spatial resolution that does not permit localized investigations.

The details of the spatial epidemiological analysis are beyond the scope of this chapter as it deals only with introduction/brief account of the spatial epidemiology; however, some the analytical methods are described below (Figs 1.3 to 1.5).

Disease Mapping

Aims

1. Simple description—a visual summary of geographical risk.
2. Provide estimates of risk by area to inform public health resource allocation.
3. Give clues to aetiology via informal examination of maps with exposure maps, components of spatial versus non-spatial residual variability may also provide clues to source of variability (e.g. environmental exposures usually have spatial structure). The formal examination is carried out via spatial regression.
4. In general mapping is based on count data (which is more routinely available)—may also be carried out with point data but much less common (case-control studies are explicitly carried out to examine an exposure of interest, and cannot inform on risk without additional information).
5. Provide a context within which specific studies may be placed.
   a. Example: Surveillance of disease registries will be greatly helped if we have a knowledge of the variability in residual spatial risk, and the nature of that variability (spatial versus non-spatial), i.e. what is the 'null' distribution (distribution in absence of a 'hot spot')?
   b. Regression will be aided if we have a 'prior' on the background variability.

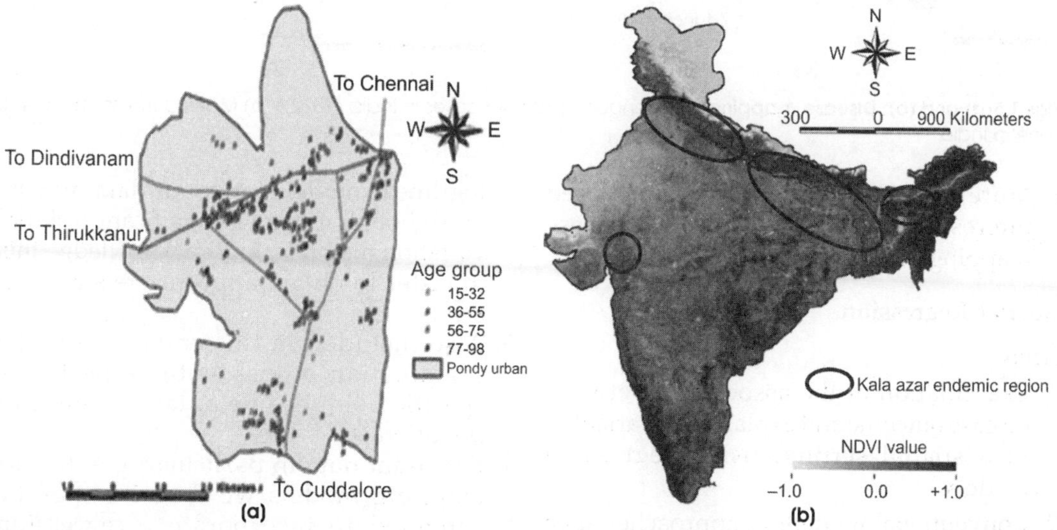

Figs 1.3(a) and (b): Disease mapping. (a) Map quantities; (b) The landscape environment of visceral leishmaniasis transmission in India

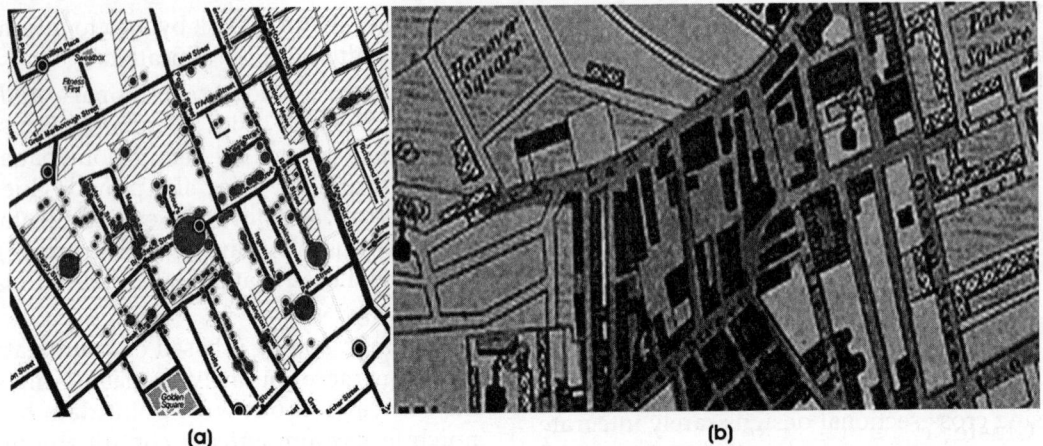

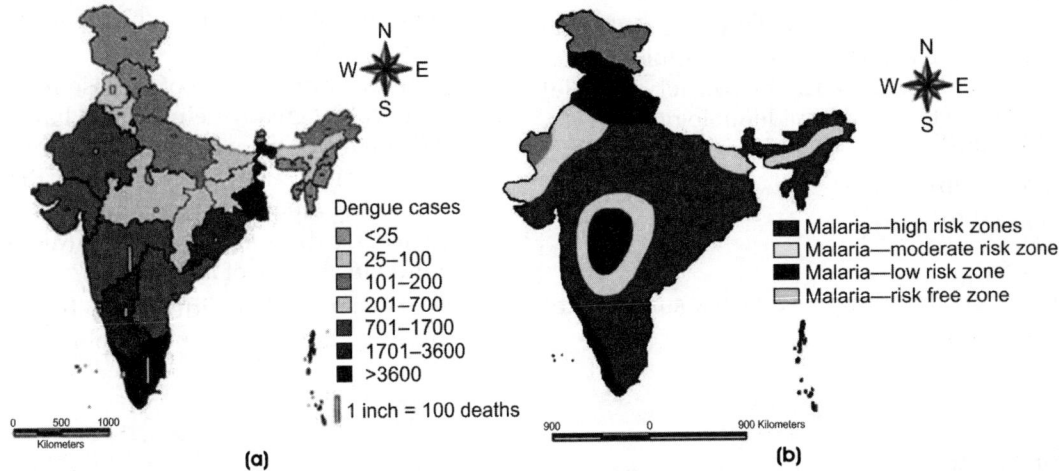

(a) (b)

Figs 1.4(a) and (b): Disease mapping. (a) John Snow—Cholera map—1850s disease clustering; (b) Edwin Chadwick (sanitation; 1832). Map locations

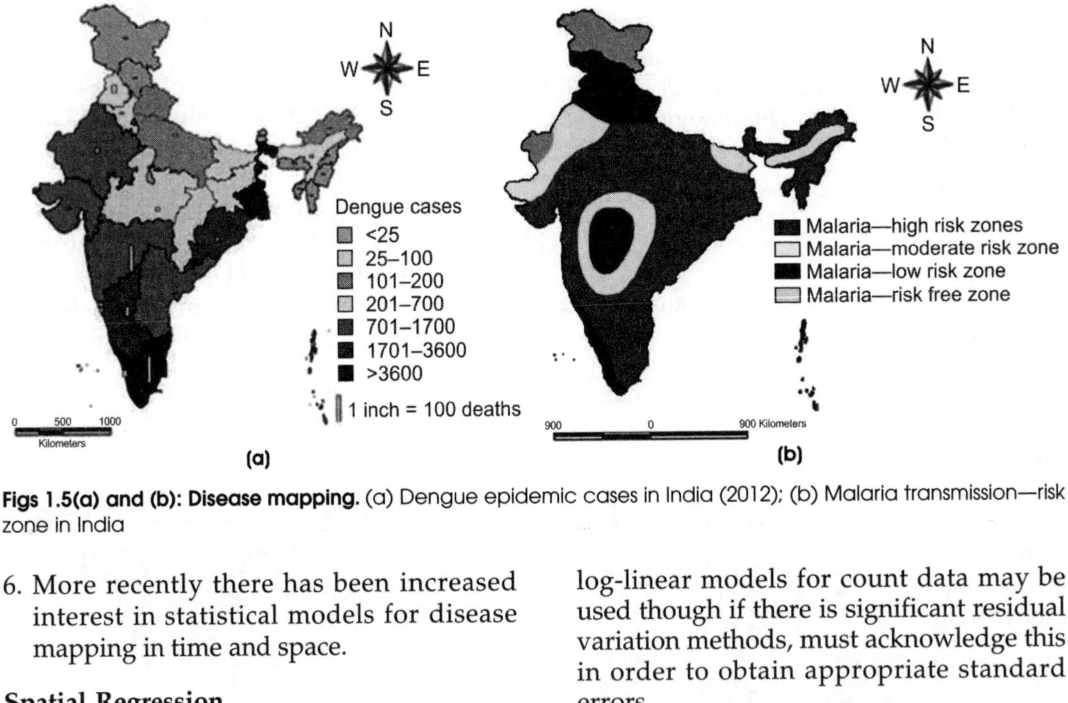

(a) (b)

Figs 1.5(a) and (b): Disease mapping. (a) Dengue epidemic cases in India (2012); (b) Malaria transmission—risk zone in India

6. More recently there has been increased interest in statistical models for disease mapping in time and space.

Spatial Regression

Aims

1. Examination of the association between disease outcome and explanatory variables, in a spatial setting, using regression models.
2. Conventional modelling approaches such as logistic regression for point data, and log-linear models for count data may be used though if there is significant residual variation methods, must acknowledge this in order to obtain appropriate standard errors.
3. Also included in this enterprise is the examination of risk with respect to a specific point or line putative source of pollution.
4. For count data in particular, the disease mapping models we describe may be extended to incorporate a regression component.

Cluster detection

Aims:

1. Cluster detection—examination of spatially-indexed data in order to detect 'clusters'. May be carried out retrospectively, or prospectively—in the latter case the operation is referred to as surveillance.
2. Surveillance may offer clues to aetiology, but also has a public health role, for example, to determine whether screening programs are being taken up universally (across space).
3. Cluster examination in response to an inquiry is subtly different because the hypothesis of increased risk may be the result of data dredging.
4. Surveillance is data dredging, but we have set the rules for dredging and so can attempt to adjust significance levels.

CONCLUSION

Spatial epidemiology has provided new opportunities to investigate the environmental, social, and behavioural factors underlying geographic variations in disease rates at small-area scale with the help of GIS and statistical methodology. Spatial epidemiological studies are useful due to instant visualization, mapping and statistical analysis. It is crucial to apply these methods for better understanding of the complex relationships between environment, health and diseases. It is also important for better planning of resources and optimal utilization of the same for best health outcome and productivity.

References

1. Walter SD. Disease mapping: A historical perspective. In: Spatial Epidemiology: Methods and Applications (Elliott P, Wakefield J, Best N, Briggs DJ, eds). Oxford: Oxford University Press. 2000;223–52.
2. Doll R. The epidemiology of cancer. Cancer 1980; 45:2475–85. [PubMed]
3. Keys A. Seven Countries—A Multivariate Analysis of Death and Coronary Heart Disease. Boston: Harvard University Press, 1980.
4. Russell S Kirby, Eric Delmelle, Jan M Eberth. Introduction Advances in spatial epidemiology and geographic information systems. Annals of Epidemiology, 27 (2017) 1e9, http://dx.doi.org/10.1016/j.annepidem.2016.12.001
5. Charles DiMaggio. Spatial Epidemiology Notes: Applications and Vignettes in R, July 25, 2014, downloaded from http://www.columbia. edu/~cjd11/charles_dimaggio/DIRE/resources/spatialEpiBook.pdf
6. Elliott P, Wakefield J, Best N, Briggs B, (ed.). Spatial epidemiology: Methods and applications. Oxford, England: Oxford University Press; 2000.
7. English D. Geographical epidemiology and ecological studies. In: Elliott P, Cuzick J, English D, Stern R, editors. Geographical and Environmental Epidemiology: Methods for Small-Area Studies. Oxford, England: Oxford University Press; 1992; pp 3e13.
8. Lawson AB. Statistical methods in spatial epidemiology. 2nd ed. New York: John Wiley & Sons; 2013.
9. Dummer TJB. Health geography: Supporting public health policy and planning. CMAJ 2008; 178(9):1177e80.
10. Kwan M-P, editor. Geographies of health, disease and well-being: recent advances in theory and method. New York, New York: Routledge. 2014.
11. Diez Roux AV. Investigating neighborhood and area effects on health. Am J Public Health 2001; 91(11):1783e9.
12. Gavin Shaddick, Spatial epidemiology. https://www.stat.ubc.ca/~gavin/SpatEpiPart1.pdf.

Chapter

2

Uses and Application of Epidemiology

Ram Chandra Goyal

The basic nature of epidemiology is inquisitiveness, therefore, it is imperative to ask questions about epidemiology itself to get through six gates to answer the uses of epidemiology. They are summarized in Table 2.1 and Fig. 2.1.

In 1955, Jerry Morris published an article 'The Uses of Epidemiology' in British Medical Journal later in 1957, it was expanded and published a book on the same topic. He mentioned seven uses of epidemiology: historical study, community assessment, working of health services, individual risks and chances, completing the clinical picture, identification of syndromes, and the search for causes (Box 2.1).[1–4]

HISTORICAL STUDY OF PAST, CURRENT AND FUTURE TRENDS IN HEALTH AND DISEASE

The study of the changed scenario in health and diseases and comparing data over a period of time (secular trend) is known as historical study. It helps to answer the all questions related to determinants of health, health status/event and plan appropriately to improve the situation for future. If we analyze the data closely, unexpected trends appear (Figs 2.1 to 2.5).

Table 2.1: Questions to get answer for uses of epidemiology

Past	*Current*	*Future*
History of the health of population	Learn from the past, understand present, implement and evaluate diagnosis of the health of the community, and the working of health services	Future planning for diagnosis of the health of the community, and the working of health service
What was it?	What is it?	What will it be?
Whom was more?	Whom is it more?	Whom will it be more?
Who was suffering?	Who is suffering?	Who will be suffering?
Why were they suffering?	Why are they suffering?	Why will they be suffering?
Where were sufferers?	Where are sufferes?	Where will be more sufferers?
How were they suffering?	How are they suffering?	How will they be suffering?

Box 2.1: Seven uses of epidemiology (as described by Jerry Morris)

The epidemiological method is the only way of asking some questions in medicine, one way of asking others, and no way at all to ask many. Several uses of epidemiology have been described as follows:

1. To study the ***history of the health of populations,*** and of the rise and fall of diseases and changes in their character. Useful projections into the future may be possible.
2. To ***diagnose the health of the community*** and the condition of the people, to measure the true dimensions and distribution of ill-health in terms of incidence, prevalence, disability, and mortality; to set health problems in perspective and define their relative importance; to identify groups needing special attention. Ways of life change, and with them the community's health; new measurements for monitoring them must therefore constantly be sought.
3. To study ***the working of health services*** with a view to their improvement. Operational research translates knowledge of (changing) community health and expectations in terms of needs for services and measure [sic] how these are met. The success of services delivered in reaching stated norms, and the effects on community health and its needs have to be appraised, in relation to resources. Such knowledge may be applied in action research pioneering better services, and in drawing up plans for the future. Timely information on health and health services is itself a key service requiring much study and experiment. Today, information is required at many levels, from the local district to the international.
4. To estimate from the group experience what are the ***individual risks*** on average of disease, accident and defect, and the chances of avoiding them.
5. To ***identify syndromes*** by describing the distribution and association of clinical phenomena in the population.
6. To ***complete the clinical picture*** of chronic diseases and describe their natural history by including in due proportion all kinds of patients, wherever they present, together with the undemanding and the symptomless cases who do not present and whose needs may be as great; by following the course of remission and relapse, adjustment and disability in defined populations. Follow-up of cohorts is necessary to detect early subclinical and perhaps reversible disease and to discover precursor abnormalities during the pathogenesis, which may offer opportunities for prevention.
7. To ***search for causes*** of health and disease by computing the experience of groups defined by their composition, inheritance and experience, their behaviour [sic] and environments. To confirm particular causes of the chronic diseases and the patterns of multiple causes, describing their mode of operation singly and together, and to assess their importance in terms of the relative risks of those exposed. Postulated causes will often be tested in naturally occurring experiments of opportunity and sometimes by planned experiments.

Source: Reprinted from Morris JN. *Uses of Epidemiology*. 3rd ed. Edinburgh, UK: Churchill Livingstone, 262–63.

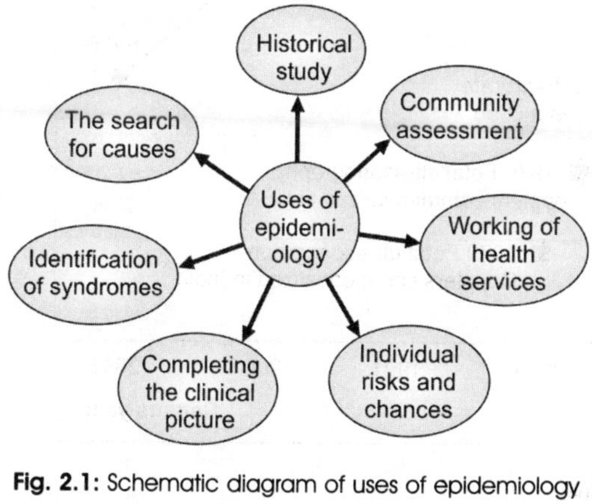

Fig. 2.1: Schematic diagram of uses of epidemiology

The trends help to understand the current status, the strategies, strength and weakness to overcome in future. The Indian scenario/ historical review show the following.

Situation in 1947: According to the 1951 Census, India's population was 36.1 crores. Only 18.33% of the total population was literate then, of which female literacy was 8.86%; only one out of every 11 women was able to read and write. The overall life expectancy was 32 years. The infant mortality rate (IMR) was 145.6/1000 live births. Maternal mortality ratio (MMR) in the 1940s was 2000/100,000 live births, which apparently came down to 1000 in the 1950s. There were only 50,000 doctors across the country. The number of primary healthcare centers in the country was only 725.

In 2017, India has progressed immensely across several sectors in the past 70 years. Today, India's population is over 1.32 billion (2016 estimate). Our literacy rates have risen to a total of 74%, with male and female literacy being 82% and 66%, respectively. MMR steeply declined from 2000 (1940s) to 174 (2015) for every 100,000 live births and IMR has dropped down from 145.6 to 38/1000 live births over 70 years.

Figures 2.2a to d and Tables 2.2 to 2.4 show examples of various trends.

Top 10 causes of death (*Source:* WHO Country Health Profile 2012: India)[6]

1. Ischaemic heart disease (12%)
2. Chronic obstructive pulmonary disease (11%)
3. Stroke (9%)
4. Diarrhoeal disease (6%)
5. Lower respiratory infections (5%)
6. Preterm birth complications (4%)
7. Tuberculosis (3%)
8. Self-inflicted injuries (3%)
9. Falls (3%)
10. Road injury (2%)

Changing Trends

Although, the history is important as guidelines, but we must analyze with a caution of change determinants over the period of time, there trends should not be taken as absolute truth for the present time. According to MacMahon and Pugh, these determinants are variation in diagnosis, reporting, case fatality, or some other circumstance other than a true change of incidence.

Specific examples follow:

1. Lack of comparability over time due to altered diagnostic criteria, procedure, and coding.
2. Demographic changes in terms of age, social class, education, occupation, etc.

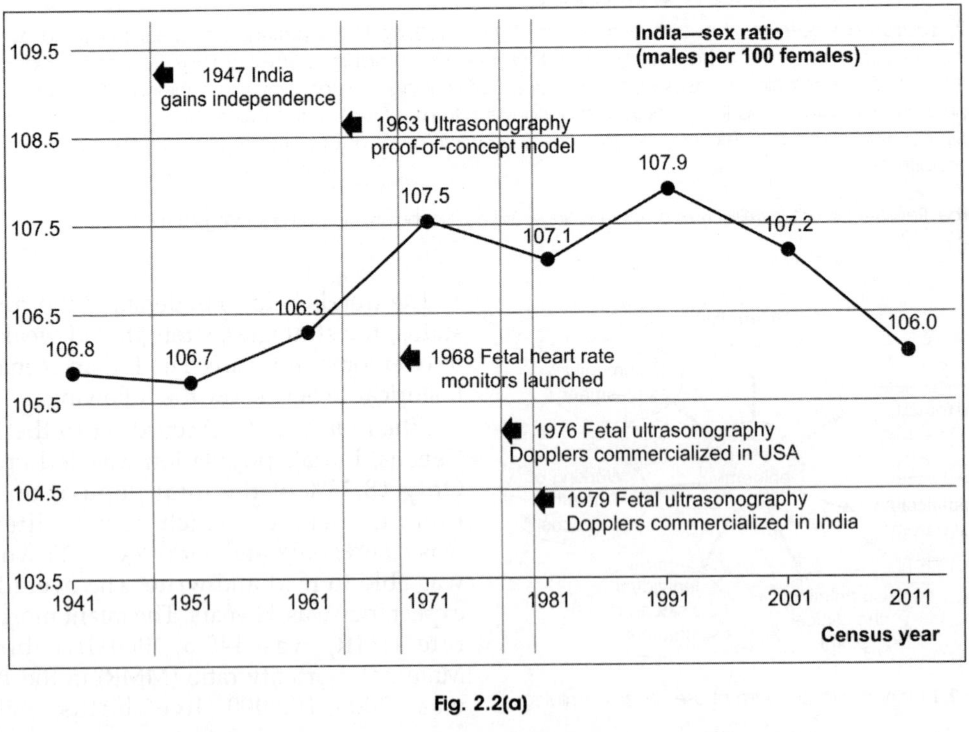

Fig. 2.2(a)

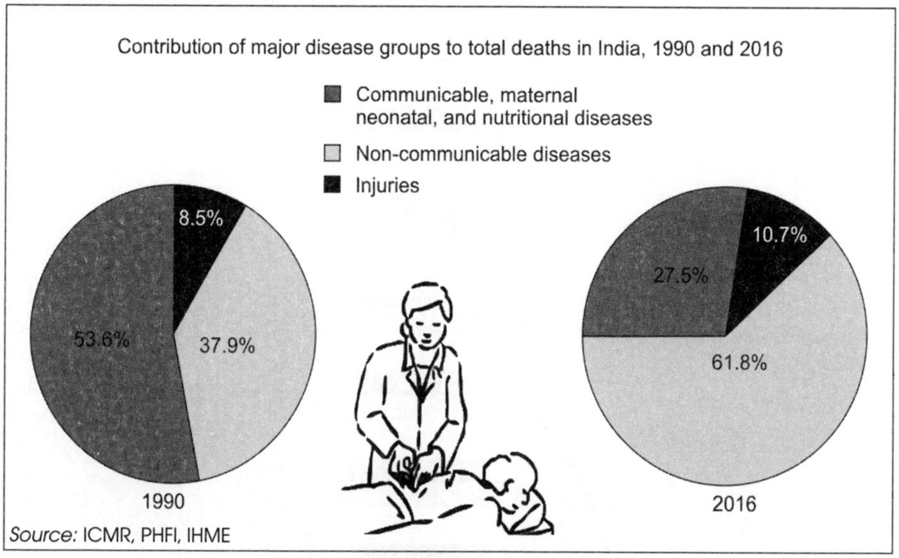

Fig. 2.2(b): Health of the states

Table 2.2: Size and growth of population in India: 1901 to 2001

Census year	*Total (in crores)*	*Average annual exponential growth (%)*	*Decadal growth rate (%)*
1901	23.84	—	—
1911	25.20	0.58	2.75
1921	125.13	(–) 0.03	(–) 0.31
1931	27.89	1.04	11.00
1941	31.86	1.33	14.22
1951	36.10	1.25	13.31
1961	43.92	1.96	21.51
1971	54.82	2.20	24.80
1981	38.33	2.22	24.66
1991	84.63	2.14	23.85
2001	102.70	1.93	21.34

Table 2.3: Birth and death rates in India (per 1000 population) (1901 to 2001)

Years	*Birth rate*	*Death rate*	*Natural increase*
1901–1910	49.2	42.6	6.6
1911–1920	48.1	47.2	0.9
1921–1930	46.4	36.3	10.1
1931–1940	45.2	31.2	14.0
1941–1950	39.9	27.4	12.5
1951–1960	41.7	22.8	18.9
1961–1970	41.2	19.0	22.2
1971–1980	37.2	15.0	22.2
1981–1990	32.5	11.4	21.1
1991–2001	25.0	8.0	17.0

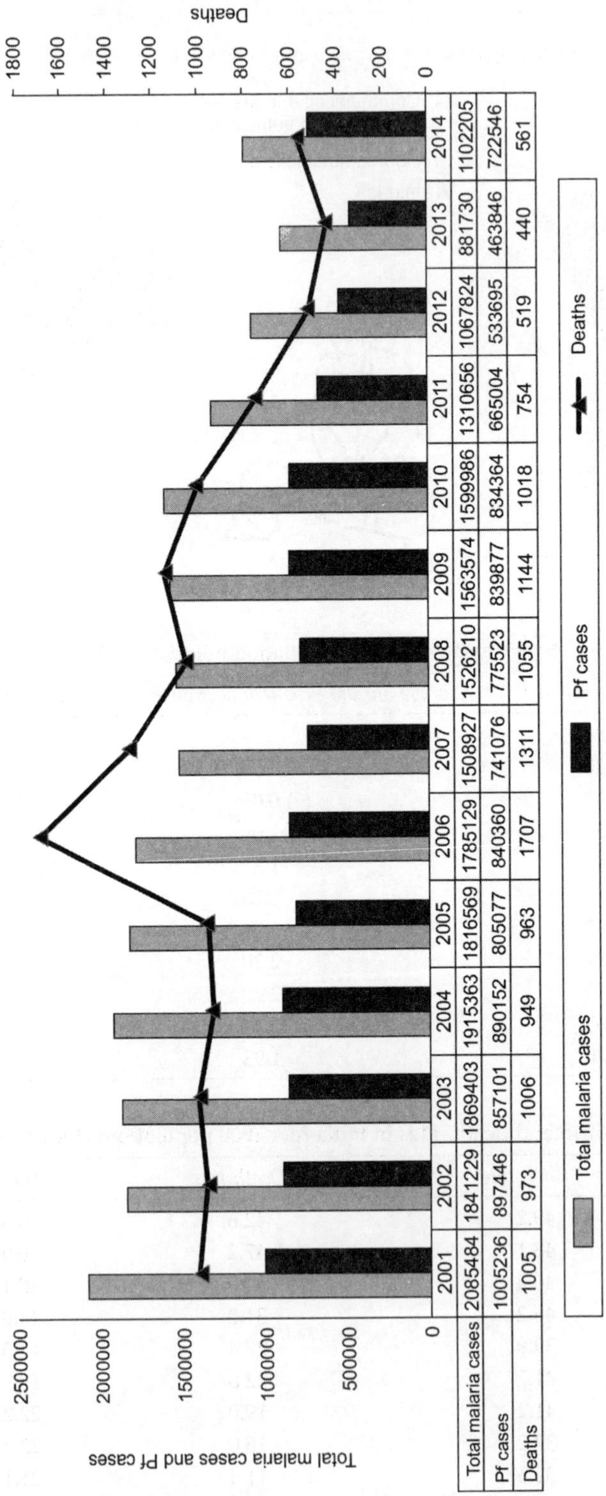

	2001	2002	2003	2004	2005	2006	2007	2008	2009	2010	2011	2012	2013	2014
Total malaria cases	2085484	1841229	1869403	1915363	1816569	1785129	1508927	1526210	1563574	1599986	1310656	1067824	881730	1102205
Pf cases	1005236	897446	857101	890152	805077	840360	741076	775523	839877	834364	665004	533695	463846	722546
Deaths	1005	973	1006	949	963	1707	1311	1055	1144	1018	754	519	440	561

Fig. 2.2(c)

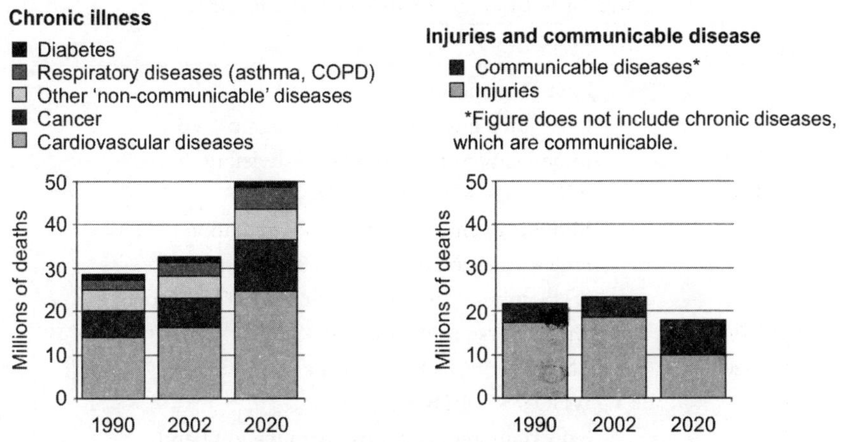

(**Source:** Yach D, et al. JAMA 2004;291:2616–22.)

Fig. 2.2(d): Annual global mortality by category

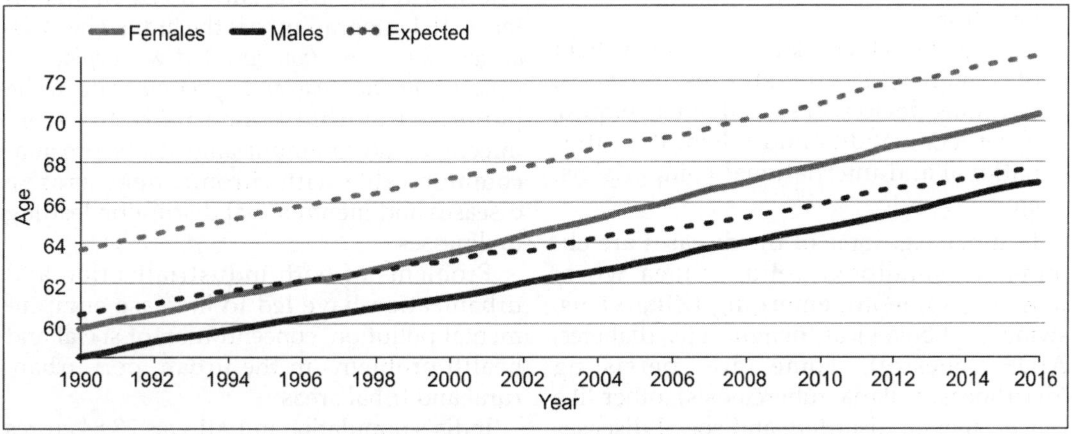

Fig. 2.3: Life expectancy (http://www.healthdata.org/india)[5]

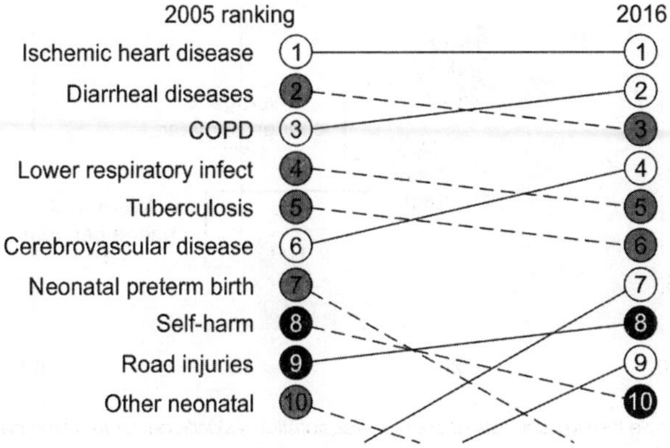

Fig. 2.4: Causes of deaths (http://www.healthdata.org/india)[5]

Table 2.4: A brief history of TB control in India

Years	*Event*
1906	First TB sanatoria
1929	India joins international union against TB
1949	Indian Government opens TB division
1944–50	ATT drugs—SM, PAS, INH, Th
1951–65	Millions of children got BCG vaccination
1956	First estimation of TB cases: 8 million
1961–78	NTP-ambulatory program in 390 (89%) districts
1983–86	Short course chemotherapy (SCC)
1993–2006	RNTCP with DOT—biweekly
2006	WHO's STOPTB program
2017	Now daily regimen, dose with weight bands

3. Changes in the natural history of diseases due to better preventive and control measures.
4. Changes in technical know-how in the field of genetics, family studies, surveys, screening devices, observation techniques, observers' validity and reliability, intra-national and international comparisons, etc.[7]

In India, e.g. some of the diseases are eliminated (smallpox, polio, guinea worm disease), some are emerging (Zika virus, swine flu, Ebola virus, dengue, etc., diabetes, AIDS, obesity), some are persisting (diarrhoeas, malaria, tuberculosis), other like cancer, mental disorders and social diseases are still beyond control.

What We Learnt from Past for Better Future

The world has undergone a sea change in terms of demography so is the India. The *socio-demographic transition* coupled with *epidemiological transition has an impact on* shift in the pattern of morbidity and mortality from infectious and communicable diseases to non-communicable with chronic, degenerative diseases and mento-social disruption leading to illnesses.

Problems of both industrialization and urbanization have led to increase environmental pollution, concentration of social and health problems in the urban, peri-urban, rural and tribal areas.

India's population in 1901 was 23.84 crores and in 2017 was 130.2 crores, with this huge

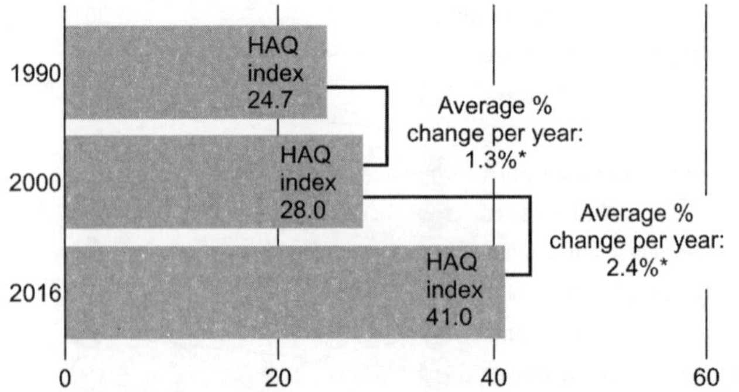

** indicate the average rate of change was statistically significant for that time period.*

Fig. 2.5: Health access and quality index, 2016 (http://www.healthdata.org/india)

population, it is obvious that resources, if not increased proportionately, bound to result in problems like low health access, persistence of malnutrition, infectious diseases, etc. We need to study other determinant of health than focusing only on morbidity and mortality patterns as epidemiology is beyond the boundary of this.

COMMUNITY ASSESSMENT[8–12]

What actual and potential health problems are there? It is identification and quantification of the health issues in the community. It is also called community diagnosis.

Health is facing a paradigm shift from planning service delivery for an individual to population-based community health services planning and delivery of services with client satisfaction.

Simply we ask people about the health services available, types of needs, types of diseases, who need the most, satisfaction regarding the services, how to find out resources, how to monitor, supervise and evaluate the services.

Comprehensive community health services planning is a two-step process: Community assessment and community action, in that order. Assessment identifies community problems and resources; action follows planning, which determines which of those problems should be addressed with which resources are linked (Figs 2.6 and 2.7).[8]

A community health assessment (CHA) or community health needs assessment (CHNA), refers to health assessment that identifies key health needs and issues through systematic, comprehensive data collection and analysis. Community health assessments use such principles as

- Multi-sector collaborations that support shared ownership of all phases of community health improvement, including assessment, planning, investment, implementation, and evaluation
- Proactive, broad, and diverse community engagement to improve results

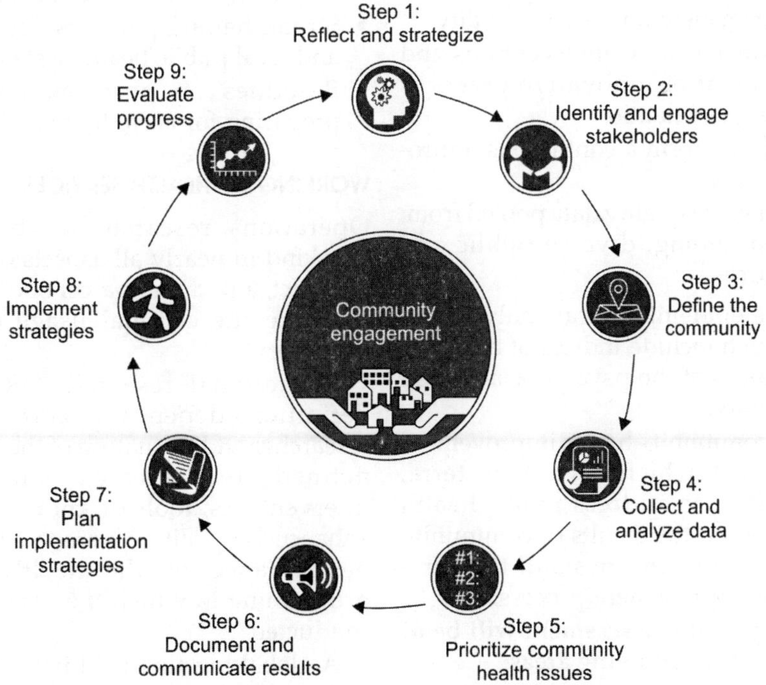

Fig. 2.6: Community health assessment cycle[12]

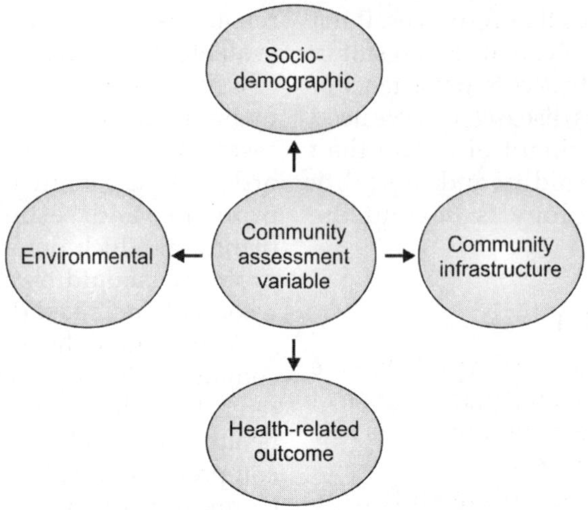

Fig. 2.7: Community assessment variable

- A definition of community that encompasses both a significant enough area to allow for population-wide interventions and measurable results, and includes a targeted focus to address disparities among subpopulations
- Maximum transparency to improve community engagement and accountability
- Use of evidence-based interventions and encouragement of innovative practices with thorough evaluation
- Evaluation to inform a continuous improvement process
- Use of the highest quality data pooled from, and shared among, diverse public and private sources.[11]

A complete epidemiological analysis will be needed which include indices of health as well as indicators of the psychosocial milieu of the community.

Develop a community health improvement plan (or CHIP) which is a long-term, systematic effort to address public health problems based on the results of community health assessment activities and the community health improvement process.

Community health assessment will be of greater help in the following areas.

- Benchmarking for public health needs and practice improvements
- Identifying strengths and weaknesses of the health services to address in quality improvement
- Improving organizational and community coordination and collaboration
- Increasing knowledge about public health and the interconnectedness of activities
- Strengthening partnerships within state and local public health systems
- Baselines on performance to use in preparing for accreditation.[9,10]

WORKING OF HEALTH SERVICES

Operations research has benefited the mankind in nearly all aspects of his life. OR is in fact, a part and parcel of our life. It tries to make the optimal usage of available resources.

Operational research (OR) has many definitions depending on the setting, the researcher and the nature of the research. It is defined as "research into strategies, interventions, tools or knowledge that can enhance the quality, coverage, effectiveness or performance of the health system or programme in which the research is being conducted".[13]

A global meeting held in Geneva in April 2008 resulted in a consensus definition of OR in context to public health as "any research producing practically usable knowledge (evidence, findings, information, etc.) which can improve program implementation (e.g. effectiveness, efficiency, quality, access, scale up, sustainability) regardless of the type of research (design, methodology, approach) falls within the boundaries of operations research".

Supporting this practical definition are three basic steps to guide operational research:

1. Spell out well-defined goals and objectives of the health programme or system in question
2. Identify, prioritize and articulate constraints and obstacles that prevent these objectives being achieved
3. Develop research questions that address the constraints.

To successfully undertake relevant operational research, it is necessary to have a common understanding of what is meant by operational research as well as agreement on the key principles.

Operational research is different from clinical or epidemiological research in that it examines a system (healthcare system) rather than focusing on an individual or a group of individuals (as in clinical or epidemiological research where patients are examined).[14]

The usual epidemiologic approaches—descriptive, analytic, and experimental—are all used in health services research and, in addition, methods of evaluation have been expanded through their application to problems in health services.

Operation research is crucial with its useful modelling techniques, it helps to identify, quantify and solve problems related to healthcare system like resource allocation, congestion/queuing problems, risk analysis, assessment of healthcare projects, disease prevention, etc.[15]

Many studies pointed out the new ways of dealing with problems, services at the door step rather than in hospital, simple technologies at low cost, how to deal with health workforce issues, etc. through operational research (Table 2.5).

Triangulation operations research studies can integrate, harmonize and optimize the working of healthcare services at all levels. It can help in optimal use of health workforce, funds, infrastructure, supplies, and continuity of services with high efficiency and services security. Broad areas of operational research are mentioned in Table 2.6.

The community-based approach will have wider impact on health status of individuals, families and community as a whole.

INDIVIDUAL'S RISK AND CHANCES OF ILL-HEALTH[18,9]

WHO defined risk factor as "any attribute, characteristic or exposure of an individual that increases the likelihood of developing a disease or injury". Some examples of the more important risk factors are underweight, unsafe sex, high blood pressure, tobacco and alcohol consumption, and unsafe water, sanitation and hygiene.

To prevent disease and injury, it is necessary to identify and deal with their causes—the health risks that underlie them. Each risk has its own causes too, and many have their roots in a complex chain of events over time, consisting of socio-economic factors, environmental and community conditions, and individual behaviour. The causal chain offers many entry points for intervention.

Some risks located further back in the causal chain act indirectly through intermediary factors. These risks include physical inactivity, alcohol, smoking or fat intake. For the most distal risk factors, such as education and income, less causal certainty can be attributed to each risk. However, modifying these background causes is more likely to have amplifying effects, by influencing multiple proximal causes; such modifications therefore have the potential to yield fundamental and sustained improvements to health. In addition to multiple points of

Table 2.5: Few examples of operations research studies from India[13]

Authors (Ref.)	*Type of study*	*Objective*	*Results relevance*	*Programme/policy*
Babu *et al.*	Cross-sectional	To evaluate reasons for treatment non-initiation in smear-positive pulmonary TB patients diagnosed and reported as initial defaulters (ID) in 20 districts of Andhra Pradesh	Of 1304 reported ID, 619 (47.5%) had been placed on treatment. Out of total confirmed (695) ID, 51% were untraceable, 22% had died before treatment initiation, 5.5% were treated privately, and 13.5% had other reasons	Inadequate documentation of referrals, delays in treatment initiation, and registration along with deficiencies in address documentation were highlighted areas for programme improvement
Jha *et al.*	Case control (through record reviews)	To assess the timing, characteristics, and risk factors for default among re-treatment TB cases	Defaults occurred early, before start of continuation phase. Being male, previous history of default during ATT, previous treatment from non-RNTCP providers or DOT at public health facility were key risk factors identified	The study pointed out to strengthen efforts to improve pretreatment counselling, retrieval mechanisms of interrupters and to increase the proportion of patients treated by community DOT providers
Varkey *et al.*	Non-equivalent control Quasi-experimental	To investigate the feasibility, acceptability, and cost of a new, more comprehensive model of maternity care that encouraged husbands' participation in their wives' antenatal and postpartum care in Employee State Insurance Corporation (ESIC) dispensaries in Delhi	Significant changes were noted in family planning knowledge and behaviours of both men and women in intervention group. Significant higher client-provider discussions occurred during maternity care in the intervention group. The marginal cost of implementing the intervention per dispensary per year was ₹ 50,000 (approx. US$ 1,000)	On the basis of the results, the model was scaled in all the ESIC dispensaries in Delhi
Tripathy *et al.*	Cluster-randomized trial	To assess the effect of community mobilization through participatory women's group in improving birth outcomes in underserved tribal clusters of Jharkhand and Odisha	Neonatal mortality rate (NMR) was 32% lower in intervention clusters after adjustments	The study underscored the importance of involving women groups as an alternative to just having health worker led interventions for improving NMR.
Patel *et al.*	Economic analysis	To ascertain the efficiency of zinc and copper supplementation in the treatment of acute diarrhoea under 5 years	The study demonstrated lowers cost of treating acute diarrhoea, lowers cost per unit health and incremental cost effectiveness ratio	Cost savings as evidenced by the study makes a stronger case for micronutrients supplementation as an adjunct therapy to ORS management

Table 2.6: Broad areas of operational research in healthcare system[16,17]

Healthcare services analysis	*Economic analysis*	*Public policy*	*Clinical applications*
• Scheduling and workforce planning • Inventory management • Supply chain management • Logistics planning and modelling • Equipment planning • Planning facility, location and layout • Workforce and workload models • Decision support systems • Performance measurement and modelling • Queuing models • Quality management	• Equipment evaluation and selection models • Optimal pricing and costing models • Demand forecasting and planning models • Impact of policies on healthcare demand • Technology assessment	• Regional planning and network models • Access and availability population models • Technology diffusion models • Disease prevention • Healthcare coverage • Vaccine modelling • Organ allocation models • Disease screening • Resource allocation • Drug policies • Blood supply management policies	• Risk assessment and analysis • Clinical diagnosis and decision making • Decision support systems • Disease modelling (individual level) • Treatment design and planning • Drug selection models • Optimal dosing models • Vaccine models • Clinical qualities

intervention along the causal chain, there are many ways that populations can be targeted (Fig. 2.8).

The two major approaches to reducing risk are:
- Targeting high-risk people, who are most likely to benefit from the intervention

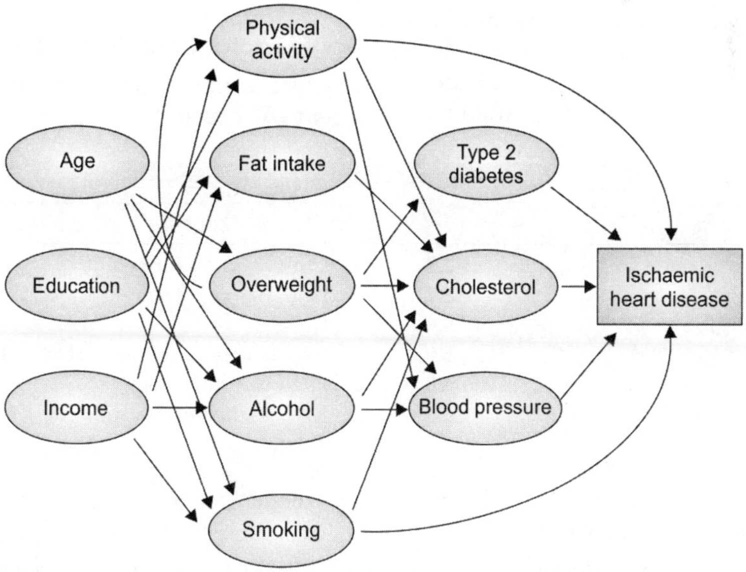

Fig. 2.8: The causal chain. Major causes of ischaemic heart disease are shown. Arrows indicate come (but not all) of the pathways by which these causes interact.

- Targeting risk in the entire population, regardless of individual's risk and potential benefit.

World Health Organization reported some of the risk for factors as an individual risk and community risk for various morbidity and mortality (Table 2.7).

Some of examples are given below.

- High blood pressure is the leading risk factor for mortality, responsible for 13% of deaths globally
- Childhood underweight is the leading risk factor for burden of disease and is responsible for over 2 million children dying per year, mainly in low-income countries
- Environmental risks such as unsafe water, sanitation and hygiene and indoor smoke from solid fuels cause around 2 million children deaths per year.
- Low fruit and vegetable intake, lack of exercise, alcohol and tobacco use, high body mass index, high cholesterol, high blood glucose, and high blood pressure are risk factors responsible for more than half of the deaths due to heart disease, the leading cause of death in the world.
- Unsafe sex, which leads to transmission of human papillomavirus, is responsible for virtually all deaths due to cervical cancer. Cervical cancer is responsible for 11% of global unsafe sex deaths and is the leading cause of cancer death in Africa.
- Tobacco is a leading risk factor for mortality, responsible for 5.1 million deaths. Almost 1 in 8 deaths of adults over the age of 30 is due to smoking.
- Being overweight or suffering from obesity is the fifth leading risk for death. It is responsible for 7% of deaths globally—8% in high income countries and 7% in middle income countries.

The risk transition: In developing countries, risk factors are also changes, the types of diseases that affect a population shift from primarily infections, such as diarrhoea and pneumonia, to primarily non-communicable, such as cardiovascular disease and cancers.

This shift is caused by:

- **Improvements in medical care**, which mean that children no longer die from easily curable conditions such as diarrhoea.
- **The ageing of the population**, because non-communicable diseases affect older adults at the highest rates
- **Public health interventions** such as vaccinations and the provision of clean water and sanitation, which reduce the incidence of infectious diseases.

Single Factor Causation of Diseases

It was thought merely presence of a disease agent will cause the disease like *Mycobactirium*

Table 2.7: Leading causes of attributable global mortality and burden of disease, 2004

Attributable mortality	%	*Attributable DALYs*	%
1. High blood pressure	12.8	1. Childhood underweight	7.8
2. Tobacco use	8.7	2. HIgh blood pressure	7.5
3. High blood glucose	5.8	3. Unsafe sex	6.6
4. Physical inactivity	5.5	4. Unsafe water, sanitation, hygiene	6.1
5. Overweight and obesity	4.8	5. High blood glucose	4.9
6. High cholesterol	4.5	6. Indoor smoke from solid fuels	4.8
7. Unsafe sex	4.0	7. Tobacco use	3.9
8. Alcohol use	3.8	8. Physical inactivity	3.8
9. Childhood underweight	3.8	9. Suboptimal breastfeeding	3.7
10. Indoor smoke from solid fuels	3.3	10. High cholesterol	3.3
59 million total global deaths in 2004		1.5 billion total global DALYs in 2004	

http://who.int/healthinfo/globen_burden_disease/GBD2004ReportFigure.ppt

tuberculosis only was responsible for tuberculosis, in such circumstances, everyone should get the tuberculosis, but in reality does not happen. This has led to multi-factorial causation of illnesses.

Multi-factorial Causation of Diseases

Many diseases are caused by more than one risk factor, and thus may be prevented by reducing any of the risk factors responsible for them. As a result, the sum of the mortality or burden of disease attributable to each of the risk factors separately is often more than the combined mortality and burden of disease attributable to the groups of these risk factors. For example, of all infectious and parasitic child deaths (including those caused by acute lower respiratory infections), 34% can be attributed to underweight; 26% to unsafe water, hygiene and sanitation; and 15% to smoke from indoor use of solid fuels. The joint effect of all three of these risk factors is, however, 46%.

The association of the causality must have the following criteria to prove the causality Table 2.8.

Epidemiological studies conducted groups of individuals (case-control/cohort studies); the studies provide evidence that groups with particular exposures or lifestyle characteristics are more or less likely to develop disease than groups of individuals with or without the exposures. Extrapolation based on observations of groups to the individual should be viewed seriously.

We know that hypertension may cause IHD, epidemiological studies can find out whether the sole cause is hypertension or some other associated factors are also present and what is the level of contribution of each factor? Another application of epidemiology is predicting the individual's prognosis and likelihood of survival if afflicted by a serious medical condition.

Table 2.8: Aspects of an association that suggest causality

1. Strength	2. Consistency
3. Specificity	4. Temporality
5. Biological gradient	6. Plausibility
7. Coherence	8. Experiment
9. Analogy	

Source: Data from Hill AB. The environment and disease: association or causation? *Proceedings of the Royal Society of Medicine,* 1965; 58:295–300.

COMPLETING THE CLINICAL PICTURE/ COMPLETING THE NATURAL HISTORY OF THE DISEASES

Natural history of any disease defines "the natural course of a disease from the time immediately prior to its inception, progressing through its pre-symptomatic phase and different clinical stages to the point where it has ended and the patient is either cured, chronically disabled, or dead without external intervention" (Figs 2.9 to 2.11).

Or natural history of disease refers to the progression of a disease process in an individual over time, in the absence of treatment. In other words, a natural history study is a way to:

- Track the course of a disease over time
- Identify demographic, genetic, environmental, and other variables that correlate with disease and outcomes in the absence of treatment
- Document changes in severity over time, occurrence of concomitant conditions, usual treatment patterns, and survival

To complete the clinical picture of a disease and describe its natural history: By including in due proportion all kinds of patients, wherever they present, together with the undemanding and the symptomless cases who do not present and whose needs may be as great; by following the course of remission and relapse, adjustment and disability in defined populations. Follow-up of cohorts is necessary to detect early subclinical and perhaps reversible disease and to discover precursor abnormalities during the pathogenesis, which may offer opportunities for prevention.

The epidemiological methods can identify spectrum of diseases (subclinical infections to

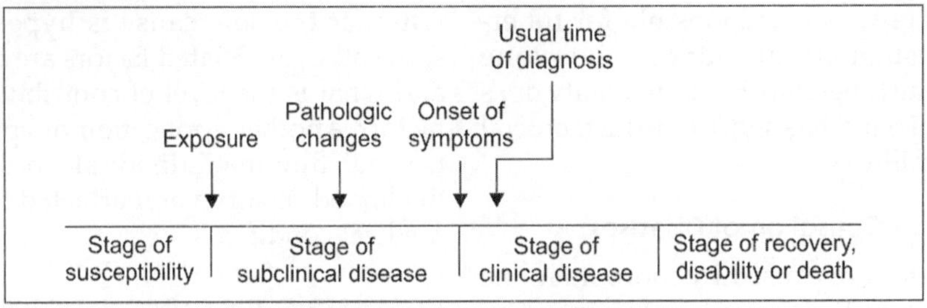

Fig. 2.9(a): Stages in natural history of disease

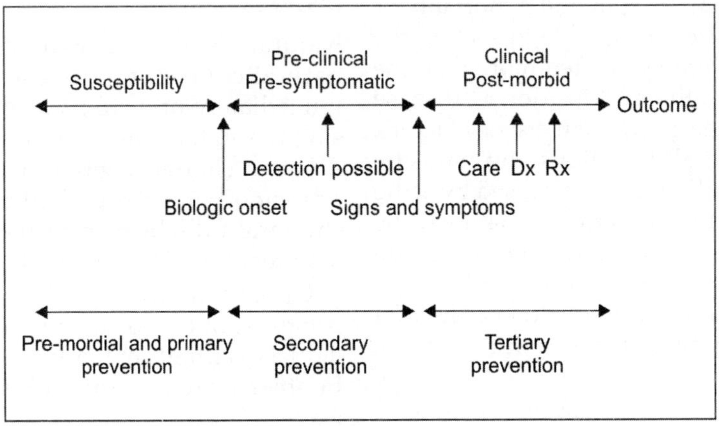

Fig. 2.9(b): Natural history of disease

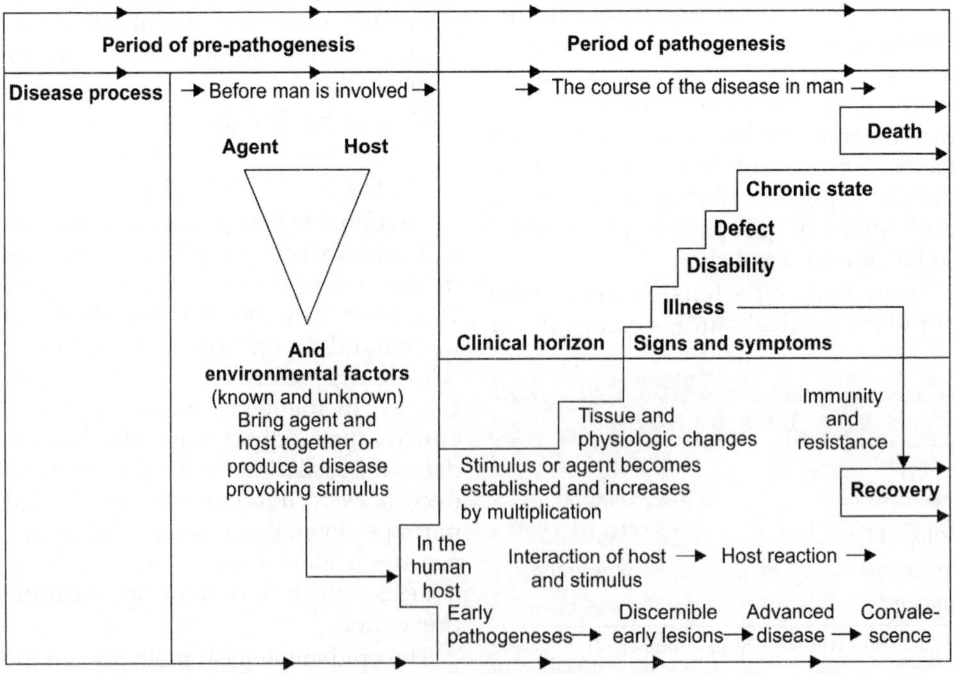

Fig. 2.10: Stages in natural history of disease with phases and level of prevention

full blown diseases pattern). Understanding of natural history of diseases helps to take corrective intervention at an appropriate time. The intervention ranges from health promotional activities to rehabilitation activities.

IDENTIFICATION OF SYNDROMES

Syndrome comes from a Greek word that combines the root 'to run' (dramein) with the prefix 'together' (sun-). When many or all of the symptoms for a disease 'run together,' that is a syndrome.

A **syndrome** is a set of *medical signs* and *symptoms* that are correlated with each other and, often, with a particular *disease* or disorder.

Morris states that "the mode of occurrence of clinical phenomenon in the population, their distribution among different social groups or during different period of times may indicate that some clinical phenomenon are different and distinct from others and therefore should not be lumped together; some have important affinity with others, and therefore may be. That is to say that the epidemiological behaviour of the clinical

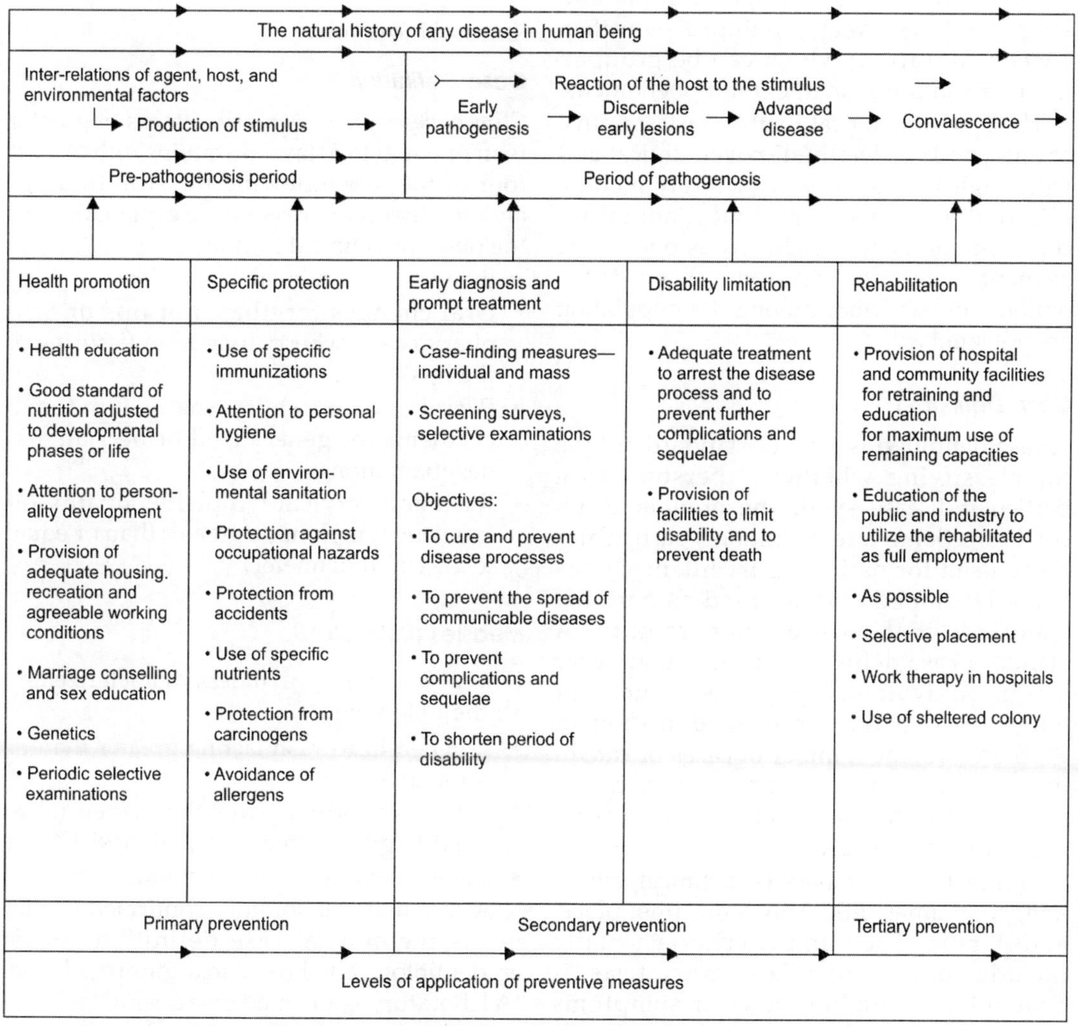

Fig. 2.11: Stages in natural history of disease with phases, level of prevention and detailed action plan

phenomenon may help in identifying the syndrome".

Morris gave an example of cardiovascular disease. The common lumping together of coronary and cerebrovascular lesions as 'atherosclerosis' is not very strongly justified in clinical or pathological terms. Nor do the two conditions always behave similarly epidemiologically.

Epidemiological studies make it possible to group together various differing manifestations of a condition or to separate seemingly identical diseases into more than one category.

Tuberculosis has a range of signs and symptoms (fever, cough, sputum of more than 2 weeks duration) which can be grouped together and called an integrator phenomena.

The epidemiological methods (descriptive or analytical) generally discover clinical and pathological categories which may include different elements. Sometimes laboratory confirmation is also included as one of the element to describe syndrome. Their distribution and behaviour among the population are not similar.

Case Definition

A case definition is a set of standard criteria for classifying whether a person has a particular disease, **syndrome**, or other health condition. Some case definitions, particularly those used for national surveillance, have been developed and adopted as national standards that ensure comparability. A standard case definition ensures that every case is equivalent, regardless of when or where it occurred, or who identified it. Furthermore, the number of cases or rate of disease identified in one time or place can be compared with the number or rate from another time or place.

A case definition consists of clinical criteria and, sometimes, limitations on time, place, and person. The clinical criteria usually include confirmatory laboratory tests, if available, or combinations of symptoms (subjective complaints), signs (objective physical findings), and other findings. Case definitions used during outbreak investigations are more likely to specify limits on time, place, and/or person than those used for surveillance.

There are thousands of the syndromes indentified worldwide; some of the examples are acute respiratory distress syndrome, Budd-Chiari syndrome, carcinoid syndrome, cardiovascular syndrome, carpal tunnel syndrome, Carpenter syndrome, cat eye syndrome, Cushing's syndrome, Down's syndrome, etc.

Examples with description are as under.

Kawasaki Syndrome

Case Definition

Clinical description: A febrile illness of greater than or equal to 5 days' duration, with at least four of the five following physical findings and no other more reasonable explanation for the observed clinical findings:

- Bilateral conjunctival congestion
- Oral changes (erythema of lips or oropharynx, strawberry tongue, or fissuring of the lips)
- Peripheral extremity changes (edema, erythema, or generalized or peri-ungual desquamation)
- Rash and cervical lymphadenopathy (at least one lymph node greater than or equal to 1.5 cm in diameter)

Measles (Rubeola)

Clinical description: An illness characterized by all the following.

- A generalized rash lasting greater than or equal to 3 days
- A temperature greater than or equal to 101.0°F (greater than or equal to 38.3°C)
- Cough, coryza, or conjunctivitis

A case that is laboratory confirmed or that meets the clinical case definition and is epidemiologically linked to a confirmed case. (A laboratory-confirmed case does not need to meet the clinical case definition.)

THE SEARCH FOR THE CAUSE(S)

Through epidemiological studies, we can find out the proportion of the people suffering from the disease, death rates—high or low, fertility rates—more or less.

While doing so, one must try to answer, why is it so? Is there any pathological or nutritional or changes by an individual or community behavioural and practice?

Ideally, the goal is to identify a cause so that appropriate public health action might be taken.

Observations on the nutritional deficiencies (scurvy, beriberi, pellagra and goitre), the geographical study of cancer (especially of the skin and liver); the industrial cancers (bladder, for instance); and industrial accidents (of coalminers or railway workers).

In India, various socio-cultural practices (useful, harmful, and harmless) were responsible for many diseases like applying *kajal* (carbon powder) in eyes led to trachoma, use of rock salt enhanced the chances of goitre, avoidance of nutritious food during pregnancy. Similarly, growing concern over non-communicable diseases due to physical inactivity, high fatty diet, smoking, etc. is a new dynamics in epidemiology.

Epidemiologist analyzed the increasing deaths due to road traffic accidents and found non-usage of seat belt was major cause of death, recently other causes have also been added like use of mobile phone while driving, drink and drive, non-adherence to traffic rules, under stressful conditions, etc.

So, epidemiological tools help to identify causative factors and also proving the association between diseases and causative factor(s).

USES OF EPIDEMIOLOGY IN SUPPORT OF PUBLIC HEALTH

Epidemiology is an integral part of public health system which helps to focus not only individuals but community as whole. Following are some of the areas for the uses of epidemiology in public health.

- **Describe the spectrum of the disease:** Spectrum of disease can guide to design more effective intervention strategies.
- **Describe the natural history of the disease:** Epidemiological studies describe the natural history of disease, to elucidate the specific manipulations in the host, and to improve diagnostic accuracy. The field of 'clinical epidemiology' applies research on the natural history of disease to improving the diagnostic accuracy of doctors in their clinical practice.
- **Identify factors that increase or decrease the risk of acquiring disease:** These 'risk factors' may be social (smoking, drinking), genetic (ethnicity), dietary (saturated fats, vitamin deficiencies), and so on. Knowing these risk factors can often provide public health professionals with the necessary tools to design effective programs to intervene before disease occurs.
- **Predict disease trends:** Knowledge of these disease patterns has been useful in designing the public health programs to prevent and control diseases.
- **Test the efficacy of intervention strategies:** Wide-spread use of an intervention not subjected to epidemiological studies of efficacy may result in implementation of an ineffective intervention program at great public expense and may actually result in greater morbidity and mortality because of an increased reliance on the favoured but unproved intervention and a reduced use of other strategies which are thought to be less effective but which are actually more effective.
- **Evaluate intervention programs:** Another problem of inferring public health efficacy from small vaccine trials is that volunteers for vaccine trials may not be representative of the general public which needs to be protected against a specific disease. Thus broad-based intervention trials also need to be carried out, to demonstrate the acceptability and public health efficacy of a vaccine or other intervention to the population in need of protection.

- **Identify the health needs of a community:** Descriptive, i.e. cross-sectional, co-relational and ecological studies reveal the magnitude of the problems/burden of the diseases in the community as well as in specific subgroups of the population, while surveillance programs can identify trends in disease, infection, and/or health status overtime.
- **Evaluate public health programs:** Ongoing monitoring and evaluation of health programs is necessary to ensure the effectiveness and efficiency. Periodic review can provide information to modify the programs so as to get maximum benefit.

References

1. Morris JN. Uses of epidemiology. International Journal of Epidemiology 2007;36(6):1165–72, https://doi.org/10.1093/ije/dym227
2. Davey Smith. The uses of 'uses of epidemiology'. The International Journal of Epidemiology 2001;30:1146–56. http://www.med.mcgill.ca/epidemiology/hanley/c609/material/Davey Smith Uses Of Uses OfEpi2001.pdf
3. Uses of Epidemiology, Ch 2. Practical applications of Epidemiology 3rd ed. pp 1975, Elsevier _CH02_Pass3.indd 56 I... including in due proportion all kinds of continues 51589_CH02_Pass3.indd 57 58, samples.jbpub.com/9781449665494/Chapter2.pdf
4. MaxcyRosenauLast's Public Health and Preventive Medicine, 13th edn. First published: July-Aug 1992. https://doi.org/10.1016/0091-2182(92)90134-O.
5. Country Profile, India | Institute for Health Metrics and Evaluation. http://www.healthdata.org/india, accessed on 22/7/2018.
6. WHO-Country Health Profile, India, 2012. Who.int/gho/countries/ind.pdf. accessed on 22/7/2018
7. MacMahon B, Pugh TF. Epidemiology Principles and Methods. Boston, MA: Little, Brown; 1970.
8. HYPERLINK "https://www.ncbi.nlm.nih.gov/pubmed/?term=Rice% 20JA%5BAuthor%5D&cauthor=true&cauthor_uid=10130406" Rice JA. Community health assessment. The first step in community health planning. (HYPERLINK "https://www.ncbi.nlm.nih.gov/pubmed/10130406" Hosp Technol Ser. 1993;12(13):1–32.
9. Sara Rosenbaum JD. Principles to Consider for the Implementation of a Community Health Needs Assessment Process. https://nnphi.org/.../PrinciplesToConsiderForTheImp... Accessed on 24/7/2018
10. Sharma Aprana BS, et al. A community need assessment guide: A brief guide on how to conduct needs assessment. https://cyfar.org/sites/default/.../Sharma%202000.pd. Accessed on 25/7/2018
11. HYPERLINK "https://www.cdc.gov/stltpublichealth/cha/plan.html" CDC - Assessment and Plans - Community Health Assessment - STLT ... https://www.cdc.gov/stltpublichealth/cha/plan.html
12. Community Health Assessment Toolkit. Association for Community Health Improvement. (2017). Accessed at HYPERLINK "http://www.healthycommunities.org/assesstoolkit" www.healthycommunities.org/assesstoolkit
13. Malhotra S, Zodpey SP. Operational research in public health. Indian J Public health(serial online) 2010 [cited 2018 Jul];54:145–50. Available from http://www.ijph.in, text.asp010/54/3/145/75737
14. Country Profile, India | Institute for Health Metrics and Evaluation. http://www.health data.org/india, accessed on 22/7/2018
15. Priyan S. Operations Research in Healthcare: A Review. JOJ Pub Health 1(3): pp 001–007. JOJPH.MS.ID.555561 (2017). DOI: 10.19080/JOJPH.2017.01.555561. Accessed on 22/7/2018
16. Rakesh kumar. Operations Research Applications in Healthcare. www.pezzottaitejournals.net/index.php/IJASMP/.../0; . http://www.accman.in/images/jan10/OR%20IN%20HEALTH%20CARE.doc.accessed on 24/7/2018
17. Sara Rosenbaum, J.D. Principles to Consider for the Implementation of a Community Health Needs Assessment Process. https://nnphi.org/.../PrinciplesToConsiderForTheImp... Accessed on 24/7/2018
18. Sharma Aprana BS et al. A community need assessment guide: A brief guide on how to conduct needs assessment. https://cyfar.org/sites default/.../Sharma%202000.pd. Accessed on 25/7/2018

Chapter

3

Basics of Communicable Diseases Epidemiology

Mohan K Doibale

We need to understand the following before application of principles of epidemiology to communicable diseases.

COMMUNICABLE DISEASE

An illness is due to a specific infectious agent or its toxic products capable of being directly or indirectly transmitted from man to man, animal to animal, or from the environment (through air, dust, soil, water, food) to man or animal.[1] Most of the communicable diseases follow the epidemiological triad (Fig. 3.1).[2] Communicable diseases continue to present as the most important acute health problem overall worldwide.

NATURAL HISTORY OF DISEASE

Natural history of disease refers to the progression of a disease process in an individual over time, in the absence of treatment or any intervention, e.g. typhoid fever. After the infecting, the organism enters our body by feco–oral contamination, there is an incubation period of about 14 days after which we have clinical manifestations in the form of headache, remittent fever which rises in a step

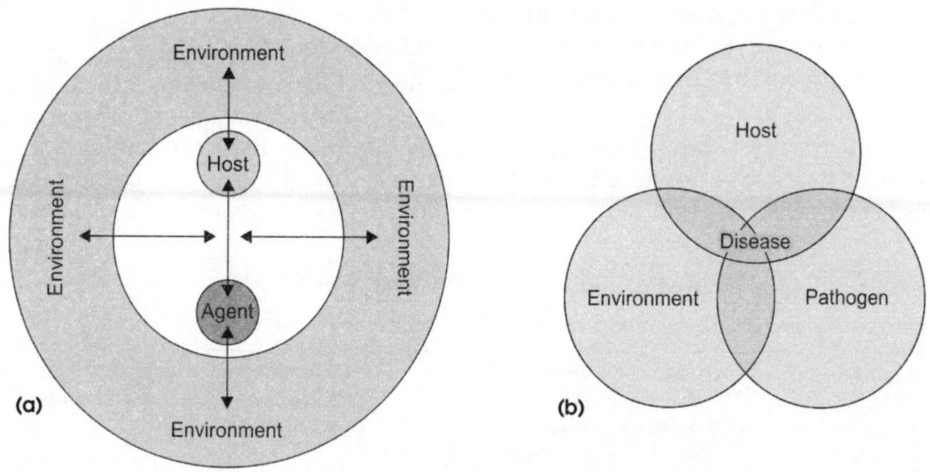

Fig. 3.1: Epidemiological triad of communicable disease[2]

ladder pattern initial constipation followed by pea-soup stools. Some patients may recover spontaneously by 3 weeks; others develop complications in the third week in the form of intestinal haemorrhage, perforation and peritonitis, with high mortality. Another small percentage may pass on to a chronic carrier state after an apparent clinical recovery.

LEVELS OF PREVENTION

Activities designed to protect patients and other members of the public from actual or potential health threats and their harmful consequences.[3]

The natural history of disease lays the basic foundation for planning of preventive measures. Prevention can be done at four basic levels (Table 3.1 and Fig. 3.2).[4]

1. Primordial prevention
2. Primary prevention
3. Secondary prevention
4. Tertiary prevention.

Primordial prevention: Nowadays, there is a growing recognition of concept of primordial prevention in contemporary health state. It mainly aims at non-communicable diseases and endeavours to prevent the very creation of such environment or the establishment of such conditions that are conducive to the development of the disease prior to arrival of risk actors of the disease process, e.g. counselling for lifestyle modification to lower cholesterol levels in an 8-year-old child.

Two main approaches of primordial prevention are:

a. *Population strategy*—counselling for lifestyle modification to lower cholesterol levels in an 8-year-old child.
b. *High risk strategy*—high risk groups are detected by screening procedure and counselled accordingly.

Primary revention: Measures taken in pre-pathogenesis phase, i.e. before starting of the disease process. It involves two sub-steps—health promotion and specific protection.

Health promotion: It includes all steps undertaken to improve the level of general health and well-being, so as to prevent initiation of disease process. The various methods included are:

- Health education for personal hygiene and improving environmental sanitation
- Sex education
- Adequate nutrition
- Breastfeeding promotion and proper weaning practices
- Family planning practices
- Efficient antenatal and post-natal care

Specific protection: Include measures to prevent the initiation of specific diseases, e.g.

- Immunization
- Use of condom to protect against HIV and STIs
- Wearing helmets, earplugs and masks
- Supplementary nutrition (vitamin A for night-blindness, iodised salt for goitre)
- Sterilization process for surgical instruments
- Quality control of food

Secondary prevention: It includes actions undertaken at the stage of early pathogenesis (asymptomatic disease) with a view to halt the progress of disease at its earliest, incipient stage, by "*early diagnosis and prompt treatment*".

Table 3.1: What happens when an agent enters the host?

Pre-pathogenesis phase	*Early pathogenesis phase*	*Phase of full blown disease*	*Phase of termination*
Silent period—no signs/symptoms—disease cannot be detected	No signs or symptoms of the disease, but can spread the disease; and certain specialized procedures can detect the disease	Typical manifestations of the disease	Recovery, complication, residual disability/chronicity

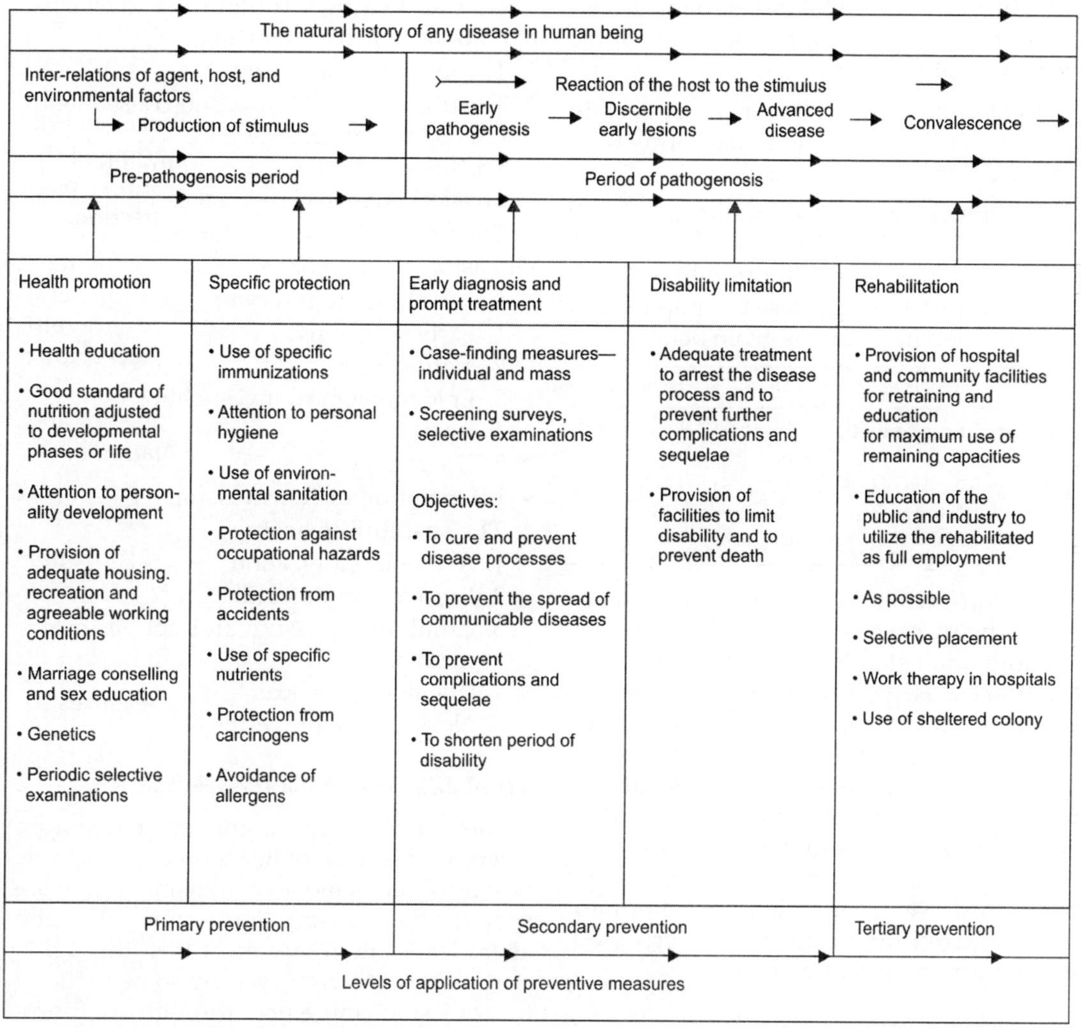
The natural history of any disease in human being
Inter-relations of agent, host, and environmental factors
Production of stimulus
Reaction of the host to the stimulus
Early pathogenesis
Discernible early lesions
Advanced disease
Convalescence
Pre-pathogenosis period
Period of pathogenosis
Health promotion
Specific protection
Early diagnosis and prompt treatment
Disability limitation
Rehabilitation
• Health education
• Good standard of nutrition adjusted to developmental phases or life
• Attention to personality development
• Provision of adequate housing. recreation and agreeable working conditions
• Marriage conselling and sex education
• Genetics
• Periodic selective examinations
• Use of specific immunizations
• Attention to personal hygiene
• Use of environmental sanitation
• Protection against occupational hazards
• Protection from accidents
• Use of specific nutrients
• Protection from carcinogens
• Avoidance of allergens
• Case-finding measures—individual and mass
• Screening surveys, selective examinations
Objectives:
• To cure and prevent disease processes
• To prevent the spread of communicable diseases
• To prevent complications and sequelae
• To shorten period of disability
• Adequate treatment to arrest the disease process and to prevent further complications and sequelae
• Provision of facilities to limit disability and to prevent death
• Provision of hospital and community facilities for retraining and education for maximum use of remaining capacities
• Education of the public and industry to utilize the rehabilitated as full employment
• As possible
• Selective placement
• Work therapy in hospitals
• Use of sheltered colony
Primary prevention
Secondary prevention
Tertiary prevention
Levels of application of preventive measures

Fig. 3.2: The natural history of disease in human being[5]

Treatment modalities include chemotherapy, radiotherapy, immunotherapy, surgery, hormonal therapy, etc.

Early diagnosis is helpful in:

- Recovery from disease
- Reduce duration of illness
- Prevents development of complications and further spread in the community

Tertiary prevention: It includes all measures undertaken when the disease has clinically manifested or advanced, so as to prevent or delay death, reduce or limit the impairments and disabilities, minimize suffering and to promote adjustment to irremediable conditions.

The two modalities included here are—disability limitation and (b) rehabilitation.

Disability limitation: This means halting further development of complications, impairments, disabilities and handicaps or even death.

The sequence of events in a disease process is:

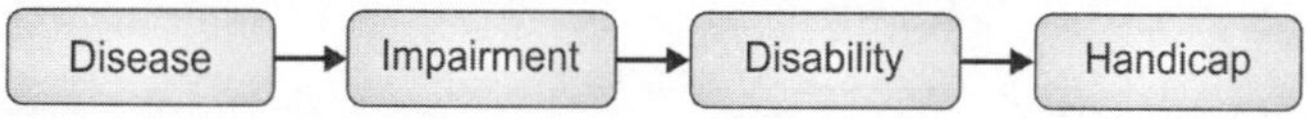
Disease
Impairment
Disability
Handicap

Impairment: The actual loss or damage of a part of body anatomy or an aberration of the physiological functions.

Disability: Inability to carry out certain routine activities which are otherwise expected normal for that age/sex.

Handicap: Disadvantages in life as a result of impairment/disability which makes the person ineligible to fulfill the role which is expected from him, e.g. disease, impairment disability and handicap as given below.

Disease	*Impairment*	*Disability*	*Handicap*
Accident	Loss of foot	Inability to walk	Loss of job
Leprosy	Nerve involvement	Inability to work due to clawhand	Unemployment

Rehabilitation: This measure is untaken when the disease is very much advanced. Rehabilitation stands for the combined and coordinated usage of all the available medical, social, educational and vocational measures, for training and retraining the person to the highest level of functional ability. We identify the remaining capabilities of the individual and adopt measures to make him fit, independent, productive and useful in family/community, e.g. establishing school for blinds, providing crutches to crippled, reconstructive surgery in leprosy.

DISEASE CONTROL

Disease control is reducing the transmission of disease agent a low level that it ceases to be a public health problem. It describes operations aimed at reducing:

1. The incidence of disease.
2. The duration of disease, and consequently the risk of transmission.
3. The effects of infection, including both the physical and psycho-social complications.
4. The financial burden of the community.

Disease control involves:

- **Controlling the reservoir**
  1. Early diagnosis
  2. Notification
  3. Epidemiological investigations
  4. Isolation
  5. Quarantine
- **Interruption of transmission**
- **The susceptible host**
  1. Active immunization
  2. Passive immunization
  3. Combined passive and active immunization
  4. Chemoprophylaxis
  5. Non-specific measures

DYNAMICS OF DISEASE TRANSMISSION

Communicable diseases are transmitted from reservoir or source of infection to susceptible host by different modes of transmission. More specifically, transmission occurs when the agent leaves its reservoir or host through a portal of exit, is conveyed by some mode of transmission, and enters through an appropriate portal of entry to infect a susceptible host. This sequence is sometimes called the chain of infection (Fig. 3.3).

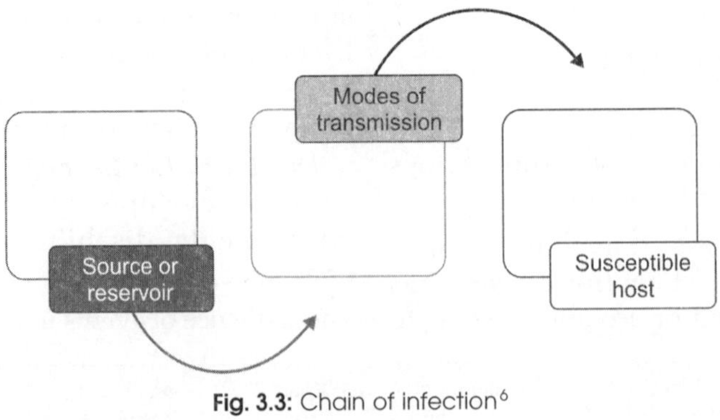

Fig. 3.3: Chain of infection[6]

Source or Reservoir

The source of infection is defined as the person, animal, object or substance from which an infectious agent passes or disseminated to the host. It is primary habitat of any infectious agent.

The reservoir of an infectious agent is the habitat in which the agent normally lives, grows, and multiplies. The reservoir may or may not be the source from which an agent is transferred to a host. For example, the reservoir of *Clostridium botulinum* is soil, but the source of most botulism infections is improperly canned food containing *C. botulinum* spores.

The reservoirs are:
1. Human reservoirs
2. Animal reservoirs
3. Environmental reservoirs.

Human Reservoirs

Many common infectious diseases have human reservoirs. Diseases that are transmitted from person to person without intermediaries include the sexually transmitted diseases, measles, mumps, streptococcal infection, and many respiratory pathogens. Because humans were the only reservoir for the smallpox virus, naturally occurring smallpox was eradicated after the last human case was identified and isolated. Human reservoir can be cases and carriers.

A. Cases: Case is defined as a person in the population identified as having the particular disease, health disorder or condition under investigation.

***Clinical cases*:** Depending upon extent of involvement, cases may be mild or moderate, typical or atypical, severe or fatal. Mild cases being ambulatory are of major concern as they can go from places to places and spread the infection, however severe cases are mostly confined to bed.

Subclinical cases: These are also referred as unapparent, covert, missed or abortive cases. In them the agent multiplies but does not show sign and symptoms. They play a pivotal role in maintaining the chain of infection in the community. As such they are a major public concern.

Latent cases: In such cases, the host does not sheds the agent rather the agent lies in dormant stage inside the host, e.g herpes simplex, Brill- Zinsser disease, etc.

Primary case: The first case of a communicable disease in the community.

Index case: The first case that comes to the investigator/healthcare agencies. It may or may not be primary case.

Agent characteristics with reference to disease production: Disease production by an agent is determined by:
1. Infectiousness: It is the ease with which agent is transmitted to the host. It mainly depends on environmental factors.
2. Infectivity: The ability of an agent to cause infection, i.e. entry, survival and multiplication inside the host. It is measured by secondary attack rate (SAR).

$$\text{SAR} = \frac{\text{No. of persons developing disease following exposure}}{\text{Total no. of exposed persons or susceptibles}} \times 100$$

3. Pathogenicity is the ability of agent to manifest disease out of those who are infected.
4. Virulence is the ability of an agent to cause severe disease. It is measured in terms of death.

B. Carriers: An infected person or animal that harbours a specific infectious agent in the absence of discernible clinical disease and serves as a potent source of infection[1] (Park), e.g. typhoid carriers (Table 3.2).
1. Incubatory carriers: They spread disease during incubation period, e.g. measles, mumps, pertussis, influenza.
2. Convalescent carriers: A person who acts as a carrier during recovery from the disease, i.e. the individual is clinically cured but not

Table 3.2: Classification of carriers by type, duration and portal of entry

1. Type	a. Incubatory, e.g. measles, mumps, pertussis, influenza
	b. Convalescent, e.g. typhoid fever, dysentery, cholera
	c. Healthy, e.g. polio, meningococcal meningitis, salmonellosis
2. Duration	a. Temporary, includes incubatory, convalescent and healthy carriers
	b. Chronic
3. Portal of entry	a. Urinary—typhoid
	b. Intestinal—amebiasis
	c. Respiratory—nasal diphtheria
	d. Others—cutaneous: *Staphylococcus*, genital—gonorrhoea, AIDS

bacteriologically, e.g. typhoid fever, dysentery, cholera.

3. Healthy/contact carriers: Individuals with subclinical infection, who act as a source of infection for others, e.g. polio, meningococcal meningitis, and salmonellosis.
4. Temporary carriers: They act as carrier and spread infection for a short period of time (several days), it includes incubatory, convalescent and healthy carriers.
5. Chronic carriers: They spread infection for longer time period (several weeks to months), e.g. Typhoid Mary, hepatitis B.

Mary Mallon was born in 1869 in Ireland and emigrated to the US in 1884. She was a 'healthy carrier' of *Salmonella typhi* in the United States. From March 1907, Mary was transmitting disease and death by her activity. That year, about 3,000 New Yorkers had been infected by *Salmonella typhi*, and probably Mary was the main reason for the outbreak. Immunization against *Salmonella typhi* was not developed until 1911, and antibiotic treatment was not available until 1948. Thus, a dangerous source like Mary had to be restrained. She was forced into quarantine on two separate occasions on North Brother Island for a total of 26 years and died alone without friends, having evidently found consolation in her religion to which she gave her faith and loyalty.[7]

Animal Reservoirs

Humans are also subject to diseases through animal reservoirs. Many of these diseases are transmitted from animal to animal, with humans as incidental hosts (Table 3.3).

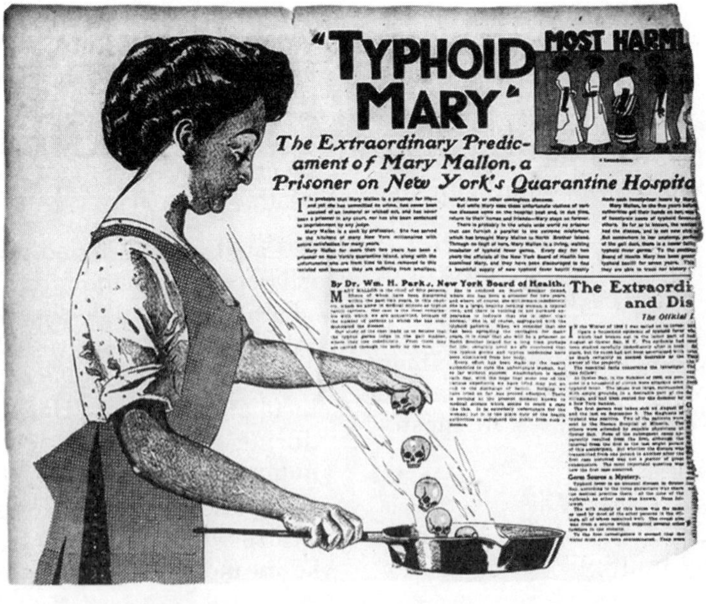
"TYPHOID MARY"
MOST HARML
The Extraordinary Predicament of Mary Mallon, a Prisoner on New York's Quarantine Hospita
By Dr. Wm. H. Park., New York Board of Health.
The Extraordi
and Dis

Table 3.3: Animal reservoirs and transmitted diseases

Animal reservoir	*Disease transmitted*
Cattle	Bovine tuberculosis, salmonellosis, tetanus, *T. saginata*, brucellosis
Horses	Tetanus
Dogs	Rabies, hydatid disease
Monkeys	Yellow fever, dengue, KFD
Sheep	Anthrax, liver fluke
Pigs	*T. solium*, Japanese encephalitis
Birds	Psittacosis, histoplasmosis, ornithosis
Rodents	Plague, leptospirosis, endemic typhus

The term zoonosis (zoo = animal, nosis = diseases) refers to an infectious disease that is transmissible under natural conditions from vertebrate animals to humans and vice versa.

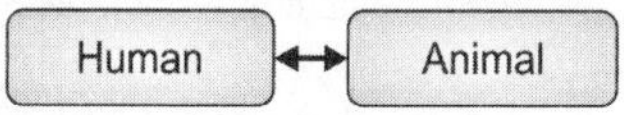

Long recognized zoonotic diseases include brucellosis (cows and pigs), anthrax (sheep), plague (rodents), trichinellosis/trichinosis (swine), tularemia (rabbits), and rabies (bats, raccoons, dogs, and other mammals). Zoonoses newly emergent in North America include West Nile encephalitis (birds), and monkeypox (prairie dogs).

Many newly recognized infectious diseases in humans, including HIV/AIDS, Ebola infection and SARS, are thought to have emerged from animal hosts, although those hosts have not yet been identified.

These are of three types:

a. *Anthropozoonosis:* Diseases transmitted from animal to human beings, e.g. rabies from dogs, plague from rats, kyasanur forest disease from monkeys, brucellosis from cattle.
b. *Zooanthroponoses:* Diseases transmitted from human beings to animals, e.g. brugiamalayi filariasis from man to cats and dogs.
c. *Amphixenoses:* Diseases occurring in both humans and lower vertebrates and can be transmitted in either direction, e.g. Chaga's disease, schistosomiasis.[8]

Environmental Reservoirs

Plants, soil, and water in the environment are also reservoirs for some infectious agents. Many fungal agents, such as those that cause histoplasmosis, live and multiply in the soil. Outbreaks of Legionnaires disease are often traced to water supplies in cooling towers and evaporative.

MODES OF TRANSMISSION

Communicable disease may spread from source or reservoir to susceptible host via different ways. Mode of transmission also provides basis for prevention of disease process. The modes of transmission may be classified as given in Table 3.4.

Host

The final link in the chain of infection is a susceptible host. Susceptibility of a host depends on genetic or constitutional factors, specific immunity, and non-specific factors that affect an individual's ability to resist infection or to limit pathogenicity.

Characteristics of host that affect the probability of infection: It includes the following.

Age: People at extremes of age are at greater risk of developing infection. Children have a habit of oral exploring while elderly have reduced defence mechanism.

Sex: Females are more exposed to urinary tract infections than males due to anatomical built-up.

Socio-economic status: Poverty and poor living conditions go hand in hand with disease occurence.

Genetic make-up: Poor immunity is harbinger of infections.

Table 3.4: Classification of modes of infection

A. Direct transmission	1. Direct contact	Skin-to-skin: Scabies Sexual contact: HIV, STDs
	2. Droplet infection	Aerosol: Common cold, influenza
	3. Soil transmission	Bare foot walking: Hookworm, tetanus
	4. Transplacental	Mother to child: HIV, rubella, CMV
B. Indirect transmission	5. Vector borne	a. Mechanical: Houseflies—*Cholera*, dysentery b. Biological: Propogative—plague in rat flea; cyclo-propogative—plasamodium in mosquito; cyclo-developmental: filarial in mosquito
	6. Vehicle borne	a. Waterborne: *Cholera, Shigella* b. Foodborne: Salmonellosis c. Airborne: TB, measles d. Unsafe injection: Hepatitis B, HIV

Host can be:

a. *Definitive host (primary host; final host):* The parasite undergoes sexual phase and attains maturity inside the host, e.g. dog—hydatid disease, *Anopheles* mosquito—malaria.

b. *Intermediate host (secondary host; alternate host):* The parasite undergoes asexual phase of its life cycle inside them, e.g. man—malaria and hydatid disease, female *Culex*—filariasis.

c. *Obligate host (compulsory host):* The only host status available, e.g. human—measles, polio.

d. *Transport host (mechanical host):* The host in which the organism remains alive but does not undergo multiplication or development, e.g. housefly.

INCUBATION PERIOD

The **incubation period** is the time from exposure to the causative agent until the first symptoms develop and is specific for each disease agent (Flowchart 3.1).

Example: Shiga toxin—producing *E. coli*, has an average incubation period of 3–4 days with a range from a minimum of 2 days to a maximum of 10 days.[9]

Flowchart 3.1: Events occurring during incubation period

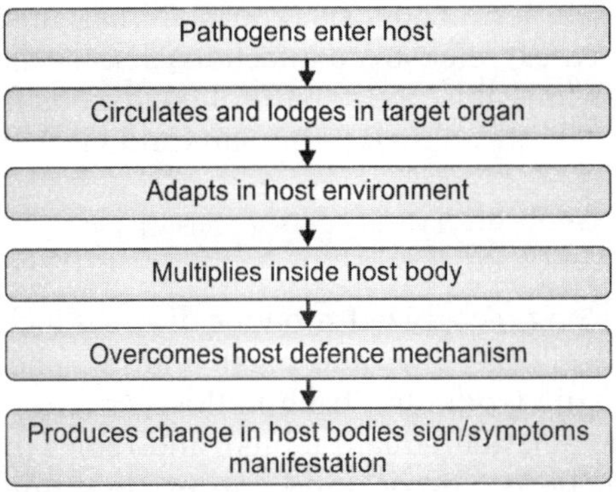
Pathogens enter host
Circulates and lodges in target organ
Adapts in host environment
Multiplies inside host body
Overcomes host defence mechanism
Produces change in host bodies sign/symptoms manifestation

Factors Influencing Incubation Period

1. Virulence of pathogens
2. Infective dose
3. Susceptibility of host

Virulence: Refers to the proportion of clinically apparent cases that are severe or fatal.[10]

Infective dose: That amount of a pathogenic agent that will cause infection in susceptible subjects/host.

Susceptible host: A person who is likely to develop disease. For a disease to occur there must be a portal of entry, a site of election and defence mechanism.

Portal of entry: It may be respiratory route, alimentary route, percutaneous and genital route. If there is no portal of exit then host is called dead-end host.

Site of election: The site where pathogen finds optimum favourable condition for its growth, development, multiplication and survival—target organ.

Defense mechanism: It can be achieved at three levels:

1. Anatomical protection by intact skin
2. Chemical protection by gastric acid
3. Biological by immunity

Related Terms

Extrinsic incubation period: The period between the entry of a pathogen inside an arthropod till the arthropod becomes infective.

Serial interval: The period between onset of the first or index case and the secondary case.

Generation time: The period between the onset of infection and the maximum infectivity. This may be shorter than incubation period, (e.g. mumps) or longer, (e.g. measles).

Latent period: Similar to incubation period but used for non-communicable disease mostly.

Window period: The period between entry of the pathogen and the production of the antibodies. The infected person is infectious to other persons during this period.

Prepatent period: The interval between the entrance of parasite and its first appearance in blood.

Median incubation period: The time required for 50% of cases to occur after an exposure to disease agent.

Communicable period: The period during which the reservoir is infectious to others. The indicator to measure communicability of the disease is 'secondary attack rate' (SAR). Higher the SAR, so higher will be the communicability of the disease.

Uses of incubation period:

1. Making diagnosis
2. Helps in tracing contacts or the source of infections
3. Quarantine purposes
4. Immunization purpose
5. Assessment of prognosis

OCCURRENCE OF COMMUNICABLE DISEASES

The communicable diseases occur in various modes.

ENDEMIC

An endemic is a disease or condition that is regularly found in a community or in a geographical region. The disease is said to be endemic to an area or community, when the incidence and prevalence for the said disease are maintained at an expected level. Although seasonal variations may be observed, the disease is ever present. The disease persists if the factors and conditions conducive to the survival of infectious agent of the disease are always favourable and the disease transmission continues. Examples of endemic diseases include chickenpox that occurs at a predictable rate among young school children in the United States and *malaria* in some areas of Africa.[11]

Hyperendemic: A *hyperendemic* disease is one that is constantly present at a high incidence and/or prevalence rate and affects all groups equally.[12]

Holoendemic: Holoendemic means that the disease appears early in life and affects most of the population, as in malaria or hepatitis A and B in some regions.

Level of endemicity: The level of endemicity varies geographically. It is high in some areas while low in others. For example, Haryana has low level of endemicity for leprosy, while Odisha, Uttar Pradesh, Bihar, and Maharashtra have high prevalence rates.[8] The level of endemicity can be determined by the incidence (newly diagnosed cases) and prevalence (old cases) rates. An epidemic of the endemic disease may breakout when the conditions for disease transmission become favourable or the number of the susceptible hosts goes up. It is for this reason that the outbreak of typhoid breakout during rainy seasons, floods, etc.

Epidemic

The unusual occurrence of cases of disease, health-related behaviour, or health-related events than expected in a given area or among a specific group of people, over a particular period of time is defined as an epidemic.[13] Epidemicity depends upon the normally observed number of cases in the area in a specified population in the same season. Therefore, even a single case of a disease of an unknown disease, or one that has been absent from the community for a long time is an epidemic. Similarly a single case of typhoid in a country like USA is designated as a epidemic as the disease is not routinely encountered in the population, meanwhile that is not the case in countries like India where the disease is endemic. A limit to standard errors from the endemic frequency is used to define the threshold for epidemics. The term epidemic also encompasses in it the modern era, slowly propagating diseases of non-communicable diseases like cardiovascular diseases, and diabetes mellitus which grow slowly over years to decades.

Epidemics of communicable diseases occur in the following ways.

Point source epidemic: The susceptible hosts are exposed to the infectious agent more or less simultaneously leading to a rapid increase in the number of cases in few hours or days post-exposure.[14] The commonest example is food poisoning, where all those having ingested the contaminated food are exposed simultaneously and there is a abrupt rise in the number of cases. Given below is the graphical representation of a point source epidemic, with the number of cases on the y-axis and time on the x-axis (Fig. 3.4).[15] The time gap between the exposure and appearance of cases is the incubation period and the peak of the curve coincides with the 'median incubation period' of the disease. This curve rises and falls rapidly (Fig. 3.4).

Common source epidemic with continued exposure: When the infectious agent persists in the source for some time, the susceptible hosts coming in contact with it keep getting exposed and developing disease. The epidemic spreads slowly and persists until either the source is eradicated or all the susceptible hosts are infected. Examples of

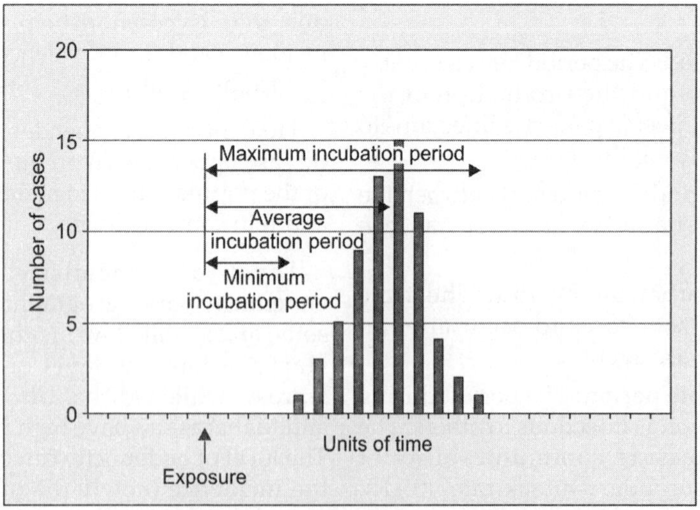

Fig. 3.4: Point source outbreak with no propagation

this type of spread are seen due to infected water sources or foodhandlers, who are themselves carriers and propagate the disease to the community. The curve of this epidemic is slow rising, and without a distinct peak, but more like a plateau. It is spread wide over the time axis and falls gradually.

Propagated epidemic: In this epidemic, disease is contacted from one person to another. The rise in the number of cases is initially slow, in waves, reaches a plateau, and then gradually declines (Figs 3.5 and 3.6).[15,16] An infected person passes on the disease to the susceptible hosts that come in contact with him. The cycle continues and the epidemic spreads. The example of chickenpox spreading in school children can be considered. An infected child passes on the infection to say two other children. They in turn propagate to four more and so on. The first case in this

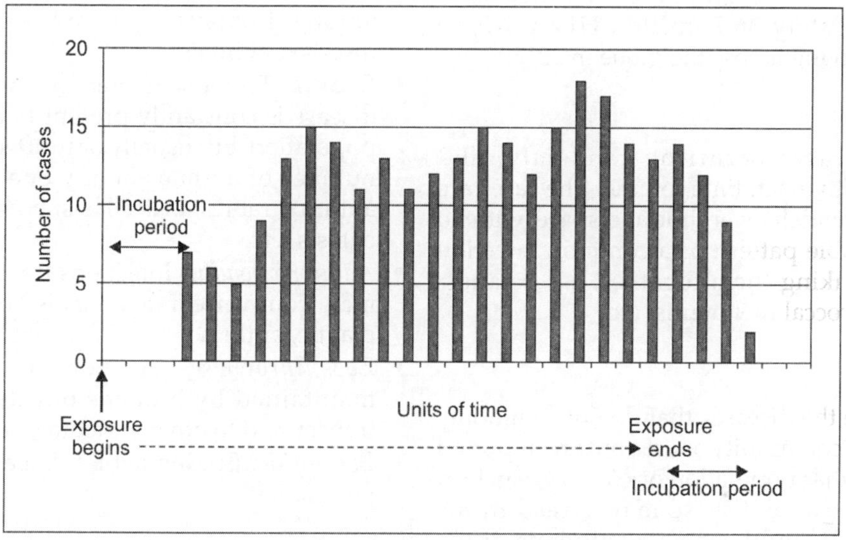

Fig. 3.5: Continuing source outbreak

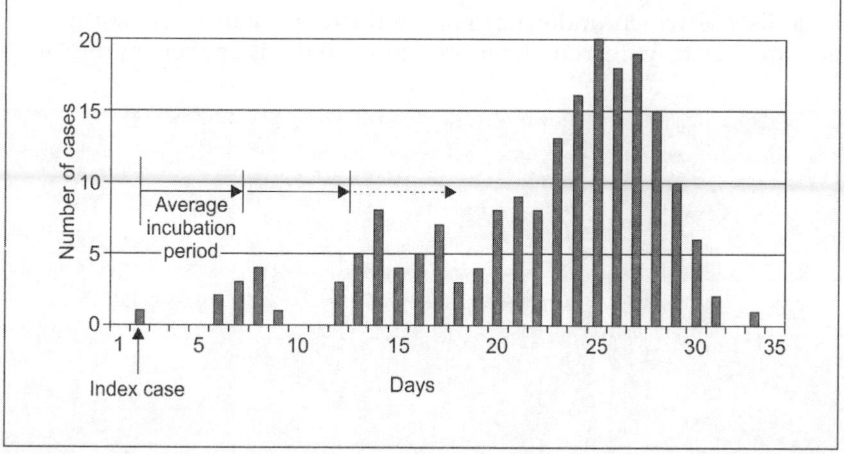

Fig. 3.6: Disseminated outbreak originating from an index case with propagated spread

scenario is called the 'index case'. The epidemic eventually declines because of the development of herd immunity, or no more susceptible hosts being present for infection (Fig. 3.6).

Pandemic

It is an epidemic that is wide-spread in a large chunk of the total population or spreading over vast geographical area. A disease with a global outbreak is a pandemic. For example, HIV AIDS is a global pandemic, with approximately 36.7 million HIV positive patients living across the globe in 2016.[17]

Sporadic

Disease cases occurring randomly, and infrequently from time to time. The cases are scattered widely over time and space, with no recognizable pattern or a common infection source linking them together, e.g. tetanus, meningococcal meningitis, etc.

Exotic

These are the diseases that do not commonly occur in a community or area but are imported from another population or country, e.g. bird flu.[18] An exotic disease may spread in the community and become a epidemic, if the factors for its spread are favourable.

Zoonosis

An infectious disease which under normal conditions can be transferred from a vertebrate animal to a human susceptible host is called zoonotic infection (Fig. 3.7).

It may be further classified in following types.

- *Epizootic:* These diseases break out as epidemics among the animal population but may also affect the human population. For example, rift valley fever (RVF) primarily affects livestock and can cause disease in a large number of domestic animals—an 'epizootic'—and the presence of an RVF epizootic can lead to an epidemic among humans who are exposed to diseased animals.
- *Enzootic*: Endemic in animals. An enzootic disease is constantly present in an animal population, but usually only affects a small number of animals at any one time, e.g. anthrax, rabies, brucellosis, bovine tuberculosis, etc.
- *Anthropozoonosis*: Infections transmitted to man from vertebrate animals,[8] e.g. rabies, plague, anthrax.
- *Zooanthropnoses:* A zoonosis normally maintained by humans but that can be transmitted to other vertebrates (Fig. 3.7).[19]
- *Epornithic*: Epidemic of a disease in bird population.

Nosocomial infection: Nosocomial infection or hospital acquired infections are those that patients acquire during the course of receiving treatment for other conditions within a healthcare setting. These are unrelated to the patient's original condition for

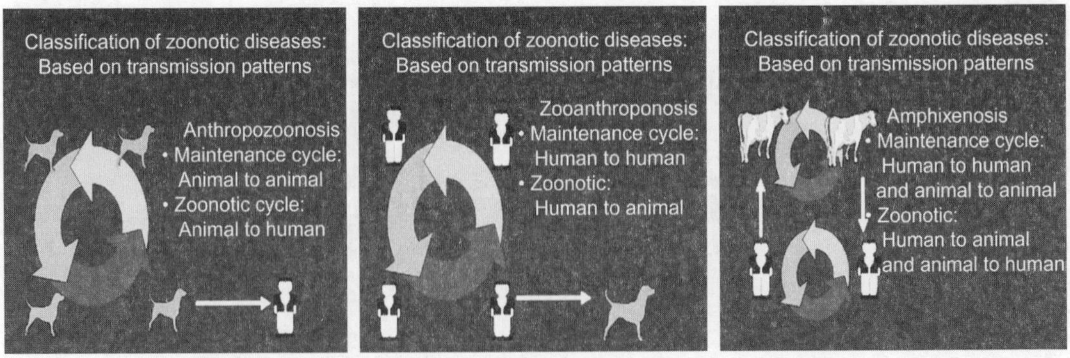

Fig. 3.7: Classification of zoonotic diseases based on various patterns

which patient was hospitalized. The infection must not have been present or incubating at the time of admission. It could however have been acquired during the hospital stay and manifesting after discharge. Nosocomial infections also include those in the hospital staff. Common types of HAIs include catheter-associated urinary tract infections, surgical site infections, bloodstream infections, pneumonia, and *Clostridium difficile*.[20]

Opportunistic infections: An *infection* by a microorganism that normally does not cause disease but becomes pathogenic when the body's immune system is impaired and unable to fight off *infection*, as in AIDS and certain other diseases. Examples include herpes simplex, cytomegalovirus, toxoplasma, etc.

INVESTIGATION OF AN EPIDEMIC

(Details are discussed in Chapter 6.)

Investigation of an epidemic is carried out for the following reasons:

1. To define the total magnitude of the epidemic outbreak over time, place, and person.
2. To determine the factors responsible for the outbreak
3. To identify the source of infection and modes of transmission
4. To identify the methods that can be used to break the chain of transmission.
5. To recommend preventive methods to avoid recurrence.

STEPS FOR INVESTIGATING AN EPIDEMIC

Verification of Diagnosis

The initial reporting of an outbreak could be spurious, or false. Also most times the reporting is done by lay people in form of a collection of symptoms like vomiting, diarrhea, fever. The epidemiologist then needs to diagnose and verify cases, by clinical, laboratory and epidemiological parameters.[21]

Confirmation of Existence of an Epidemic

The incidence rate for the current outbreak is calculated and compared to the rate in the population, in the same season in the past 3 years. An epidemic is said to be present if the number is 'clearly in excess' as compared to the normal expectations. In certain cases however, even single case of the disease may be regarded as an epidemic. Such as a single case of polio, or plague.

Developing a Line Listing of Cases

A line listing is produced by epidemiologists in outbreak investigations. A line listing allows information about time, person, and place to be organized and reviewed quickly. It is also a good way to keep track of different categories of cases. For example, cases can be entered into the line listing as possible, probable or confirmed (laboratory confirmed, clinically confirmed or both). The designation can easily be updated as the investigation progresses. A line list helps in defining the disease, and identifying the population at risk.

Defining Population at Risk

A detailed map of the area may be obtained from engineering and local administrative authorities.

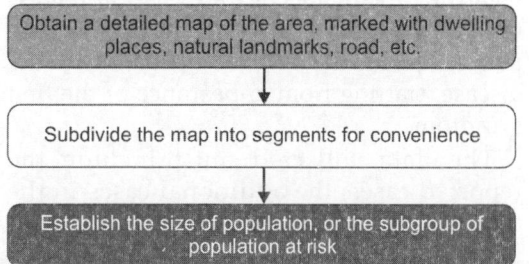

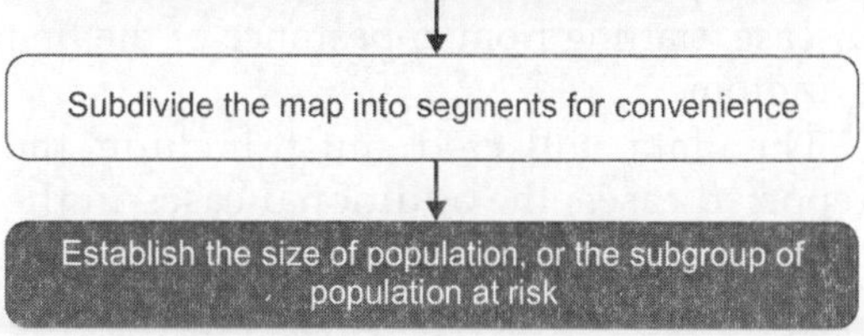

Developing Valid Case Detection

Medical surveys: Surveys carried out in defined areas to identify cases, and also those exposed to risk. Valid criteria for case detection must be pre-decided and communicated to all the health personnel and para-medical staff.

Preparing an epidemiological case sheet: in addition to the data normally present on a clinical case sheet, an epidemiological case sheet must also have relevant data regarding to the factors of modes of transmission, details about exposure, socio-economic class, occupational history, history of contact, travel, attending social gathering, ingestion of food or drink, clinical history, and all other factors relevant to the disease under investigation.

Searching for secondary cases: The identified case should be asked if he knows any other cases in his knowledge with the same symptoms in the same incubation period. Also the people who have been in contact with the case need to be followed and secondary cases need be found. This process should continue till the decline of the epidemic.

Laboratory Diagnosis

This includes collection, storage and transport of the body sample. Environmental sample, entomological samples, and animal samples. A joint effort with close coordination between a pathologist, microbiologist and epidemiologist is required.

Collection of information: The investigator must record all the relevant information regarding the modes of transmission related to the disease under investigation, for a time period equal to the range of incubation for the disease, starting from appearance of the first symptom.

The data collected must include the reported cases, the additional cases in the community, and the concerning environmental information relating to the disease (e.g. food, water supply and sanitation and waste disposal systems of the concerned area in faco–oral diseases).

In addition information about the people who were present in the population at risk, but did not suffer from the disease must also be collected in order to formulate a hypothesis at a later date.

Description of the Epidemic

Overall attack rate: The total number of new cases divided by the total population at risk.

Time: An epidemic curve is prepared with the number of cases on y-axis and time on x-axis. It helps in identifying the temporal relation between exposure to the source of infection, and clustering of cases. It also helps in identifying the type of epidemic, i.e. point source, propogated, etc. seasonal variations, or temporal patterns of the disease, if any can also be studied.

Place: The geographical distribution of cases, and their possible relations with the source of infection are plotted on a map called the spot map. A spot map can identify the cases with a high density of cases, and possible common source of infection.

Person: Distribution of the disease in relation to age, sex, occupation, marital status, etc. probable risk factors.

Formulation of Hypothesis

A tentative hypothesis regarding the infection source, causative agent, possible modes of transmission, and related environmental factors is formulated after analysing the data collected regarding the time, place, and person variables with respect to the agent host and environment epidemiological model.

Testing the Hypothesis

The cases and the controls (people from the exposed population who did not develop the disease) are compared in respect to each and every formulated theory. Odds ratio for each exposure is calculated, and test for statistical significance (chi square test) are performed to narrow down which of all the exposures in cases and controls is likely to the source of the outbreak. Further research is made to explore the factors for disease transmission and spread.

Measures for Control and Prevention

These are both immediate and long-term measures that need to be implemented immediately and simultaneously as the investigation proceeds.

Measures of control of source of infection:
1. Detection treatment of cases and carriers
2. Isolation
3. Control of zoonotic reservoirs

Measures of controlling the modes of transmission:
1. Clean water supply
2. Food hygine
3. Vector control
4. Waste disposal
5. Sanitation
6. Disinfection of contaminated substances.

Protection of population at risk:
1. Immunisation
2. Immunoprophylaxis
3. Chemoprophylaxis
4. Personal protective measures.

Long-term strategies:
1. Launching a surveillance system
2. Early warning systems about impending outbreaks.

USES OF EPIDEMIOLOGY IN COMMUNICABLE DISEASE[22]

Details of uses of epidemiology are given in Chapter 2.

Study of Natural History of the Disease

The progression of a disease from start to end in absence of medical or public health intervention is called natural history of the disease. The goal of therapeutic and preventive interventions is to alter the natural history of the disease in favourable way, i.e. to prevent the disease from happening or make its course less sever and less eventful.

Stages of disease: All cases of a disease do not take a uniform course. This diversity in the course of a particular disease could take a wide range from very mild and even unnoticeable cases to very sever and fatal cases. In fact, in many diseases, especially the infectious diseases, a majority of cases of the disease are subclinical or asymptomatic and therefore not noticed. This is called iceberg phenomenon. The following stages of disease are described:

1. *Pre-disease stage*: At this stage the disease has not yet affected the individual directly, i.e. the pathologic process has not begun in his/her body. The aim of health services at this stage is to prevent occurrence of the disease.
2. *Latent stage*: The pathologic process of the disease has begun, but the disease is still asymptomatic. In infectious disease like measles, the infection has begun in the individual, but the person is still asymptomatic. In non-infectious diseases such as coronary atherosclerosis, the changes have started in the coronary vessel, but the patient has not yet developed any symptoms. The aim of the health services in this stage is to identify people with the disease in order to start treatment as soon as possible and prevent spread in case of infectious disease.
3. *Symptomatic stage*: After a variable period of latent stage, signs and symptoms of the disease become manifest. For example, in case of measles when fever, rash and other symptoms become apparent. The aim of the health services in this stage is to treat the patients adequately and prevent complications and death.

Outcome of disease: All disease do not end in the same way in terms of its effect on the life of the patient. Diseases differ in their severity and the end result. The outcome of a disease process could be any of the following:

1. *Recovery*: When the patient recovers fully and re-enters the healthy population. He may be protected from the disease in the future (immune) like in some infectious diseases such as measles; or he may not be

protected and could get the disease again (susceptible) like in most other diseases, e.g. common cold, minor accidents, etc.

2. *Complications*: Many disease lead to complications during the course of the disease, some of which could recover by itself or be controlled by treatment. For example, common cold could be complicated by sinusitis which could be treated. Infarction could be complicated by arrhythmia and fractures could be complicated by bleeding.
3. *Disability*: Lasting disability happens in some diseases which may require rehabilitation later on. For example, poliomyelitis and stroke may cause weakness of lower legs, diabetes may cause impairment of vision, and meningitis may cause brain damage and mental retardation.
4. *Death*: Many diseases could lead to death if proper management is not provided such as fatal accidents, infarction and cholera.

This includes the relationship between the agent, host and environmental factors, and the further evolution of disease from its inception to ultimate resolution in the form of recovery, or death, in the absence of any preventive, or curative interventions.

Magnitude of the Problem

Measurement of various morbidity and mortality rates measure the extent of a nation's health and provision of health facilities. These data could be used to measure the extent to which medical facilities are utilized. They could help, too, in the investigation of the patterns of occurrence of illness, assessment of the health needs of the community, planning of health related interventions and programmes, monitoring the efficacy of the health services, prioritization of health problems and needs, and allocation of appropriate funds and health personnel.

Community Diagnosis

Community diagnosis (community assessment) is the foundation for improving and promoting the health of community members. The role of community assessment is to identify, and quantifying the health problems of the community factors that affect the health of a population and determine the availability of resources within the community to adequately address these factors (Fig. 3.8).

Planning and Evaluation

Distribution of health problems across the community over time and place can be used as an template for formulation of health programmes and recognizing the need of health services. The socio-demographic factors of the community need to be reviewed regarding the acceptability the health interventions being proposed. Epidemiology

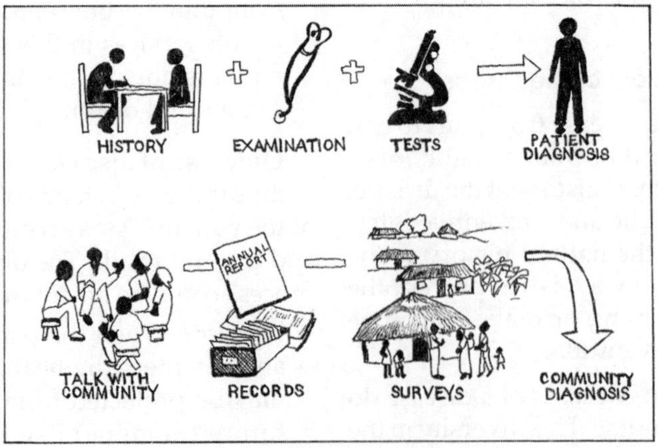

Fig. 3.8: Community diagnosis factors[10]

can be used to evaluate the existing health services and compare newer methods with each other in terms of cost effectiveness.

Aetiological Hypothesis

Descriptive epidemiology searches for patterns by examining characteristics of **person, place, and time**. These characteristics are carefully considered when a disease outbreak occurs, because they provide important clues regarding the source of the outbreak. Hypotheses about the determinants of disease arise from considering the characteristics of person, place, and time and looking for differences, similarities, and correlations.

Evaluation of Individual Risk

Epidemiology can be used to assess the degree of risk for the population.

Absolute risk: It is a measure of the risk of a certain event happening. For example, a woman of 35 years of age, with no known risk factors for breast cancer, has an absolute risk of getting breast cancer over a lifetime of 90 years of about 13.5%, meaning one out of every seven women will develop breast cancer.

Relative risk: In statistics and epidemiology, relative risk or risk ratio (RR) is the ratio of the probability of an event occurring (for example, developing a disease, being injured), in an exposed group to the probability of the event occurring in a comparison, non-exposed group.

Attributable risk of a factor: The contribution of a risk factor to a disease or a death is quantified using the population attributable fraction (PAF). PAF is the proportional reduction in population disease or mortality that would occur if exposure to a risk factor were reduced to an alternative ideal exposure scenario.

Study of Historical Trends in Communicable Disease

Epidemiology can be used to track the health trends over long or short periods of time. As time passes by diseases emerge, undergo fluctuations and wax and wane. The diseases that had once been under control reappear. For example, in India smallpox and guinea worm disease have been eradicated from the country; polio is on the verge of being eradicated; leprosy, kala azar, and filariasis can be expected to be eliminated in the coming few years, while rickettsial infections are caused by a different obligate intracellular, gram-negative bacteria (*Rickettsia, Orientia, Ehrlichia, Neorickettsia, Neoehrlichia,* and *Anaplasma*) are re-emerging. We can make useful projections into the future and identifying emerging health problems and their correlates.

Identifying Syndromes

'Syndromic surveillance' applies to surveillance using health-related data that precede diagnosis and signal a sufficient probability of a case or an outbreak to warrant further public health response. Syndromic surveillance is based on non-specific health-related data including clinical signs, symptoms, absenteeism, number of trips to the nurses station in schools, etc.[23]

This data is usually collected for purposes other than surveillance and, where possible, is automatically generated for allowing collection, analysis, interpretation, and dissemination of health-related data to enable the early identification of potential human or veterinary public health threats. For example, the abnormal increase in the number of young homosexual men infected by *Pneumocystis carinii* in Los Angeles between 1980 and 1981, prompted the discovery of the HIV virus in 1983. Similarly, the outbreak of a severe respiratory illness of unknown origin that affected 180 people who had attended a state American Legion convention in Philadelphia in July 1976, allowed the identification of *Legionella* pneumophila.

CONTROL OF AN EPIDEMIC

The main concept behind controlling epidemic is breaking the chain of transmission. It targets the weakest link in the chain.[24] It includes three steps in the light of epidemiological triad, i.e. agent, host and environment—

1. Eliminating the reservoir of infection
2. Breaking the channels of transmission
3. Protection of susceptible

Measures for Elimination of Reservoir

This is a difficult step to cope up with, as it is impossible to eliminate air, water, soil reservoirs. Then comes elimination of animal reservoirs which can be attempted but not completely done, e.g. cattles, pigs, birds, etc. eliminating human reservoirs means stopping them from acting as a source of infection. This can be done by:

Early diagnosis: An early diagnosis ensures early treatment which prevents further spread of infection. It is also helpful in tracing the source of infection so that they can be treated. Needed for:

1. Treatment of patient
2. Epidemiological investigation to trace the source of infection from the known or index case to the unknown
3. To study the time, place and person distribution
4. For the institution of prevention and control measures, e.g. STDs, food poisoning, etc.

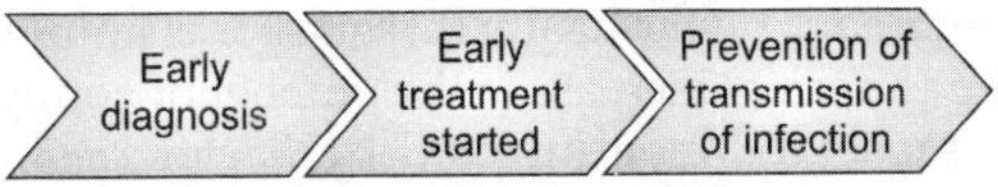

Notification: It means giving an official report to the concerned authorities so that they can take essential measures to control further spread of infection. Reporting can be done by medical personnel, paramedical staffs even lay persons, e.g. polio (Box 3.1).

Epidemiological investigation: It helps:

- In knowing the detailed information regarding distribution of disease with reference of time, person and place.

Box 3.1: Notifiable disease to WHO under international health regulation (IHR)

Yellow fever

Cholera

Plague

Diseases under international surveillance

Poliomyelitis

Rabies, relapsing fever

Malaria

Influenza, louseborne typhus

- To track the source of infection, causative agent, mode of transmission and influencing factors
- Finally to know the magnitude of problem (from calculating attack rate, case fatality rate

Isolation: Separating the sick individual/animals from healthy ones till it becomes non-infectious to others (Table 3.5). In cases of diphtheria, plague and SARS, it is of great significance. This has a limited significance in case of diseases with huge number of

Table 3.5: Epidemic diseases and period of their isolation[10]

Disease	*Period of isolation*
Chickenpox	6 days after onset of rash
Measles	Onset of catarrhal to 3rd day of rash/7 days after onset of rash
German measles	None (except first trimester)
Influenza	3 days after onset of rash
Tuberculosis	Until 3 weeks of chemotherapy
Herpes zoster	6 days after onset of rash
Pertussis	3–4 weeks or until paroxysm ceases
Meningococcal meningitis	Until first 6 hr antibiotics completed
Mumps	Until swelling subsides

sub-clinical and carrier states, e.g. typhoid, viral hepatitis A.

Isolation can also be achieved by 'ring immunization', i.e. encircling infected person/house by a barrier of immunized individuals, e.g. practiced in case of smallpox eradication.

Types of isolation:

1. Standard isolation
2. Strict isolation
3. Protective isolation
4. High security isolation

Disinfection (concurrent disinfection): It includes disinfecting body discharge as sputum, urine and stool of the patient.

Terminal disinfection: It is done for leftover articles of the patients.

Precurrent (prophylactic) disinfection: Pasteurization of milk, water disinfection by chlorine, handwashing.

Treatment: Done to kill the infective agent while still inside the reservoir so as to make the infectious person non-infective to others. In high endemic areas, we target at mass treatment. 'Blanket treatment' is done in case of scabies, where we treat the whole family.

Quarantine (absolute quarantine): It is confinement of those healthy individuals who are suspected to have been exposed to a communicable disease for a period equivalent to the maximum incubation period of the disease. This is done to prevent international spread of an infection, e.g. yellow fever, plague, etc.

Modified quarantine (partial quarantine) is selective limitation of the freedom of movement, e.g. preventing children from attending school in case of chickenpox.

Measures for Breaking the Channel of Infection

The chain of infection requires transmission of disease agent to susceptible host. The link between agent and host may be direct or indirect.

Direct: This mode of transmission can be broken by:

- Avoiding close contact with the infectious agent.
- Aaerosol infection can be prevented by covering the mouth while sneezing, coughing.
- Preventing soil-borne infection by avoiding bare-foot walking.
- Prevention of animal bites.
- Preventing vertical transmission by giving treatment to mothers.

Indirect: An indirect mode of transmission can be defined as one in which its infectious agent requires an 'intermediary agency' to convey it from the source of infection to the susceptible host. This can be prevented by:

- Chlorination of water.
- Pasteurization of milk.
- Screening of blood prior to transfusion.
- Controlling air pollution levels.
- Fomite-borne infections can be prevented by proper disinfection of fomites.
- Contamination via dirty hands and fingers can be prevented by adopting personal hygiene measures.

Measures for Protection of Susceptible Hosts

Susceptible population can be protected from infection by:

1. Specific measures like immune-prophylaxis, chemoprophylaxis
2. General measures like improving quality of life, implementing legislative measures, ESI Act, FSSAI Act, Epidemic Diseases Act, 1897, the Transplantation of Human Organs Act, 1994, the International Health Regulation Act.

Immunization: One of the most satisfactory control measures is that it renders the host immune from infectious disease by an infectious agent. Active immunization is a cornerstone of public health measures for the control of many infectious diseases and is considered one of the most cost-effective methods of individual, institutional, and community protection from many infectious diseases. Immunization may be:

1. Active immunization
2. Passive immunization
3. Combined active and passive

Active immunization: It is an effective way of controlling the spread of infection by strengthening host's immunity. It is cost-effective method of reducing the number of susceptible in the community (herd immunity = immunizing a group of people provides protection to those who are not immunized, OPV), e.g. national immunization schedule. The planning of an immunization schedule should be:

1. *Epidemiologically relevant,* i.e. it should only include vaccines that are against diseases which are of public health concern and should have an effective vaccine against them.
2. *Immunologically effective:* Vaccine should be given at an age from which the individual is benefitted maximally, e.g. a child should be immunized after it has lost the maternal antibodies and before it is exposed to possible infection.
3. *Operationally feasible:* It should be cost effective, high in coverage, less number of visits.
4. *Socially accepted:* It should take in consideration the local customs, beliefs, work pattern of community, seasonal factors, and reduce duration of visit.

Passive immunization: It is for short term when the exposure has just occurred. It confers limited immunity and is recommended for special circumstances only. Passive immunity is induced by:

1. Administering antibody containing preparation/immunoglobulin
2. Maternal antibodies are across placenta

Combined active and passive immunization: *It is recommended for certain infections, e.g. diphtheria, tetanus, rabies, hepatitis.* The site of administration should be different for both to achieve optimum benefit.

Chemoprophylaxis: Chemoprophylaxis is the prevention of infection or its progression to clinically manifest disease through the administration of chemical substances, including antibiotics (Table 3.6). Chemoprophylaxis may be specifically directed against a particular infectious agent or it may be non-specifically directed against many infectious agents. The use of antibiotics before surgical procedures is an example of non-specific chemoprophylaxis to prevent wound infections in the post-operative period. Chemoprophylaxis may be:

1. Causal prophylaxis—completely preventing infection by early elimination of agent, e.g. malaria.
2. Clinical prophylaxis—merely preventing clinical symptoms.

Table 3.6: Epidemic diseases and their chemoprophylaxis

Disease	*Chemoprophylaxis*
Cholera	Tetracycline
Bacterial conjunctivitis	Erythromycin eye ointment
Influenza	Oseltamavir
Meningococcal meningitis	Ciprofloxacin
Plague	Tetracycline
Diphtheria	Erythromycin
Filaria	DEC and albendazole

Epidemiological principles are to wisely use in community diagnosis, prevention and control strategies of communicable diseases. The distribution characters of communicable disease help in identification of weaker links which helps in prevention and control. Searching for determinants of communicable diseases by adopting epidemiological tools and techniques forms the foundation for launching programme of prevention and control at community as well as at individual level.

NON-SPECIFIC MEASURES FOR THE PREVENTION AND CONTROL OF COMMUNICABLE DISEASES

- Mainly interrupt pathways of transmission.
- Improvements on the quality of life, (e.g. better housing, water supply, nutrition, education)
- Formulation of legislative measures and integrated program.
- Have played a dominant role in decline of diseases like TB, cholera, leprosy and child mortality.

Surveillance

- Surveillance must follow control measures.
- Defined as "the continuous scrutiny of all aspects of occurrence and spread of disease that are pertinent to effective control."
- The ultimate objective of surveillance is 'Prevention'.

References

1. Park K. Park's Textbook of Preventive & Social Medicine 24th edn. Bhanot Publishers, Jabalpur, India. 2017.
2. Canada P. Introduction: The Chief Public Health Officer's Report on the State of Public Health in Canada 2013—Canada.ca. [online] Canada.ca. Available at: https://www.canada.ca/en/public-health/corporate/publications/chief-public-health-officer-reports-state-public-health-canada/chief-public-health-officer-report-on-state-public-health-canada-2013-infectious-disease-never-ending-threat/introduction.html [Accessed 13 Jul. 2018].
3. Mosby's Medical Dictionary. 8th edn. St. Louis: Mosby Elsevier. 2008.
4. Beaglehole R, Bonita R. Basic epidemiology, World health organisation. Madras: Orient Longman Limited. 1993.
5. Natural history of disease in human being—bing images [Internet]. Bing.com. 2018 [cited 18 Jul 2018]. Available from: https://www.bing.com/images/search? view=detail V2&ccid=3Pe4Z29G&id=E5758E3883E15E791ACB6F3FFC6563DDE0044015&thid=OIP.3Pe4Z29GFCeM25_l2Tx6hgHaFj&mediaurl=https%3a%2f%2fimage.slidesharecdn.com%2ffinalnaturalhistory-140602135457-phpapp02%2f95%2fnatural-history-of-disease-60-638.jpg%3fcb%3d1401717625&exph=479&expw=638&q=natural+history+of+disease+in+human+being&simid=608026686468851220&selectedIndex =20&ajaxhist=0
6. Bing [Internet]. Bing.com. 2018 [cited 18 Jul 2018]. Available from: https://www.bing.com/images/search?view=detailV2&ccid=aWWZozwL&id=56B58005376965BB0CE05EFBA7418E5D9CCDBDA2&thid=OIP.aWWZozwLW_N498iy5MiH5AHaFj&mediaurl=https%3a%2f%2fimage.slideshare cdn.com%2finfectionpreventionandsafetymeasures-160204173732%2f95%2finfection-prevention-and-safety-measures-9-638.jpg%3fcb%3d1454607619&exph=479&expw=638&q=Chain+of+infection+park&simid=607988585852896864&selectedIndex=8&ajaxhist=0
7. Marineli F, Tsoucalas G, Karamanou M, Androutsos G. Mary Mallon (1869–1938) and the history of typhoid fever. Annals of Gastroenterology/: Quarterly Publication of the Hellenic Society of Gastroenterology.[internet] 2013;26(2): 132–34. Available from:https://www.ncbi.nlm.nih.gov/pmc/articles/PMC3959940/
8. Suryakantha AH. Community Medicine with Recent Advances 2nd edition. India: Jaypee, New Delhi 2010.
9. Centers for Disease Control and prevention. https://www.cdc.gov/training/QuickLearns/exposure/2.html browsed on 21st july 2018
10. Centers for Disease Control and Prevention. Principles of epidemiology in public health practice, 3rd edn. An introduction to applied epidemiology and biostatistics https://www. cdc.gov/ophss/csels/dsepd/ss1978/browsed on 21st July
11. MedicineNet.com. Medical definition of endemic [internet] cited on 30th June 2018. Available at: https://www.medicinenet.com/chickenpox_varicella/article.htm#what_is_chickenpox_what_causes_chickenpox.
12. Glossary of epidemiology terms—Columbia CS. [internet] cited on 22nd July 2018.
13. Available at: http://www.cs.columbia.edudigigov/LEXING/CDCEPI/gloss.html d3
14. Dr (Brig.) Sunder Lal. Textbook of Community Medicine. CBS Publishers and Distributors, New Delhi. 2007.
15. Outbreaks unpacked-recent tutorial material [Internet]. Microbiology and Infectious Diseases postgraduate teaching. 2016 [cited 23 Jul 2018]. Available from: https://idmic.net/2016/10/05/outbreaks-unpackedrecent-tutorial-material/
16. Komjathy J. (2016). Why the whole world has seen Gangnam style – The Network Pages. [online] Networkpages.nl. Available at: https://www.

networkpages.nl/why-the-whole-worldhas-seen-gangnam-style/ [Accessed 23 Jul 2018].

17. Centers for Disease Control and Prevention (CDC) Basic Statistic/HIV basics. [Internet]cited on 29th June 2018. Available at: https://www.cdc. gov/hiv/basics/statistics.html
18. Craighead JE. Pathology and Pathogenesis of Human Viral Disease, 1st edn. San Diego: Academic Press, 2000.
19. Internet]. Pitt.edu. 2018 [cited 23 Jul 2018]. Available from: http://www.pitt.edu/~super1/lecture/lec0302/009.htm http://www.pitt.edu/~super1/lecture/lec0302/010.htm http://www.pitt.edu/~super1/lecture/lec0302/010.htm
20. Centers for Disease Control and Prevention (CDC) Healthcare Associated Infections. [internet] cited on 28th June 2018. Available at: https://www.cdc.gov/hai/infectiontypes.html
21. Bhalwar R. Textbook of Community Medicine. 2nd edn. India: Wolters Kluwer. 2018
22. Morris JN. Uses of Epidemiology, 2nd edn. Edinburgh and London: E and S Livingstone Ltd. 1964.
23. Wood CH, et. al. Individual and community diagnosis. [Internet]. Flickr. 1989 [cited 23 Jul 2018]. Available from: https://www.flickr.com/photos/communityeyehealth/5 687626220
24. Manual of epidemiology for district health management. WHO, 1989. [internet] cited on 29th June 2018. Available at: http://helid.digicollection. org/en/d/Jwho31e/3.4.html#Jwho31e.3.4

Chapter 4

Basics of Non-Communicable Diseases Epidemiology

Ram Chandra Goyal

INTRODUCTION

Non-communicable diseases (NCDs), also known as chronic diseases, tend to be of long duration and are the result of a combination of genetic, physiological, environmental and behavioural factors.

NCDs are chronic diseases that develop progressively, impacts on functional health with the passing of time, and need sustained health services for a prolonged period.

As the burden of communicable/infectious diseases started decreasing, the focus on non-infectious/non-communicable diseases started growing. The concept of communicability, however, is not fundamentally a concept of infection but natural course of disease in community, which is an epidemiological concept. For example, rheumatic heart disease, cancer cervix, in spite of its microbial origin, these are not communicable.

The low- and middle-income countries (LMICs) are ageing, the communicable diseases and economic 'development,' and they will become 'old before they are rich' (WHO, 2016).

Developing countries (LMICs) are at a cross road: The demographic transition has opened up the opportunity of reaping 'demographic dividend' due to less children and elderly to be cared for by the income-earning population. On the other hand, epidemiological transition (from communicable to pre-dominantly non-communicable diseases), the 'double burden' has thrown up a challenge to the mostly unprepared health system of these countries.[1]

The challenge for the LMICs is that most of the health systems, plausibly so, are geared to address the communicable diseases and mainly targets children and reproductive age women. The challenge is also compounded by the fact that experiences from the high income countries (HICs), may not be valid, since the cultural values and norms between HICs and LMICs varied widely, need a culture-sensitive approach to tackle the situation.[1]

Non-communicable diseases (NCDs) represent the largest and even growing proportion of the global burden of disease. In addition to their mortality burden, NCDs have major economic consequences worldwide. Premature deaths from NCDs are largely preventable, and many are mainly driven by four big risk factors: Physical inactivity, unhealthy diets, tobacco use, and the harmful use of alcohol. These risk factors are interrelated, and rooted in social, political, economic, cultural, environmental and commercial factors that are often outside of an individual's control.[2–4]

Underfunding, lack of social mobilization, and conflicts of interest with the private sector make NCDs a challenging public health problem, but also creates an interesting opportunity for coordinated and multi-sectoral action.

Magnitude of Problem: Global Burden

Non-communicable diseases (NCDs) are the leading causes of death globally, killing more people each year than all other causes combined (Table 4.1). Contrary to popular opinion, available data demonstrate that nearly 80% of NCD deaths occur in low- and middle-income countries. Despite their rapid growth and inequitable distribution, much of the human and social impact caused each year by NCD-related deaths could be averted through well-understood, cost-effective and feasible interventions.

Of the 57 million deaths that occurred globally in 2008, 36 million—almost two-thirds—were due to NCDs, comprising mainly cardiovascular diseases, cancers, diabetes and chronic lung diseases. The combined burden of these diseases is rising fastest among lower-income countries, populations and communities, where they impose large, avoidable costs in human, social and economic terms. About one-fourth of global NCD-related deaths take place before the age of 60 (WHO-GHR-2010).[5]

The human, social and economic consequences of NCDs are felt by all countries but are particularly devastating in poor and vulnerable populations. Reducing the global burden of NCDs is an over riding priority and a necessary condition for sustainable development. As the leading cause of death globally, NCDs were responsible for 38 million (68%) of the world's 56 million deaths in 2012. More than 40% of them (16 million) were premature deaths under age 70 years. Almost three-quarters of all NCD deaths (28 million), and the majority of premature deaths (82%), occur in low- and middle-income countries (WHO-GHR-2014).

Developing populations have long been troubled by poverty, malnutrition, infectious diseases, and disorders related to pregnancy and childbirth, but now face a new challenge.

Since 2012, the burden of these traditional diseases in developing populations has decreased from 49% to 38%, whereas the burden of non-communicable diseases has increased from 40% to 51%, measured in disability-adjusted life years relative to all causes of disease.

Likewise, the number of deaths due to the traditional diseases has decreased from 37% to 27%, whereas the number of deaths due to non-communicable diseases has increased from 53% to 63% of all deaths. Most of the burden and deaths because of

Table 4.1: Leading causes of attributable global mortality and burden of disease, 2004[8]

Attributable mortality	%	*Attributable DALYs*	%
1. High blood pressure	12.8	1. Childhood underweight	7.8
2. Tobacco use	8.7	2. HIgh blood pressure	7.5
3. High blood glucose	5.8	3. Unsafe sex	6.6
4. Physical inactivity	5.5	4. Unsafe water, sanitation, hygiene	6.1
5. Overweight and obesity	4.8	5. High blood glucose	4.9
6. High cholesterol	4.5	6. Indoor smoke from solid fuels	4.8
7. Unsafe sex	4.0	7. Tobacco use	3.9
8. Alcohol use	3.8	8. Physical inactivity	3.8
9. Childhood underweight	3.8	9. Suboptimal breastfeeding	3.7
10. Indoor smoke from solid fuels	3.3	10. High cholesterol	3.3
59 million total global deaths in 2004		1.5 billion total global DALYs in 2004	

http://who.int/healthinfo/globen_burden_disease/GBD2004ReportFigure.ppt

non-communicable diseases are caused by cardiovascular diseases, cancer, chronic respiratory diseases, and diabetes, together accounting for 636 million disability-adjusted life years and 23 million deaths per year. Currently, the burden of non-communicable diseases is more than 3.5 times higher and the number of deaths due to non-communicable diseases is more than 2.5 times higher as compared with Western populations.[7]

Indian Scenario

India's population is around 1.32 billion and expected to overtake China before 2030 (Table 4.2 and Fig. 4.1). At the same time, elderly population is also increasing (8.0%) and more sedentary.

NCDs now account for the majority of death and disability in the country and affect in particular adults in the productive years between 30 and 69. Most of these conditions are caused by underlying (and often inter-related) risk factors such as smoking, high blood pressure, obesity and lack of exercise. 15% of Indian females and 12% of males are classified as overweight or obese and about 30% have high blood pressure (hypertension). Rates of hypertension are generally higher in urban areas, an important factor as more and more people are moving to cities from the countryside.

Non-communicable diseases (NCDs) contribute to around 5.87 million deaths that account for 60% of all deaths in India. India shares more than two-third of the total deaths

Table 4.2: Total population (estimates)—in millions

	1950	*2017*	*2030*	*2050*	*2100*
World	2536	7550	8551	9771	11184
China	554	1410	1441	1364	1021
India	376	1339	1513	1656	1517

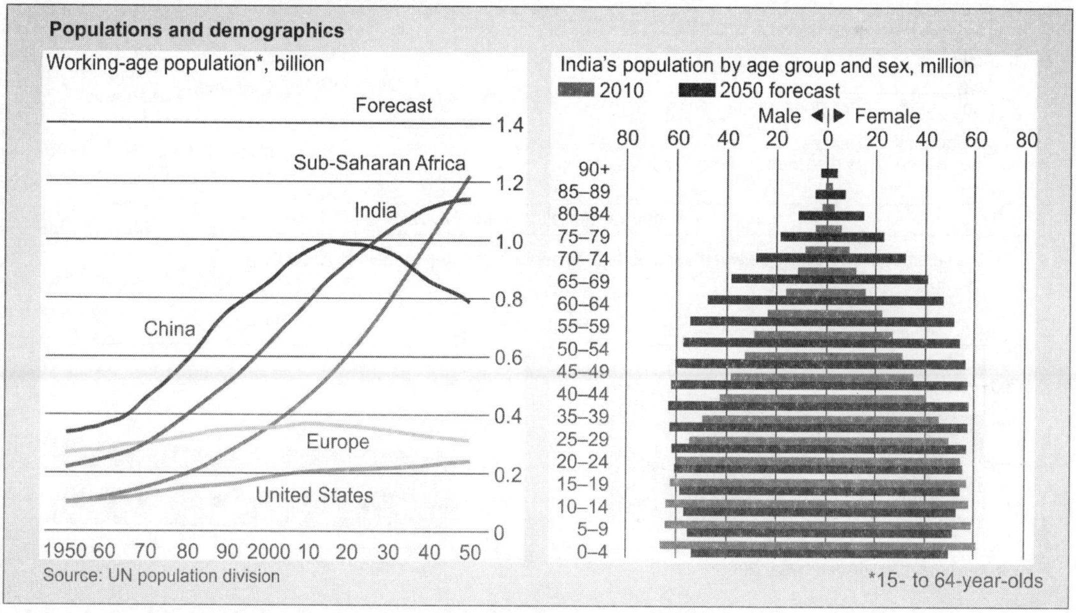

* http://economist.com/graphicdetail

Fig. 4.1: Population estimates of India

due to NCDs in the South-east Asia region (SEAR) of WHO.[6]

- **Four types of NCDs**—cardiovascular diseases, cancer, chronic respiratory diseases and diabetes make the largest contribution to morbidity and mortality due to NCDs (Figs 4.2 and 4.3).
- **Four behavioural risk factors** are responsible for significant proportions of these diseases—tobacco use, unhealthy diet, physical inactivity and harmful use of alcohol. Major metabolic risk factors are obesity, raised blood pressure, raised blood glucose and raised blood total cholesterol levels.
- Cardiovascular diseases (coronary heart disease, stroke, and hypertension) contribute to 45% of all NCD deaths followed by chronic respiratory disease (22%), cancers (12%) and diabetes (3%).
- The probability of dying between ages 30 and 70 years from four major NCDs is 26%, which means that a 30-year-old individual has a one-fourth chance of dying from these diseases before the age of 70 years.

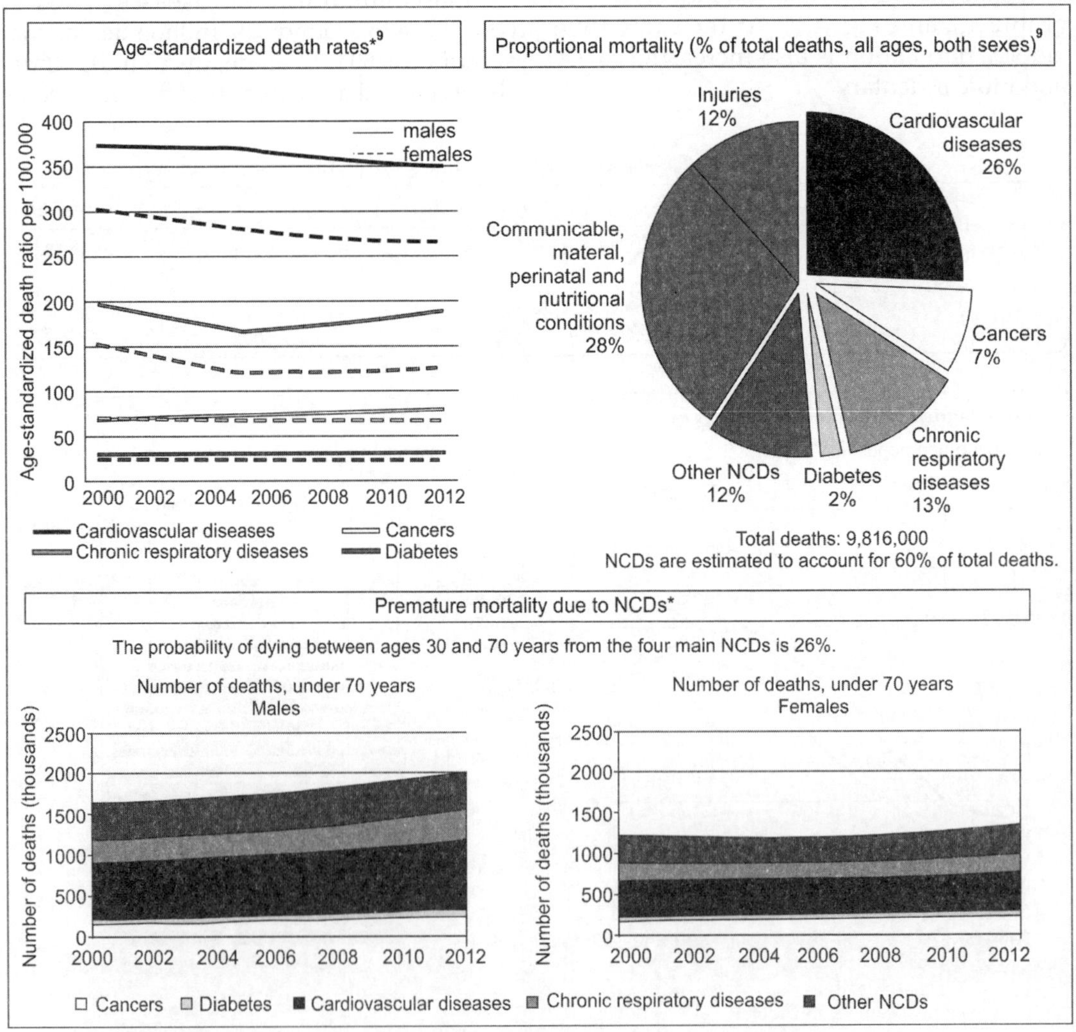

Fig. 4.2: Probability of dying between ages 30 and 70 years due to four main NCDs

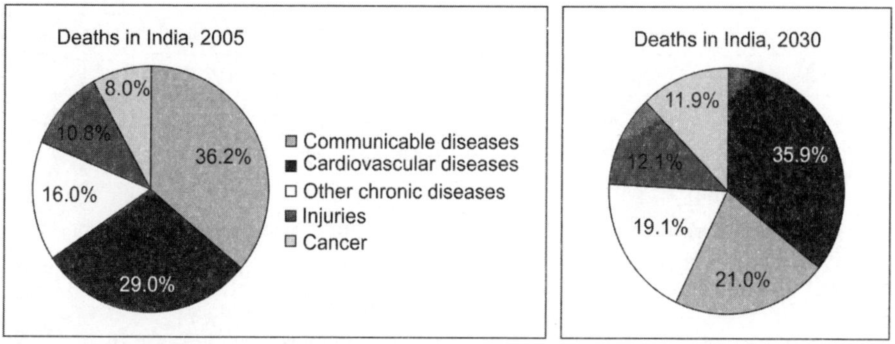

Fig. 4.3: Percentages of cause of death in the year 2005 and estimated death in the year 2030[10]

- The prevalence of current tobacco smoking has shown a slight decline in males but the prevalence (23.6%) is still higher than the global prevalence of current tobacco smoking (22%). Tobacco use has been identified as single largest risk factor attributable to NCDs.
- The prevalence of obesity and overweight is also showing a rapid increase in trends. Age-standardized prevalence of obesity (BMI ≥30) has increased by 22% in the span of four years (2010–2014).
- Nearly one out of every 10 persons aged 18 years and above in India has raised blood glucose, which poses extra financial and service burden on health systems. The age-standardized prevalence of raised blood glucose is 9.0% for both sexes.
- Every fourth individual in India aged above 18 years has raised blood pressure (hypertension) and the prevalence has increased by 10% from 2010 to 2014.
- The per capita consumption of pure alcohol (age +15) in India is estimated to be 5.2 litres per year. In 2010, the corresponding figure was 4.3 liters per year, which was significantly higher than the average consumption in the SEAR (3.2 liters per year).
- More than two-thirds of the adolescents aged 11–17 years are physically inactive in India as per WHO standards. The level of physical inactivity among adults is around 13% (excerpts from WHO: Global health report 2014).

CHARACTERISTICS OF NON-COMMUNICABLE DISEASES

Non-communicable diseases are altogether different in many ways than communicable diseases. Some of characteristics are as under (Table 4.3).

Variations on Causal Models[11]

Beyond differences in procedures for reaching conclusions about causation, differences in concepts or models of causation must also be recognized. These can be appreciated, and causation of NCD can be better understood, by considering several contrasts:

- One cause, or many?
- One outcome, or many?
- Immediate causes or 'fundamental causes'?
- All causes or only a few?
- Causes of cases, or causes of incidence?

Aetiological factors: Non-communicable diseases are driven by seemingly unrelated causes such as rapid unplanned urbanization, globalization of unhealthy lifestyles and population ageing. Apparent causes such as raised blood pressure, increased blood glucose, elevated blood lipids and obesity may be representations of deep lying lifestyle habits.

Multiple risk factors: There are a number of risk factors that lead to the onset and development of NCDs. The various types of risks can be divided into three primary risk sets—modifiable behavioural risk factors, non-modifiable risk factors and metabolic risk

Table 4.3: Characteristics of communicable and non-communicable diseases

Communicable diseases	*Non-communicable diseases*
No gap in natural history of disease	Natural history of NCD is not certain (gaps exists)
Rapid onset	Gradual onset
Single cause (fundamental)	Multi-factorial
Short natural history/short incubation period	Long natural history/long latency period
Short period of treatment	Long period of treatment (generally life-long)
Single outcome	Multiple outcomes
Generally cures, if treated	Care dominates
Involves single discipline	Multidisciplinary in nature
Short follow-up	Long follow-up
Normalcy achieved	Quality of life compromised

factors, many of which are common for a number of diseases.

Long latency period for non-communicable diseases: This stage is asymptomatic (no symptoms) or inapparent. This period may be as brief as seconds for hypersensitivity and toxic reactions to as long as decades for certain chronic diseases (CVD, diabetes, cancer, etc.). There may be some changes at cellular level which might be detected by screening test (blood sugar test for diabetes or markers in cancers).

Non-contagious origin (non-communicable): NCDs are not communicated from one person to another, so it is given that these diseases develop in a person from non-contagious origins.

Prolonged course of illness: NCDs are chronic in nature and thus the course of illness, if often prolonged and takes years before a patient may be forced to opt for medical care or intervention.

Multidisciplinary in nature of management: Since the NCDs are chronic, the management of these diseases are possible only with involvement of various discipline like medicine, physiotherapist, counsellors, etc.

Multiple Morbidity

In contrast to communicable diseases, where only single morbidity (most of the time) is seen but in NCD multiple morbidity may be possible, e.g. diabetes is associated with CVD, eye problems or neuro/nephropathy. This leads to long management and need multi-sector involvement for prevention and control.

Quality of Life

Majority of NCDs are related to functional impairment or that make patients to lead a normal life. Some patients may develop compromised activity of daily living (ADL) which leads to dependency. Various types of non-communicable diseases are given in Table 4.4.

RISK FACTORS IN NON-COMMUNICABLE DISEASES[13–16]

NCDs are caused by many risk factors but to a large extent by four behavioural risk factors that are pervasive aspects of underlying determinants like globalization, rapid urbanization, ageing population, socio-economic transition, and 21st-century lifestyles—tobacco use, unhealthy diet, physical inactivity and the harmful alcohol consumption. The low- and middle-income countries, and on poorer people within all countries affected the most. The immediate risk factors are raised blood sugar, raised blood pressure, dyslipidemia (Fig. 4.4), obesity (Fig. 4.6) and abnormal pulmonary functions.

Table 4.4: Types of common non-communicable diseases[12]

The WHO list of the most common non-communicable diseases—worldwide	
1. Asthma	7. Diseases of the digestive system (e.g. peptic ulcers)
2. Cancers	8. Eye conditions
3. Cardiovascular diseases (CVDs)	9. Genito-urinary conditions (prostate disorders, nephritis)
4. Chronic obstructive pulmonary diseases (COPDs)	10. Neuro-psychiatric conditions (mental disorders, epilepsy, Alzheimer's disease)
5. Congenital conditions	11. Skin and musculo-skeletal conditions (e.g. arthritis)
6. Diabetes	12. Skin diseases
The Indian list of the most common non-communicable diseases	
1. CVD including ischaemic heart disease	7. Mental disorders
2. Diabetes	8. Chronic kidney disease
3. COPD, asthma	9. Congenital defects
4. Cancer	10. Rheumatic heart disease
5. Accidents	11. Self-harm and drowning
6. Sense organ disease	12. Musculo-skeletal disorders

(*Source:* www.thelancet.com, Vol 390 December 2, 2017)

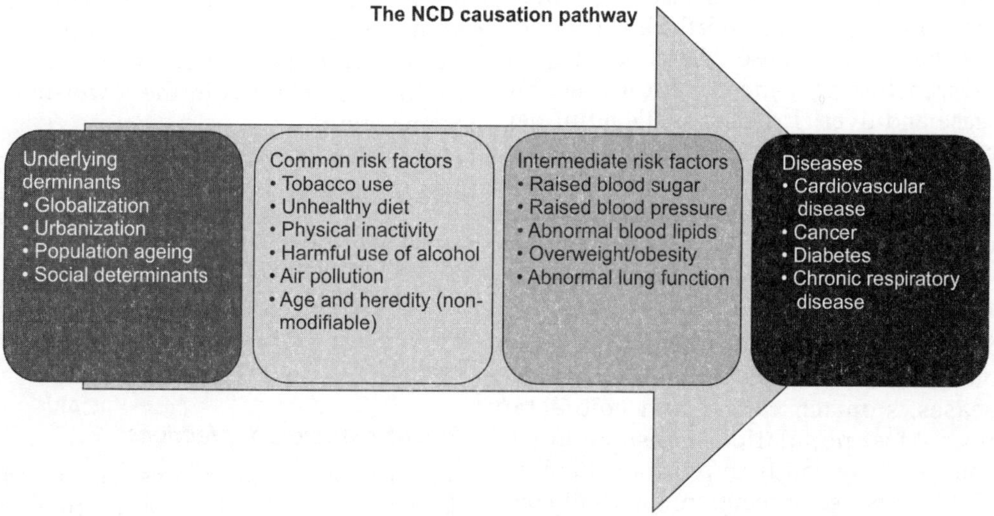

Fig. 4.4: The NCD pathways from main risk factors to intermediate to diseases progression. Adapted from WHO (2005). Preventive chronic disease a vital investment.

A large percentage of NCDs are preventable through the reduction of their four main behavioural risk factors—tobacco use, physical inactivity, harmful use of alcohol and unhealthy diet. The influences of these behavioural risk factors, and other underlying metabolic/physiological causes, on the global NCD epidemic include the following.

Global Situation

Tobacco

Almost 6 million people die from tobacco use each year, both from direct tobacco use and second-hand smoke. By 2020, this number will increase to 7.5 million, accounting for 10% of all deaths.

Smoking is estimated to cause about 71% of lung cancer, 42% of chronic respiratory disease and nearly 10% of cardiovascular disease. The highest incidence of smoking among men is in lower-middle-incomecountries; for total population, smoking prevalence is highest among upper-middle-income countries.

Insufficient Physical Activity

Approximately 3.2 million people die each year due to physical inactivity. People who are insufficiently physically active have a 20% to 30% increased risk of all-cause mortality. Regular physical activity reduces the risk of cardiovascular disease including high blood pressure and diabetes.

Harmful Use of Alcohol

Approximately 2.3 million people die each year from the harmful use of alcohol, accounting for about 3.8% of all deaths in the world. More than half of these deaths occur from NCDs including cancer, cardiovascular disease and liver cirrhosis. While adult per capita consumption of alcohol is highest in high-income countries, it is nearly as high in the populous upper-middle-income countries.

Unhealthy Diet

Adequate consumption of fruit and vegetables reduces the risk for cardiovascular diseases, stomach cancer and colorectal cancer. Most populations consume much higher levels of salt than recommended by WHO for disease prevention; high salt consumption is an important determinant of high blood pressure and cardiovascular risk. High consumption of saturated fats and trans-fatty acids is linked to heart disease. Unhealthy diet is rising quickly in lower-resource settings.

Available data suggest that fat intake has been rising rapidly in lower-middle-income countries since 1980s.

Raised Blood Pressure

Raised blood pressure is estimated to cause 7.5 million deaths, about 12.8% of all deaths. It is a major risk factor for cardiovascular disease. The prevalence of raised blood pressure is similar across all income groups, though it is generally lowest in high-income populations.

Overweight and Obesity

At least 2.8 million people die each year as a result of being overweight or obese. Risks of heart disease, strokes and diabetes increase steadily with increasing body mass index (BMI). Raised BMI also increases the risk of certain cancers. The prevalence of overweight is highest in upper-middle-income countries but very high levels are also reported from some lower-middle-income countries. In the WHO European region, the Eastern Mediterranean region and the region of the America, over 50% of women are overweight. The highest prevalence of overweight among infants and young children is in upper-middle-income populations, while the fastest rise in overweight is in the lower-middle-income group.

Raised Cholesterol

Raised cholesterol is estimated to cause 2.6 million deaths annually; it increases the risks of heart disease and stroke. Raised cholesterol is highest in high-income countries.

Cancer-associated Infections

At least 2 million cancer cases per year, 18% of the global cancer burden, are attributable to a few specific chronic infections, and this fraction is substantially larger in low-income countries. The principal infectious agents are human papillomavirus, hepatitis B virus, hepatitis C virus and *Helicobacter pylori*. These infections are largely preventable through vaccinations and measures to avoid transmission, or treatable. For example, transmission of hepatitis C virus has been largely stopped among high-income populations, but not in many low-resource countries.

Indian Situation

Tobacco

19.0% of men, 2.0% of women and 10.7% (99.5 million) of all adults currently smoke tobacco. 29.6% of men, 12.8% of women and 21.4% (199.4 million) of all adults currently use smokeless tobacco. 42.4% of men, 14.2% of women and 28.6% (266.8 million) of all adults currently use tobacco (smoked and/or smokeless tobacco).

38.7% of adults were exposed to second hand smoke at home. 30.2% of adults who work indoors are exposed to second-hand smoke at their workplace. 7.4% of adults were exposed to second hand smoke at restaurants. 92.4% of adults believed that smoking causes serious illness and 95.6% of adults believed that use of smokeless tobacco causes serious illness (Fig. 4.5).[17]

Tobacco use also entails huge economic costs. The cost of treating three major tobacco-related diseases (cancer, heart disease and COPD) alone is colossal and in 2002–2003 was estimated to be 308.3 billion rupees, which was substantially more than the revenue received by the government from tobacco sales.

Use of Alcohol[18-20]

India is one of the fastest growing alcohol markets in the world. Rapid increase in urban population, increased middle class population with rising purchasing power, and better economy are significant caused for increase in consumption of alcohol.

The Indian alcohol industry is segmented into IMFL (Indian made foreign liquor), IMIL (Indian made Indian liquor), wine, beer and imported alcohol. Imported alcohol has a meager share of around 0.8% in the Indian market. The heavy import duty and taxes levied raise the price of imported alcohol to a large extent. Alcohol is exempted from the taxation scheme of GST.

The Indian alcohol market is growing at a CAGR of 8.8% and it is expected to reach 16.8 billion liters of consumption by the year 2022.

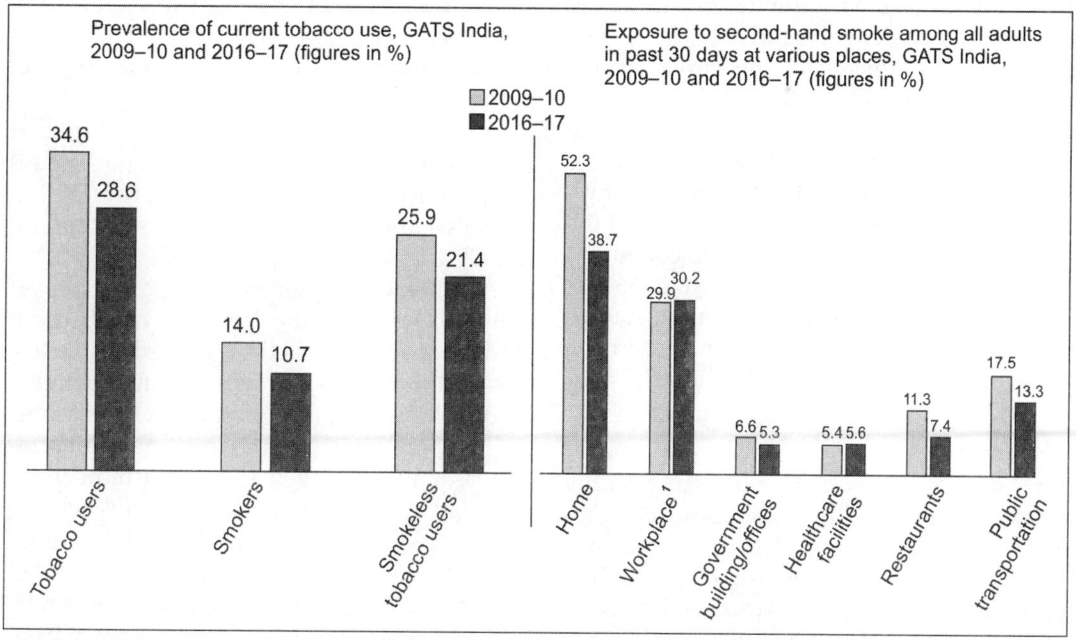

(http://www.who.int/tobacco/surveillance/survey/gats/GATS_India_2016-17_FactSheet.pdf. accessed on 28/7/2018)

Fig. 4.5: Situation of tobacco use in India

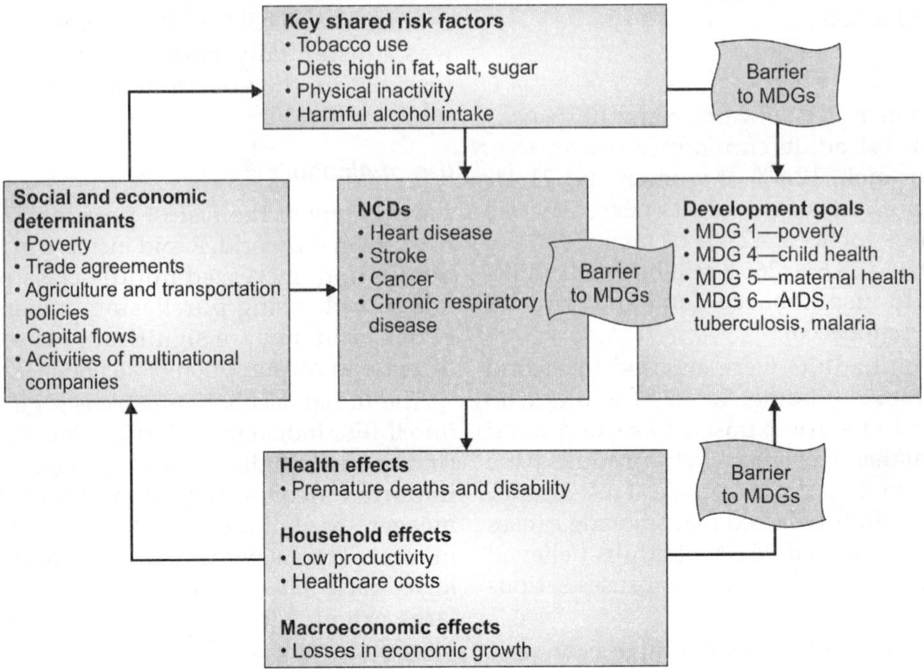

Fig. 4.6: Effect of NCDs to achieve MDGs

The popularity of wine and vodka is increasing at a remarkable CAGR of 21.8% and 22.8%, respectively. India is the largest consumer of whiskey in the world and it constitutes about 60% of the IMFL market.

Though India is one of the largest consumers of alcohol in the world owing to its huge population, the per capita alcohol consumption of India is very low as compared to the Western countries. The per capita consumption of alcohol per week for the year 2016 was estimated at 147.3 ml and it is expected to grow at a CAGR of 7.5% to 227.1 ml according to our estimates (Figs 4.7 and 4.8).

Insufficient Physical Activity

WHO defines physical activity as any bodily movement produced by skeletal muscles that requires energy expenditure—including activities undertaken while working, playing, carrying out household chores, travelling, and engaging in recreational pursuits.

According to phase 1 of the ICMR-INDIAB study conducted in four regions of India with a combined population of 213 million people, shows that 54.4% (n = 7737) were inactive (male: 41.7%), while 31.9% (n = 4537) were active (male: 58.3%) and 13.7% (n = 1953) were highly active.[21]

Population-based data on physical inactivity levels are sparse in India. The Indian component of the World Health Survey (WHS), the only national level survey thus far, found that 29% of the adult population had inadequate physical activity levels. A quarter of men (24%) and one-third of women (34%) had inadequate physical activity levels (defined as one to 149 minutes of activity in the week before the survey). Physical in activity was higher in urban than rural people and increased in those aged 45 years or more with over half of them being in adequately active.[22]

In a study conducted by Patil *et al.* noted that 59% were having a sedentary lifestyle, 27% were having a moderately active lifestyle and 14% were having a vigorously active lifestyle. A statistically significant increasing trend for sedentary study subjects (p = 0.002

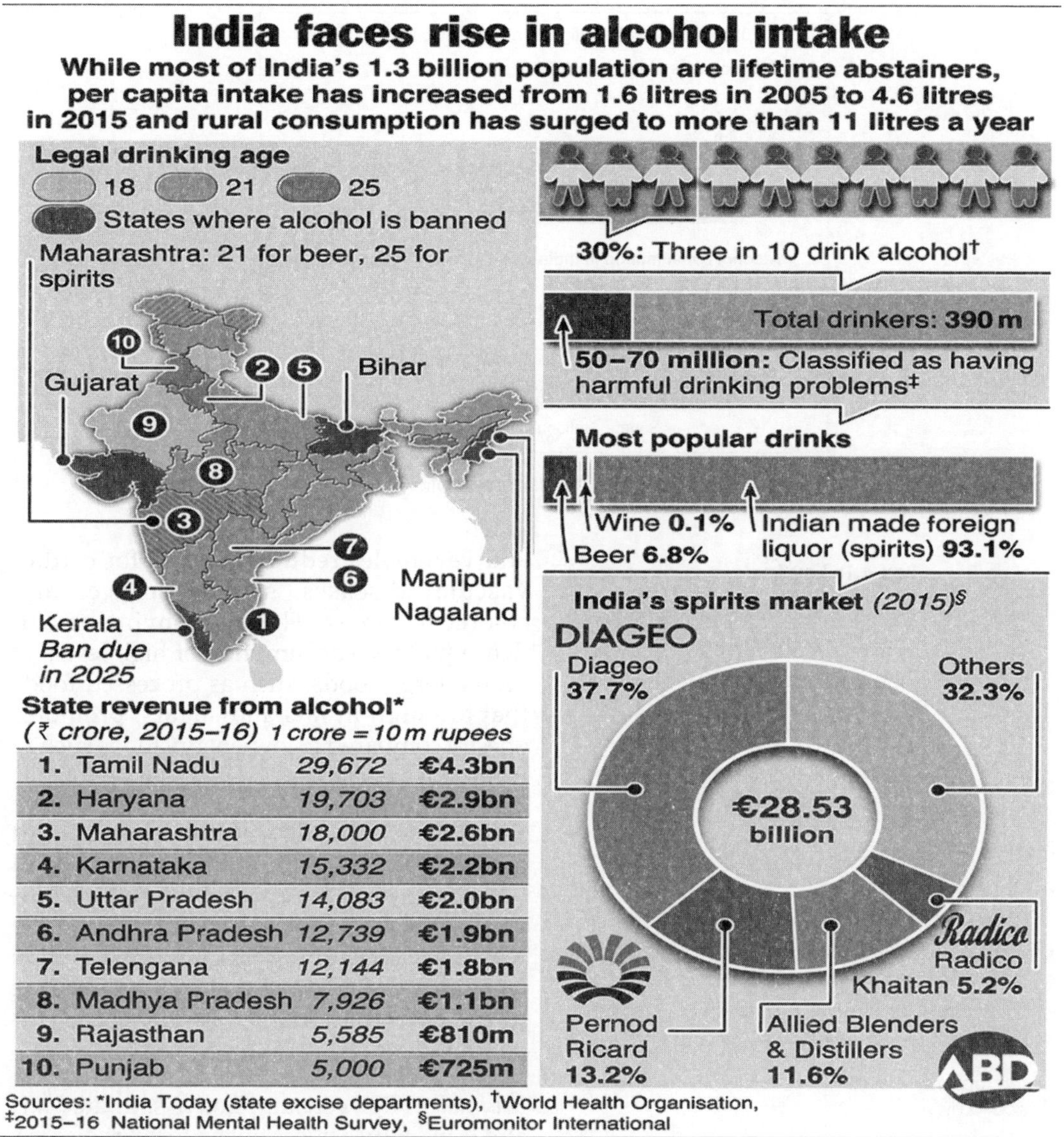

Fig. 4.7: Rise in alcohol intake in India

with age was found. Those who reported sedentary physical activity levels had 3.42 odds of being hypertensive, 7.44 times odds of being diabetic, 3 times odds of being overweight and 241 odds of being obese.[23]

The study shows that a large percentage of people in India are inactive with fewer than 10% engaging in recreational physical activity. Therefore, urgent steps need to be initiated to promote physical activity to stem the twin epidemics of diabetes and obesity in India. Some of the important key facts are given in Box 4.1.

Unhealthy Diet

An unhealthy diet is one of the major risk factors for a range of chronic diseases, including cardiovascular diseases, cancer, diabetes

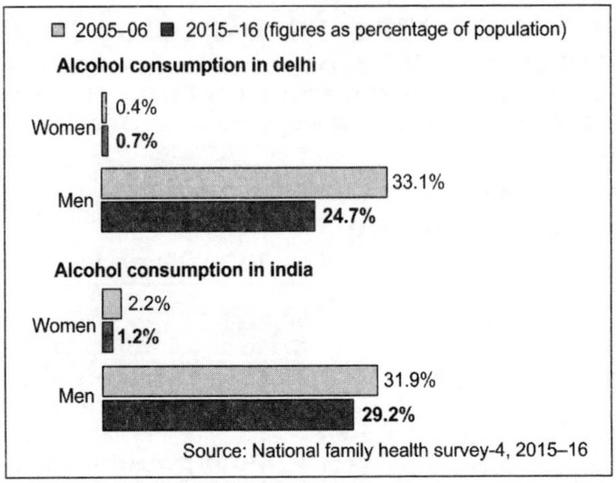

Fig. 4.8: Alcohol consumption

Box 4.1: Key facts[24]

- Insufficient physical activity is one of the leading risk factors for death worldwide.
- Insufficient physical activity is a key risk factor for non-communicable diseases (NCDs) such as cardiovascular diseases, cancer and diabetes.
- Physical activity has significant health benefits and contributes to prevent NCDs.
- Globally, 1 in 4 adults is not active enough.
- More than 80% of the world's adolescent population is insufficiently physically active.
- Policies to address insufficient physical activity are operational in 56% of WHO Member States.
- WHO Member States have agreed to reduce insufficient physical activity by 10% by 2025.

Source: http://www.who.int/news-room/fact-sheets/detail/physical-activity

and other conditions linked to overweight and obesity. Specific recommendations for a healthy diet include—eating more fruit, vegetables, legumes, nuts and grains; cutting down on salt, sugar and fats. It is also advisable to choose unsaturated fats, instead of saturated fats and towards the elimination of trans-fatty acids.

Fruit and vegetable consumption: Around 1.7 million (2.8%) of deaths worldwide are attributable to low consumption of fruit and vegetable. Adequate consumption of fruit and vegetables reduces the risk for cardiovascular diseases, stomach cancer and colorectal cancer. There is convincing evidence that the consumption of high levels of high-energy foods, such as processed foods that are high in fats and sugars, promotes obesity compared to low-energy foods such as fruits and vegetables.

Salt intake: The amount of dietary salt consumed is an important determinant of blood pressure levels and overall cardiovascular risk. Various countries around the world are consuming much more salt than recommended (5 grams per day) and reached to the current global levels of 9–12 grams per day.

Fat intake: High consumption of saturated fats and trans-fatty acids is linked to heart disease; replacement with polyunsaturated vegetable oils lowers coronary heart disease risk. Higher unsaturated fatty acids from vegetable sources and polyunsaturated fatty acids have also been shown to reduce risk of type 2 diabetes.

There were large variations across WHO regions in the amount of total fats available for human consumption. The lowest quantities available were recorded in the South-east Asia region, and the highest availability in the European region. For saturated fatty acids (SFA), the lowest rates were in the African region, and the highest was in the European region and the American region, with very high values observed in some of the Pacific islands. Energy from SFA usually accounts for a third of the energy from total fat, with the notable exception of the South-east Asia region, where SFAs account for over 40% of total fat intake.

The Food and Agriculture Organisation of the United Nations (FAOSTAT) analysed the consumption patterns of countries across the world over a period of 50 years (1961–2011).

In 1961, the average **Indian** had a daily calorie intake of 2,010. Their daily diet consisted of 43% grains (378 g), 23% produce (199 g), 12% dairy and eggs (108 g), 12% sugar and **fat (108 g),** 2% meat (17 g) and 8% as other (68 g) (Fig. 4.9).

While in 2011, the average Indian had a daily calories intake of **2,458**. Their daily diet consisted of 34% produce (450 g), 32% grains (416 g), 18% eggs and dairy (235 g), 10% sugar and **fat (129 g)**, 2% meat (29 g) and 4% as other (58 g) (Fig. 4.10[25] and Table 4.6).

In a recent data, the average daily protein consumption has risen from 55 g per day to 59 g per day in the past 25 years (from 1990–2015) with the protein from animal consumption increasing from 9 g per day to 12 g.

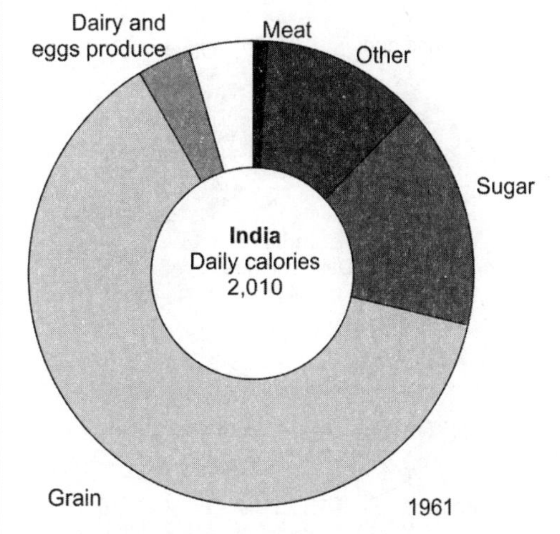

Figs 4.9: Daily calories intake in 1961

The share of dietary energy supplied from cereals and roots has decreased from an average of 66 g per day to 59 g.[26]

A study by the World Health Organization (WHO) reported that 8.7% of the world's diabetes sufferers (or 69.2 million people) live in India. Nowadays, Indian diet is full of junk and 'superfoods' which will harm in days to come.

Improving dietary habits is a societal, not just an individual problem. Therefore, it

Table 4.5: Consumption of edible oil, all-India[26]

Edible oil	*Per capita consumption in 30 days*				*% of consuming/hhs* (in 7 days)*	
	quantity (g)		*value (₹)*			
	R	*U*	*R*	*U*	*R*	*U*
(1)	(2)	(3)	(4)	(5)	(6)	(7)
Vanaspati, margarine	20	21	1.47	1.59	6.0	5.0
Mustard oil	304	242	25.07	20.20	52.7	34.1
Coconut oil	15	16	1.36	1.57	3.5	3.5
Groundnut oil	40	81	3.68	7.53	6.0	8.5
Refined oil	227	400	17.19	32.62	35.7	51.7
Edible oil—others	69	94	4.66	6.52	11.3	12.3
Edible oil—sub-total	674	853	53.44	70.03	98.3	92.6

* Note that these are the percentages of households reporting *items* of edible oil and exclude households whose members consumed edible oil only as part of meals prepared outside the households (in restaurants, in other households, etc.)

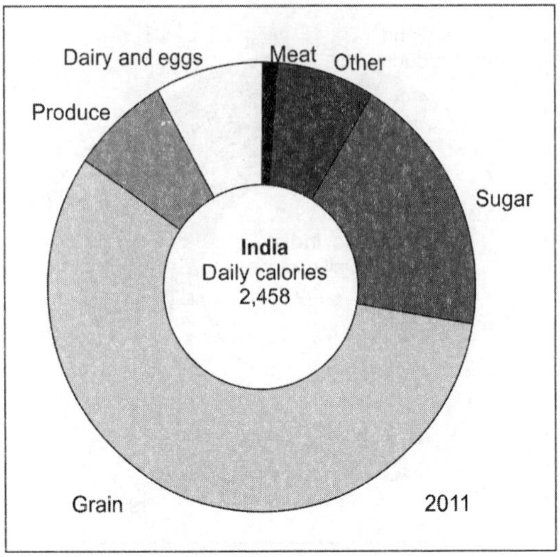

Figs 4.10: Daily calories intake in 2011

demands a population-based, multi-sectoral, multi-disciplinary, and culturally relevant approach. Some of the tips for healthy diet are given in Box 4.2.

OTHER RISK FACTORS

Raised Fasting Blood Glucose

Diabetes was directly responsible for 1.5 million deaths in 2012. The risk of cardiovascular disease increases continuously with rising fasting blood glucose levels, even below levels diagnostic of diabetes. Higher-than-optimal blood glucose was responsible for an additional 2.2 million deaths, due to increased risk of cardiovascular and other diseases, for a total of 3.7 million deaths related to blood glucose levels.

In addition to increasing cardiovascular risk, diabetes can damage the kidneys, nerves and eyes, leading to other complications. An estimated 80% of end-stage renal disease is caused by diabetes, hypertension or a combination of the two. Lower-limb amputations—necessitated by infected, non-healing ulcers—are 10 to 20 times more common among people with diabetes than among those without the disease.

Diabetic retinopathy is estimated to be the cause of 1.9% of moderate or severe visual impairment and 2.6% of blindness worldwide. The direct annual cost of diabetes is estimated to total more than US $ 827 billion. Research in developing countries has found that people with diabetes are significantly more likely to incur catastrophic medical expenditure than similar individuals without diabetes.

The prevalence of hyperglycemia depends on the diagnostic criteria used in epidemiological surveys. Defined as a fasting plasma

Box 4.2: Key facts of healthy diet

- A healthy diet helps protect against malnutrition in all its forms, as well as non-communicable diseases (NCDs), including diabetes, heart disease, stroke and cancer.
- Unhealthy diet and lack of physical activity are leading global risks to health.
- Healthy dietary practices start early in life—breastfeeding fosters healthy growth and improves cognitive development, and may have longer-term health benefits, like reducing the risk of becoming overweight or obese and developing NCDs later in life.
- Energy intake (calories) should be in balance with energy expenditure. Evidence indicates that total fat should not exceed 30% of total energy intake to avoid unhealthy weight gain, with a shift in fat consumption away from saturated fats to unsaturated fats, and towards the elimination of industrial trans fats.
- Limiting intake of free sugars to less than 10% of total energy intake is part of a healthy diet. A further reduction to less than 5% of total energy intake is suggested for additional health benefits.
- Keeping salt intake to less than 5 g per day helps prevent hypertension and reduces the risk of heart disease and stroke in the adult population.
- WHO Member States have agreed to reduce the global population's intake of salt by 30% and halt the rise in diabetes and obesity in adults and adolescents as well as in childhood overweight by 2025.

glucose value ≥ 7.0 mmol/L (126 mg/dl) or on medication for raised blood glucose. The global prevalence of diabetes in 2014 was estimated to be 8.5% and **India—8.7%.**

Raised Blood Pressure

Raised blood pressure is a major risk factor for coronary heart disease and ischemic as well as hemorrhagic stroke. In some age groups, the risk of cardiovascular disease doubles for each increment of 20/10 mmHg of blood pressure, starting as low as 115/75 mmHg. In addition to coronary heart diseases and stroke, complications of raised blood pressure include heart failure, peripheral vascular disease, renal impairment, retinal hemorrhage and visual impairment. Treating systolic blood pressure and diastolic blood pressure until they are less than 140/90 mmHg is associated with a reduction in cardiovascular complications.

In 2015, around the **world**, the prevalence of raised blood pressure in females aged 18 and over was around 20% and males around 24%. The top five countries with the highest proportion of men with high blood pressure in 2015 were all in Central and Eastern Europe: Croatia, Latvia, Lithuania, Hungary, and Slovenia. Nearly two in five men in these countries had high blood pressure.

The top five countries with the highest proportion of women with high blood pressure in 2015 were all in Africa: Niger, Chad, Mali, Burkina Faso, and Somalia. Around one in three women in these countries had high blood pressure.

In 2015, India—prevalence of raised blood pressure was 25.8% (WHO). India has a large number of hypertensives with projections indicating nearly a doubling from 8 million in 2000 to 213 million by 2025. Hypertension prevalence in adults is between 20% and 40% in urban areas and 12% and 17% in rural areas. An earlier meta-analysis reported 25% prevalence among urban adults and 10% among rural adults.

Raised Cholesterol

Globally, one-third of ischaemic heart disease is attributable to high cholesterol. Overall, raised cholesterol is estimated to cause 2.6 million deaths (4.5% of total) and 29.7 million disability adjusted life years (DALYs), or 2.0% of total DALYs. Raised total cholesterol is a major cause of disease burden in both the developed and developing world as a risk factor for ischaemic heart disease (IHD) and stroke. A 10% reduction in serum cholesterol in men aged 40 has been reported to result in a 50% reduction in heart disease within 5 years; the same serum cholesterol reduction for men aged 70 years can result in an average 20% reduction in heart disease occurrence in the next 5 years. In Ireland, a 30% reduction in the heart disease death rate has been attributed to 4.6% reduction of the population mean for total cholesterol. In Finland, 50% of the decline in IHD mortality has been explained by the reduction of population blood cholesterol level.

In 2008, the global prevalence of raised total cholesterol among adults (>5.0 mmol/L) was 39% (37% for males and 40% for females). Globally, mean total cholesterol changed little between 1980 and 2008, falling by less than 0.1 mmol/L per decade in men and women.

The prevalence of elevated total cholesterol was highest in the WHO Region of Europe (54% for both sexes), followed by the WHO American region (48% for both sexes). The WHO African region and the WHO South-east Asian region showed the lowest percentages (22.6% for AFR and 29.0% for SEAR).

Overweight and Obesity (adults aged 18+)

Research has established that overweight and obesity lead to adverse metabolic effects on blood pressure, cholesterol, triglycerides and insulin resistance. Risks of coronary heart disease, ischemic stroke and type 2 diabetes mellitus rising with increasing body mass index (BMI). Raised body mass index also increases the risk of cancer of the breast, colon, prostate, kidney and gallbladder. Mortality rates increase with morbid obesity and overweight, risk of co-morbidities body mass index 30 or more.

Globally in 2016, 39% men and 39% of women aged 18+ were overweight (BMI

≥25 kg/m²) and 11% of men and 15% of women were obese (BMI ≥30 kg/m²). Thus, nearly 2 billion adults worldwide were overweight and, of these, more than half a billion were obese. Both overweight and obesity have shown a marked increase over the past four decades. Obesity rates in men have risen from around 3% in 1975 and in women from just over 6% in 1975, while overweight has risen over this same time period from 20% in men and from just under 23% in women.

In India, prevalence of obesity is 19.7%. Overweight and obesity in adolescent ranged from 2.2 to 25.8% and 0.73 to 14.6% respectively. The prevalence was comparatively higher in urban areas than in rural areas and males were more preponderate to get overweight/obese.[27]

The pooled data after 2010 estimated a combined prevalence of 19.3% of childhood overweight and obesity, which was a significant increase from the earlier prevalence of 16.3% reported in 2001–2005.[28]

Recent estimates reveal that >12% of the entire population is overweight or obese and India, after China, has the highest number of people with diabetes in the world. Rapid economic development has seen dietary patterns shift towards energy-dense foods which together with increased urbanization and an associated sedentary lifestyle have contributed to the rise in overweight/obesity.[29]

Of the 956 studies screened, 18 met the eligibility criteria. The pooled odds ratio between obesity and hypertension was 3.82 (95% CI: 3.39 to 4.25). The heterogeneity around this estimate (I2 statistic) was 0%, indicating low variability. The pooled odds ratio from the included studies showed a statistically significant association between obesity and T2DM (OR = 1.14, 95% CI: 1.04 to 1.24) with a high degree of variability.[30]

In 2016, in India, the leading risk factors responsible for DALYs due to NCD for more than 5% of the total DALY each were child and maternal malnutrition (under nutrition; 14.6%), air pollution (9.8%), dietary risks (unhealthy diet; 8.9%), high systolic blood pressure (8.5%), high fasting plasma glucose (6%), and tobacco use (includes smoking, second-hand smoke, and smokeless tobacco; 5.9%). Dietary risks, systolic blood pressure, high total cholesterol, tobacco, and alcohol were common risk factors.

STRATEGIES FOR PREVENTION AND CONTROL OF NON-COMMUNICABLE DISEASES

Application of levels of prevention and control of communicable diseases are easier as there is a definitive natural history as contrast to NCD, where natural history is obscure with distinctive characteristics. However, basic levels of diseases prevention can also be applied to NCD (Table 4.6).

Non-communicable diseases cannot be prevented without the concerted and coordinated efforts, globally major approaches to be adopted are as follows with its vision and goals:

Vision: A world free of the avoidable burden of non-communicable diseases.

Goal: To reduce the preventable and avoidable burden of morbidity, mortality and disability due to non-communicable diseases by means of multi-sectoral collaboration and cooperation at national, regional and global levels, so that populations reach the highest attainable standards of health, quality of life, and productivity at every age and those diseases are no longer a barrier to well-being or socio-economic development.

The action plan relies on the following overarching principles and approaches (Fig. 4.11).

Human Rights Approach

Highest attainable standard of health is one of the fundamental rights of every human being, without distinction as enshrined in the Universal Declaration of Human Rights.

Equity-based Approach

Inequitable distribution of social determinants of health is responsible for the unequal distribution of non-communicable diseases; hence action on these determinants, both for vulnerable groups and the entire population is essential.

Table 4.6: Levels of prevention and strategies

Levels of prevention	*Strategies*	
Primary	Health promotion	Life course approach with lifestyle modifications be adopted, e.g. increased physical activity, avoidance of tobacco and alcohol, increase intake of fruits and vegetable, reduction of salt, etc. Practice on yoga.
	Prevention	• Policies on tobacco and alcohol control (taxation, regulation, production, pricing, ban on advertisements and access restrictions consumer education) • National transport policy, national nutrition policies, etc. • School-based programs for healthy life education
Secondary	Screening and early diagnosis	Screening for high risk factors like history, blood sugar level, lipid profile, pap smear/cancer markers, kidney function tests, pulmonary function test, body mass index, ECG, X-rays, etc.
	Treatment	Preparation and application of standard management protocols for IHD, stroke, DM, malignancies, dyslipidemia, obesity control, etc.
Tertiary	Disability limitation	Adequate treatment to halt further development of complications, impairments, disabilities and handicaps or even death
	Rehabilitation	Tobacco cessation for users, monitoring of BP and DM control, post-stroke rehabilitation

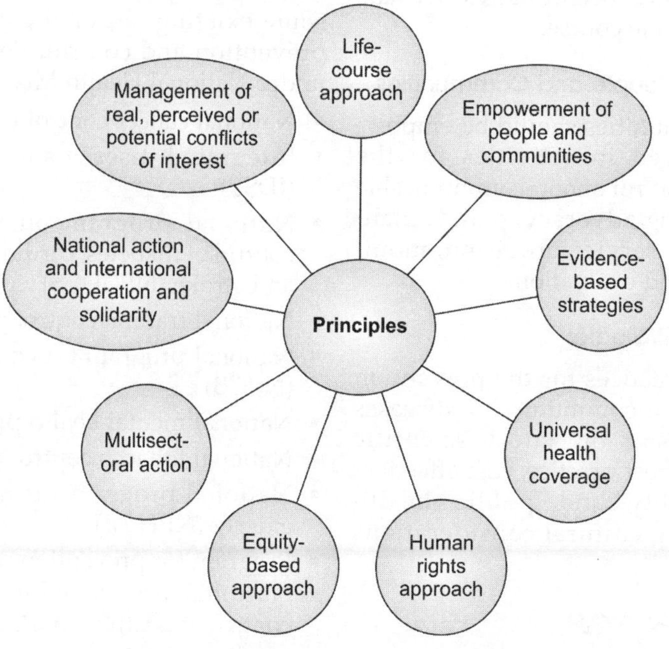

Fig. 4.11: Overarching principles and approaches

National Action, International Cooperation and Solidarity

The primary role and responsibility of governments in responding to the challenge of non-communicable diseases should be recognized, together with the important role of international cooperation in assisting member states, as a complement to national efforts.

Multi-sectoral Action

An appropriate health-in-all policies and whole-of-government approach across sectors (health, agriculture, communication, education, employment, energy, environment, finance, food, foreign affairs, housing, justice and security, legislature, social welfare, social and economic development, sports, tax and revenue, trade and industry, transport, urban planning and youth affairs and partnership with relevant civil society and private sector entities) are needed for prevention and control of NCD.

Life-course Approach

Since the NCDs are lifestyle diseases, the control lies in life-course approach at multiple stages of life; interventions in early life often offer the best chance for primary prevention. Policies,plans and services for the prevention and control of non-communicable diseases need to take account of health and social needs at all stages of the life course.

Empowerment of People and Communities

People and communities should be empowered and involved in activities for the prevention and control of non-communicable diseases, including advocacy, policy, planning, legislation, service provision, monitoring, research and evaluation.

Evidence-based Strategies

Strategies and practices for the prevention and control of non-communicable diseases need to be based on latest scientific evidence and/or best practice, cost-effectiveness, affordability and public health principles, taking cultural considerations into account.

Universal Health Coverage

All people should have access to nationally determined sets of the needed promotive, preventive, curative and rehabilitative basic health services and essential, safe, affordable, effective and quality medicines. At the same time it must be ensured that the use of these services does not expose the users to financial hardship, with a special emphasis on the poor and populations living in vulnerable situations.

Management of Real, Perceived or Potential Conflicts of Interest

Public health policies, strategies and multisectoral action for the prevention and control of non-communicable diseases must be protected from undue influence by any form of vested interest. Real, perceived or potential conflicts of interest must be acknowledged and managed.

Global objectives and targets, and best interventions for prevention and control of non-communicable diseases are mentioned in Tables 4.7 and 4.8.

STRATEGIES FOR PREVENTION AND CONTROL OF NON-COMMUNICABLE DISEASES IN INDIA

Existing program for NCDs, the country has some existing national program for NCD prevention and control. Following include under National Health Mission.

- National cancer control program (NCCP)
- Integrated disease surveillance project (IDSP)
- National program on prevention and control of diabetes, cardiovascular diseases and stroke (NPCDCS)
- National trauma control program
- National program for control of blindness (NPCB)
- National mental health program (NMHP)
- National tobacco control program (NTCP)
- National program for healthcare of the elderly (NPHCE)
- Program for prevention of burn injuries
- National program for prevention and control of deafness (NPPCD)
- National oral health program (NOHP)
- National program for palliative care.

Progress and Highlights of NPCDCS

During the period 2010–2012, the program was implemented in 100 districts across

Table 4.7: Global objectives and targets

Global objectives	*Voluntary global targets for prevention and control of non-communicable diseases to be attended by 2025*
1. To raise the priority accorded to the prevention and control of non-communicable diseases in global, regional and national agendas and internationally agreed development goals, through strengthened international cooperation and advocacy. 2. To strengthen national capacity, leadership, governance, multi-sectoral action and partnerships to accelerate country response for the prevention and control of non-communicable diseases. 3. To reduce modifiable risk factors for non-communicable diseases and underlying social determinants through creation of health-promoting environments. 4. To strengthen and orient health systems to address the prevention and control of non-communicable diseases and the underlying social determinants through people-centered primary healthcare and universal health coverage. 5. To promote and support national capacity for high-quality research and development for the prevention and control of non-communicable diseases. 6. To monitor the trends and determinants of non-communicable diseases and evaluate progress in their prevention and control.	1. A 25% relative reduction in the overall mortality from cardiovascular diseases, cancer, diabetes, or chronic respiratory diseases. 2. At least 10% relative reduction in the harmful use of alcohol, as appropriate, within the national context. 3. A 10% relative reduction in prevalence of insufficient physical activity. 4. A 30% relative reduction in mean population intake of salt/sodium. 5. A 30% relative reduction in prevalence of current tobacco use. 6. A 25% relative reduction in the prevalence of raised blood pressure or contain the prevalence of raised blood pressure, according to national circumstances. 7. Halt the rise in diabetes and obesity. 8. At least 50% of eligible people receive drug therapy and counselling (including glycogenic control) to prevent heart attacks and strokes. 9. An 80% availability of the affordable basic technologies and essential medicines, including generics, required to treat major non-communicable diseases in both public and private facilities.

21 states. Review of the initial phase of program implementation helped to identify the bottle-necks and accordingly the program was re-strategized and scaled-up. Till March, 2020, there are 665 district NCD cells, 637 district NCD clinics, 4472 CHC NCD clinics, 181 cardiac care units and 218 daycare units functional in the country.

Around 6.61 crore persons attended NCD clinics and were screened for common NCDs like diabetes, hypertension, CVDs and common cancers during 2019–20. More than 1.1 crore population has been covered under population-based screening so far. In addition, during outreach activities, 5.6 crore NCD check up were conducted (Fig. 4.12).

Place of screening	*No. of people screened*
Screened at NCD clinics	6.61 crore
Population-based screening	1.1 crore
During outreach activities	5.6 crores

The modified strategies are:

i. Health promotion through behaviour change with involvement of community, civil society, community-based organizations, media, etc.

Table 4.8: Best buy interventions[31]

Risk factor/disease	*Interventions*
Tobacco use	• Tax increases • Smoke-free indoor workplaces and public places • Health information and warnings • Bans on tobacco advertising, promotion and sponsorship
Harmful alcohol use	• Tax increases • Restricted access to retailed alcohol • Bans on alcohol advertising
Unhealthy diet and physical inactivity	• Reduced salt intake in food • Replacement of trans fat with polyunsaturated fat • Public awareness through mass media on diet and physical activity
Cardiovascular disease (CVD) and diabetes	• Counselling and multi-drug therapy for people with a high risk of developing heart attacks and strokes (including those with established CVD) • Treatment of heart attacks with aspirin
Cancer	• Hepatitis B immunization to prevent liver cancer (already scaled up) • Screening and treatment of pre-cancerous lesions to prevent cervical cancer

Source: http://www.who.int/nmh/publications/best_buys_summary

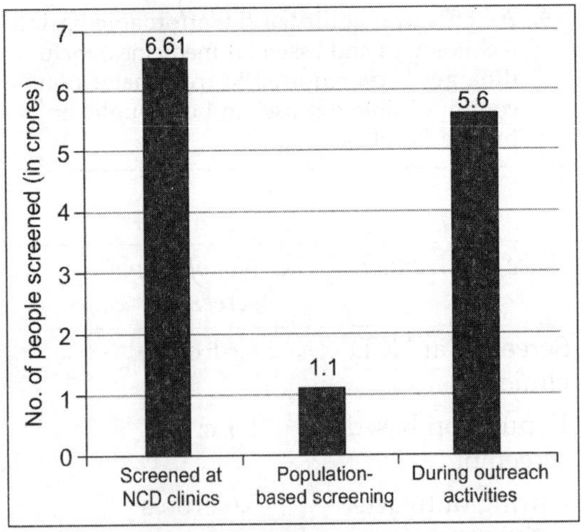

Fig. 4.12: Number of people screed for common NCDs during 2019–2020

ii. Outreach camps are envisaged for opportunistic screening at all levels in the healthcare delivery system from sub-centre and above for early detection of diabetes, hypertension and common cancers.

iii. Management of chronic non-communicable diseases, especially cancer, diabetes, CVDs and stroke through early diagnosis, treatment and follow-up through setting up of NCD clinics.

iv. Build capacity at various levels of health care for prevention, early diagnosis, treatment, IEC/BCC, operational research and rehabilitation.

v. Provide support for diagnosis and cost-effective treatment at primary, secondary and tertiary levels of healthcare.

vi. Provide support for development of database of NCDs through a robust surveillance system and to monitor NCD morbidity, mortality and risk factors.

Total cost of the program for period 2012–2017 is ₹ 8,096 crore (share of Government of India is ₹ 6,535 crore and that of State

Governments is ₹ 1,561 crore). The funds are being provided to the States under NCD Flexi-Pool through State PIPs of respective States/UTs, with the Centre to State share in ratio of 60:40 (except for NE and Hilly States, where the share is 90:10).

Program Performance (as on March 2016)

The program is under implementation in all 36 States/UTs. A total of 298 district NCD cells and 293 district NCD clinics have been established in the country. Also, there are 103 functional cardiac care units for emergency cardiac care and 64 day-care centers for cancer care at the district levels in the country.

During 2015–2016, more than 1.29 crore persons have been screened in the designated NCD clinics. Among these NCD clinic attendees, around 8% were diagnosed to be diabetics and 12% were hypertensive. Also,

Table 4.9: Targets for NCDs prevention and control in India[32]

S.No.	*Framework element*	*National NCD TARGETS*		
		Outcome	*2020*	*2025*
1.	Premature mortality	Relative reduction in overall mortality from cardiovascular disease, cancer, diabetes, or chronic respiratory disease	10%	20%
2.	Alcohol use	Relative reduction in alcohol use	5%	10%
3.	Obesity and diabetes	Halt the rise in obesity and diabetes prevalence	No mid-term target set	Halt the rise in obesity and diabetes prevalence
4.	Physical inactivity	Relative reduction in prevalence of insufficient physical activity	5%	10%
5.	Raised blood pressure	Relative reduction in prevalence of raised blood pressure	10%	25%
6.	Salt/sodium intake	Relative reduction in mean population intake of salt, with aim of achieving recommended level of less than 5 g per day	20%	30%
7.	Tobacco use	Relative reduction in prevalence of current tobacco use	15%	30%
8.	Drug therapy to prevent heart attacks and strokes	Eligible people receiving drug therapy and counselling (including glycemia control) to prevent heart attacks and strokes	30%	50%
9.	Essential NCD medicines and basic technologies to treat major NCDs	Affordability of quality, safe and efficacious essential NCD medicines including generics, and basic technologies in both public and private fucilities	60%	80%
10.	Household indoor air pollution	Relative reduction in household use of solid fuels as a primary source of energy for cooking	25%	50%

around 90,000 persons were diagnosed to be suffering from cardiovascular diseases and over 13,000 persons were detected to be having common cancers (including oral, cervical and breast cancers) among them (Fig. 4.11).

During 2015–2016, around 96 lakh persons were screened under various outreach activities for common NCDs (in camps and PHC/SC), and they were referred to higher centres for diagnosis and management.

Recent Initiatives Under NPCDCS

1. Inclusion of guidelines for prevention and management of chronic obstructive pulmonary disease (COPD) and chronic kidney disease (CKD) under NPCDCS, to prevent and manage the chronic respiratory and kidney diseases respectively, which are also major causes of death due to NCDs.
2. For early detection of diabetes, hypertension and common cancers in the community, guidelines are being issued to the states for initiating 'population-based screening of common NCDs' utilising the services of the frontline-workers and health-workers under the existing primary healthcare system.
3. Pilot project on 'integration of AYUSH with NPCDCS' has been initiated in six districts

Table 4.10: India's NCD progress[33]

1,309,000,000 Total population	*61%—percentages of deaths from NCDs*	*5, 817, 000—total number of NCD deaths*	*23%—risk of premature death from target NCDs*
1. National NCD targets			●
2. Mortality rates			◐
3. Risk factor surveys			◐
4. National integrated NCD policy/strategy/action plan			○
5. Tobacco demand-reduction measures:			
a. Increased excise taxes end prices			○
b. Smoke-free policies			◐
c. Large graphic health warnings/plain packaging			●
d. Bans on advertising, promotion and sponsorship			◐
e. Mass media campaigns			◐
6. Harmful use of alcohol reduction measures:			
a. Restrictions on physical availability			◐
b. Advertising bans or comprehensive restrictions			○
c. Increased excise taxes			○
7. Unhealthy diet reduction measures:			
a. Salt/sodium policies			◐
b. Saturated fatty acid and trans-fat policies			●
c. Marketing to children restrictions			○
d Marketing of breast-milk substitutes restictions			●
8. Public education and awareness campaign on physical activity			○
9. Guidelines for management of cancer, CVD, diabetes and CRD			●
10. Drug therapy/counselling to prevent heart attacks and strokes			◐

● fully achieved ◐ partially achieved ○ not achieved

World Health Organization—non-communicable disease progress monitor, 2017

in the country. AYUSH facilities and methodologies are being integrated with NPCDCS services for prevention and management of common NCDs, wherein the practice of Yoga is an integral part of the intervention.

4. Pilot intervention has been initiated for the prevention and control of rheumatic fever and rheumatic heart disease under the platforms of NPCDCS and RBSK (Rashtriya Bal Swasthya Karyakram), in three selected districts (Gaya—Bihar, Firozabad—Uttar Pradesh and Hoshangabad—Madhya Pradesh). This intervention would be scaled up to other districts in a phased manner.
5. Another initiative is the integration of RNTCP with NPCDCS, wherein the 'National Framework for Joint Tuberculosis–Diabetes collaborative activities' has been developed to articulate a national strategy for 'bi-directional screening', early detection and better management of tuberculosis and diabetes comorbidities in India.

Targets for NCD prevention and control are summarized in Table 4.9 and NCD progress in India is shown in Table 4.10.

References

1. Malabika Sarker, et al. Non-communicable diseases in Bangladesh: Current scenario and future directions. Bangladesh Health Watch Report 2016. Published by Bangladesh Health Watch Secretariat, James P Grant School of Public Health, BRAC University, 2017.
2. Thippeswamy T, Chikkegowda P. Basic Risk Factors Awareness in Non-communicable diseases (BRAND) Study Among People Visiting Tertiary Care Centre in Mysuru, Karnataka. Journal of Clinical and Diagnostic Research/:JCDR. 2016; 10(4):OC04-OC07.doi:10.7860/JCDR/2016/19041.7556.
3. Nethan S, Sinha D, Mehrotra R. Non-communicable Disease Risk Factors and their Trends in India. Asian Pacific Journal of Cancer Prevention: APJCP.2017;18(7):2005–2010.doi:10.22034/APJCP.2017.18.7.2005.
4. Shah B, Mathur P. Surveillance of cardiovascular disease risk factors in India: The need & scope. The Indian Journal of Medical Research. 2010;132(5): 634-642. doi:10.4103/0971-5916.73420.
5. Dr Ala Alwan (Ed). Global status report on non-communicable diseases 2010. Published by WHO Press, World Health Organization, 20 Avenue Appia, 1211 Geneva 27, Switzerland. HYPER LINK "http://www.who.int" www.who.int accessed on 25.7.2018
6. Shanthi Mendis (lead auth). Global status report on noncommunicable diseases 2014. Published by WHO Press, World Health Organization, 20 Avenue Appia, 1211 Geneva 27, Switzerland. HYPERLINK "http://www.who.int" www.who.int accessed on 25.7.2018
7. Koopman, et al. Am J Trop Med Hyg, 2016;94(6): 1189–92. doi:10.4269/ajtmh.15-0715
8. WHO. Global burden of diseases 2004 update: selected figures & tables, Health statistics and Informatics department. Who.int/healthinfo/global_burden_diseases/GBD2004 reports figureppt.
9. World Health Organization – Non-communicable Diseases (NCD) Country Profiles, 2014. HYPER LINK "http://www.who.int" www.who.int accessed on 26.7.2018.
10. Sailesh Mohan K, Srinath Reddy D, Prabhakaran. Chronic non-communicable diseases in India reversing the tide, September 2011, PHFI, accessed from http://www.indiaenvironmentportal.org.in/files/file/PHFI_NCD_Report_Sep_2011.pdf
11. Tabish SA. Lifestyle Diseases: Consequences, Characteristics, Causes and Control. J Cardiol Curr Res 2018;9(3):00326.
12. Dandona L. Nations within a nation: variations in epidemiological transition across the states of India, 1990–2016 in the Global Burden of Disease Study. Lancet 2017;390:2437–60 www.thelancet.com Vol 390 December 2, 2017. Published Online November 14, 2017. http://dx.doi.org/10.1016/S0140-6736(17)32804-0
13. Deepa M, Pradeepa R, Anjana RM, Mohan V. Noncommunicable Diseases Risk Factor Surveillance: Experience and Challenge from India. Indian J Community Med [serial online] 2011 [cited 2018 Jul 27];36, Suppl S1:50-6. Available from: http://www.ijcm.org.in/text.asp?2011/36/5/50/94709.
14. HYPERLINK https://www.cdc.gov/globalhealth/healthprotection/fetp/training_modules/1/intro-to-epi_ppt__final_09252013.pdf Introduction to NCD Epidemiology Presentation - CDC. HYPERLINK "https://www.cdc.gov/.../intro-to-epi_ppt__final_092..%20Accessed%20on%2027/7/2018" https://www.cdc.gov/.../intro-to-epi_ppt__final_092.. Accessed on 27/7/2018
15. Hunter David J, Reddy K Srinath. HYPERLINK "Noncommunicable Diseases". N Engl J Med 2013; 369:1336–43. DOI: 10.1056/NEJMra1109345 Non-communic able Diseases. N Engl J Med 2013;369:

1336-43.DOI: 10.1056/NEJMra1109345 https://www.nejm. org/doi/pdf/10.../nejmra1109345

16. Venkatachalam J, Purty, Anil Jacob and Singh, Zile and Abraham, Sherin, Narayanan S and Gr, Sathya and Bhumika, Nateshan and Bazroy, Joy. 2013 Prevalence of Non Communicable Diseases (NCDs) in a Rural Population of South India. Indian journal of public health and development. January-June 2014;2(1):55.10.5958/j.2321-1032. 2.1.012.
17. GATS 2-Global Adult Tobacco Survey. Factsheet-India 2016-17.http://www.who.int/tobacco/surveillance/survey/gats/GATS_India2016-17.
18. Indian Alcohol Consumption Report 2017-Focus on the Changing Behavior - Research and Markers https://www.businesswire.com/news/home/20171122005374/en/
19. Global Alcohol Report–2011. http://www. who. int/substance_abuse/publications/global_alcohol_report/msbgsruprofiles.pdf
20. Manimunda SP, Sugunan AP, Thennarasu K, Pandian D, Pesala KS, Benegal V. Alcohol consumption, hazardous drinking, and alcohol dependency among the population of Andaman and Nicobar Islands, India. Indian J Public Health 2017;61:105–11.
21. Anjana, et al. International Journal of Behavioral Nutrition and Physical Activity 2014, 11:26 Page 3 of 11 http://www.ijbnpa.org/content/11/1/26 (male: 61.3%).
22. Patil C, et al. Int J Community Med Public Health. 2017 Apr;4(4):1154-1158. DOI: http://dx.doi.org/10.18203/2394-6040.ijcmph20171341, http://www.ijcmph.com PISSN 2394) accesses on 28/7/2018.
23. http://www.who.int/news-room/fact-sheets/detail/physical-activity
24. Annual Report 2016–17. Government of India, Ministry of Statistics and Programme Implementation, Sardar Patel Bhawan, Sansad Marg , New Delhi-110001 http://www.mospi.gov.in
25. NASSO report on Household Consumption of Various Goods and Services in India. NSS 68th Round, (JULY 2011 - JUNE 2012) . Report No. 558 (68/1.0/2) published by National Sample Survey Office, Ministry of Statistics and Programme Implementation, Government of India, June 2014.
26. Nirpal Kaur Shukla et al. Prevalence of overweight and obesity among adolescentsin india: a systematic review. HYPERLINK "http://www. scopemed. org/?jtt=International%20Journal%20of%20 Current%20Research%20and% 20Review" IJCRR. 2016; 8(18): 21–25).
27. Ranjani H, et al. Epidemiology of childhood overweight and obesity in India: A systematic review. Indian J Med Res 2016;143:160–74.
28. Khandelwal S, Reddy S. Eliciting a policy response for the rising epidemic of overweight-obesity in India. Obesity Reviews 2013;14:114–25.
29. Babu GR, et al. Association of obesity with hypertension and type 2 diabetes mellitus in India: A meta-analysis of observational studies. World J Diabetes 2018;9(1):40–52.
30. Global action plan for the prevention and control of noncommunicable diseases 2013–2020). Published by WHO Press, World Health Organization, 20 Avenue Appia, 1211 Geneva 27, Switzerland. HYPERLINK "http://www. who.int" www.who.int accessed on 25.7.2018.
31. WHO. From Burden to "Best Buys":Reducing the Economic Impact of Non-Communicable Diseases in Low- and Middle-Income Countries. The Global Economic Burden of Non-communicable Diseases–prepared by the World Economic Forum and the Harvard School of Public Health (2011). Available through: http://www.weforum.org/Economics OfNCD. http://www.who.int/nmh/publications/ best_buys_summary.pdf
32. Non-communicable Diseases Progress Monitor, 2017. Geneva: World Health Organization; 2017. License: CC BY-NC-SA 3.0 IGO.
33. World Health Organization—non-communicable disease progress monitor, 2017, https://www.who.int/nmh/publications/ncd-progress-monitor-2017/en/

Chapter

5

Applied Epidemiology: An Overview

Social, Clinical, Molecular, Genetic and Pharmacoepidemiology

Pradeep Deshmukh, Ram Chandra Goyal and Mabashshera Firdos Khan

SOCIAL EPIDEMIOLOGY

Introduction

WHO defined the health as, "it is a state of complete physical, mental and social-well being, not merely the absence of disease or infirmity." Now, it also include spiritual health" so as to lead a socially and economically productive life.

Social health is a life cycle approach which depends on various social determinants of health (SDH). SDH, in which people are born, grow, work, live, and age, and the wider set of forces and systems shaping the conditions of daily life (Fig. 5.1). These forces and systems include economic policies and systems, development agendas, social norms, social policies and political systems. The SDGs provide a comprehensive blueprint for human development and for systematically addressing the social determinants of health.[1]

Definition of Social Epidemiology

1. Social epidemiology is a branch of epidemiology that studies the distribution and determinants of health and disease in populations.
2. Social epidemiology is defined as "the branch of epidemiology that studies the social distribution and social determinants of states of health.[2]"

— *Berkman and Kawachi*

Social Determinants

The unsatisfactory health condition of the economically and socially deprived sections of the communities is caused by unequal distribution of income, goods and services. Their vulnerability makes it difficult for them to achieve satisfactory health status since they are continuously affected by poor social policies and programs, unfair economic arrangements and decades of economic and social deprivation. Their health condition can be substantially altered only by a social determinants approach, which improves their daily living conditions, help to tackle inequitable distribution of power and resources and adequate state policies to address their multiple development challenges adequately (Fig. 5.2).[3]

Historical Background of Social Epidemiology

Social epidemiology is not an entirely new discipline. About 2,400 years ago, Hippocrates, recorded his observations about how climate, living conditions, and people's professions affected the people with various

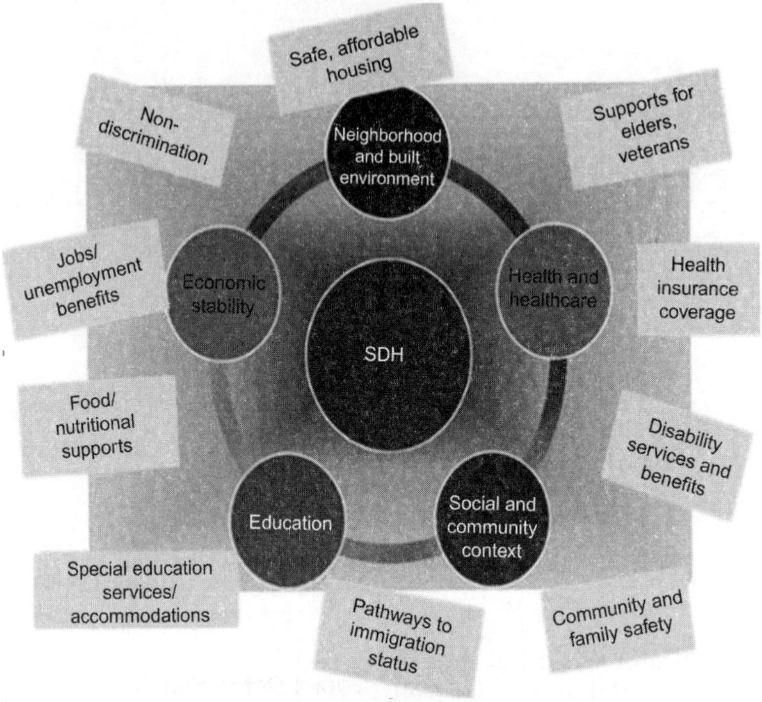

(a)

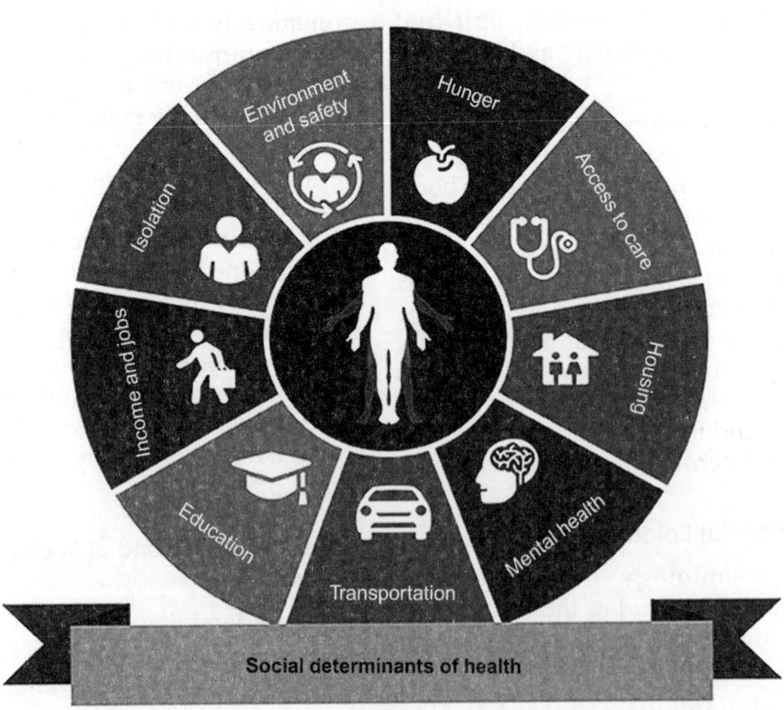

(b)

Fig. 5.1: Components of social determinants of health[3]

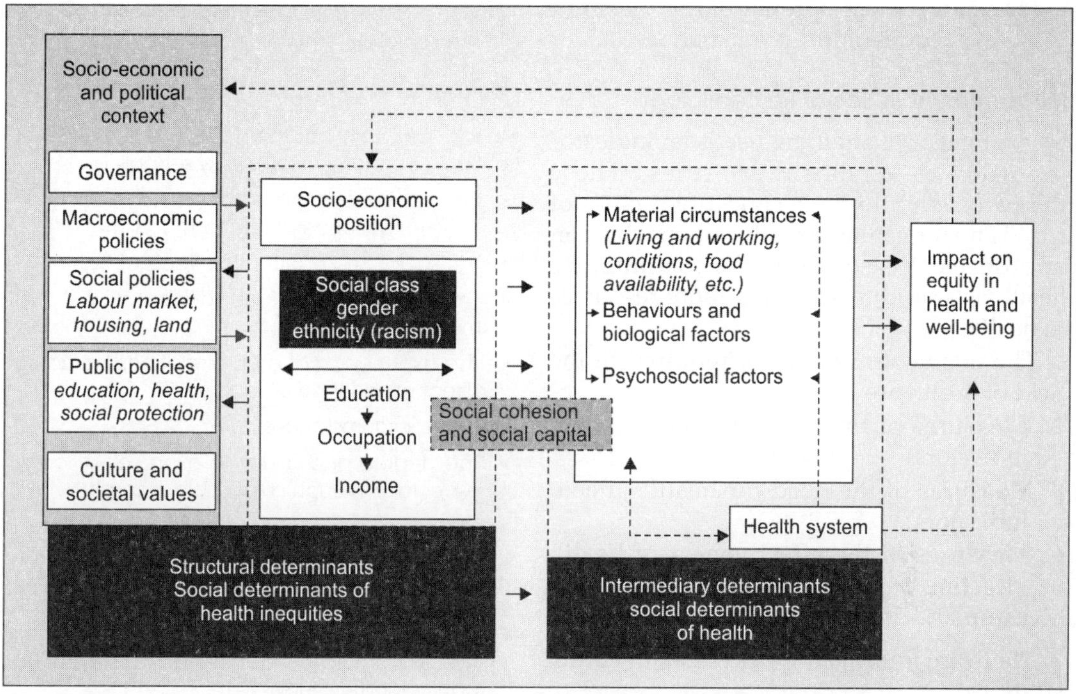

Fig. 5.2: Components of social determinants of health

types of illnesses as he saw in his practice. In his writings 'On Airs, Waters and Places' he implicated the seasons, winds, sources and quality of drinking water, and behaviour of the locals in the determination of health status **(Hippocrates 460–370 BC).**

In the middle of the 19th century, Chadwick reported that unsanitary soil, air, and water were major causes of diseases and promoted sanitation measures to improve the health of the poor. Clearly, studies in the beginning and middle of the 19th century were conducted with the assumption that societal conditions affect physical health.[4]

In the early 20th century, the idea of a single individual risk factor, including germs that led to disease; however, with the rise of infectious diseases multiple individual risk factors, the so-called 'web of causation,' were epidemiological theories.

Social Epidemiological Theory

A theory in the social sciences is defined as "a set of interrelated constructs or concepts, definitions, and propositions that present a systematic view of phenomena by specifying relations among variables, with the purpose of explaining and predicting the phenomena" (Kerlinger 1986:9). In epidemiology, following theories were put forth.

1. **Bio-psychosocial paradigm:** The bio-psychosocial paradigm assumes that population is not merely the sum of its individuals; rather, every population has its own history and culture, which determine how and why people are exposed to specific individual risk factors.
2. **Population perspective:** Geoffrey Rose pointed out that an individual's risk of disease cannot be isolated from the disease risks of the population to which she belongs. This is Rose's population perspective, which has a crucial meaning in social epidemiology.
3. **Multi-level statistical analysis:** This multilevel approach allows epidemiologists to develop quantitative and structural analyses of social factors as they affect health, and has contributed significantly to the development of social epidemiology.

However, social epidemiology does not always require multi-level analysis.

Measurement in Social Epidemiology

Measurement of anything needs an indicator in order to establish priorities. These indicators should have conceptual basis of social and humanitarian value upon which an improvement is sought in the community's health as a result of devoting more resources to health.

The main social indicator required in the field of health are:

A. Measures of the state-of-health ('state' indicators)
B. Measures of the need-for-health ('need' indicators)
C. Measures of the effectiveness of health affecting activities ('effectiveness' indicators).

There are four main types of health equity stratifies:

1. Socio-economic groups—education; occupation; income/consumption/expenditure/wealth/assets
2. Gender
3. Ethnic groups—ethnic, racial, tribal, caste, religious and national origin groups
4. Place of residence—urban *vs* rural, northern *vs* southern regions.

Currently there are multiple indicators which measure social determinant of health like GDP, human poverty index, human development index, human suffering index, PQLI, quality of life, etc. However, most composite index is multi-dimensional poverty index (MPI), employment and financial protection, political participation and environment [nitrogen dioxide (NO_2), sulphur dioxide (SO_2), particulate matter (PM10)]. The core candidate indicators for measurement of social determinants are given in Box 5.1.

Box 5.1: Core-candidate indicators with respect to the social determinants of health

- Poverty, hunger
- Gender equity and equality
- Socio-economic status and schooling
- Occupational exposure to hazards, occupational experience of relations at work
- The social and economic effects of aging
- The experience of gender relations and marital status
- The experience of ethnic relations including direct experience of racism
- Home circumstances
- The degree and ability to exert self-efficacy especially through disposable income
- Dietary intake
- Habitual behaviours relating to food, alcohol, tobacco and exercise
- Position now and in the past in the life course
- The accumulated deficits associated with particular life courses

Multi-dimensional Poverty Index (MPI)[5–7]

Multi-dimensional poverty index (MPI) is a composite indicator of several social determinants of health. This index weights ten indicators across three dimensions as given in Table 5.1.[5]

Other SDH

Employment and financial protection: The proportion of households with any household member receiving any employment-based financial protection.

Political participation: The proportion of candidates by gender and caste (voter participation by gender and caste)

Environment—air and water quality monitoring: The proportion of stations with pollutant levels above set thresholds. Nitrogen dioxide (NO_2), sulphur dioxide (SO_2), and particulate matter less than 10 micrograms in diameter (PM10).

Water quality is also measured nationwide by the central pollution control board (CPCB) in India. It has set targets for levels of biochemical oxygen demand (BOD), total coliform concentration, and faecal coliform concentration in each type of water sources.

Table 5.1: Ten indicators across three dimensions that comprise the multi-dimensional poverty index (MPI)

Dimension	*Indicator*	*Definition*
Health	Child death	One or more children born in the household in the last 5 years have died
	Child undernutrition	At least one child in the household under the age of 3 is underweight
Education	Adult education	No household member has completed 5 or more years of schooling
	Child not in school	At least one school-aged child is not enrolled in school
Standard of living	Unimproved water	The drinking water source does not meet the WHO/UNICEF joint monitoring programme (JMP) criteria for 'improved' drinking water source
	Unimproved sanitation	The sanitation facilities do not meet the WHO/UNICEF JMP criteria for 'improved' sanitation
	Indoor biomass fuel use	The household cooks food with biomass fuels, as defined in the MDGs
	Low quality housing	The main housing material is kachha or semi-pucca
	No electricity	The household has no electricity
	Limited assets	The household has no car or truck and owns at most one of these bicycle, motorbike, radio, refrigerator, or television

Definitions presented here are those used in this as analysis. The original MPI indications and detailed descriptions of the rationale and methodology for each adaptation are included in additional file 1: "Adaptions to the MPI methodology".

In UK, the New Economics Foundation (NEF), proposed five indicators in 2015, they are:

1. **Good jobs:** Employment statistics tell us what proportion of people have jobs. They don't tell us what proportion of those with jobs are paid too little to afford a decent standard of living, or worry about whether they'll still have work next month.
2. **Well-being: Apart from GDP,** the well-being is also measured by asking people about their life satisfaction on 10 point scale.
3. **Environment:** The NEF proposed a national indicator of lifestyle-related carbon emissions, relative to an allocation calculated from global targets for avoiding dangerous levels of climate change.
4. **Fairness:** Research increasingly shows that high income inequality has negative social consequences, while casting doubt on the idea that it incentivizes hardwork.
5. **Health:** The NEF proposes 'avoidable deaths' as a simple, easily-understandable measure that captures the quality of health interventions—not only treatment, but also prevention.

United Nations 14 categories of social indicator are mentioned in Table 5.2.

Table 5.2: Categories of social indicator	
1. Population	8. Social security and welfare services
2. Family formation	9. Health services and nutrition
3. Families and household	10. Housing and its environment
4. Learning and educational service	11. Public order and safety
5. Earning activities	12. Time use
6. Distribution of income	13. Leisure and culture
7. Consumption and accumulation	14. Social stratification and mobility

References

1. Commission on Social Determinants of Health: Closing the Gap in a Generation: Health Equity through Action on the Social Determinants of Health. Geneva: World Health Organization. 2008.
2. Honjo Kaori. Social Epidemiology: Definition, History, and Research Examples. Environmental Health and Preventive Medicine 2004;9:193–99.
3. WHO. Social determinants of health. https://www.who.int/social_determinants/en/
4. Berkman LF, Kawachi I. A historical framework for social epidemiology. In: Berkman LF, Kawachi I, eds. Social epidemiology. New York; Oxford university press, 2000;3–12 (cross ref.).
5. Cowling, et al. Social determinants of health in India: progress and inequities across states. International Journal for Equity in Health 2014;13:88. doi:10.1186/s12939-014-0088-0.
6. World Economic forum, Five measures of growth that are better than GDP. https://www.weforum.org/agenda/2016/04/five-measures-of-growth-that-are-better-than-gdp/
7. Alkire S, Santos M. Acute Multidimensional Poverty: A New Index for Developing Countries. Oxford Poverty and Human Development Initiative; 2010. Working Paper No. 38.

CLINICAL EPIDEMIOLOGY

Epidemiological thinking differs conceptually from clinical thinking. Epidemiology can be defined as the study of disease and other health related phenomena in groups of persons. The word derives from the Greek *epi* (upon) and *demos* (people). The epidemiologist thus thinks in terms of groups, not individuals, and asks whether a group of patients with a given demographic, clinical, and psycho-social characteristics will be fair better, average or just OK, with a particular medical theory. He will then advocate that the patient receive the treatment with the higher average rate of success.

A clinical caring for an individual patient needs to consider published data based on groups of patients with knowledge of factors about the particular case at hand. He must make decisions for that patient, not for some hypothetical group of patients, however similar to the members of the group may appear to be his patient. And his decision are mostly based on clinical judgment—whether to order a certain diagnostic test, whether to recommend surgery or medication, whether to continue or discontinue life-support measures. Since, in order to be effective, the clinician must believe that each of his decisions is best for his patient. Although he may be aware of the uncertainty, he cannot afford to act indecisively. Consequently, he views the range of choices as right ones and wrong ones.

The epidemiologist is not obliged to make decisions for individual patients, he can live with uncertainty. He focuses on improving the health of populations and is less interested in the outcome of individuals within these populations; he prefers to think probabilistically.

It is important to emphasize that some fundamental clinical facts can be observed only in groups. No amount of patho-psychologic, mechanistic reasoning would reveal that the sex ratio at birth is not 50:50, but 51:49, or that males have a higher overall mortality rate than females. Predicting the sex of an individual newborn or whether prediction of mortality in women verses man may lead to considerable error. But the sex ratio among the next 1000 newborns or the comparative mortality of a large representative group of men and women can be predicted within a fairly narrow range.

In the past, these two different approaches, individualized on the one hand, group-oriented and probabilistic on the other, have had little in common. Unlike the laboratory base sciences, epidemiology tended to remain far from beside. Epidemiologists concerned themselves almost exclusively with investigating the aetiology of infectious and chronic diseases, and clinicians consequently found epidemiology to be of little relevance to their roles as caretakers and decision makers. Medical, dental, or nursing school courses in epidemiology were viewed with an attitude ranging from indifference to contempt.

Recently, however, the essential compatibility and mutual benefit of the two approaches have become more evident, and this has given rise to the term 'clinical epidemiology'. Although all epidemiology is clinical in a broad sense, since it concerns diseases and other health related phenomena, 'classical epidemiology' has usually concerned itself with disease aetiology, but are equally interested in diagnosis, prognosis, therapy, prevention, evaluation of healthcare services, and analysis of risks and benefits. Clinical epidemiology can be defined as study of variation in the outcome of illness and of reasons for that variation.

SCOPE OF CLINICAL EPIDEMIOLOGY

The main areas of interest within clinical epidemiology are aetiology, diagnosis, prognosis, treatment, prevention, analysis of the risks and benefits of diagnostic and therapeutic interventions, and evaluation of healthcare services.

1. **Aetiology:** What are the causes of coronary artery disease (CAD)? Most of what, we know about this condition derives from long term, population-based epidemiologic studies. For example, in the well-known Framingham study, a two-third sample of the 30- to 60-year-old population of that Massachusetts town was examined at the inception of the study and periodically thereafter to identify socio-demographic and clinical risk factors for CAD. As a result of this and other similar studies, it is now widely acknowledged that smoking, hypertension, high blood cholesterol levels, insufficient exercise, and a high-stress (so called type-A) personality significantly increase the risk of heart attack.
2. **Diagnosis:** How is CAD diagnosed? A variety of invasive and non-invasive diagnostic tests have been developed in an attempt to assess the anatomical state of the coronary arteries, the derangement in blood supply to the heart muscle, and the resulting tissue damage. These include blood tests, roentgenographic studies, electrocardiograms (at rest and during exercise), and radioisotopic tracer uptakes. Before such tests achieve wide application, they should be subjected to appropriate epidemiologic study to ascertain their ability to discriminate accurately between individuals with and without CAD or its sequelae. That is, what is the specificity and the sensitivity of such investigations? What are the likelihood ratios of the test?
3. **Prognosis:** What is likelihood that patient with CAD will be alive in 5 years? That is, epidemiology related to future morbidity and mortality. These prognostic factors are analogous to the risk factors discussed above in reference to aetiology, but include, in addition, various indicators of the extent and severity of the underlying disease in question. Some prognostic factors are casually related to the outcome (morbidity or mortality) of interest; others serve merely as markers of the underlying disease or other casual factors. Fortunately, prognosis is a dynamic, rather than static, process that can be influenced by treatment and prevention. In other words, therapeutic and prevention interventions can themselves be prognostic factors.

4. **Treatment:** Most questions about therapeutic efficiency (surgical *vs* medical, drug *vs* placebo, drug A *vs* drug B, treatment *vs* no treatment) are best answered by means of experimental epidemiologic studies, also called clinical trials. In the past, many treatments that were recommended for patients with CAD, based on 'clinical experience' and 'cumulative wisdom' rather than well-designed clinical trials, were successfully shown to be useless or even harmful. Intra-myocardial implantation of the internal mammary artery, for example, became a popular surgical treatment in the 1950s and 1960s following the enthusiastic, but uncontrolled, experiences of its developers. Later studies with longer-term follow-up showed far less impressive results, and the procedure was subsequently abandoned. By contrast, coronary artery by-pass grafting using a portion of the saphenous vein from the leg has been the subject of several well-designed clinical trials. These trials have provided much useful information about its merits and limitations for specific groups of patients.
5. **Prevention:** How can CAD be prevented? Some epidemiologists distinguish here between primary prevention (preventing the disease from developing in the first place) and secondary prevention (preventing progression or complication of the disease already present). In fact, many 'experts' believe recent changes in smoking, and exercise behaviour and improved control of hypertension are responsible for the clearly perceptible decline in morbidity and mortality from CAD.
6. **Evaluation of health services:** Here we have the provision of a service (a certain mode of providing healthcare for coronary patients), rather than a specific treatment, but many of the epidemiologic methods (especially clinical trials) for evaluating such a service are similar to those used to study efficacy of treatment. Older epidemiologic evidence suggests the coronary care units (CCUs) are not effective in reducing post-infarction mortality, but new trials are required to assess the potential benefit of more recent monitoring and therapeutic techniques.
7. **Analysis of benefits and risks:** Suppose it could in fact shown that CCUs result in a slightly lower rate of post-infarction mortality. Suppose, however, that the constant noise, light, and tension of such units kept most patients away from sleeping and resulted in developing stress ulcer. How great a reduction in cardiac mortality would be necessary to justify this increase in non-cardiac morbidity? Or, suppose it costs one million dollars in CCU expenses for each 10 years of life saved by the unit. Is it worth it? Since financial resources are limited, can a greater reduction in cardiovascular mortality be realized by spending that one million dollars on mobile emergency rescue vehicles? Or an anti-smoking campaign? Weighing the potential benefits, risks and cost of diagnostic, therapeutic and healthcare approaches comprises a set of activities including decision analysis, cost-benefit analysis, and cost-effectiveness analysis. With the growing recognition that no course of action is without adverse consequences and that choices are inevitable, these activities are receiving increased attention from clinical epidemiologists (as well as from economists and ethicists).

To conclude, clinical epidemiology helps to generate evidence on multiple issues discussed above. This evidence is used to advance clinical practice for the betterment of patients.

GENETIC EPIDEMIOLOGY

In classical epidemiology, we study association of different factors with disease outcomes. However, when we study disease causation, there is always a 'black-box' which remains unexplained. Because of the 'black-box', we never completely understand causation and precise roles of different factors. Molecular and genetic epidemiology has potential to open the 'black-box' and tell us precise roles of the causative factors.

Understanding of precise roles of these factors are crucial to develop approaches for disease prevention.

GENETIC EPIDEMIOLOGY

Genetic epidemiology is a combination of the scientific disciplines of human genetics, epidemiology and biometry. Genetic epidemiology studies the genetic components that contribute to the development or the course of a disease, or in general terms to a phenotype, i.e. the observed trait.

As per Morton and Chung (1978), genetic epidemiology is defined as the science which deals with the aetiology, distribution, and control of disease in groups of relatives and with inherited causes of disease in populations.

According to Thomas (2004), the process of defining the genetic basis of the diseases usually follows the progression as descriptive epidemiology, familial aggregation, segregation analysis, linkage analysis, fine mapping, association, cloning and characterization.

General epidemiology study the distribution in terms of time, place, and person and also measures the frequency of diseases and familial aggregation of genetic risk factors, whereas genetics tends to focus on the genotype-phenotype correlation without studying the environment.

Aims of Genetic Epidemiology[1]

- To describe the genetic influence of phenotypes or diseases.
- To detect the inheritance pattern of a particular disease.
- To identify/localize the gene/risk factors associated.
- To construct modelling of the role of these genetic risk factors.
- To find a marker associated with disease susceptibility.

Genetic epidemiology is highly dependent on the direct incorporation of family structure and biology. The structure of families and chromosomes leads to major dependencies between the data and thus to customized models and tests. In many studies only indirect evidence can be used, since the disease-related gene, or more precisely the functionally relevant DNA variant of a gene, is not directly observable. In addition, the data sets to be analyzed can be very complex.

Genetic epidemiological investigations are conducted in following situations.

- *Positive family history* as a risk factor for disease indicating possible genetic or environmental factors.
- When the *relative risk for relatives of affected individuals* in relation to the general population is strong.

To investigate further familial aggregation, a *segregation analysis, linkage analysis and association analysis should* be done to establish the hypothesis.[1–3]

Familial Aggregation

Familial aggregation may be defined as the aggregation of disease appear in families more often than one would expect if diseased cases were spread uniformly and randomly over individuals—"it runs in the family". Actual approaches for detecting aggregation depend on the nature of the phenotype, but the common factor in existing approaches is that they are taken without any specific genetic model in mind.

Segregation Analysis

It is precisely identification of the factors responsible for familial aggregation. It may find the aggregation due to environmental, cultural or genetic factors, proportion of the trait due to genetic factors, mode of inheritance which represents the genetic factors and genetic heterogeneity.

Linkage analysis: It is the co-segregation between marker and disease is investigated in related individuals. The aim is to find evidence for linkage and often to estimate the recombination rate.

The classical linkage analysis method is the *lod score method* (Morton 1955). This is a test for linkage between a susceptibility gene locus and a marker locus (null hypothesis $H_0{:}\theta = 0.5$ versus alternative $H_1{:}\theta < 0.5$) in combination with the estimation of the recombination rate.

Association Studies

It is the study of association of allele with the disease susceptibility. The principle is the coexistence of the same marker on the same chromosome in affected individuals (due to linkage disequilibrium). Association studies may be family-based (TDT) or population-based. Alleles or haplotypes may be used. Genome-wide association studies (GWAS) are increasing in popularity.

There are two types of association:

a. The positively (or negatively) associated allele is the susceptibility allele itself. If so, this association is expected to occur in all populations harbouring this allele.
b. The positively (or negatively) associated allele is in linkage disequilibrium with the susceptibility allele at the disease locus. If this is the case, then different associations can occur in different populations due to different haplotype frequencies of the allele combinations of both marker and susceptibility locus.

Some common genetic models for conducting genetic studies

- Single major locus: Simple traits/diseases
  - o Dominant model
  - o Recessive model
  - o Additive
  - o Multiplicative
- Multi-factorial/polygenic: Complex traits/diseases
  - o Multi-factorial (many factors)
  - o Polygenic (many genes)
  - o General assumption: Each of the factors and genes contribute a small amount to phenotypic variability
- Mixed model—single major locus with a polygenic background

Examples genetic epidemiology

1. Gene expression profiling to assess prognosis and guide therapy, e.g. breast cancer
2. Genotyping for stratification of patients according to risk of disease, e.g. myocardial infarction
3. Genotyping to elucidate drug response, e.g. antiepileptic agents
4. Designing and implementing new drug therapies, e.g. imatinib for hypereosinophilic syndrome
5. Functional understanding of disease causing genes, e.g. obesity

Conclusion: It is only a brief introduction to genetic epidemiology. It studies role of genetic factors in disease occurrence in population. It deals with aetiology, distribution and control of diseases in families. It is concerned with inherited diseases in population and utilizes statistical techniques to evaluate the genetic aspects of chronic diseases. It involves linkage analysis, family-based association studies, and outcome is gene discovery.

References

1. Van Steen K. Introduction to genetic epidemiology (presentation). http://www.montefiore.ulg.ac.be/~kvansteen/GeneticEpi-PublicHealth/ac0910/Chapter7/Slides%20geneticepi_PH_Chapter7.pdf
2. Heike Bickeböller. Genetic Epidemiology (author). Wolfgang Ahrens, Iris Pigeot (Eds). Handbook of Epidemiology, Ch-III.7 pp 1140–65. https://publichealthdentistryindia.files.wordpress.com/.../wolfgang ahrens, irispigeot
3. Burton P, Tobin M, Hopper J. Key concepts in genetic epidemiology. The Lancet. 2005.

MOLECULAR EPIDEMIOLOGY

INTRODUCTION

Revolution in molecular biology has revolutionized the science, medicine, epidemiology and society at large (Fig. 5.3). The contribution of traditional epidemiological studies has tremendous effect on the prevention and control of diseases. However, some questions are still bothering and scientists are striving hard to search the answer for the same. Some of areas of concern are:

- Exact causes and pathogenesis of an infectious disease and non-infectious diseases,
- Every individual respond differently to a specific pathogen, therapy, or vaccine,

- Developing primary prevention to control, eliminate and eradicate diseases and so on.[1]

To address these issues study, one need to solemnize marriage between traditional epidemiology and molecular epidemiological (ME).

Historically, it seems that Kilbourne had used the term molecular epidemiology, in 1973 to describe influenza subtype distribution around the world, Hingginson in 1977 in his paper on 'role of pathologist in environmental medicine and public health,' the term 'molecular epidemiology' was first introduced by Lower *et al.* in 1979 introduced genetic effects modifiers in terms of phenotype markers, external exposure and individual susceptibility. In 1982, Parera and Weinstein coined the term molecular cancer epidemiology. Since then, a tremendous rise in the number of molecular epidemiological studies in various research areas.

As we know that results of genetic epidemiology are not generalizable to the population at large. Hence, molecular epidemiology is required which deals with contribution of genetic and environmental risk factors identified at the molecular and biochemical level, to the aetiology, distribution and control of diseases in families and population. Molecular epidemiology poses itself as a critical link between human genome project and its public health utility.

The molecular epidemiology helped to conduct aetiologic research, increase knowledge base regarding determinants of disease, contribute to the development of approaches for disease prevention and improve public health (Table 5.3).[2]

DEFINITION OF MOLECULAR EPIDEMIOLOGY

There is no consensus on definition of molecular epidemiology as on today. As per Centers for Disease Control and Prevention (CDC), it is defined as "the various biochemical and molecular techniques used to type and subtype pathogens" (CDC 1994).

J Dorman defined molecular epidemiology as 'A science that deals with the contribution of genetic and environmental risk factors identified at the molecular and biochemical level, to the aetiology, distribution and control of disease in families and populations'.[3]

Molecular epidemiology involves use of biological markers of exposure, susceptibility and outcome in epidemiologic research. The markers are either molecular or biochemical

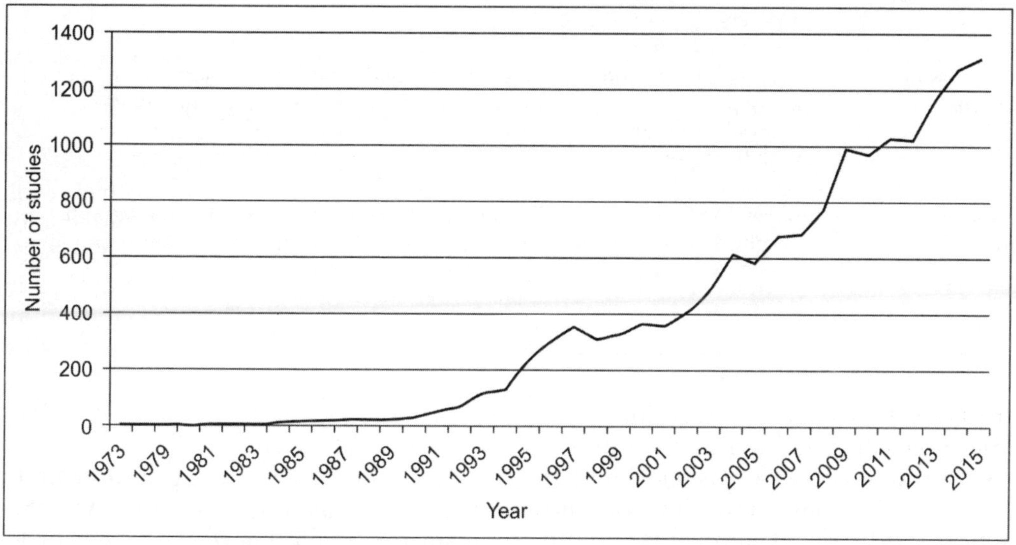

Fig. 5.3: Number of molecular epidemiological studies published

Table 5.3: Methodological overview and rationale for some ME methods used in the field of infectious disease[2]

Domain	*Study design or analysis method*	
Causation of infectious disease	Case-control	Cases: Patients with clinical manifestations of the disease; Controls: Patients without clinical manifestations of the disease; Exposure: Genetic material of pathogens
	Nested case-control/ cohort	Exposed: Individuals infected with the pathogen; Unexposed: Individuals not infected with the pathogen; Outcome: Disease onset
Pathogenesis of infectious disease	Case-control	Cases: 1. Severe, fatal, drug-resistant patients; 2. Patients with a disease or an especial clinical symptom; Controls: 1. Mild, non-fatal, drug-sensitive patients, 2. Patients without a disease or an especial clinical symptom Exposure: 1. Pathogen's genetic sequence, 2. Metagenome in a specific body site
	Genome wide association studies	Cases: Patients with the disease or disease susceptibility Controls: Patients without the disease or disease susceptibility Exposure: Millions of SNPs along human genome
Sources/reservoirs	Phylogenetic analysis	Sampling from suspected sources and infected individual
Circulation pattern	Molecular surveillance	Routine, population-based genotyping of circulating pathogens
Transmission probability	Cross-sectional studies using phylogenetic analysis	Pathogen's genetic sequence isolated from temporally and epidemiologically related individuals
Transmission patterns	Cross-sectional studies using phylogenetic analysis in combination with behavioural data	Pathogenic genetic material is isolated from infected individuals within or between communities
Transmission order	Bayesian phylogeographic studies	The order of virus spread across large geographic distances is estimated using information accumulated in the virus genome. Viral genomes are used to reconstruct a family tree showing the relationships between these viral samples

that play role in disease causation. These studies unearth gene–environment interactions and gene–disease associations and outcome is gene characterization. The most practical and useful molecular typing methods for both large and small scale epidemiologic studies are the DNA-based methods of REAP and PFGE.

Omics in molecular epidemiology: A neologism for the constellation of an organism's **'-omic'** information. They include the genome itself (genomic), transcription

Box 5.2: Some measures used in molecular epidemiologic studies for specific biological materials[4]

Biological material: Measures

1. **DNA**
   a. Genomic DNA
      Single nucleotide polymorphisms (SNPs) (>1% prevalence)
   b. Tumour DNA
      Mutations (<1% prevalence)
   c. Mitochondrial DNA
      Insertions, deletions
2. **RNA**
   RT-PCR [reverse transcriptase polymerase chain reaction (PCR)]
   Microarray chips for expression of RNA
3. **Whole Cells**
   a. Lymphocytes
      Incorporation of damaged plasmid [host cell reactivation assay (HCRA)], Comet assay
   b. Chromosomes (cytogenetic assays to assess mutagen sensitivity)
      Chromosome breaks and deletions
      Sister chromatid exchanges (SCEs)
   c. Shed cells
      1. Exfoliated bladder cells
         Measures of damage and repair (Comet assay)
      2. Oral buccal cells
         Measures of DNA adducts
      3. Broncho lavage
      4. Micronuclei
   d. Adducts (i.e. exogenous chemicals bound to DNA)
4. **Plasma serum**
   Measurement of biochemical, i.e. vitamin E
   Tumour and genomic DNA in plasma and serum
5. **Red blood cells**
   Hemoglobin, hemoglobin adducts, biochemical content, i.e. folate
6. **Urine**
   a. Urinary metabolites
      Biochemical assays
   b. Exfoliated bladder cells (see above)
7. **Hair**
   Chemicals, i.e. arsenic
8. **Finger nails, toe nails**
   Chemicals, i.e. mercury

products (transcriptomic), protein products (proteomic) and metabolic products (metabolomic) (Figs 5.4 and 5.5).

FUNCTIONS OF GENETIC AND MOLECULAR EPIDEMIOLOGY

1. Validation of biomarkers;
2. Studying gene–disease associations;
3. Studying gene–gene/gene-environment interactions.

Validation of biomarkers are done in three steps. First is analytic validity, which is expressed in terms of sensitivity, specificity and predictive values (positive and negative) along with likelihood ratios (positive and negative) of a biomarker to detect a particular disease. These are typically done in laboratory settings. Clinical validity is studied using conventional and non-conventional epidemiological designs. We can find out the risk of disease among those who are positive for a biomarker as compared to those who are negative for the biomarker, typically in terms of odds ratio or risk ratio. Before we start using the biomarker in practice, its clinical utility needs to evaluated using controlled trials. Whether the interventions using biomarker are more beneficial than without the use of biomarker needs to be answered. Definite clinical advantage in prevention, treatment, prognosis or quality of life has to be there for use of a biomarker. Conventional epidemiological studies used are cross-sectional, case-control and cohort studies in addition to randomized clinical trials.

To study gene–disease association linkage analysis and segregation analysis is used. Linkage analysis identifies regions of the genome that contain genes that predispose a person to a particular disease. Linkage is the tendency of genes to be inherited together because of their location on the same chromosome. After studying familial aggregation of disease, which is assessed by recurrence risk ratio and interfamily correlation coefficient, linkage analysis is carried out to identify location of causative gene. Linkage analysis is the analysis of co-segregation of

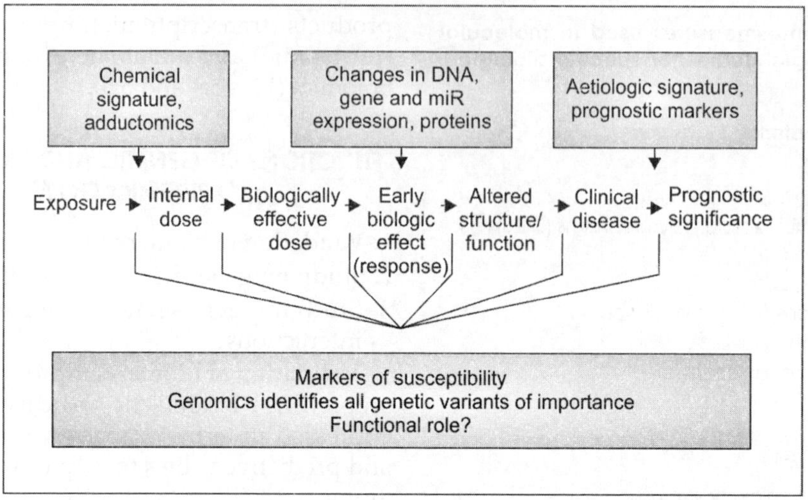

Fig. 5.4: Omics in molecular epidemiology[5]

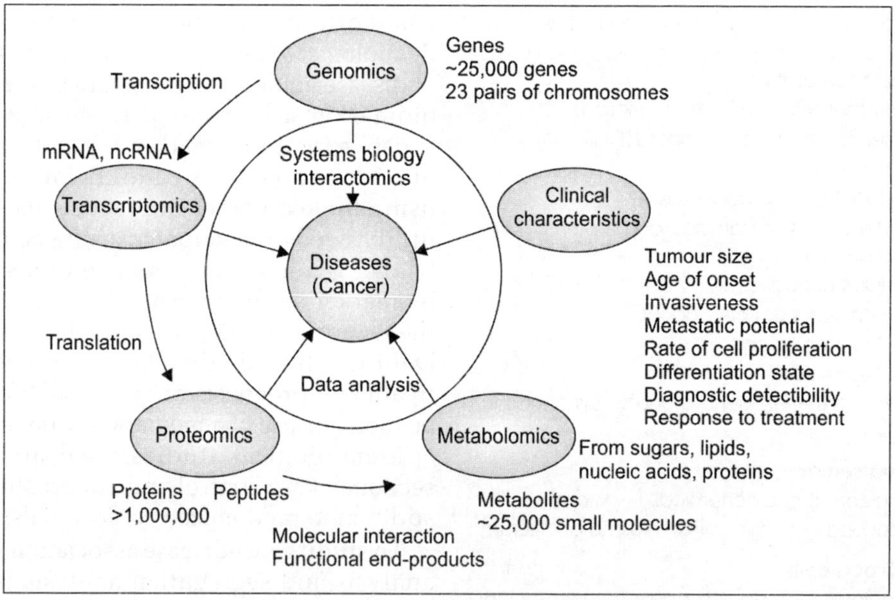

Fig. 5.5: Omics in cancer molecular epidemiology[6]

genetic loci in pedigree. Loci that are close enough together on the same chromosome segregate together more often than loci on different chromosomes. Logarithm of the odds score assesses the probability of co-segregation of disease and marker in a given pedigree. A score of three is regarded as significant evidence of linkage. Mendelian disorders can be modelled using aggregation and segregation studies. They are usually the first step in genetics. Aggregation analysis examines whether there is familial aggregation of the trait. Questions asked are the relatives of diseased individuals more

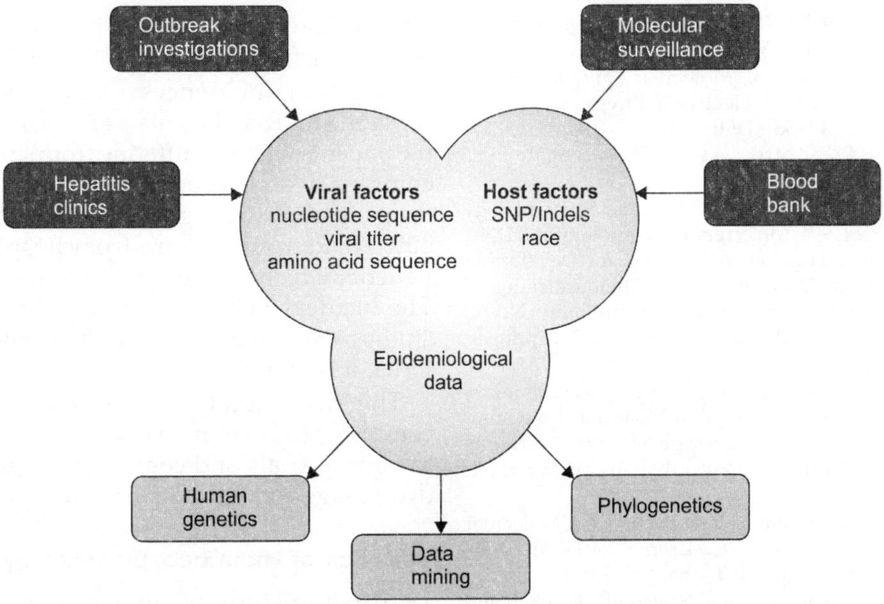

Fig. 5.6: The main components required for advanced molecular surveillance of HCV[7]

likely to have the disease than the general population or is the clustering of disease in families more than expected in a general population. The segregation analysis moves beyond the aggregation analysis and looks for the reasons for aggregation. Is the aggregation due to environmental, social or genetic factors? What proportion of it is due to genetic factors?

Some non-conventional studies used are case-only studies and case-parents studies, which are useful to study gene–gene interaction or gene–environment interactions. These studies have internal control group. Case-only studies also help scan for contribution of complex genotypes and assess heterogeneity in outcomes.

FUTURE OF MOLECULAR EPIDEMIOLOGY

Technological progress is continuing at a greater pace. However, advances are more subtle in chronic diseases than infectious diseases. Along with molecular and genetic technological advances, we must also focus on cost-effectivity, accessibility, availability and equity. In future, well planned study designs to address confounders and generation of authentic and adequate data through metagenomic and metatranscriptomic (study of whole transcripts present in a specific environment) studies provide a snapshot of whole genetic materials present at each time in an environment, having chronological information of changes in genes or transcript composition in a body site can provide great knowledge about the pathogenesis of infections. It requires holistic approach and integration with molecular data (genome, transcriptome, proteome, metabolome) with clinical and epidemiological data, assisted by geographic information systems (GIS).

In general, as the time goes by, the "Omics" area (the field of study in biology ending in omics, such as genomics, transcriptomics, proteomics, etc.), continues to progress rapidly by development of more sensitive techniques, databases that store omics data, and bioinformatics tools that can efficiently handle such data.

References

1. Michel Tibayrenc, Molecular Epidemiology and Evolutionary Genetics of Infectious Diseases. Chapter 3 in S. Morand, et al. (Eds.), New Frontiers of Molecular Epidemiology of Infectious Diseases,

29 DOI 10.1007/978-94-007-2114-2_3, © Springer Science + Business Media BV. 2012.
2. Eybpoosh Sana, et al. Molecular epidemiology of infectious diseases. Electronic Physician. August 2017;9(8):5149–58, DOI: http://dx.doi.org/10.19082/5149. https://www.researchgate.net/publication/319628316
3. Dorman J.S., International Molecular Epidemiology Task Force (1994) Molecular Epidemiology and DNA Technology Transfer: A Program for Developing Countries. In: Dorman J.S. (eds) Standardization of Epidemiologic Studies of Host Susceptibility. NATO ASI Series (Series A: Life Sciences), vol 270. Springer, Boston, MA.
4. Wolfgang Ahrens, Iris Pigeot (Eds). Handbook of Epidemiology. Chapter III. 6 Molecular Epidemiology. Paolo Vineis, Giuseppe Matullo, Marianne Berwick (Auth). 2004 published by Springer, Germany.
5. Smith MT, et al. Future perspectives on Molecular Epidemiology. <file:///C:/Users/user Downloads/IARC 20Sci%20Pub20163_Chapter 27.pdf>
6. Zhan, Xianquan and Long, Ying and XH, Zhan and Mu, Yun. (2017). Consideration of Statistical vs. Biological Significances for Omics Data-Based Pathway Network Analysis. Med One. 1. 10.20900/mo.20170002.
7. Rossi, Livia and Escobar-Gutierrez, Alejandro and Rahal, Paula. (2015). Advanced Molecular Surveillance of Hepatitis C Virus. Viruses. 7. 1153–88. 10.3390/v7031153.

PHARMACOEPIDEMIOLOGY

"A desire to take medicine is, perhaps, the great feature, which distinguishes man from other animals."

— *Sir William Osler, 1891*

INTRODUCTION

Safety is a major issue in all countries specially in low- and middle-income group countries as the market of spurious drugs has mushroomed even in the presence of drug regulations. Drug regulations in many countries have the aim of ensuring safe and efficient drug provision with the participation of all stakeholders like community, healthcare agencies, researchers, pharmaceutical industries and governments.

All drugs have therapeutic effects and none are absolutely devoid of adverse effects and prescription of them should be judicious and with a satisfactory risk/benefit ratio.

Common incidences of adverse drug reaction (ADR) in hospitals are recognized in the patients who are suffering from severe and complex disease process or are on multiple drugs, leading to drug interactions. About 10–20% ADRs reported are from hospitalized patients which lead to prolongation of stay. The incidence of ADR reported by various studies across the world is 6–20%, whereas in India, it is up to 3%.[1]

The drug safety can be enhanced by complete study from invent of drug molecule to clinical trials and continuous vigil of the drug usage and effect in long run.

Definition of Pharmacoepidemiology[2]

1. "It is the study of the use and effect of medicine in large number of people."

— *'Strom'*

2. It can be defined as the study of the therapeutic effect(s), risk and use of drugs, usually in large populations, using epidemiological methods and/or reasoning.
3. "The application of epidemiologic knowledge, methods, and reasoning to the study of the effects (beneficial and adverse) and use of drugs in human populations."

— *'Porta and Hartzema'*

4. "The study of drugs as determinants of health and disease in the general unselected population."

— *'Spitzer'*

The most important purpose of pharmacoepidemiology is to define populations in specific times and places and identify and explain drug treatments and make estimations about their uses and effects.

NEED FOR PHARMACOEPIDEMIOLOGY

The drugs and medical devices developed are tested rigorously for safety and efficacy using controlled environment. However, the controlled environment may be technically very sound but has limitations of its own and many times are away from real life settings. The gap between controlled setting and real life settings pose limitations to evaluating the real risks and benefits of pharmaceuticals. Pharmacoepidemiology gives an opportunity to study the additional risk and benefits when drugs and medical devices are used in real settings. Pharmacoepidemiologists use epidemiologic principles to study effects of medications in human population. They study drug use pattern and adverse drug effects. They are interested in understanding the patterns of drug prescriptions, adherence to medication, and the identification of predictors for medication use. Drugs and other products need to be monitored closely following their introduction in the market to find out added benefits and the risks.[3]

We need to understand that if stringent actions are devised like regulation, marketing protocols, legal binding and proper clinical studies and application, only then in real sense development of pharmacoepidemiology can be possible (Table 5.4).

Table 5.4: Possible areas for requirement of pharmacoepidemiology

Sections	*Sub-sections*
Regulatory	1. Requirement 2. To obtain earlier approval for marketing 3. As a response to question by regulatory agency 4. To assist application for approval for marketing elsewhere
Marketing	1. To assist market penetration by documenting the safety of the drug 2. To increase name recognition 3. To assist in re-positioning the drug a. Different outcomes, e.g. quality of life and economic b. Different types of patient, e.g. the elderly c. New indications d. Less restrictive labelling 4. To protect the drug from accusations about adverse effects
Legal	In anticipation of future product liability litigation
Clinical	Hypothesis testing

Relationship between Pharmacoepidemiology and Other Disciplines

Although many disciplines are related to pharmacoepidemiology like law, public health, economics, medicine, biotechnology, management, etc. (Fig. 5.7).

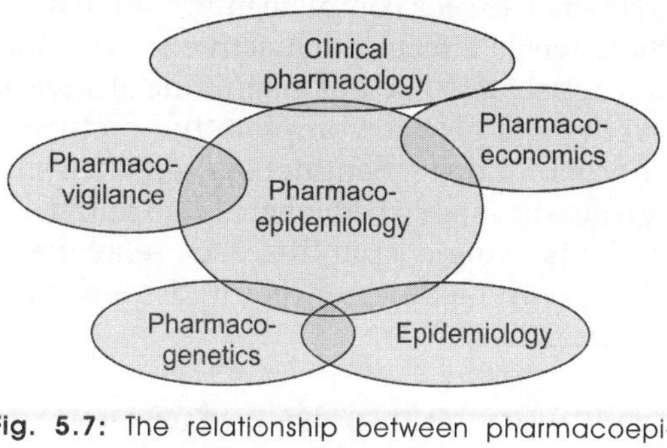

Fig. 5.7: The relationship between pharmacoepidemiology and core disciplines

STUDY DESIGNS IN PHARMACOEPIDEMIOLOGY[4,5,7–9]

In Indian scenario research in pharmacoepidemiology, an important medical specialty has suffered due to shortage of financial support, difficulty in procuring and maintaining experimental animals or patients/ healthy volunteers, political will, complete technological know-how, are the few reasons to take up only observational studies.

All sorts of epidemiological designs and surveillance mechanisms are used in pharmacoepidemiology starting from case reports to experimental designs. Case report is a description of single case who was exposed to a specific drug and experienced a particular unexpected event, generally an adverse event. This is generally taken as a warning signal for the further systematic enquiry.

Case series is a collection of people who were exposed to a specific drug and outcomes are described. However, causation cannot be interpreted from case-series due to lack of control group.

Case-control designs are more robust and causality of a drug for a specific drug can be interpreted using the case-control designs. Cohort studies are even more robust than the case-control designs as they are prospective in nature. It not only quantifies the strength of association (risk or benefit), it is also helpful in measuring incidence of the event.

Experimental studies are helpful in assessing risks and benefits of an exposure in the population groups, which were not adequately represented in pre-marketing trials. These are called phase-IV trials. Additionally, they can be used for assessing risks and benefits of long-term drug use as pre-marketing trials are of limited periods. Since, there is no proper randomization in these studies; they are of quasi-experimental in nature.

Active surveillance is an important pharmacoepidemiological exercise in which patients on a drug or a disease are registered and followed periodically on a pre-decided frequency to seek complete information on all the adverse effects. Such active surveillance can be useful to find out magnitude of adverse events and also to complete the picture of effects of a drug. Sentinel surveillance sites can also be established where large number of patients using a drug/disease are available along with facilities of required specialized investigations.

CONCLUSION AND FUTURE DEVELOPMENT

Pharmacoepidemiology has started to grow and flourish within academia, industry and government. This will be facilitated by methodological advances as well as integration of risk management programs and pharmacogenetics with pharmacoepidemiology.

The areas which need to be explored are drug utilization review, hospital pharmacoepidemiology, pharmacoeconomics, medication adherence, patient safety, and intermediate surrogate markers will empower the decision-making process.[4–6]

Pharmacoepidemiology is considered to have a very important role in increasing individual life quality by improving drug use across society. Therefore, it is expected that the interest for the discipline of pharmacoepidemiology will increase in the future.

References

1. Singh P, Agrawal M, Hishikar R, Joshi U, Maheshwari B, Halwai A. Adverse drug reactions at adverse drug reaction monitoring center in Raipur: Analysis of spontaneous reports during 1 year. Indian J Pharmacol [serial online] 2017 [cited 2018 Sep 20]; 49:432-7. Available from: http://www.ijp-online.com/text.asp?2017/49/6/432/228452
2. Hennessy Sean. Pharmacoepidemiology: Goals and Methods presentation downloaded from dimacs. rutgers.edu/Workshops/.../Hennessy.ppt
3. Strom BL, Kimmel SE, Hennessy S, Pharmacoepidemiology, 3rd edn, Wiley-Blackwell; 2000.
4. Saket J Thaker, Nithya J Gogtay, Urmila M Thatte. Pharmacoepidemiology: The essentials clinical epidemiology and global health 3rd edn. 2015; 52(5):7.
5. Bergman U, Pharmaco-epidemiological perspectives, Pharmaceutical Weekblad 1989;11(5):151–54.
6. Briggs AH, Levy AR. Pharmacoeconomics and Pharmacoepidemiology: Curious Bedfellows or a Match Made in Heaven? Pharmacoeconomics 2006; 24(11):1079–86.
7. Patil JS. Pharmacoepidemiology and Drug Safety Concept: Indian Scenario. Adv Pharmacoepidemiol Drug Saf 2015;4:e130. doi:10.4172/2167-1052. 1000e130
8. Andrews E, Gilsenan A, Cook S. Therapeutic risk management interventions: Feasibility and effectiveness. J Am Pharm Assoc 2004; 44(4):491e500.
9. Onder G, Landi F, Cesari M, Gambassi G, Carbonin P, Bernabei R, Investigators of the GIFA Study. Inappropriate medication use among hospitalized older adults in Italy: Results from the Italian Group of Pharmacoepidemiology in the Elderly. Eur J Clin Pharmacol. 2003;59(2):157e162.

Chapter

6

Field Epidemiology* Including Investigation of an Epidemic

Ram Chandra Goyal

All scientific work is incomplete—whether it be observational or experimental. All scientific work is liable to be upset or modified by advancing knowledge. That does not confer upon us a freedom to ignore the knowledge we already have, or to postpone the action that it appears to demand at a given time.

— Sir Austin Bradford Hill

INTRODUCTION

Epidemiology is not a new branch and is being applied to all concerned areas of health and diseases to understand internal and external environment of the human being. We are witnessing the epidemiological and demographic transition, as result, there are emergence of new diseases and re-emergence of previously controlled diseases. This type of epidemiological challenge has to be dealt urgently and adequately to save the human lives.

Since 1970, more than 1,500 new pathogens were discovered, of which 70% proved to be of animal origin—a connection that deserves renewed scrutiny. Not all of them have had a public health impact, but some of them have become famous. They included the Ebola virus, in 1976, and the human immunodeficiency virus (HIV), in 1983. HIV has infected about 70 million people in just 35 years, and killed an estimated 35 million people in the same period. In the last 40 years, Ebola has surfaced in almost 25 separate and deadly outbreaks, often after long dormant stage. Other new communicable diseases include COVID-19 (Corona virus -19), SARS—severe acute respiratory syndrome, H1N1, MERS—Middle East respiratory syndrome, zika virus infection, bird flu, etc. and old diseases continues like cholera, dengue, chikenguinea, plague (in Madagascar), yellow fever, etc. These diseases are spreading very rapidly through out the world as facilities for transport are available in abundance (Fig. 6.1).[1]

In view of the above, we are sitting on the volcano of emergencies, which not only affect human life but the whole bio-life along with a serious impact on travel and trade; local–global economy, infrastructure, etc.

The term 'emergencies' encompasses all situations in which large populations are in need of urgent humanitarian relief.

****Synonyms for*** field epidemiology are: Intervention epidemiology/applied epidemiology/shoe leather epidemiology/consequential epidemiology.

Emergencies include complex emergencies ("situations of war or civil strife affecting large civilian populations with food shortages and population displacement, resulting in excess mortality and morbidity") and natural disasters (e.g. floods and earthquakes). Emergencies due to communicable diseases outbreaks and epidemics are a major cause of mortality and morbidity and particularly in complex emergencies, where collapsing health services and disease control programs, poor access to healthcare, malnutrition, interrupted supplies and logistics, and poor coordination among healthcare agencies.[2]

Recent Major Health Emergencies

The South-east Asia region is considered a '**hotspot**' for emerging infectious diseases, including those with pandemic potential. Some of the major public health emergencies that occurred in last two decades in the region are listed below (Table 6.1).[3]

India: The geographical statistics of India shows that almost 58% of the land is vulnerable to earthquake, 68% of cultivable area to drought, 8% to cyclones and 12% to floods. Indian population of 1.25 billion is also highly vulnerable to diseases outbreak. On an average, 30–40 outbreaks are reported every week across 36 states and Union Territories; of which outbreaks of acute diarrheal diseases, acute respiratory infections, food poisoning, measles and vector-borne diseases (malaria, dengue, chikungunya, scrub typhus, Japanese encephalitis) are most frequent. In addition, there are new challenges such as air pollution, heat waves, toxic exposures from industrial, chemical and radiation leaks.[3]

This field epidemiology chapter will have broader aim to apply principles of general epidemiology in relation to emergencies management.

'Field epidemiology' can be described as "the practice of **epidemiology in real time and real place**, which in turn involves both

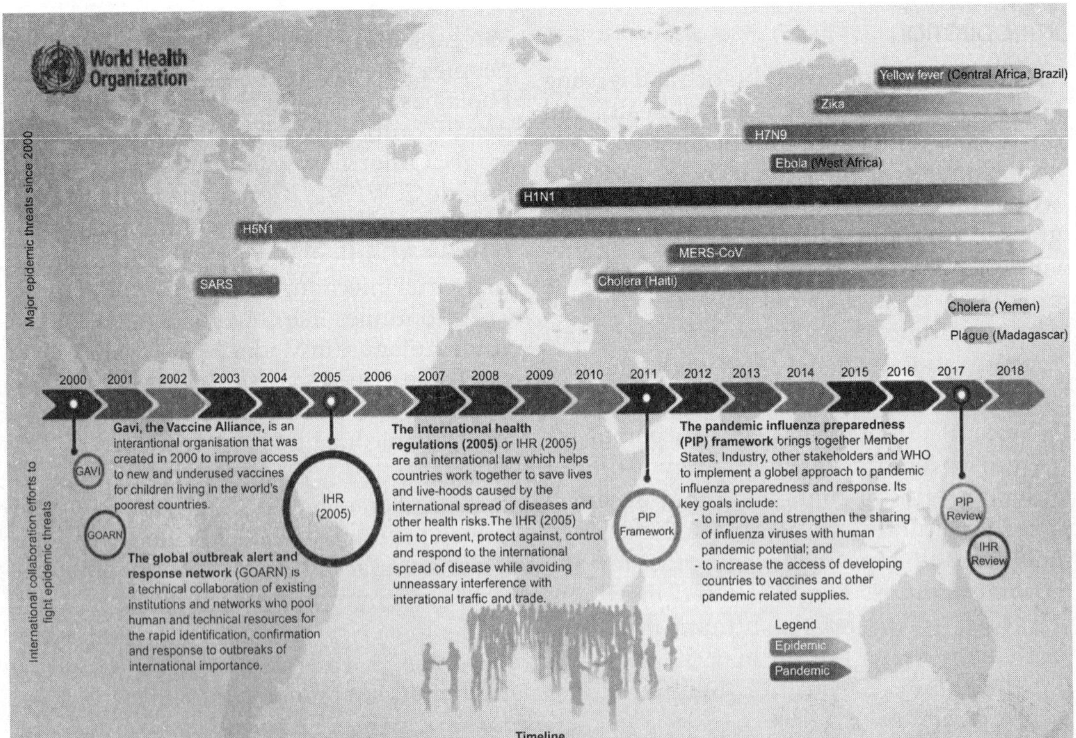

Fig. 6.1: Major infections threats in the 21st century and collaboration mechanisms to fight against them[1]

Table 6.1: Major public health emergencies in the South-east Asia region[3]

Year	*Public health emergency*	*SEA countries affected*	*Morbidity*	*Mortality*
2001	Gujarat earthquake (Richter scale 7.7) on 26 January	India	167,000 injured 6.3 million affected	25,000 deaths
2003–2004	Avian influenza H5N1	Bangladesh, Myanmar, Indonesia, Thailand	228 cases	181 deaths
2004	Indian ocean tsunami	Indonesia, India, Bangladesh, Sri Lanka, Thailand	125,000 injured	>230,210 deaths
2005	Kashmir earthquake (Richter scale 7.6) on 8th October	India	4 million become homeless	86,000 deaths
2006	Chikungunya outbreak	India	1.39 million cases	2,944 deaths
2006	Yogyakarta earthquake (Richter scale 6.4) 27th May	Indonesia	37,000 injured	>5700 deaths
2007	Cyclone Sidr	Bangladesh	7.5 million affected	>5,000 deaths
2007	Cyclone Alia	India (Sunderbans) and Bangladesh	3.8 million affected	190 deaths
2008	Cyclone Nargis	Myanmar	2.4 million affected	138,000 deaths
2008–2009	Conflict/Civil war	Sri Lanka	60,000 wounded	>20,000 deaths
2009	Chikungunya	Thailand	42,000 cases	
2010	Dengue outbreak	Indonesia, Thailand, Sri Lanka, India	>20,000 cases	1,500 deaths
2011	Floods	Thailand	13.6 million affected	815 deaths
2012–2015	Middle-east respiratory syndrome—coronavirus (MERS-CoV)	Thailand	3 lab-confirmed cases	
2015	Earthquake (Richter scale 7.8) on 25 April	Nepal	22,303 injured, 41,199 hospitalized, 462 health facilities completely damaged, 765 partially damaged	9,000 deaths
2015	H1N1 outbreak	India	33,000 cases	>2,000 deaths
2015	Flood	India (Chennai)	1.8 million IDP	>500 deaths
2015	Floods	Myanmar	1 million people affected	103 deaths
2016	Flood/landslides	Sri Lanka	52,500 people affected	>100 deaths
2016	Floods/Typhoon Lionrock	DPR Korea	100,000 became homeless	138 deaths
2016	Cyclone Roanu	Sri Lanka, Bangladesh	300,000 people affected	204 deaths (Sri Lanka) and 26 deaths in Bangladesh
2016	Cyclone Roanu	Sri Lanka, Bangladesh	300,000 people affected	204 deaths (Sri Lanka) and 26 deaths in Bangladesh

Contd...

Table 6.1: Major public health emergencies in the South-east Asia region[3] (*Contd...*)

Year	*Public health emergency*	*SEA countries affected*	*Morbidity*	*Mortality*
2016	Mount Sinabung eruption	Indonesia	28,536 IDPs (203 pregnant women, 869 babies and 1573 pregnant ladies)	20 deaths
2016	Aceh earthquake (Richter scale 6.5) on 7th December	Indonesia	1,000 injured	100 deaths
2016	Zika Grade 2 (20th Jan) declared PHEIC* on 1st February and graded down to endemic status on 18th November	Bangladesh, Thailand Indonesia, India, Maldives	Bangladesh: 1 case Thailand: >360 cases, 2 microcephaly India: 4 cases	None
2017	Cyclone Storm Mora (May)	Bangladesh	3.3 million people affected, 60,000 IDPs, 17,000 houses damaged	
2017	H1N1 outbreak	Myanmar	166 confirmed cases	17 deaths
2017	H1N1 outbreak	Maldives	222 confirmed cases	3 deaths
2017	Flood and landslides (May)	Nepal	21,391 IDPs, 41,893 house totally damaged	161 deaths (including 25 children)
2017	Flood and landslides (May–June)	Sri Lanka	683,821 people affected 15,897 houses damaged	224 deaths
2017	Dengue outbreak	Sri Lanka	170,075 cases from January to November	400 deaths
2017	Drought	DPR Korea	18 million people food insecure, 200,000 children with acute malnutrition	
2017	Rohingya refugees conflict	Myanmar/Bangladesh	620,000 Rohingya people displaced to Bangladesh since 25th August, 2017 Public health risk of outbreaks of cholera, measles, tuberculosis, malnutrition. Many cases of gender and sexual violence	199 deaths (including 78 children under 5 years of age) as on 18th November, 2017
2019–2020	COVID-19 (Corona virus)**	Almost all countries are affected. Worst affected countries as on date are—USA, Brazil, India, Russia (till 17 Aug. 2020)	Globally, as of 3:16 pm CEST, 20 Aug. 2020, there have been 22,256,220 confirmed cases of COVID-19, including 782,456 deaths, reported to WHO	Globally as on 20 Aug. 2020—782,456 deaths

IDPs = Internally displaced peoples;
*PHEIC (Public Health Emergency of International Concern);
Source: **Coronavirus disease 2019 (COVID-19) Situation Report—52. March 12, 2020 https://www.who.int/docs/default-source/coronaviruse/20200312-sitrep-52-covid-19.pdf?sfvrsn=e2bfc9c0_2

science and art, and applies when the **problem is unexpected**. A timely response is required—public health epidemiologists must travel to and work in the field to solve the problem and extent of the investigation is likely to be limited because of the imperative for timely intervention".[4]

Thus field epidemiology is all about applying epidemiological methods to identify and respond to emerging situations in order to support rapid public health actions, and to provide the evidence for future guidance. The field epidemiology work is carried out in varied and very complex situations which require excellent effective communication and negotiation skills in addition to technical expertise.

"Moving practice of epidemiology from knowledge based to competency based and from four walls to actual field".

The field epidemiology is multi-disciplinary and multi-sectoral in nature and it involves experts from medicine (clinicians), public health epidemiologist, laboratory and behavioural sciences, management, finance, media and telecommunication, sociology, political science, etc. Basic domains of field epidemiology are mentioned in Box 6.1 and differences between traditional and field epidemiology are mentioned in Table 6.2. Role of field epidemiologists is critical and comprehensive (Box 6.4).

Field epidemiological investigation for an emergency situation may be warranted under following circumstances.

1. When there is sudden increase in cases of specific disease as reported by clinicians in the area or new diseases or rare case reporting.
2. Health surveillance system may detect sudden increase in cases.
3. Outbreak/epidemic as result of natural/man-made disasters/calamity.
4. As obligation under national programs like polio eradication, measles eradication, full investigation is done even for a single case to contain the epidemic/outbreak.
5. Community may report some unusual cases or diseases which may be a rumour or a real information, needed to be investigated.
6. Sometimes, there may be pressure from politicians to investigate even a single case for the larger social interest, but in reality do not need to do it.

Box 6.1: Basic domains of field epidemiology[5]

A. Fundamental of epidemiology and biostatistics
B. Diseases surveillance
C. Outbreak investigation and response
D. Laboratory in public health systems
E. Emerging and re-emerging infectious diseases
F. Communication and health promotion
G. Management and leadership
H. International health regulations
I. Basic computer applications
J. Field practice/visits/investigation
K. Teaching and mentoring

Table 6.2: Difference between traditional and field epidemiology

Traditional epidemiological investigation	*Field epidemiological investigation*
It is more of passive type of epidemiology	It is real time and place epidemiology and more of action oriented.
It takes into account of all situations	It usually applied during humanitarian emergencies situations
All types of study designs are used	Do not have clear hypotheses and required to generate hypothesis through descriptive studies
Generally planning of action done after full study including finalization of report	Requires preparation for public health action along investigation immediately with waiting for final data analysis

Why We Need Field Epidemiology?[4,6,7]

Delay in the detection of outbreaks and inadequate preparedness and response aggravates the impact of communicable diseases, leading to increased numbers of cases, increased duration of epidemics, excess mortality and the potential for spread to other areas nationally, regionally, or globally to understand ground realities and reduce/contain such situations.

Setting up early warning surveillance systems, preparing for investigating and responding to priority communicable diseases is critical in reducing morbidity and mortality in vulnerable populations affected by humanitarian emergencies, but also in protecting global health security.

Other methods of data collection in humanitarian emergencies such as surveys, as well as monitoring and evaluation of programs are vital to prioritization and the efficient allocation of resources as well as strengthening interventions.

The use of epidemiologic skills to identify public health problems, measure risk factors, and design and evaluate public health programs contributes to improving the health of the public.

The practice of field epidemiology will enhance/strengthened the following.

- Response to humanitarian emergencies/ acute problems
- The scientific basis for program and policy decisions
- Diseases surveillance systems
- The communication of epidemiologic information
- Research and learning opportunities
- Generated training needs in emergency management.

Managing Emergencies

Epidemiological investigations meet both public service and scientific needs. An investigation may use secondary data along with primary data to gather new information.

During emergencies like epidemics, a defined response and the sequence of interventions that are necessary are as follows (Fig. 6.2).

Anticipation: An emergence of epidemic is not possible to predicted, but it can certainly be anticipated. Anticipation encompasses forecasting the most likely diseases to emerge, and the quick identification of the factors that will worsen the impact or facilitate the spread. Preparedness plans, based on lessons learned from past experiences, should ready for a reactive response to the unexpected.

Early detection: Emerging and re-emerging diseases include new ones about which there is little scientific knowledge exists. These, therefore, often require investigation into their sources at the same timeas the use of coordinated, rapid-containment measures. New diseases require new interventions, because they appear irregularly or rarely, there is a need for constant vigilance, proactive risk assessment and the development of new management tools.

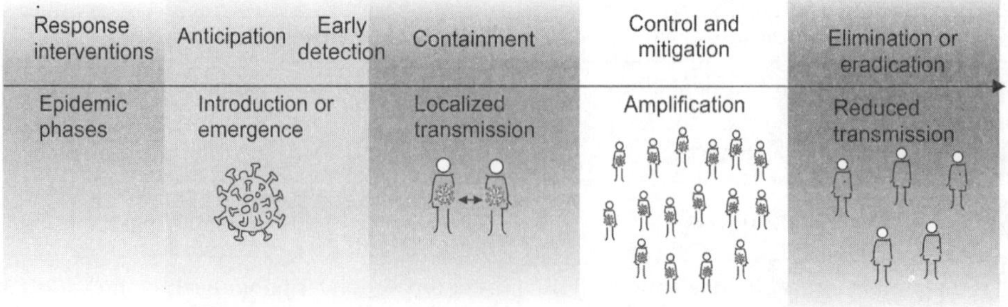

Fig. 6.2: Epidemic phases and response interventions[1]

Early detection allows the rapid implementation of containment measures, which are the key to reducing the risk of amplification and potential spread. All healthcare workers must be trained to recognize potential epidemic disease, report quickly an unusual event (such as an unusual cluster of cases or deaths). Their role is also to reduce the risk of community transmission by isolating severely-ill patients; to prevent household transmission by protecting healthcare givers at home; and to reduce the mortality rate. Healthcare workers must also know how to protect themselves and employ infection prevention and control measures and how to avoid outbreaks amplified in healthcare facilities.

Containment: Effective and rapid containment of emerging diseases is just as vital as early detection in order to avoid a large scale epidemic. Rapid containment should start as soon as the first case is detected regardless of the aetiology, which is most likely to be unknown. It requires skilled professionals to safely implement the necessary countermeasures.

Control and mitigation: Once the infectious disease threat reaches an epidemic or pandemic level, the goal of the response is to mitigate its impact and reduce its incidence, morbidity and mortality as well as disruptions to economic, political, and social systems.

Elimination or eradication: Control of a disease may lead to its elimination, which means that is sufficiently controlled to prevent an epidemic from occurring in a defined geographical area. Elimination means that the disease is no longer considered as a major public health issue. However, intervention measures (surveillance and control) should continue to prevent its re-emergence.

Eradication of a disease: Much more difficult and rarely achieved—involves the permanent elimination of its incidence worldwide. There is no longer a need for interventions measures. Three criteria need to be met in order to eradicate a disease—(i) there must be an available intervention to interrupt its transmission; (ii) there *must be available* efficient diagnostic tools to detect cases that could lead to transmission; and (iii) humans must be the only reservoir.

The fundamental principles of communicable disease control in emergencies, which are (Table 6.3):[2]

1. **Rapid assessment:** Identify the communicable disease threats faced by the emergency-affected population, including those with epidemic potential, and define the health status of the population, by conducting a rapid assessment.
2. **Prevention:** Prevent communicable disease by maintaining a healthy physical environment and good general living conditions.
3. **Surveillance:** Set up or strengthen disease surveillance system with an early warning mechanism to ensure the early reporting of cases, to monitor disease trends, and to facilitate prompt detection and response to outbreaks.
4. **Outbreak control:** Ensure outbreaks are rapidly detected and controlled through adequate preparedness (i.e. stockpiles, standard treatment protocols and staff training) and rapid response (i.e. confirmation, investigation and implementation of control measures); and
5. **Disease management:** Diagnose and treat cases promptly with trained staff using effective treatment and standard protocols at all health facilities.

BUILDING BLOCKS FOR A COMPREHENSIVE OUTBREAK RESPONSE (C-HI-C-HI)[1,8]

All steps for managing emergencies are summarized as under:

C (Coordinating responders)	HI (Health information)
C (Communicating risk)	HI (Health interventions)

Table 6.3: Steps in control of communicable diseases emergencies[2]

Conduct rapid health assessment	a. Identify main disease threats, including potential epidemic diseases b. Obtain data on geographical area and its origin c. Identify priority public health interventions d. Identify the coordinating health agency e. Establish health coordination mechanisms
Prevent communicable diseases	a. Select and plan sites b. Ensure adequate water and sanitation facilities c. Ensure availability of food d. Control vectors e. Implement vaccination campaigns (e.g. measles) f. Provide essential clinical services g. Provide basic laboratory facilities
Set up surveillance/ early warning system	a. Detect outbreaks early b. Report diseases of epidemic potential immediately c. Monitor disease trends
Control outbreaks	a. Preparation (outbreak response team, stockpiles, laboratory support, standard treatment protocols) b. Detection (surveillance/early warning system) c. Confirmation (laboratory test) d. Response (investigation, control measures) e. Evaluation

Coordinating Responders (C)

An effective coordination between various disciplines, sectors and responders needed to effectively manage the emergencies. It is the part-n-parcel of preparation for investigation. Some of the components are as under.

- Identify and intimate people, groups and organizations who will be conducting investigation
- Roles and responsibilities of each people, groups and organizations
- Identify team leader
- Prepare a rapid health assessment check-list, prepare a timetable of assessment, assign tasks
- Identification and procurement of materials needed for the investigation—obtain necessary equipment (e.g. computers, scales, stationary, laboratory supplies), other items like copies of questionnaires, spreadsheets for line lists or the coding of data, data calculation capacity, computer with internet facility, a camera, containers for laboratory specimens, etc.
- Travel planning (schedule of travel, transport, vehicles, fuel, etc.)
- Set up a communication system
- Inform the local authorities.

Health Information (HI)

Information on background geopolitical data and background health data must be collected in a systematic way, however it may not be possible all the time in epidemic investigation. A well-planned document should include following four methods of data collection.

i. Review of existing information on health status of the population, healthcare agencies available, current health program, etc.
ii. Visual inspection of the affected area—a transect walk is necessary to find out availability of local facilities, geographical information along with water source, waste disposal, schools and other shelters, etc.
iii. Interviews with key informants like village head, local health workers (ASHA,

TBA, AWW), police head, local government officials, traditional healers, prominent village persons regarding the epidemic and facilities.

iv. Rapid surveys/surveillance: Surveillance provides information on the number of cases and deaths by period and place (people, time, and place). Data on sex and age distribution of the population, the average family size, the number of people in vulnerable groups should also be obtained.

v. Information on the interventions enables knowing which ones are performed and what is their coverage and impact.

Communicating Risk (C)

Communication must be done in local language with clarity and culturally acceptable with proper channels of communication.

During the evolution of any major outbreak/epidemic, cases and deaths will inevitably increase.

There may be possibility of **'infodemic'**, i.e. the rapid spread of information of all kinds, including rumours, gossip and unreliable information. A successful management of infodemics **(infodemiology)** is based on (1) monitoring and identifying them, (2) analysis of information, and (3) control and mitigation measures.

Risk communication is an essential intervention in any response to disease outbreaks, and it involves two-way communication that is dynamic and evolving as the outbreak develops. The important components are talk, listen and manage rumours. Effective risk communication will lead to establishment of lines of dialogue with affected populations and stakeholders, and builds trust in the response which help to manage and contain epidemic/outbreak.

Guiding Principles of Risk Communication

1. When health risks are uncertain—it is uncertain that the population needs information on what is known and what is not.
2. The timely and transparent dissemination of accurate and accessible science-based information creates public trust.
3. Coordinating all of the organizations and health workers involved in creating and disseminating messages is fundamental in attempting to clear confusion.
4. Prioritize the messages. Messages should be organized in order of importance.
5. Information for the public should be accessible, technically correct but adapted to the different audiences. The messages should be translated into local languages or dialects as necessary.
6. Make preparations for social mobilization and effective community participation in activities designed to control the outbreak.
7. The information presented should leave as little room as possible for speculation, and should avoid over-interpretation of the data, as well as overly confident evaluations of public health investigation and control measures.
8. It will be important to realize that approaches and recommendations may change as more is learned about this disease.
9. Make contingency plans—establish mechanisms and actions to address possible situations involving socially sensitive actions.
10. Keep journalists constantly informed of how the situation is evolving.

Health Interventions (HI)

Health interventions depend on the type, extent and severity of the disease so as to reduce

a. Transmission,
b. Severe morbidity, mortality, disability
c. The impact on health systems
d. The political and other sectors.

FIELD INVESTIGATION OF AN OUTBREAK/ EPIDEMIC[2–4,6,9]

Most outbreaks are noticed by (i) Formal surveillance systems like integrated diseases surveillance program (IDSP), (ii) early aberration reporting system (EARS), (iii) rumours from the community, (iv) observation of unusual health events, and (v) self-reported cases.

Following steps may be taken to investigate an outbreak/epidemic:

1. Determine the existence of the epidemic
2. Confirm the diagnosis
3. Define a case and count cases
4. Describing the data in terms of time, place, and person
5. Determine who is at risk of becoming ill
6. Develop, test and compare hypothesis with the established facts.
7. Plan a more systematic advance study
8. Strategies for control and prevention of an outbreak/epidemic
9. Prepare a written report/documention of an outbreak/epidemic
10. Sharing the outbreak/epidemic report.

Determine the Existence of the Epidemic

A preliminary count of people with similar symptoms is often the first criterion for this decision. Laboratory confirmation may be absent. It may even be inappropriate because of the urgent need to begin an investigation (Appendix 6.1).

Compare current information with previous incidence in the community during the same time of year to determine if the observed number of cases exceeds the expected. Compare available information about new cases with a predetermined definition of an outbreak.

Confirm the Diagnosis

Analyze clinical histories of cases and have standard laboratory tests performed to confirm or reject the suspected diagnosis and to determine the type of agent associated with the illness.

The number of cases is sometimes too great to do a history and physical examination on every person. Collection of laboratory specimens (Appendix 6.2), must then follow quickly, although decisions about epidemic control are often made before laboratory confirmation is available. Confirming each reported case may not be possible, and laboratory specimens may be obtained on only 15–20% of the cases. In some large epidemics, a sample of cases gave the essential information about the agent, the host, the method of transmission, the portal of entry, and the environment of the disease.

Define a Case and Count Cases

A case definition is a standardized description of the disease associated with an outbreak which, for the purposes of the investigation, will be used to distinguish between cases and non-cases. The case definition should not be used as a basis for clinical diagnosis, treatment or other management of individuals (Appendix 6.3).

The primary objective in developing a case definition is to include as many individuals as possible who are likely to be part of the outbreak (sensitivity), while excluding as many as possible who are not likely to be part of the outbreak (specificity).

Surveillance case definitions should indicate, if appropriate, when a case is suspect, probable or confirmed (Table 6.4).

Case should be found out by interviewing family contacts of cases, reviewing notifiable disease reports, hospitals and general practitioners to report (retrospectively or prospectively), patients who meet the case definition, laboratories to report (retrospectively or prospectively), accident and emergency department records and reviewing data from other health agencies. Community should be encouraged to report such cases to nearby health agencies.

A **line-listing** is produced by epidemiologists in outbreak investigations. A line listing allows information about time, person, and place to be organized and reviewed quickly. It is also a good way to keep track of different categories of cases. For example, cases can be entered into the line listing as possible, probable or confirmed (laboratory confirmed, clinically confirmed or both). The

Table 6.4: Case classification

Type of case	*Criteria*
Suspect	Clinical signs and symptoms compatible with the disease in question but no laboratory evidence of infection (negative, pending or not possible) Example for cholera: Suspected case = meets clinical case definition
Probable	Compatible clinical signs and symptoms, and additional epidemiological (e.g. contact with a confirmed case) or laboratory (e.g. screening test) evidence for the disease in question For cholera: Probable case = suspected case + motile bacteria or ongoing epidemic or epidemiological link to confirmed case
Confirmed	Definite laboratory evidence of current or recent infection, *whether or not* clinical signs or symptoms are or have been present For meningococcal meningitis: Confirmed case = suspected or probable case + laboratory confirmation (*Vibrio cholerae* positive) Note that in outbreaks of certain diseases, clinical symptoms are not present in a proportion of people, however, they are counted as confirmed cases with laboratory evidence since subclinical infection is a major source of transmission

designation can easily be updated as the investigation progresses. A line list helps in defining the disease, and identifying the population at risk (Appendix 6.4).

Describing Data in Terms of Time, Place, and Person

Detailed information on all cases involved in an outbreak should be collected using a **structured interview** based on a standardized questionnaire **(epidemiological case sheet)** (Appendix 6.5).

Data on each case must include the date of onset of the illness, the place, where the person lives or work and/or became ill, and the characteristics of each individual, including age, sex, and occupation.

A simple histogram, often called 'the **epidemic curve,**' (Fig. 6.3) shows the relationship between the occurrence of cases and their times of onset. An epidemic curve depicts the time course of the onset of symptoms among cases in an outbreak.

The epidemic curve is a two-dimensional bar graph or histogram with an x- and a y-axes that helps to illustrate the dynamics of the outbreak, including the number of people affected the time course of the outbreak and whether the outbreak is continuing. It may also indicate the mode of transmission and help to relate the timing of key events (such as possible exposures and control measures) to the onset of symptoms.

The shape of the curve may indicate the mode of transmission.

Characteristically, the epidemic curve of a common event outbreak has a sharp rise in cases to apeak, followed by a fall-off that is less abrupt than the rise. The length of the curve will be approximately equal to one incubation period of the infection.

The rise in cases for a dispersed or common site outbreak may also be sharp, but will not fall off unless exposure to the source is discontinued or all susceptible individuals become infected.

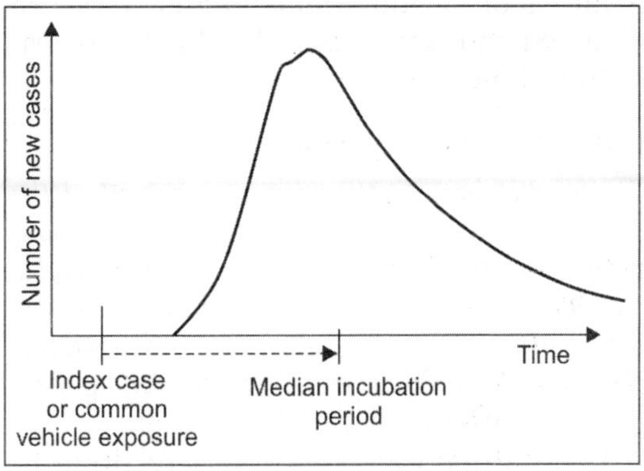

Fig. 6.3: The epidemic curve

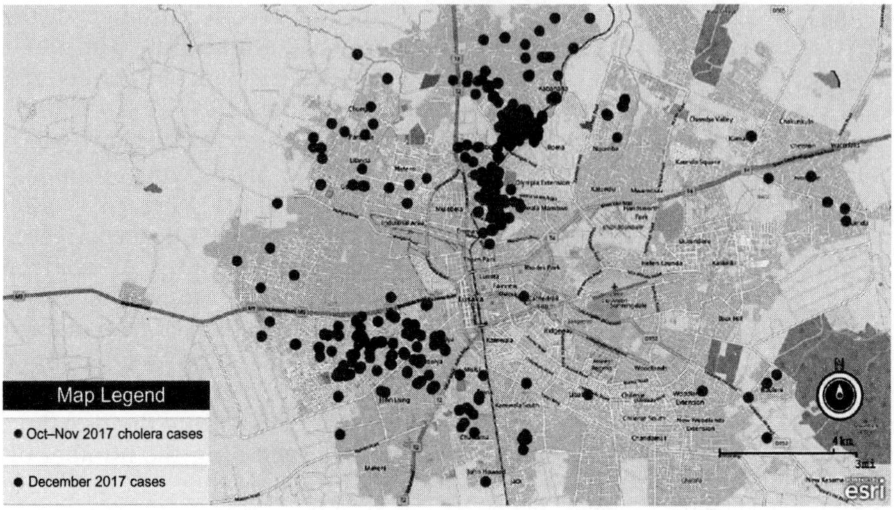

Fig. 6.4: Spot map of cases, 6 October to 31 December 2017

The spatial relationships of cases are often shown best on a **spot map** (Fig. 6.4). Maps, for instance, help show that the cases occurred in proximity to a body of water, a sewage treatment plant, or its outflow.

Environmental Investigation

Environmental investigation should be closely integrated with the epidemiological and laboratory investigations. Epidemiological information should help to focus on the environmental investigation. The major thrust of environmental investigation is risk assessment including background information, condition of physical structures, etc. by paying on-site visit by the epidemiologist. Samples of various items (water, food) to obtained and tested to find out pathological agents, if present.

Laboratory Investigation

The head of investigation team must contact the appropriate laboratory for planning the collection, preserving and shipping of the specimen for better outcome.There are different guidelines for various types of samples, e.g. water, food articles, chemicals, body fluids, etc., one must follow these guidelines while dealing with specimens.

Laboratory investigations are done to identifying and quantifying organisms and toxins mainly for identifying or confirming links between suspected contaminated substances and human illness.

Recent laboratory techniques can greatly improve the sensitivity of outbreak detection by identifying clusters of cases with a common source. Such findings may help strengthen links between outbreaks and their sources. Laboratory investigation results will help to prove the suspect cases into confirmed cases and help to take appropriate action for prevention and control of the epidemics (Appendix 6.2).

Determine Who is at Risk of Becoming Ill

One should calculate rates/ratios, at which a health problem or disease occurs, using the number of the population at risk as the denominator, while the number of those individuals with the problem form the numerator.

- **Incidence of disease** by place and population is to be calculated for occurrence of new cases.
- **Proportional morbidity** (cases of disease divided by total cases and expressed as a percentage)
- **Number of cases of any potentially epidemic disease**
- **Case fatality rates** (deaths due to specific disease or syndrome divided by total cases

of that disease or syndrome and expressed as a percentage).

- **Attack rate during outbreaks** [cumulative incidence (new cases) of epidemic disease in a population over a particular period of time, when population is known]
- **Secondary attack rate**
- **Attack ratio** among exposed to non-exposed.

Develop, Test and Compare Hypothesis with the Established Facts

Information gained from the descriptive phase, in combination with the environmental and laboratory investigation is mostly sufficient to characterize the outbreak and may also indicate the likely outbreak source and mode of transmission. Descriptive analysis is extremely valuable in generating hypotheses about the source of the outbreak that will be useful to guide a full analytic investigation.

The hypothesis that explains the epidemic must be consistent with all the facts the epidemiologist knows. If the hypothesis does not do so, then it must be re-examined. It should do more than just strengthen speculation, explaining the cases at the peak of the epidemic. The epidemiologist may need to repeat the interview of case subjects, reassess medical records, gather additional laboratory specimens, and repeat calculations.

Plan a More Systematic Advance Study

After completing the descriptive phase, next stage of the investigation is the application of intensive analytic epidemiological methods. An analytic epidemiological study is also needed to confirm the initial findings.

The situation where an analytic epidemiological investigation needed:

- Identify the transmission mechanism and/or source of infection to apply control measures
- If the characteristics of cases or their exposures suggest one or more unusual features.
- When the sample size is adequate to apply statistical power to determine exposures with an acceptable level of statistical certainty.
- When the investigation is timely done and there is less chances of recall bias.
- When epidemiological investigation will have to be focused on the environmental or laboratory investigation.

The type of analytical studies which could be undertaken as a part of advance investigation include: (i) Cross-sectional (analytical), (ii) Case-control study and (iii) Cohort studies. (Details of these study designs are described in Chapters 8, 9 and 10.)

Strategies for Control and Prevention of an Outbreak/Epidemic

Preparation for action:

- Continuation of an active surveillance system including early warning and response system.
- An outbreak response plan is prepared covering the resources, skills and activities required;
- Standard treatment protocols for the disease are prepared and made available to all health facilities and agencies and clinical workers are trained to that effect;
- Ensure stock of essential supplies for treatment, laboratory investigations and preventive activities supplies;
- **Adequate healthcare personnel**

Note: While choosing the measures for prevention and control, one must keep in mind the feasibility (technical/operational/financial), timely availability of material and man power, acceptability by the community and safety of both operators and population.

Control measures as per the chain of transmission: The most important strategy is to break the chain of transmission for further transmission of diseases so as to prevent further outbreak/epidemic. Following measures may be applied (Fig. 6.5).

Measures of control of source of infection:

1. Detection treatment of cases and carriers
2. Isolation
3. Control of zoonotic reservoirs

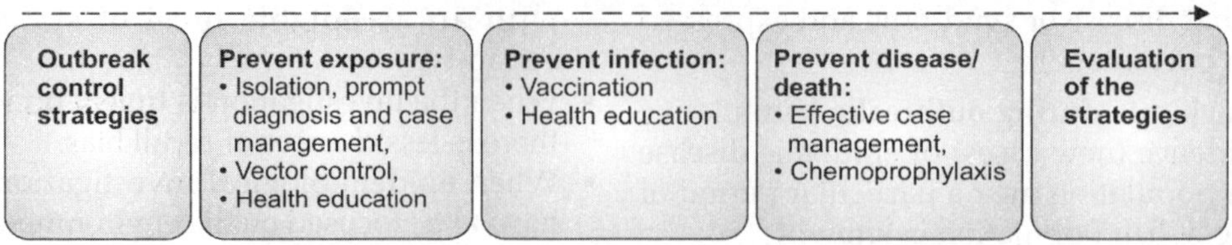

Fig. 6.5: Control measures as per the chain of transmission

Measures of controlling the modes of transmission:

1. Clean water supply
2. Food hygiene
3. Vector control
4. Waste disposal
5. Sanitation
6. Disinfection of contaminated substances.

Protection of population at risk:

1. Immunization
2. Immunoprophylaxis
3. Chemoprophylaxis
4. Personal protective measures.

Long-term strategies:

1. Launching a surveillance system
2. Early warning systems about impending outbreaks.

Boxes 6.2 and 6.3 show selected interventions for an outbreak/epidemic investigation, prevention and control.

Box 6.2: Selected public health interventions for an outbreak

Intervention efforts directed at source

- Treat infected persons/animals
- Isolate infected persons (includes cohorting)
- Quarantine exposed persons
- Quarantine contaminated sites/sources
- Implement cordon sanitaire, close public places, and prevent gatherings (to freeze/limit movement and minimize likelihood of mixing groups by exposure/infection status)
- Seize and/or destroy contaminated food, property, animals, or other sources
- Clean and disinfect contaminated surfaces and other environmental repositories
- Modify environment through vector control
- Modify environment by restricting/controlling contaminants
- Modify behaviour to reduce risks to self and/or others
- Deter through civil suits or criminal prosecution

Intervention efforts directed at susceptibles

- Administer post-exposure prophylaxis
- Immunize/vaccinate in advance
- Exclude unvaccinated persons from cohorts of vaccinated persons
- Employ barrier techniques
- Implement cordon sanitaire, close public places, and prevent gatherings (to freeze/limit movement and minimize likelihood of mixing groups by exposure/infection status)
- Modify behaviour to reduce risks to self and/or others
- Use shelter-in-place (reverse quarantine)
- Employ contact tracing, partner notification, and treatment
- Issue press releases, health alerts, and other information regarding risk reduction

Box 6.3: Steps summarization of an outbreak/epidemic investigation

Verify initial reports and thus establish whether an outbreak is occurring; personally examine cases if possible, or discuss signs and symptoms with an attending clinician:

1. Visit the household, place of work or school, and interview possible contacts of the case where appropriate;
2. Collect blood, stool and cerebrospinal fluid (CSF) samples in relevant media (e.g. on Cary-Blair medium for suspected cholera), as appropriate; perform rapid tests where indicated; order laboratory tests to confirm the diagnosis;
3. Perform environmental sampling, where appropriate;
4. Develop a case definition for the purposes of the outbreak, which should:
   - Include time, person and place;
   - Include simple and easily identified symptoms that balance sensitivity and specificity;
   - Be more specific (usually) than the case definitions used during routine surveillance;
5. Establish the extent of the outbreak by counting cases, if possible by place of residence (preferably the place of residence at the onset of disease);
6. Ensure line listing of cases by all health facilities receiving cases;
7. Expand the EWARN coverage and increase reporting as required (e.g. daily submission of line lists to the next reporting level by all health facilities receiving cases);
8. Perform descriptive epidemiology, including an epidemic curve, to determine whether cases are clustered in time, place or by person (e.g. by age and sex);
9. Develop hypotheses explaining exposure and disease (e.g. the source of the outbreak and the mode of transmission; these are often obvious from descriptive epidemiology);
10. Refine the hypothesis and carry out additional studies, including laboratory tests and environmental studies;
11. Implement control measures as soon as possible (these may change from general to specific measures as the investigation progresses and the epidemiology is refined);
12. Develop and communicate public health messages in the affected community; evaluate hypotheses (formal epidemiological studies may be needed to further define risk and refine control methods);
13. Prepare a written report;
14. Communicate the findings of the outbreak investigation to all stakeholders.

Evaluation of the Strategies (Appendix 6.4)

After cessation of an outbreak, the outbreak control team must carry out the evaluation of the following.

a. Cause of the outbreak
b. Surveillance and detection of the outbreak
c. Preparedness for the outbreak
d. Management of the outbreak
e. Control measures.

The specific issues under each heading that should be evaluated include (Appendix 6.6):

a. Timeliness of detection and response
b. Effectiveness
c. Cost
d. Lost opportunities
e. New/revised policies.

The findings of this evaluation should be documented in a written report containing clear recommendations on:

a. the epidemiological characteristics of the epidemic
b. surveillance
c. preparedness
d. control measures carried out.

Evaluation should be used for preparedness of activities for future outbreaks.

Prepare a Written Report/Documentation of an Outbreak or Epidemic

Comprehensive High quality outbreak documentation is to be prepared and shared with all stakeholders for the following.

- As a part of national/state/district surveillance system
- To convince health professionals, the community and government authorities for preventive measures
- Better understanding of emerging diseases with regards to agent, modes of transmission and risk factors
- As an educational tool for diseases and outbreak investigation
- To evaluate and improve control and prevention strategies

A complete, comprehensive detailed investigation documented report of outbreak Investigation is essential with full details of the methods, results, discussion and recommendations from the outbreak investigation in a form suitable for wider distribution and possible publication. Preparation and dissemination of an outbreak investigation report ensures that the investigation process is open for peer review, and that the findings can have an impact beyond the local circumstances.

Sharing the Outbreak/Epidemic Report

Meaningful transfer of figures, facts and their implications shapes medical and public health practice and drives the need to acquire new data. Therefore, communication is a prime function of the head of the field investigator (epidemiologist).

Through Medical Journals

Writings in medical journals can reach nationally and internationally to share, learn and practice, if similar kind of outbreaks occur and they can also share their view point. This can be written in IMRAD format or under subheadings such abstract, introduction/ background, objective, study design, setting, participants, interventions, outcome/output, results, discussion and conclusions.[2]

Through Scientific Presentation

Before preparing the presentation, one must know their audience and level of their understanding. You must choose appropriate tool of presentation with simple and culturally acceptable or internationally acceptable

Box 6.4: Role of field epidemiologist[5]

1. Detect epidemic through early warning signals.
2. Conduct epidemic investigations/field surveys.
3. Institute appropriate and timely response for prevention and control of outbreaks, health impacts of disasters and environmental health issues.
4. Collect appropriate laboratory specimens, storage and transportation of the specimens to the laboratory.
5. Provide leadership in control of endemic and epidemic-prone diseases.
6. Design, implement and evaluate disease surveillance systems.
7. Evaluate disease control/prevention measures.
8. Conduct epidemiological and statistical analysis of complex data sets.
9. Use computers effectively for data management, graphics and presentation.
10. Provide public health information to media, public and policy makers.
11. Prepare, present/publish technical reports/articles.
12. Remain prepared for any public health emergencies.
13. Train other health professionals and team members.

language. Slides should not be read rather discuss and allow audience to ask question for better transfer of figures and facts.[2]

Remember

- Be punctual in time and place.
- Do not project illegible slides/too crowded slides.
- Do not become angry or upset in front of your audience
- Avoid show-off attitudes, long words, or an air of superiority.

Other methods may be included are brief handouts, news letters, role plays at community level, rallies for preventive awareness, mouth-to-mouth propaganda for prevention activities at local answers prepared. One should also be aware and prepare for reporters' tactics by conducting quick research about the journalist (or outlet) so that the journalist's likely 'angle' can be anticipated.[4]

The problem and solution should be clearly defined, and details of the response and what others can do to be written in detail.

Through media: The media is a vehicle to deliver the single overarching communication objective (SOCO). In preparation, questions have to be anticipated and draft important to stay on message and to avoid being drawn into saying things that may impact the SOCO; it is the interviewer's job to fill the time. Bridging statements may be needed to ensure that all the key messages are delivered.[8]

Some 'golden rules' for interviews include:[8]

- Never lie
- Never say 'no comment'
- There is no such thing as 'off the record'
- Be short, to the point, and take account of the target audience
- Stay calm, confident and in charge
- Use simple language, avoid jargon
- Be human, and smile when appropriate
- It is OK to say "I don't know but I will find out"
- Do not speculate.

APPENDICES[10]

Appendix 6.1: Algorithm for alert verification and outbreak investigation for use by EWARN focal points/surveillance officers

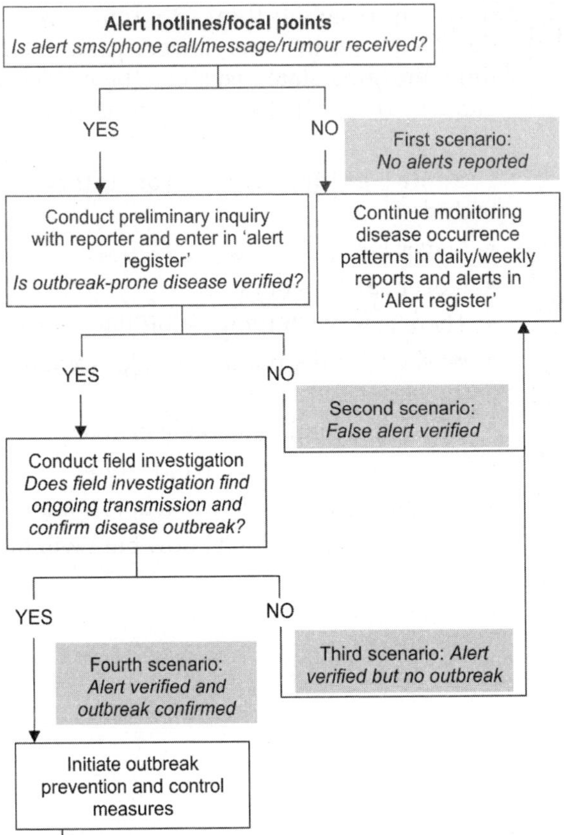

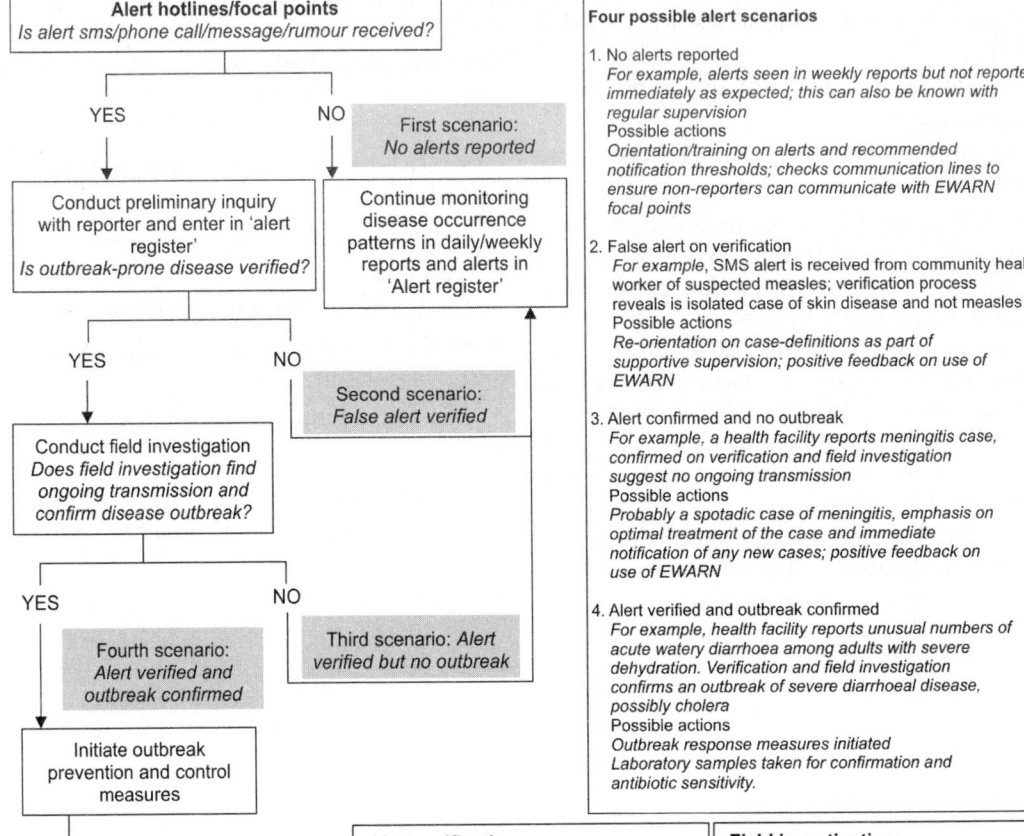

Four possible alert scenarios

1. No alerts reported
   For example, alerts seen in weekly reports but not reported immediately as expected; this can also be known with regular supervision
   Possible actions
   Orientation/training on alerts and recommended notification thresholds; checks communication lines to ensure non-reporters can communicate with EWARN focal points
2. False alert on verification
   For example, SMS alert is received from community health worker of suspected measles; verification process reveals is isolated case of skin disease and not measles
   Possible actions
   Re-orientation on case-definitions as part of supportive supervision; positive feedback on use of EWARN
3. Alert confirmed and no outbreak
   For example, a health facility reports meningitis case, confirmed on verification and field investigation suggest no ongoing transmission
   Possible actions
   Probably a spotadic case of meningitis, emphasis on optimal treatment of the case and immediate notification of any new cases; positive feedback on use of EWARN
4. Alert verified and outbreak confirmed
   For example, health facility reports unusual numbers of acute watery diarrhoea among adults with severe dehydration. Verification and field investigation confirms an outbreak of severe diarrhoeal disease, possibly cholera
   Possible actions
   Outbreak response measures initiated
   Laboratory samples taken for confirmation and antibiotic sensitivity.

Outbreak response components

- Characterize the epidemiology: *Line listing; descriptive epidemiology, epidemic curve, CFR, hypothesis regarding transmission*
- Laboratory confirmation: *Control measures should not await laboratory results; antimicrobial sensitivity should support case management.*
- Prevention: *For example, community prevention messages, immunization, prophylaxis of contacts, social mobilization*
- Control: *Interrupt transmission, isolate/manage cases*

Alert verification

By telephone, fine out about:

- Who is reporting the alert/rumour (and their contact details)
- Person/place/time
  - Number of cases/deaths
  - Age, sex, origin of cases/deaths
  - Date of onset or consultation
- Treatment and outcome
- Check case definition used and symptoms/signs exhibited
- Any healthcare staff affected
- Any clusters (by family or contacts, geographically)
- Measures taken so far
- Community reactions

Note: All the above may not be known by the person reporting the alert, but can help in deciding whether an alert is false or not, and will help orient a field investigation if needed.

Field investigation

- On-site visit, preferably within 24 hrs
- Review of cases with clinicians
- Assessment clustering of cases in time and space
- Household visit
- Examination of cases, interviews case contacts
- Interview to determine medical history, review of vaccination records
- Performance of rapid tests as indicated
- Collection samples in relevant media
- Expansion of surveillance coverage and enhancement of reporting as required

Appendix 6.2: Specimen collection

A. Blood Specimen Collection

Blood and separated serum are the most common specimens taken in outbreaks of communicable disease. Venous blood can be used for isolation and identification of the pathogen in culture by inoculation, or separated into serum for the detection of genetic material (e.g. by polymerase chain reaction), specific antibodies (by serology) and antigens or toxins (e.g. by immunofluorescence). For the processing of most specimens for diagnosis of viral pathogens, serum is preferable to unsupported, except where otherwise directed. When specific antibodies are being assayed, it is often helpful to collect paired sesa (i.e. an acute sample at the onset of illness and a convalescent sample 1–1 weeks later). Whenever possible, blood specimens for culture should be taken before antibiotics are administrated to the patient, but life-saving treatment should not be unnecessarily delayed.

Venous Blood Samples

Materials for collection

The following materials are required.

- Skin disinfection: 700% alcohol (isopropanol, ethanol) or 100% povidone iodine, swabs, gauze pads and adhesive dressings;
- Disposable latex or vinyl gloves;
- Tourniquet, Vacutainer or similar vacuum blood collection devices, or disposable syringes and needles;
- Vacutainer or sterile screw-cap tubes (or cryolubes if inculcated) and blood culture bottles (50 ml for adults, 25 ml for children) with appropriate media;
- Labels and indelible marker pen

Method of collection

Full infection control measures must be taken, with gowns, gloves, masks and boots, for suspected viral hemorrhage fever (e.g. Lassa fever or Ebola).

- Place a tourniquet above the venepuncture site. Disinfect the tops of blood culture bottles.
- Palpate and locate the vein. The venepuncture site must be meticulously disinfected with 10% povidone iodine or 70% alcohol by swabbing the skin concentrically from the centre of the venepuncture site outwards. Let the disinfectant evaporate. Do not palpate the vein again. Perform venepuncture.
- If using conventional disposable syringes withdraw 5–10 ml of whole blood from adults, 2–5 ml from children and 0.5–2 ml from infants. Using aseptic technique, transfer the specimen to the appropriate cap transport tubes and culture bottles. Secure cap tightly.
- If using a vacuum system, withdraw the desired amount of blood directly into each transport tube and culture bottle.
- Remove the tourniquet. Apply pressure to site until bleeding stops, then apply dressing.
- Label the tube, including the unique patient identification number, using indelible marker pen.
- Do not recap used sharps (e.g. needle devices, scalpels or lancets). Discard directly into the sharps disposal container.
- Complete the case investigation and the laboratory request forms using the same identification number.

Handling and transport

- Blood specimen bottles and tubes should be transported upright and secured in a screw-cap container or in a rack in a transport box. They should have enough absorbent paper around them to soak up all the liquid in case of spill.
- For serum samples (e.g. measles), the blood cells must be separated from serum. Let the clot retract for 30 minutes. then centrifuge at 2000 rpm for 10–20 minutes and pour off the serum. If no centrifuge is available, place the sample in a refrigerator overnight (at least 1–6 hours) and pour off the serum for transport in a clean glass tube.
- Do not separate blood from senun in cases of suspected viral haemorrhagic fever unless you are a clinician or laboratory technician experienced in management of the disease. Full protection and infection control measures must be taken.
- If the specimen will reach the laboratory within 24 hours, most pathogens can be recovered from blood cultures transported at ambient temperature. Keep at 4–8°C for longer transit periods, unless the bacterial pathogen is cold-sensitive.

B. Faecal Specimen Collection

Stool specimens are most useful for microbiological diagnosis if collected soon after onset of diarrhoea (for bacteria <4 days), and preferably before the initiation of antibiotic therapy. If required, two or three specimens can be collected on separate days. Stool is the preferred culture specimen for cholera or shigellosis.

Materials for Collection

- Tubes with Cary-Blair transport medium
- Clean, dry, leak-proof, screw-cap container and tape if Cary-Blair transport medium is not available.
- Appropriate bacterial transport media for transport of rectal swabs from infants (ideally Cary-Blair).
- Parasitology transport pack: 10% formalin, polyvinyl isopropyl alcohol

Note: Rapid diagnostic tests (RDTs) are available for cholera and shiga-toxin-producing *E. coli* and *Shigella*.

Method of Collecting a Stool Specimen

If Cary-Blair transport medium is available:

- Place sterile swab in freshly passed stool to allow it soak up stool.
- Place swab in the Cary-Blair transport medium inside the tube
- Break off the top part of the stick without touching the tube and tighten the screw cap firmly;
- Label the specimen tube.

If Cary-Blair transport medium is not available, collect freshly passed stool: 5 ml liquid or 5 g solid (pea-size—in a container. Label the container.

If RDTs are available, follow the manufacturer's instructions; in general, each kit contains a buffer solution in which the fresh stool is suspended immediately before testing.

Method of Collecting a Rectal Swab from Infants

To collect a rectal swab from an infant:

- Moisten a swab in sterile saline;
- Insert the swab tip just past the anal sphincter and rotate gently;
- Withdraw the swab and examine to ensure that the cotton tip is stained with faeces;
- Place the swab in a sterile tube or container containing the appropriate transport medium, unless RDTs are available (in which case, follow the manufacturer's instructions);
- Break off the top part of the stick without touching the tube and tighten the screw cap firmly;
- Label the specimen tube.

Handling and Transport

Stool specimens should be transported in a cold box at 4–8°C. Bacterial yields may fall significantly if specimens are not processed within 1–2 days of collection. *Shigella* is particularly sensitive to elevated temperatures. If transport medium is not available, do not allow specimen to dry: add a few drops of 0.85% sodium chloride solution.

C. Cerebrospinal Fluid Specimen Collection

The specimen of cerebrospinal fluid (CSF) must be taken by a physician or a person experienced in the procedure. CSF is used in the diagnosis of bacterial meningitis and encephalitis.

Materials for Collection

A lumbar puncture tray should be used that includes:

- Sterile materials—gloves, cotton wool, towels or drapes;
- Local anaesthetic, needle and syringe;
- Skin disinfectant 10% povidone iodine or 70% isopropanol;
- Two lumbar puncture needles—small bore with stylet;
- Six small sterile screw-cap tubes and tube rack;
- Water manometer (optional);
- Microscope slides and slide boxes.

Method of Collection

Only experienced personnel should be involved in the collection of CSF samples; hence, the method is not described here. CSF is collected directly into the separate screw-cap tubes. If the sample is not to be promptly transported, separate samples should be collected for bacterial and viral processing.

Handling and Transport

In general, specimens should be delivered to the laboratory and processed as soon as possible.

CSF specimens for bacteriology are transported at ambient temperature, generally without transport medium. They must never be refrigerated, because the relevant pathogens do not survive well at low temperatures.

Rapid Diagnostic Tests

Several commercial kits are available, based on the direct detection of *N. meningitidis* antigens in CSF by latex agglutination tests. Follow the manufacturer's instructions precisely when using these tests. For best results, test the supernatant of the centrifuged CSF sample as soon as possible. If immediate testing is not possible, the sample can be refrigerated (at 2–8°C) for up to several hours, or frozen at –20°C for longer periods (note: Latex suspensions should never be frozen). Reagents should be kept at 2–8°C when not in use. Product deterioration occurs at higher temperatures, especially in tropical climates, and test results may become unreliable before the expiry date of the kit. Also, some kits have a working temperature range, and tropical temperatures may be above the recommended upper limit.

Appendix 6.3: Suggested case definitions and alert thresholds

Disease	*Case definition and information*	*Alert criteria*
Suspected acute flaccid paralysis (poliomyelitis)	Any child <15 years with acute flaccid paralysis OR Any paralytic illness in a person of any age if poliomyelitis is suggested	One case
Acute haemorrhagic fever syndrome	Acute onset of fever of less than 3 weeks duration in a severely ill patient *and two* of the following signs. • Haemorrhagic or purpuric rash • Bleeding from the nose (epistaxis) • Vomiting blood (haematemesis) • Coughing up blood (haemoptysis) • Blood in stools • Other haemorrhagic symptom and absence of predisposing host factors for haemorrhagic manifestations	One case
Suspected measles	Any person with fever and maculopapular (non-vesicular) generalized rash *and one* of the following cough, runny nose (coryza) or red eyes (conjunctivitis) OR Any person in whom a clinician suspects measles	One case
Suspected cholera/ acute watery diarrhoea (AWD)	Any person 5 years or older with severe dehydration or death caused by acute diarrhoea (three or more abnormally loose or fluid stools in the past 24 hours) During a cholera epidemic, any person 2 years or older with acute diarrhoea (three or more abnormally loose or fluid stools in the past 24 hours), with or without dehydration	One case
Acute jaundice	Acute onset of jaundice (yellowing of whites of eyes or skin or dark urine) and severe illness with or without fever and the absence of any known precipiting factors	Five or more cases in one location OR Double the weekly average number of cases seen in the previous 3 weeks for a particular location

(Contd...)

Disease	*Case definition and information*	*Alert criteria*
Suspected meningitis	Any person with sudden onset of fever (>38.0°C axillary) *and one* of the following signs. • Neck stiffness • Altered consciousness • Petechial or porpural rash • Other meningeal signs (severe neck stiffness causing causing the patient's hip and knees to flex when the neck is fixed, severe stiffness of the hamstrings causing inability to straighten the leg when the hip is flexed 90°) In children <1 year, meningitis is suspected when fever is accompained by a buldging fontanel	One case in a crowed camp setting OR Population >30,000—five cases per 100,000 people per week Population <30,000—two cases per week in endemic countries of the meningitis belt of Africa
Suspected shigellosis/bloody diarrhoea	A person with diarrhoea (three or more abnormally loose or fluid stools in the past 24 hours) with visible blood in stool (preferably observed by the clinician)	Five or more cases in one location or double the weekly average number of cases seen in the previous 3 weeks for a particular location
Confirmed malaria	Positive laboratory confirmation by blood smear or rapid diagnostic test for malaria	Twice the average number of cases seen in the previous 3 weeks for a particular location
Acute haemorrhagic fever syndrome	Acute onset of fever of less than 3 weeks duration in a severly ill patient *and two* of the following signs. • Haemorrhagic or purpuric rash • Bleeding from the nose (epistaxis) • Vomiting blood (haematemesis) • Coughing up blood (haemoptysis) • Blood in stools • Other haemorrhagic symptoms and absence of predis posing host factors for haemorrhagic manifestations	One case

Appendix 6.4: Sample health facility outbreak monitoring line-listing form

Case no.	*Age*	*Address*	*Sex (M/F)*	*Date of onset (dd/mm/yy)*	*Lab specimen taken[1] and lab register number*	*Treatment given*	*Outcome[2, 3]*	*Final diagnosis*

[1] Laboratory specimens: B = Blood, S = Stool, C = CSF, U = Urine, O = Other

[2] Outcome: I = Currently ill, R = Recovering or recovered, D = Died

[3] Known contact with previously identified case (1st case no.)

Appendix 6.5: Sample outbreak investigation form

Report completed by: ....

District or area: ....

Health facility: ....

Date: ..../.........../........................

Town, village, settlement or camp:

....

Agency:

....

Name of reporting officer and when received

....

Brief summary of the initial report

....

....

....

Suspected disease or syndrome (tick one item only)	Symptoms and signs (you can tick several items)
• Suspected measles • Suspected meningitis • Acute jaundice syndrome • Acute flaccid paralysis (AFP)/suspected poliomyelitis/suspected cholera/AWD • Suspected shigellosis/bloody diarrhoea • Confirmed malaria • Other	• Fever • Rash • Other skin lesion (specify ....) • Neck stiffness • Convulsions or seizures • Altered level of consciousness • Jaundice (yellowing of eyes and/or skin) • Muscle weakness • Acute watery diarrhoea • Bloody diarrhoea • Dehydration • Vomiting • Bleeding (specify location ....) • Cough • Malaria rapid diagnostic test positive • Other (specify): .... **Total number of cases reported:** **Actions taken:**

Appendix 6.6: Evaluating public health surveillance systems

Evaluation of public health surveillance systems aims to ensure that problems are identified and addressed. It is important for ensuring data standards and that data exchange is occurring to facilitate the response of public health systems to emerging health threats. The information given below has been adapted from CDC guidelines on evaluating surveillance system.[1]

The activities include gathering credible evidence about the system's performance. The evaluation should:

- Indicate the level of usefulness by describing the actions taken in response to analysis and interpretation of the data from the public health surveillance system;
- Characterize the implementing partners that have used tile data to make decisions and take actions;
- Describe each of the following system attributes:
  - *Simplicity*
    Does the system's structure and ease of operation meet the objectives? Create a chart describing the flow of data and the lines of response.
  - *Flexibility*
    Can the system adapt to changing inflammation needs or operating conditions with little additional time, personnel or allocated funds'?
  - *Data quality*
    Are data complete and valid? Examining the percentage of 'unknown' or 'blank' responses to items on surveillance forms provides a straightforward measure of data quality.
  - *Acceptability*
    Are staff and NGOs willing to participate in the surveillance system?
  - *Sensitivity*
    At the level of case reporting, what proportion of cases of a disease is detected by the surveillance system? At the system level, can the system detect outbreaks, including monitoring changes in the number of cases over time?
  - *Predictive value positive*
    What is the proportion of reported cases that actually have a disease of outbreak potential?
  - *Representativeness*
    Is the system describing the outbreak over time and its distribution in the population by place and person?
  - *Timeliness*
    How fast is the transfer of information between steps in the alert and surveillance system?
    Does it meet the decision-making timeline demands for the emergency?
  - *Stability*
    Is the system reliable (i.e. can it collect, manage and provide data properly without failure) and available (can it be operational when it is needed)?

References

1. Managing epidemics: Key facts about major deadly diseases. Geneva: World Health Organization; 2018. License: CC BY-NC-SA 3.0 IGO. CIP data are available at http://apps.who.int/iris.
2. Connolly MA (Ed). Communicable disease control in emergencies—A field manual. WHO, 2005 (http://www.who.int/diseasecontrol_emer gencies/publications/9241546166/en/index.html,.
3. WHO–SEAR. Regional Framework on Operational Partnerships for Emergency Response (South-East Asia Region), November 2017. http://www.searo.who.int/entity/emergencies/regionalframe work.pdf
4. Michael B Gregg (Ed). Field epidemiology, (3rd edn.) 2008, Published by Oxford University Press, Inc.198 Madison Avenue, New York 10016.
5. Government of India. Regional Field Epidemiology Training Programme for Health Personnel of South-east Asia Region, National Centre for Disease for Control (Directorate General of Health Services) 22-Shamnath Marg, Delhi 110 054 India.
6. WHO. Disease control in humanitarian emergencies: Outbreak surveillance and response in humanitarian emergencies: WHO guidelines for EWARN implementation.2012. WHO/HSE/GAR/DCE/2012.1. available at http://apps.who.int/iris/bitstream/handle/10665/70812/WHO_HSE_GAR_DCE_2012_1_eng.pdf;
7. Field epidemiology Training program development Handbook. Atlanta, GA: US Centers for Disease Control and Prevention. 2006. https://www.cdc.gov/globalhealth/healthprotection/fetp/pdf/fetp_development_handbook_508.pdf
8. Government of India. National Risk Communication Plan, 2016. Epidemiology Division, National Centre for Disease Control Directorate General of Health Services, Ministry of Health and Family Welfare, New Delhi.
9. Guidelines for the Investigation and Control of Disease Outbreaks. Porirua: Institute of Environmental Science and Research Limited; Updated 2011, published in 2012 available at www.esr.cri.nz.
10. Outbreak surveillance and response in humanitarian emergencies: WHO guidelines for EWARN implementation 2012.

Chapter
7

Measures in Epidemiology

Ram Chandra Goyal

"I often say that when you can measure what you are speaking about, and express it in numbers, you know something about it; but when you cannot express it in numbers, your knowledge is of a meager and unsatisfactory kind; it may be the beginning of knowledge, but you have scarcely, in your thoughts, advanced to the stage of Science, whatever the matter may be."

— Lord Kelvin (quoted in Kenneth Rothman, Modern Perspectives in Epidemiology, 1st edn. Boston, Little Brown, 1986, pg 23)

Measure is a number or quantity, size, amount that records a directly observable value or performance by using an instrument or device marked in standard units.

There are two critical areas in measurement. First, measurement allows researchers to quantify abstract constructs and variables. Second, the level of statistical sophistication used to analyze data derived from a study is directly dependent on the scale of measurement used to **quantify the variables of interest**.

There are two basic categories of data—non-metric and metric. **Non-metric data** (also referred to as **qualitative data**) are typically attributes, characteristics, or categories that describe an individual and cannot be quantified. **Metric data** (also referred to as **quantitative data)** exist in differing amounts or degrees, and they reflect relative quantity or distance. Metric data allow researchers to examine amounts and magnitudes, while non-metric data are used predominantly as a method of describing and categorizing.

Variables or events can also be classified in **dichotomous and polytomous. Dichotomous** has only two category, e.g. population with disease and without diseases or exposed and non-exposed; whereas **polytomous** has more than two categories, such as occupation, income, religion, blood groups. A polytomous can be again divided into **nominal and ordinal.**

A careful and accurate measurement of disease occurrence (morbidity and mortality) is fundamental basis of studies. Studies are designed to describe and compare disease trends; identify disease determinants; and evaluate public health interventions aimed at prevention and health problems. The measure in epidemiology depends on purpose of the measurement, availability of data and the phenomenon under study. Figure 7.1 shows outcomes of a phenomenon under the epidemiological study.

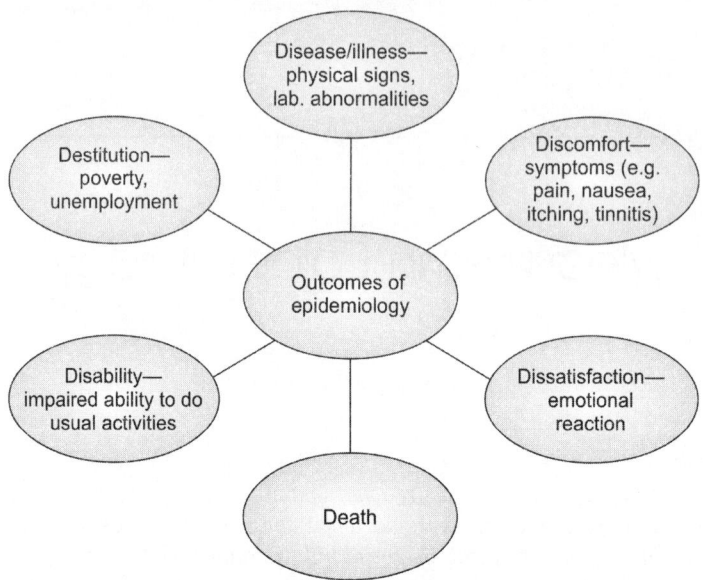

Fig. 7.1: Outcomes of epidemiology

Types of the epidemiological measure:
- Measures of frequency
- Measures of association
- Measures of impact

Measurement of Frequency

Measures of disease frequency in mathematical quantity can be analyzed in terms of count, proportion (percentage), rate and ratio. Incidence, prevalence, and mortality rates are three frequency measures that are used to characterize the occurrence of health events in a population.

Counts are the most basic measure and easy to calculate, it is an absolute number of persons who have disease or characteristic of interest. It is helpful for health planners and administrators for allocation of resources. It is used for surveillance of infectious disease for early detection of epidemics/outbreaks.

RATIO, RATE AND PROPORTION (PERCENTAGES)[1]

The rate, ratio and proportion compares one part of the distribution/frequency to another part of the distribution/frequency, or to the entire distribution/some of frequency (Fig. 7.2, Box 7.1 and Table 7.1).

RATIO ('part-to-part' and 'part-to-whole')

It can be obtained by dividing the frequency of one event, characteristic part by the frequency of another event, characteristic, parts or it is the relative magnitude of two quantities or a comparison of any two values. It is calculated by dividing one interval- or ratio-scale variable by the other. Therefore, one could compare like with unlike, e.g. male–female ratio, doctor–population ratio, child–women ratio, etc. Remember, in a ratio, numerator is not a part of denominator and no multiplier is used.

$$\text{Method for calculating a ratio} = \frac{\text{Number or rate of events, items, persons, etc. in one group}}{\text{Number or rate of events, items, persons, etc. in another group}}$$

After the numerator is divided by the denominator, the result is often expressed as the result 'to one' or written as the result. For example, 2:1, 1:1, 20:80, 50:50, etc.

What do the numbers in fractions mean?

Let's have a look at our pie again:

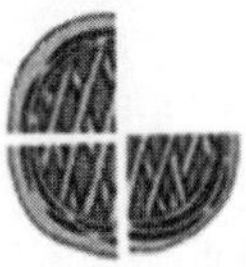

$\frac{3}{4}$

The top number shows how many pieces we have of the whole pie. Here, we have 3 pieces or parts. this is called the numerator.

The bottom number shows how many pieces there are in the whole pie. Here the whole is split into 4 pieces or parts. This is called the denominator.

$$\frac{\text{Numerator}}{\text{Denominator}} \times 10^n$$

Numerator = Upper portion of a fraction (how many parts you have)

Denominator = Lower portion of a fraction (how many total parts)

The fraction (numerator/denominator) can be multiplied by 1, 10, 100, so on.

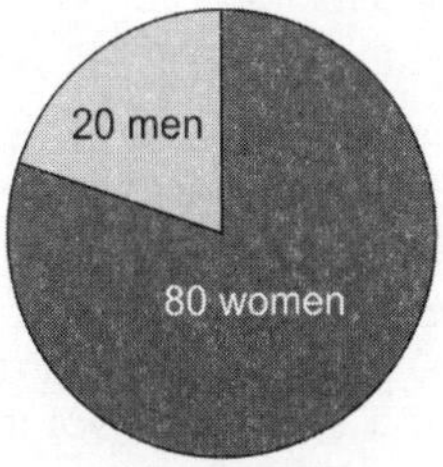

Ratio = 20:80

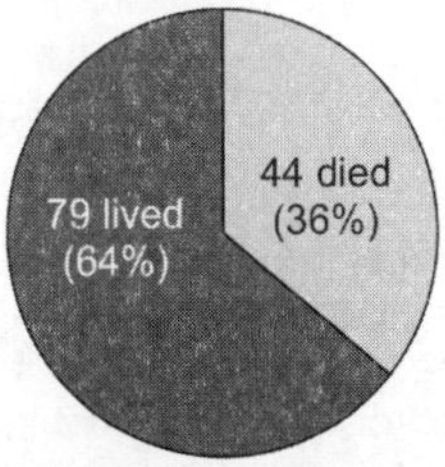

Proportions of lived = 0.64

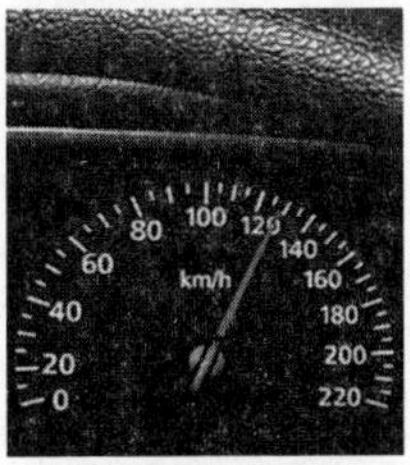

Rate = 130 km/h

Fig. 7.2: Numerator and denominator

Table 7.1: Epidemiologic measures categorized as ratio, proportion, or rate[2]

Condition	*Ratio*	*Proportion*	*Rate*
Morbidity (disease)	Risk ratio (relative risk) Rate ratio Secondary attack rate Odds ratio Period prevalence	Attack rate (incidence proportion) Point prevalence Attributable proportion	Person-time incidence rate
Mortality (death)	Death-to-case ratio	Proportionate mortality	Crude mortality rate Case-fatality rate Cause-specific mortality rate Age-specific mortality rate Maternal mortality rate Infant mortality rate
Natality (birth)			Crude birth rate Crude fertility rate

Example A: Calculating a ratio—different categories of same variable

In 2017, a village survey on diabetes was done among 25–60 years of age group 2000 persons and they categorized as diabetics and non-diabetics. The results are summarized as follows.

Total diabetics were 200 and non-diabetics 1800.

Ratio between diabetics to non-diabetics = 1800/200 = 9:1

Example B: Calculating ratios for different variables

In Nagpur (India), infant mortality rate in 2015 was 25 per 1,000 live births. Goa (India), infant mortality rate in 2015 was 10 per 1,000 live births. Calculate the ratio of the infant mortality rate in Nagpur to that in Goa.

25/10 = 2.5:1, Thus, Nagpur's infant mortality rate was 2.5 times as high as Goa's infant mortality rate in 2015.

Box 7.1: Measures of disease frequency at a glance[2]

Count

The number of individuals who meet the case definition, e.g. 400 cases of malaria in a PHC in 2015. Calculating the magnitude of disease occurrence with a count is simple and useful for certain purposes, such as allocating health resources. For other purposes, it is more helpful to have a denominator under the count that indicates the size of the study population. The remaining four measures address this.

Proportion (A/(A + B))

The fraction in which the numerator (A) includes only individuals who meet the case definition and the denominator totals the numbers of individuals who meet the case definition plus those in the study population who do not meet the case definition and are at risk. A proportion is not dependent upon time. It may be expressed as a fraction or a percentage. A proportion indicates the fraction of the population that is affected by the disease or condition. It is linked to estimating risk. For example, 60% of females over 30 years of age have been screened for breast cancer.

Ratio (A/B)

A special fraction in which the numerator includes only individuals who meeting one criterion (e.g. the case definition) and the denominator includes only individuals in the study population who meet another criterion (e.g. do not meet the case definition but are at risk). A ratio is not dependent upon time. A ratio as a measure of disease frequency is used infrequently, in special situations. (Not to be confused with an odds ratio or risk ratio).

Rate

A fraction in which the numerator includes only individuals who meet the case definition and the denominator includes individuals in the study population who do or do not meet the case definition but could meet the case definition (at risk). A rate is dependent upon time. In other words, a proportion over a particular period of time. An epidemiologic rate will contain the following—disease frequency (numerator), unit of population size, and the time period during which the event occurred. For example, 65 cases of breast cancer per 10,000 populations in a district 'A' during 2016.

Risk

The probability of an individual meeting the case definition (person-time rate). Risk is dependent upon time. For example, 0.0065 breast cancer cases per person-year (typically derived from a cohort study in which each at risk person is followed over time until he/she is no longer at risk).

Uses of Ratios

- In epidemiology, ratios are generally used to describe the event, e.g. women child ratio, dependent *vs* independent elderly.
- It is also used in analytical epidemiology to calculated for occurrence of illness, injury, or death between two groups—odds ratio (OR), relative risk (RR).
- Ratio is also in demography to describe various situations.

Types of Ratios

There are various types of ratio used in health economics, e.g. profitability ratios, coverage ratios, turnover ratios, financial ratios, compounded ratio, duplicate ratio (the ratio of two equal ratios), triplicate ratio (the ratio of three equal ratios), sub-duplicate ratio, sub-triplicate ratio, reciprocal ratio, ratio of equalities, etc. However, ratios in epidemiology are **proportions and rates**.

Proportions are ratios in which the numerator is 'contained in' or 'part of' the denominator. The statement that 10% of the population of age 60 or above expresses a proportion, since people age 60 and above are a fractional component of the population. Because the numerator is a fractional component of the denominator, a proportion can range only between 0 and 1, inclusive. Proportions are often expressed as percentages, but any **scaling factor** can be used for better expression and better to express. For example, the proportion 0.00010 would often be expressed as 1.0 per 10,000 or 10 per 100,000.

RATE

Rate is basically a proportion. It is an expression of a change in one quantity to a change in another quantity, with the time as denominator.

Types of rates:

i. Crude rates (unstandardized rates): Actual observed frequency of an event is expressed in terms of rates, e.g. crude birth rate, crude death rate, etc.
ii. Specific rates: Observed frequency is expressed in terms of rate due to:
   a. Specific cause (TB, typhoid)
   b. Specific sex (male, female)
   c. Specific age (under 5 years, 5–15 years, 15–45 years),
   d. Specific time period (annual, monthly, weekly).
iii. Standardized rates: These rates are obtained by direct or indirect method of standardization or adjustment by age, sex, and called age and sex standardized rates.

Rate is a measure, quantity, or frequency, typically one measure against another measure or quantity with time. In epidemiology, a rate is defined as a measure of the frequency with which an event occurs in a defined population over a specified period of time. Rates are particularly useful for comparing disease frequency in different locations, at different times, or among different groups of persons with potentially different sized populations. A rate is also called a measure of risk.

The basic formula for a rate is as follows:

$$\text{Rate} = \frac{\text{Population at risk during the same time period}}{\text{Number of cases or events occurring during a given time period}} \times 10^n$$

PROPORTION

Proportion is the relation of frequency of one part to the frequency of the whole (total). A proportion also has a numerator and a denominator; however, in contrast to ratio, the numerator is also include in the denominator in a proportion. The 'proportion' gives the idea of an important measure in research methodology—the 'probability'.

In epidemiology, proportions are frequently used as descriptive measures, e.g. in a research study, one could calculate the proportion of study subjects enrolled among all those who qualify eligibility criteria.

Proportions are also used to describe the magnitude of the problem or amount of disease that can be attributed to a particular exposure.

A proportion may be expressed as a decimal, a fraction, or a percentage (proportions multiplied by 100 to make it percentage).

Method for calculating a proportion:

$$\text{Proportion} = \frac{\text{Number of persons or events with a particular characteristic}}{\text{Total number of persons or events, of which the numerator is a subset}} \times 10^n$$

For a proportion, 10^n is usually 100 (or n = 2) and is often expressed as a percentage

$$\text{Proportion} = \frac{\text{Number of under-nourished children at a certain time}}{\text{Total number of children in an area at the same time}} \times 100$$

STANDARDIZATION OF RATES AND RATIOS[3–6]

Virtually every large population is heterogeneous in regard to socio-demographic (e.g. age, gender, education, religion), geographic, genetic, occupational, dietary, medical history, and innumerable other personal attributes and environmental factors related to health. A population can be viewed as a composite of diverse subgroups (ultimately, subgroups of size one, i.e. individuals, but epidemiologic measures break down at that point). Any overall measure or statistic reflects the value of that measure for each of the subgroups comprising the population.

An overall measure that does not take explicit account of the composition of the population is called **crude**. Its value will be an average of the values for the individual subgroups, weighted by the irrelative sizes. The larger the subgroup, the more influence it will have on the crude measure (i.e. 'democracy'). Thus, the death rate for a population is a weighted average of the death rates for its component subgroups.

Suppose, we consider a population of size N as consisting of five age groups, or **strata**. Each age **stratum** will have a specific number of people, say n_i (i = 1 to 5).

During the following year, each stratum will experience some number of deaths, say *di*. The total population size, N, is therefore Σn_i, the total number of deaths, D, is Σd_i, and the crude mortality rate is D/N, which can also be written as a weighted average of the **stratum-specific mortality rates**, d_i/n_i.

$$\frac{D}{N} = \frac{\Sigma d_i}{N} = \frac{\Sigma n_i (d_i / n_i)}{N}$$

$$= \Sigma\,(n_i/N)\,(d_i/n_i) = \Sigma w_i\,(d_i/n_i)$$

where w_i are the weights (note that $\Sigma w_i = \Sigma(n_i/N) = (\Sigma n_i)/N = \Sigma n_i/\Sigma n_i = 1$).

The crude rate is the simplest summary of the population experience. But mortality is strongly related to age, so the stratum-specific mortality rates will differ greatly from one another. The summary provided by the crude rate glosses over this heterogeneity of stratum specific mortality rates. This issue is particularly relevant when we compare rates across populations or time periods, because if the populations differ in composition, then at least some of what we observe may be attributable to these differences.

ADJUSTMENT AND STANDARDIZATION

The terms 'adjustment' and 'standardization' both refer to procedures for facilitating the comparison of summary measures across groups. Such comparisons are often complicated by differences between the groups in factors that influence the measures of interest but which are not the focus of attention. Adjustment attempts to remove the effects of such 'extraneous' factors that might prevent a 'fair' comparison.

'Adjustment', the more general term, encompasses both standardization and other procedures for removing the effects of factors that distort or *confound* a comparison. Standardization refers to methods of adjustment based on weighted averages in which the weights are chosen to provide an 'appropriate' basis for the comparison (i.e. a 'standard'), generally the number of persons in various strata of one of the populations in the comparison, an aggregate of these populations, or some external relevant population.

Two populations may have the same overall size and identical age-specific death rates, but different total numbers of deaths and different overall death rates, due to differences in their age distributions. Standardization (and other adjustment procedures) seeks to provide numbers and comparisons that minimize the influence of age and/or other extraneous factors.

There are several techniques for adjusting age-specific rates. Among them are direct and indirect standardization (Wolfenden, 1923), the geometric mean (Schoen, 1970), equivalent average death rates (Hill, 1977), life table rates, Yerushalmy's index (Yerushalmy, 1951), cumulative death rates (Breslow and Day, 1981), absolute probabilities of death and the comparative mortality index (Peto *et al.*, 1994; Breslow and Day, 1980, 1981, 1987; Esteve *et al.*, 1994).

There are two most common approaches to standardizing a rate:

1. Direct standardization
2. Indirect standardization.

HISTORY OF DIRECT STANDARDIZATION[7]

By the middle of the nineteenth century, public health practitioners in England had began to recognize that simple crude rates were inappropriate summary measures for comparing population health when the age distribution of the geographic areas were markedly different. Discussions centered around the development of a summary mortality index free from the effect of age differences. In a paper he read to the Statistical

Society of London, Sir Edwin Chadwick, one of the early public health reformers in England, proposed the use of 'the mean age at death' as a summary measure for comparing the health condition of the various 'sanitary districts' around London (Finer, 1952; Lewis, 1991). This index, he argued, represented a true summary of the age-specific risks of dying. In response, Neison, a practicing actuary, disagreed with Chadwick's underlying logic. He argued that since mortality increased with age, Chadwick's mean age at death for geographic areas with a relatively older population would tend to overstate excess mortality. In a subsequent article, Neison demonstrated the fallacy in Chadwick's argument by comparing the crude mean age at death with the mean age computed by a method of *direct standardization* (Neison, 1844). Neison was, thus, the first to introduce both the concepts of direct and indirect standardization, as well as the term standard population.

The Registrar General's report of 1883 was the first reported use of Neison's direct standardization method, using the 1881 population census of England and Wales as the standard (most current at the time). In subsequent reports, the standard was changed each time there was a new census, i.e. every 10 years (Woolsey *et al.*, 1959; Benjamin *et al.*, 1980). These frequent changes of the standard were cumbersome since historical rates had to be recalculated each time in order to assess current trends. As a solution, the 1901 population census was eventually adopted as a general standard in England and Wales, and remained unchanged even when a new census became available.

In order to facilitate comparison with mortality rates in England and Wales, the United States adopted the 1901 British standard. This practice continued until the early 1940s when it was decided that the difference between the US population at the time and the 1901 English population was significant enough to warrant a change in standard. As a result, the US adopted its 1940 census population (the most current at the time) as the new standard. Recently, however, there has been growing concern that the 1940 standard no longer reflects the increasingly older US age structure. In response, the National Center for Health Statistics sponsored two national workshops in 1991 and 1997 on the issue of a new US standard. The final report of these workshops recommended the adoption of a new standard based on the projected 2000 population age distribution (NCHS, 1998).

Frequently used standard populations include (Table 7.2):

1. The Segi world population
2. The European standard population based on the Swedish population
3. The WHO world standard population, which is based on world overall average projected populations 2000–2025.

Table 7.2: Standard population distribution (%)[7]

Age group (years)	*Segi ('world') standard*	*Scandinavian ('European') standard*	*WHO world standard* (average 2000–2025)*
0–4	12.00	8.00	8.86
5–9	10.00	7.00	8.69
10–14	9.00	7.00	8.60
15–19	9.00	7.00	8.47
20–24	8.00	7.00	8.22
25–29	8.00	7.00	7.93
30–34	6.00	7.00	7.61
35–39	6.00	7.00	7.15
40–44	6.00	7.00	6.59
45–49	6.00	7.00	6.04
50–54	5.00	7.00	5.37
55–59	4.00	6.00	4.55
60–64	4.00	5.00	3.72
65–69	3.00	4.00	2.96
70–74	2.00	3.00	2.21
75–79	1.00	2.00	1.52
80–84	0.50	1.00	0.91
85+	0.50	1.00	0.63
Total	**100.00**	**100.00**	**100.00**

* For purposes of comparison, the WHO Standard age group 85+ is an aggregate of the age groups 85–89, 90–94, 95–99 and 100+.

Table 7.3: Crude and age-standardized death rates (per 100,000) for heart disease in 3 selected countries (men and women combined), 2002

Country	*Crude death rate*	*Age-standardized death rate*
Brazil	79	118
Finland	240	120
USA	176	105

The age-standardization of rates eliminates the influence of different age distributions on the morbidity or mortality rates being compared. For example, there is great variation between countries in the reported crude mortality rates for heart disease as shown in Table 7.3. Finland has a crude heart disease death rate approximately three times that of Brazil, but the standardized rate is the same.

DIRECT STANDARDIZATION

Direct standardization, more commonly used, creates a summary disease rate for a population that would be expected if the study population had a *population distribution* identical to that of an arbitrarily chosen standard population. A reference population is used as the standard population. The standardized rate is the sum of weighted group-specific rates, with weights derived from the standard population. The weights sum to 1.0. A standardized rate is essentially a weighted average of the age-specific rates.

Computationally, direct standardization of rates is straightforward.

Important Consideration

There are several things to consider about the above formula and computation. First, the directly standardized rate is a weighted average. Since each W_k is the proportion that the k-th stratum is of the total standard population, the weights are simply the proportional age distribution in the standard population. The crude death rate in a population, which represents the total number of deaths divided by the total number of persons, can be regarded as an average of the population's stratum-specific death rates (R_k) weighted by its own age distribution (Box 7.2).

Similarly, a directly standardized rate corresponds to the crude rate that would be observed in the standard population if the standard population had the same stratum-specific rates as does the study population. Distribution of population and deaths for India is mentioned in Tables 7.4 and 7.5.

Reasons for Standardizing Rates

Firstly, summary indices from two or more populations are more easily compared than multiple strata of specific rates. This becomes especially important when comparing rates from several populations or when each population has a large number of strata.

Secondly, small numbers in some strata may lead to unstable specific rates. When sample populations are so small that their

Table 7.4: Indian population distribution (%) 2011 census[8]

Age group (years)	*Numbers*	*Percentages*
0–4	11,28,06,778	9.32
5–9	12,69,28,126	10.48
10–14	13,27,09,212	10.96
15–19	12,05,26,449	9.95
20–24	11,14,24,222	9.20
25–29	10,14,13,965	8.38
30–34	8,85,94,951	7.31
35–39	8,51,40,684	7.03
40–44	7,24,38,112	5.99
45–49	6,23,18,327	5.15
50–54	4,90,69,254	4.05
55–59	3,91,46,055	3.23
60–64	3,76,63,707	3.11
65–69	2,64,54,983	2.18
70–74	1,92,08,842	1.59
75–79	92,32,503	0.77
80+	1,12,89,005	0.93
Age not stated	44,89,802	0.37
All ages	**1,21,08,54,977**	**100**

Table 7.5: Distribution of deaths by age and gender in India: 2004–2006[8]

Age group	*No. of deaths*					
	Male	*%*	*Female*	*%*	*Person*	*%*
0–1	10,350	14.2	9,009	15.9	19,359	14.9
1–4	2,702	3.7	3,073	5.4	5,775	4.5
0–4	13,052	17.9	12,082	21.3	25,134	19.4
5–14	2,132	2.9	2,097	3.7	4,229	3.3
15–29	4,930	6.8	3,847	6.8	8,777	6.8
30–34	2,105	2.9	1,252	2.2	3,357	2.6
35–44	5,444	7.5	2,711	4.8	8,155	6.3
45–54	7,172	9.8	3,921	6.9	11,093	8.6
55–69	17,099	23.4	11,693	20.6	28,792	22.2
70+	21,034	28.8	19,132	33.7	40,166	31.0
Total	**72,968**	**100.0**	**56,735**	**100.0**	**1,29,703**	**100.0**

Box 7.2: Calculation of directly standardized rate

$$\text{Directly standardized rate } (R_s) = \frac{\Sigma \text{ (stratum-specific rates} \times \text{standard weights)}}{\Sigma \text{ (standard weights)}}$$

$$\text{Directly standardized rate } (R_s) = \frac{(r_1 N_1 + r_2 N_2 + r_3 N_3 + \ldots 4+ r_n N_n)}{(N_1 + N_2 + N_3 + \ldots + N_n)}$$

$$R_s = \frac{\Sigma (r_k \times N_k)}{\Sigma (N_k)} = \Sigma (r_k \times \frac{N_k}{\Sigma (N_k)} = \Sigma (r_k \times \frac{N_k}{N})$$

$$R_s = \Sigma (r_k W_k)$$

where:

r_k = rate in k-th stratum of the *study* population

N_k = number of persons in k-th stratum of the *standard* population

N = total number of persons in the *standard* population (ΣN_k)

W_k = weight for each stratum (equal to N_k/N)

Σ means summation over the k strata.

This formula shows that, when the same standard is used, if two study populations have the same age-specific rates (i.e. for each *k* their R_k's are equal), then their directly standardized rates will be identical, independent of the age distributions in the study populations.

strata contain mostly unstable rates and zeroes, the direct standardization procedure may not be appropriate and an alternate procedure becomes desirable.

Standardized Ratios and Differences

Rates that have been standardized by the direct method, using the same standard population, may be compared in relative or absolute

Example

The hypothetical data of two cities A and B corresponding to the number of deaths occurred for different age groups are given below. Compute CDR, standardized age specific death rates.

Age group	*City A*		*City B*	
	No. of death	*Population*	*No. of death*	*Population*
Under 10	645	25,000	542	30,000
10–20	262	15,000	382	28,000
20–40	1,340	56,000	1,450	81,000
40–60	1,145	35,000	1,235	39,000
Above 60	521	12,000	613	16,000

terms (i.e. as a ratio or as a difference). A 'standardized rate ratio (SRR)' can be obtained by dividing the (directly) standardized rate for place 'X' by that of place 'Y'. Using the values computed above.

SRR = directly standardized rate for place 'X'÷ directly standardized rate for place 'Y'

Similarly, the difference of the two rates would be a 'standardized rate difference'

[SRD = Place'X'– Place 'Y' (per 1,000)—the ratio has no need for the scaling factor, but the difference does].

Since the rates are virtually identical, the SRR is close to 1.0, and the SRD is close to zero, indicates that mortality experience in place 'X', place 'Y' and standard population all about the same when the differences due to age structure are eliminated.

Directly standardized rate can also be compared to the crude rate in the population from which the weights were drawn (the 'standard population') because the crude rate for a population can be expressed as a weighted average of the population's stratum-specific death rates (R_k) weighted by its own age distribution. Therefore, the crude rate and the directly standardized rates are all weighted averages based on the same set of weights (the proportional age distribution in the standard population).

SRR = Directly standardized rate for place 'X' ÷ directly standardized rate for standard population

INDIRECT STANDARDIZATION

When stratum-specific numbers are small state/city), stratum-specific rate estimates are too susceptible to be influenced by random variability for such situation an 'indirect' standardization methods are used and a 'standardized mortality ratio' ('SMR') is calculated.

The standard mortality difference = indirectly standardized rate **minus** the crude rate from the standard population.

In *direct standardization*, the study population provides the rates and the standard population provides the weights and in *indirect standardization*, the standard population provides the rates and the study population provides the weights.

Estimating Indirect Standardization

Indirect standardization can be estimated by the comparing the **'observed'** number of deaths or events in the study population to an **'expected'** number of deaths, i.e. the number of deaths that would be expected in the study population, if its mortality experience (its stratum-specific rates) were the same as for the standard population.

The **ratio of observed to expected deaths** is termed the **standardized mortality ratio** (SMR) or **standardized morbidity ratio** (SMR) (if disease, rather than death, is the outcome). The SMR indicates the relative excess or decrement in the actual mortality experience in the study population with respect to what might have been expect had it experienced the force of mortality in the standard (or reference) population (Box 7.3).

The **SMR** is usually scaled up by multiplying it by 100. An SMR over 100 indicates that more deaths were observed than expected (i.e. the study population had a relatively poor outcome). An SMR less than 100 means that fewer deaths were observed than expected (i.e. the study population had a relatively favourable outcome). Obviously, the value of the SMR will depend on the choice of the reference population used for the comparison mortality rates. If the reference population is healthy, they will have low mortality rates and thereby increase the SMR. Conversely, if the reference population is unhealthy, they will have high mortality rates and thereby decrease the SMR. It is therefore crucial to choose an appropriate reference population or at least to know in which direction the reference population differs from an appropriate one.

An indirectly standardized rate can be obtained from an SMR as follows:

Indirectly-standardized rate = SMR × (Crude death rate in the standard population)

The logic for this relationship is that the SMR gives a standardized comparison of the mortality experience in a study population compared to that in the standard population. So, if the study population has twice the mortality rate of the standard population, the standardized rate for the study population should be twice the observed (crude) death rate in the standard population.

Box 7.3: Calculating standardized mortality ratio (SMR)

We need to find out (i) expected value and (ii) observed value of death/disease, so,

i. **Expected number of deaths**
 = Σ ((Stratum-specific rates from the standard population) × (stratum sizes from the study population)) = $\Sigma (R_k \times n_k)$

ii. **Observed number of deaths** = Σd_k

Standardized mortality ratio (SMR) = Observed deaths/Expected deaths = $\Sigma d_k / \Sigma (R_k n_k)$

where d_k = number of deaths in the k-th stratum of the *study* population **(observed deaths)**

n_k = size of the k-th stratum of the *study* population

R_k = death rate in the k-th stratum of the *standard* population

Points to be Noted

Healthy worker effect: The SMR is frequently used to examine mortality in an industrial plant or industry. However, when workers are compared to the general population, it is common to find lower mortality rates in the workers (SMR less than 100). The reason is thought to be that the general population includes people who are too sick to work. The elevated mortality in such people raises the mortality rate of the general population, so that mortality in the general worker population is lower. This phenomenon is called the healthy worker effect. The healthy worker effect is an important consideration primarily for mortality from diseases, such as cardiovascular disease, where an extended period of physical limitation or disability frequently precedes death and thus affects entrance into and remaining in the workforce.

Care to be Taken While Using of SMR

- An SMR is an indirect standardization procedure and, therefore, two SMRs cannot be compared, unless their respective populations have the same age. *(If the age distributions are not markedly different or the relationships in mortality rates between the populations are similar across age strata, then the damage is not great. The latter possibility can only rarely be checked, of course, since SMRs are typically computed in situations where there are too few deaths in each stratum to calculate meaningful stratum-specific rates.)*
- SMRs do not readily translate into life-expectancy (though recent work provides an approximation).
- As length of follow-up increases, an SMR based on cumulative mortality tends toward 100.

MEASURES OF MORBIDITY

Morbidity has been defined as any departure, subjective or objective, from a state of physiological or psychological well-being. Nowadays departure from sociological well-being is also considered as social morbidity. In practice, morbidity encompasses disease, injury, and disability. In addition, it can also be used to describe the periods of illness that these persons experienced, or the duration of these illnesses. The various measures of morbidity are mentioned in Table 7.6.

Incidence

Refers to the occurrence of new cases of disease or injury in a population over a specified period of time or incidence is a measure of the number of new cases of disease that develop overtime. Persons having disease are not included in numerator. Two types of incidence are commonly used—**incidence proportion** and **incidence rate**. There are two definitions of incidence, differing only by the choice of the denominator:

$$\text{Incidence proportion} = \frac{\text{Number of new cases of disease or injury during specified period}}{\text{Population without disease at baseline (size of population at start of period)}}$$

$$\text{Incidence rate (incidence density)} = \frac{\text{Number of new cases of disease or injury during a specified period of observation}}{\text{Total person time at risk for each of the subjects observed*}}$$

* Person time is the sum of the periods of time at the time of risk for each of the subjects observed

Incidence Proportion or Risk

Incidence proportion is the proportion of an initially disease-free population that develops disease, becomes injured, or dies during a specified (usually limited) period of time. **Synonyms** include attack rate, risk, probability of getting disease, and cumulative incidence.

Incidence proportion is a proportion because the persons in the numerator (those who develop disease) are also included in the denominator (total population).

Incidence proportion measures the proportion of people who develop new disease during a specified period of time.

Calculating an Example of Incidence Proportion (risk)

There was an outbreak of food poisoning among inmates of a hostel after consuming food at a party. Table 7.7 shows the information collected after the outbreak about various foods consumed by the inmates. Find out which food item might have caused the outbreak.

a. **Attack rate:** It measures the frequency of new cases when the population is exposed to an agent for a limited period of time, such as during an epidemic. It measures the extent or magnitude of the disease during an epidemic (Fig. 7.3).

$$\text{Attack rate} = \frac{\text{Number of cases of the disease during an epidemic period}}{\text{Total people at risk of developing the disease during the same epidemic period}} \times 100$$

Table 7.6: Measures of morbidity

Measure	*Numerator*	*Denominator*
Incidence proportion (or attack rate or risk)	Number of new cases of disease during specified time interval	Population without diseases at start of time interval
Secondary attack rate	Number of new cases among contacts	Total number of contacts
Incidence rate or person time rate or incidence density	Number of new cases of disease	Person time at risk
Point prevalence	Number of current cases (new and old) at a specified point in time	Population at the same specified point in time
Period prevalence	Number of current cases (new and old) over a specified period of time	Average or mid-interval population

Table 7.7: Calculating incidence proportion (risk)

Food items	*Persons who ate*		*FSAR (a)*	*Persons who did not eat*		*FSAR (b)*	*a–b*
	Ill	*Well*	*No. of ill/total no. × 100*	*Ill*	*Well*	*No. of ill/total no. × 100*	
1. Eggs	8	4	8/12 × 100 = 66.6%	15	21	15/36 × 100 = 41.6%	+ 25%
2. Fried chicken	19	13	19/32 × 100 = 59.3%	5	13	5/18 × 100 = 27.7%	+ 31.6%
3. Chicken kheema	10	33	10/43 × 100 = 23.2%	4	2	4/6 × 100 = 66.6%	– 43.4%
4. Paneer	17	1	17/18 × 100 = 94.4	3	27	3/30 × 100 = 10.0%	+ 84.4%
5. Mashroom	12	13	12/25 × 100 = 48.0%	12	10	12/22 × 100 = 54.5%	– 6.5%
6. Potato curry	17	20	17/37 × 100 = 45.9%	8	6	8/14 × 100 = 57.1%	– 11.2%
7. Cucumber salad	9	15	9/24 × 100 = 37.5%	15	10	15/25 × 100 = 60.0%	– 22.5%
8. Rice	8	9	8/17 × 100 = 47.0%	18	13	18/31 × 100 = 58.0%	– 11%
9. Ice cream	1	2	1/3 × 100 = 33.3%	21	21	21/42 × 100 = 50.0%	–16.7%

Steps:

1. Calculate food specific attack rate (FSAR) for each item = Number of ill persons/total number of persons × 100 for those who ate food and did not ate food
2. Find-out difference between FSAR in two groups (a–b)
3. Find-out the food item for which difference is maximum, i.e. the food item which may have caused outbreak.

Note: In this case Paneer is responsible for outbreak since FSAR difference is maximum, i.e. 84%.

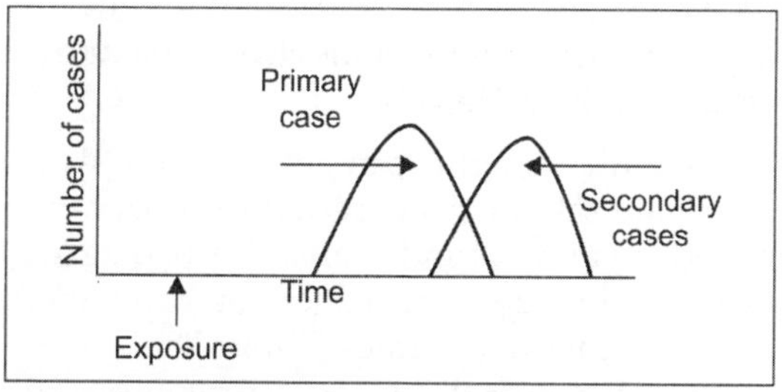

Fig. 7.3: Exposure to a factor and development of cases

b. Secondary attack rate (SAR): It is the number of exposed susceptible persons developing the disease within the range of one incubation period following exposure to the primary case.

SAR is estimated for infectious diseases (measles, influenza) in which primary case is infective only for a short period of time. It also measures the communicability of a disease.

Often, the total number of contacts in the denominator is calculated as the total population in the households of the primary cases, minus the number of primary cases. For a secondary attack rate, 10^n usually is 100%.

$$SAR = \frac{\text{Number of exposed susceptible persons developing the disease within the range of one incubation period}}{\text{Total number of exposed susceptible contacts}} \times 10^n = 100$$

Uses of SAR

- To measure the spread or communicability of an infection within family or in a closed group, e.g. hostel inmates.
- To know the communicability of a new disease.
- To evaluate the control and preventive measures, e.g. vaccination, isolation, etc.

Examples: Calculating secondary attack rates

- In an orphanage with 20 children aged 5–15 years, 2 children were protected from chickenpox as they had suffered the same before they joined the orphanage. This year, 1 child got infected with V-Z virus and suffered from chickenpox. Within 3 weeks of this incident, 15 other inmates of the orphanage got the infection and suffered from chickenpox. Calculate the secondary attack rate (SAR) of chickenpox.

$$\text{(a) SAR} = \frac{\text{No. of exposed persons developing the disease within one incubation period following exposure to primary case}}{\text{Total no. of exposed (susceptible) persons}}$$

(b) SAR = 15/17 × 100 = 86% (20−2 = 18−1 or Primary case = 17)

- Consider an outbreak of shigellosis in which 18 persons in 18 different households all became ill. If the population of the community was 1,000, then the overall attack rate was 18/1,000 × 100% = 1.8%. One incubation period later, 17 persons in the same households as these 'primary' cases developed shigellosis. If the 18 households included 86 persons, calculate the secondary attack rate.

Secondary attack rate = [17/(86−18)] × 100% = (17/68) × 100% = 25.0%

Incidence Rate or Incidence Density or Person-time Rate

Incidence rate or person-time rate is defined as a measure of incidence that incorporates time directly into the denominator. A person-time rate is generally calculated from a long-term cohort follow-up study, wherein enrollees are followed over time and the occurrence of new cases of disease is documented. Typically, each person is observed from an established starting time until one of four 'end-points' is reached: Onset of disease, death, migration out of the study ('lost to follow-up'), or the end of the study. Similar to the incidence proportion, the numerator of the incidence rate is the number of new cases identified during the period of observation.

However, the denominator differs, it represents the person time is the sum of the periods of time at the time of risk for each of the subjects observed. Thus, the incidence rate is the ratio of the number of cases to the total time the population is at risk of disease.

$$\text{Incidence rate (incidence density)} = \frac{\text{Number of new cases of disease or injury during specified period of observation}}{\text{Total person time at risk observed}}$$

* Person time is the sum of the periods of time at the time of risk for each of the subjects observed.

Choosing between Cumulative Incidence and Incidence Density

It depends on the purpose of the study (estimate rate or risk), period of observation (fixed or variable) and availability of data (e.g. fixed cohort, dynamic cohort or population, different follow-up times (Table 7.8).

Prevalence: Is the most basic of epidemiologic measures. It is like a 'still photograph'. Prevalence focuses on disease status.

Table 7.8: Two complementary measures of incidence: CI and ID

Cumulative incidence (CI) or incidence proportion	*Incidence density (ID) or incidence rate*
1. CI increases with period of observation (i.e. it is 'cumulative')	1. ID suggests ability to extrapolate over time—'duration free'
2. CI has problems with multiple events in one subject and it has variable follow-up times for subjects	2. ID accommodates multiple events in one subject and different follow-up times for subjects
3. It is not necessary to know exact time of onset of the disease	3. ID does not require a cohort to estimate or interpret
4. CI directly estimates risk	4. ID is more appropriate for aetiologic inference

Factors influencing prevalence are mentioned below.

(a)

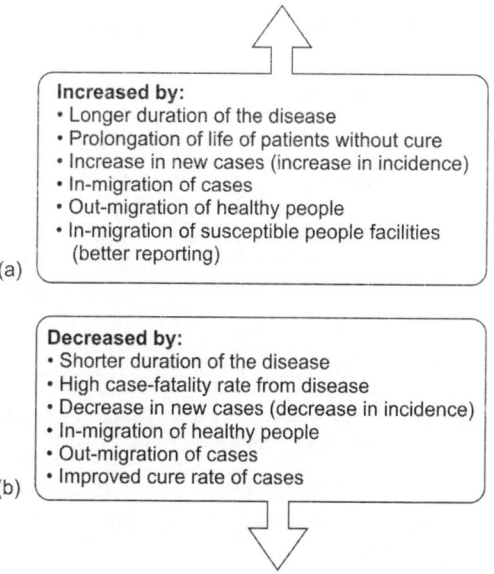

Increased by:
- Longer duration of the disease
- Prolongation of life of patients without cure
- Increase in new cases (increase in incidence)
- In-migration of cases
- Out-migration of healthy people
- In-migration of susceptible people facilities (better reporting)

(b)

Decreased by:
- Shorter duration of the disease
- High case-fatality rate from disease
- Decrease in new cases (decrease in incidence)
- In-migration of healthy people
- Out-migration of cases
- Improved cure rate of cases

Prevalence rate (PR): Measures the total number of cases (new + old) present in a specified population at a given point of time (means total case load at a specific time/period).

Types of prevalence rate: (a) Point prevalence rate, (b) period prevalence.

a. **Point prevalence rate (prevalence rate):** It is defined as the total number of all cases (new + old) of a disease/attribute in a specified population, at a given point of time. The given point, in point prevalence rate may be of one day, several days, few weeks depending upon the time survey takes to examine/interview/enumerate (count) the population/sample. **When the term 'prevalence rate' is used, without any further qualification, it means 'point prevalence rate'** only

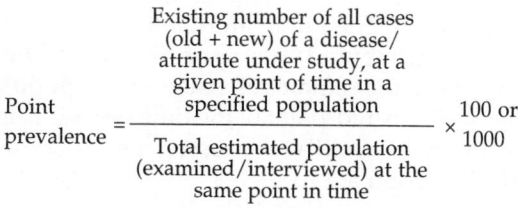

$$\text{Point prevalence} = \frac{\text{Existing number of all cases (old + new) of a disease/attribute under study, at a given point of time in a specified population}}{\text{Total estimated population (examined/interviewed) at the same point in time}} \times \text{100 or 1000}$$

b. **Period prevalence rate:** This is not used frequently. It measures the total number of existing cases (new and old) existing during a defined period of time (e.g. annual prevalence, monthly prevalence, etc.

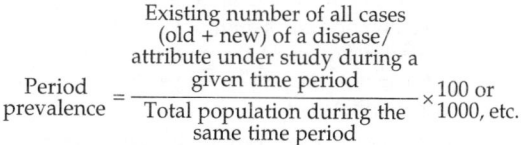

$$\text{Period prevalence} = \frac{\text{Existing number of all cases (old + new) of a disease/attribute under study during a given time period}}{\text{Total population during the same time period}} \times \text{100 or 1000, etc.}$$

Relationship of Prevalence, and Incidence

Prevalence rate of a disease depends on two factors, that is, incidence rate of a disease and duration of a disease (Fig. 7.4). If the population is stable, incidence rate and duration of a disease relationship is expressed as

Prevalence (P) = Incidence rate (I) × Duration of disease (D) or $P = I \times D$

The key difference is in their numerators.

Numerator of incidence = New cases that occurred during a given time period

Numerator of prevalence = All cases present during a given time period

Influences on the Relation of Incidence and Prevalence

The relationships among incidence, mortality, and prevalence are affected by following factors:

- Virulence of the disease.
- Healthcare available and availed
- Behaviour of people towards disease
- Competing causes of death
- Migration

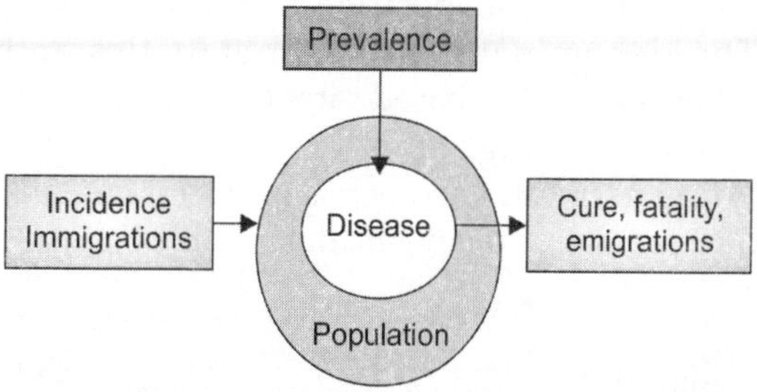

Fig. 7.4: Relationship between incidence and prevalence of disease

Table 7.9: Uses of incidence and prevalence rates

Incidence rate	*Prevalence rate*
1. To plan control and preventive measures 2. To evaluate control and preventive measures, i.e. if incidence rate of a disease is increasing after application of control and preventive measures, it indicates failure of the measures. There is a need for new measures or present measures needs modification 3. Provides research direction into a disease	1. To estimate the total magnitude of a disease in the community 2. To identify potential high-risk population 3. Useful for administrative and planning purposes. 4. To plan facilities to deal with the total magnitude of disease, e.g. number of beds, doctors, nurses, required drugs, rehabilitation facilities.

Table 7.10: Difference between incidence and prevalence

Points	*Incidence*	*Prevalence*
Numerator	Only new cases are considered	Total case load (old and new cases) forms the numerator
Denominator	Total population at risk	Total population examined
Follow-up	There is a specified time period for follow-up	No follow-up required
Rate or proportion	Rate	Proportion
Temporal relationship	Evidence of temporal relationship can be shown	No proof of temporal relationship
Money, manpower and material	Incidence more expensive	Less expensive

There are many uses of incidence and prevalence rates (Table 7.9) and difference between incidence and prevalence (Table 7.10).

MEASURES OF MORTALITY (DEATH)

A mortality rate is a measure of the frequency of occurrence of deaths in a defined population during a specified period/interval. The denominator for vital statistics and other population-based rates (e.g. death rates, birth rates, migration rates, etc.) is population estimates from the national census, SRS or other vital events data (Table 7.11).

$$\text{Mortality (death) rate} = \frac{\text{Deaths occurring during a given time period}}{\text{Size of the population among which the deaths occurred}} \times 10^n$$

Crude Mortality (Death) Rate

The crude mortality rate is the mortality rate from all causes of death in a population. It is number of deaths (from all causes, all age groups, and both sexes) in one year, in a given place/geographical area per 1000 mid-year population (means population on 1st July of that year). India's crude death rate in 2016 was 6.4/1000 mid-year population. (SRS,Vol. 51, no. 1 Sept. 2017.)

Cause-specific Mortality Rate

The cause-specific mortality rate is the mortality rate from a specified cause for a population. The numerator is the number of deaths attributed to a specific cause. The denominator remains the size of the population at the mid-point of the time period. The fraction is usually expressed per 1000 or 100,000 population.

Examples: Incidence versus prevalence

Figure represents 15 new cases of cholera over 12 months in a population of 200 persons. Each horizontal line represents one person. The down arrow indicates the date of onset of illness. The solid line represents the duration of illness. The ✹ and the ⊘ represent the date of recovery and date of death, respectively.

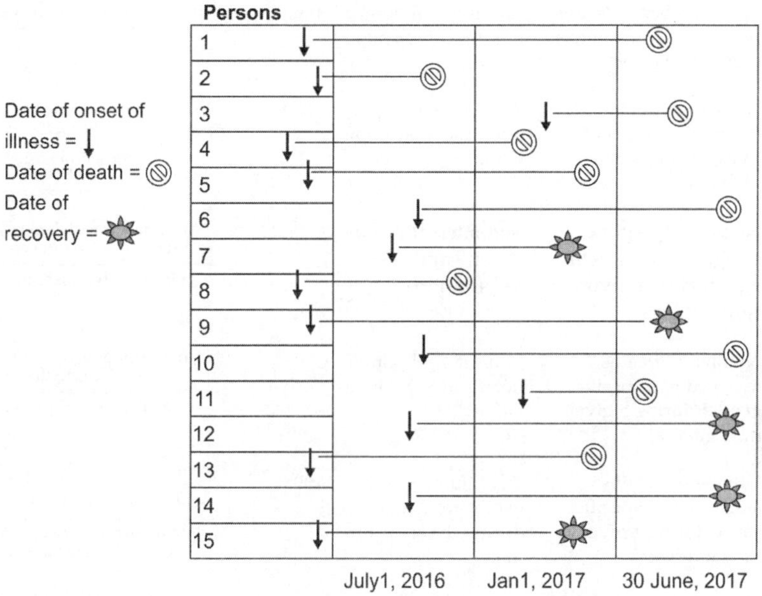

Fig. X: New cases of cholera from July 1, 2016 to June 30, 2017

Example A: Calculate the incidence rate from July 1, 2016 to June 30, 2017, using the mid-point population (population alive on Jan 1, 2017) as the denominator. Express the rate per 100 populations.

Incidence rate numerator = Number of new cases between July 1 and June 30 = 7 (the other 8 all had onsets before July 1, and are not included)

Incidence rate denominator = Jan 1, 2017 population = 198 (persons 2 and 8 died before April 1)

Incidence rate = (7/198) × 100 = 3.54 new cases per 100 population

Example B: Calculate the point prevalence on Jan 1, 2017. Point prevalence is the number of persons ill on the date divided by the population on that date. On Jan 1, 11 persons were ill.

Point prevalence = (11/198) × 100 = 5.56%

Example C: Calculate the period prevalence from July 1, 2016, to June 30, 2017. The numerator of period prevalence includes anyone who was ill any time during the period. In Fig. X, the first 10 persons were all ill at some time during the period.

Period prevalence = (15/200) × 100 = 7.5%

Age-specific Mortality Rate

An age-specific mortality rate is a mortality rate limited to a particular age group. The numerator is the number of deaths in that age group; the denominator is the number of persons in that age group in the population. Some specific types of age-specific mortality rates are neonatal, post-neonatal, infant mortality, under five mortality rates, child and adolescent mortality, etc.

Table 7.11: Frequently used measures of mortality

Measure	*Numerator*	*Denominator*	*Expressed per number at risk (10^n)*	*Formula*
Crude death (mortality) rate	Total number of deaths reported during a given time interval	Mid-interval population (mid-year population)	1000	$\frac{\text{No. of deaths during the year}}{\text{Mid-year population}} \times 1000$
Cause-specific death rate	Number of deaths assigned to a specific cause during a given time interval	Mid-interval population (mid-year population)	1000	$\frac{\text{No. of deaths assigned to a specific cause during the year}}{\text{Mid-year population}} \times 1000$
Age-specific death rates	Number of deaths assigned to a specific age during a given time interval	Mid-interval population (mid-year population)	1000	$\frac{\text{No. of deaths assigned to a specific age during the year}}{\text{Mid-year population}} \times 1000$
Gender-specific death rates	Number of deaths assigned to a specific gender during a given time interval	Mid-interval population (mid-year population)	1000	$\frac{\text{No. of deaths assigned to a specific gender during the year}}{\text{Mid-year population}} \times 1000$
Proportionate mortality	Number of deaths assigned to a specific cause during a given time interval	Total number of deaths from all causes during the same time interval	100	$\frac{\text{No. of deaths assigned to a specific cause during a given time interval}}{\text{Total number of deaths from all causes during the same time interval}} \times 100$
Death-to-case ratio	Number of deaths assigned to a specific cause during a given time interval	Number of new cases of same disease reported during the same time interval	100	$\frac{\text{No. of deaths assigned to a specific cause during a given time interval}}{\text{Total number of new cases of same disease reported during the same time interval}} \times 100$
Case fatality rate	Number of cause-specific deaths among the incident cases	Number of incident cases	100	$\frac{\text{No. of cause-specific deaths among the incident cases}}{\text{Number of incident cases}} \times 100$
Perinatal mortality rate	Number of late foetal (above 28 weeks of gestation) deaths + early neonatal deaths (0–7 days of life) during a given time interval	Total number of live births in same time interval	1000	$\frac{\text{No. of late foetal (above 28 weeks of gestation) deaths + early neonatal deaths (0–7 days of life during a given time interval}}{\text{Total number of live births in same time interval}} \times 1000$
Neonatal mortality rate	Number of deaths among children <28 days of age during a given time interval	Number of live births during the same time interval	1000	$\frac{\text{No. of deaths among children <28 days of age during a given time interval}}{\text{Number of live births during the same time interval}} \times 1000$
Post-neonatal mortality rate	Number of deaths among children 28–364 days of age during a given time interval	Number of live births during the same time interval	1000	$\frac{\text{No. of deaths among children 28–364 days of age during a given time interval}}{\text{Number of live births during the same time interval}} \times 1000$
Infant mortality rate	Number of deaths among children <1 year of age during a given time interval	Number of live births during the same time interval	1000	$\frac{\text{No. of deaths among children <1 year of age during a given time interval}}{\text{Number of live births during the same time interval}} \times 1000$

(Contd.)

Table 7.11: Frequently used measures of mortality *(Contd.)*

Measure	*Numerator*	*Denominator*	*Expressed per number at risk (10^n)*	*Formula*
Under 5 mortality rate	Number of death of children <5 years	Total number of live births in same year of age in a given time interval	1000	$\frac{\text{No. of death of children <5 years of age in a given time interval}}{\text{Number of live births during the same time interval}} \times 1000$
Maternal mortality rate	Number of deaths assigned to pregnancy-related causes during a given time interval	Number of live births during the same time interval	1000 or 100,000	$\frac{\text{No. of deaths assigned to pregnancy-related causes during a given time interval}}{\text{Number of live births during the same time interval}} \times 100{,}000$

Perinatal Mortality Rate

Perinatal period extends from 28th weeks of gestation to less than 7 days of life, after birth. This includes both late foetal deaths (stillbirths) and early neonatal deaths. The important thing to consider is the weight 1000 g and more at birth or a gestation of 28 weeks if birth weight is not available and if both weight and gestation are not available, body length (crown to heel) of at least 35 cm should be used (WHO).

The preferred criterion is birth weight. The denominator used in calculation of perinatal mortality is 1000 live births (suits nations with poor recording of still births) but for more precise comparison the denominator includes all live births weighing 1000 g or more.

Perinatal mortality is a sensitive indicator of essential maternal and newborn care provided at childbirth. The factors responsible for stillbirths and early neonatal deaths are often similar. This indicator also assumes importance in view of the fact that many of the early neonatal deaths are recorded as stillbirth in developing nations thereby inflating figures for stillbirths, but showing figures for early neonatal deaths lower than the factual. This anomaly is taken care of by perinatal mortality rate.

The perinatal period comprises just 0.5% of the average lifespan, but has more deaths in this period than next 30–40 years of life.

The national level (India), perinatal mortality rate has been estimated to be 24 per 1,000 live births and ranges from 26 in rural areas to 14 in urban areas (SRS 2017).

Neonatal Mortality Rate

The neonatal period covers birth up to but not including 28 days. The numerator of the neonatal mortality rate therefore is the number of deaths among children under 28 days of age during a given time period. The denominator of the neonatal mortality rate, like that of the infant mortality rate, is the number of live births reported during the same time period. The neonatal mortality rate is usually expressed per 1,000 live births (Table 7.12).

Post-neonatal Mortality Rate

The post-neonatal period is defined as the period from 28 days of age up to but not including 1 year of age. The numerator of the post-neonatal mortality rate, therefore, is the number of deaths among children from 28 days up to but not including 1 year of age during a given time period. The denominator is the number of live births reported during the same time period. The post-neonatal mortality rate is usually expressed per 1,000 live births.

Infant Mortality Rate

The infant mortality rate is perhaps the most commonly used measure for comparing health status among nations. It is calculated as follows.

Table 7.12: Year-wise changes in NMR, U5MR and IMR in India

Neonatal mortality rate			*Under-5 mortality rate*			*Infant mortality rate*		
Year	*Value*	*Change, %*	*Year*	*Value*	*Change,%*	*Year*	*Value*	*Change,%*
2016	25.4	– 3.79	2016	43.0	– 4.87	2016	34.6	– 4.42
2015	26.4	– 4.00	2015	45.2	– 5.24	2015	36.2	– 4.49
2014	27.5	– 3.85	2014	47.7	– 5.17	2014	37.9	– 4.53
2013	28.6	– 4.03	2013	50.3	– 5.09	2013	39.7	– 4.57
2012	29.8	– 3.56	2012	53.0	– 5.19	2012	41.6	– 4.37
2011	30.9	– 3.74	2011	55.9	– 4.93	2011	43.5	– 4.40

$$\text{Infant mortality rate} = \frac{\text{Number of deaths among children <1 year of age reported during a given time period}}{\text{Number of live births reported during the same time period}} \times 1{,}000$$

The infant mortality rate is generally calculated on an annual basis. It is a widely used measure of health status because it reflects the health of the mother and infant during pregnancy and the year thereafter. The health of the mother and infant, in turn, reflects a wide variety of factors, including access to prenatal care, prevalence of prenatal maternal health behaviours (such as alcohol or tobacco use and proper nutrition during pregnancy, etc.), postnatal care and behaviours (including childhood immunizations and proper nutrition), sanitation, and infection control.

Is the infant mortality rate a ratio? Yes. Is it a proportion? No, because some of the deaths in the numerator were among children born the previous year.

Is the infant mortality rate truly a rate? No, because the denominator is not the size of the mid-year population of children <1 year of age. India's infant mortality rate in 2016 was 34 per 1000 live births (SRS, Vol. 51, no. 1 Sept. 2017) (Table 7.12).

Under-5 Mortality Rate (U5MR) (Child Mortality Rate)

This is defined as the number of deaths in children under 5 years of age expressed as rate per 1000 live births. This rate measures the probability of dying between birth and exactly 5 years of age. This indicator is considered as the single best indicator of social development and well-being.

It has several advantages as a barometer of child well-being in general and child health in particular. First, it measures an 'outcome' of the development process rather than an 'input', such as per capita calorie availability or the number of doctors per 1,000 population—all of which are means to an end. Second, the U5MR is known to be the result of a wide variety of inputs: The nutritional status and the health knowledge of mothers; the level of immunization and oral rehydration therapy; the availability of maternal and child health services (including prenatal care); income and food availability in the family; the availability of safe drinking water and basic sanitation; and the overall safety of the child's environment, among other factors. Third, the U5MR is less susceptible to the fallacy of the average than, for example, per capita gross national income (GNI per capita) (Table 7.12).

Maternal Mortality Rate

The maternal mortality rate is really a ratio used to measure mortality associated with pregnancy. The numerator is the number of deaths during a given time period among women while pregnant or within 42 days of termination of pregnancy, irrespective of the duration and the site of the pregnancy, from any cause related to or aggravated by the pregnancy or its management, but not from accidental or incidental causes. The denominator is the number of live births reported during the same time period. Maternal mortality rate is usually expressed per 1000 or 100,000 live births. India's maternal mortality rate was 112 per 100,000 live births (NHM report 2015).

Sex-specific Mortality Rate

A sex-specific mortality rate is a mortality rate among either males or females. Both numerator and denominator are limited to the one sex.

Race-specific Mortality Rate

A race-specific mortality rate is a mortality rate related to a specified racial group. Both numerator and denominator are limited to the specified race.

Combinations of Specific mortality rates

Mortality rates can be further stratified by combinations of cause, age, sex, and/or race.

For example, in 2016, the death rate from diseases of the colon cancer among women ages 50–64 years was 50.6 per 100,000. The death rate from diseases of the colon cancer among men in the same age group was 138.4 per 100,000, or more than 2.5 times as high as the comparable rate for women.

These rates are a cause-, age-, and sex-specific rates, because they refer to one cause (diseases of the colon cancer), one age group (50–64 years), and one sex (female or male).

Age-adjusted Mortality Rate

It is defined as a mortality rate statistically modified to eliminate the effect of different age distributions in the different populations. Mortality rates can be used to compare the rates in one area with the rates in another area, or to compare rates over time. However, because mortality rates obviously increase with age, a higher mortality rate among one population than among another might simply reflect the fact that the first population is older than the second.

To eliminate the distortion caused by different underlying age distributions in different populations, statistical techniques are used to adjust or standardize the rates among the populations to be compared. These techniques take a weighted average of the age specific mortality rates, and eliminate the effect of different age distributions among the different populations. Mortality rates computed with these techniques are age-adjusted or age-standardized mortality rates (*see* under standardization of rates and ratio).

Death-to-case Ratio

The death-to-case ratio is defined as the number of deaths attributed to a particular disease during a specified time period divided by the number of new cases of that disease identified during the same time period. The death-to-case ratio is a ratio but not necessarily a proportion, because some of the deaths that are counted in the numerator might have occurred among persons who developed disease in an earlier period, and are therefore not counted in the denominator.

Example: Calculating death-to-case ratios

Between 2005 and 2015, a total of 50,000 incident cases of measles were reported. During the same decade, 10,000 deaths were attributed to measles. Calculate the death-to-case ratio.

$$\text{Death-to-case ratio} = \frac{\text{Number of deaths attributed to a particular disease during specified period}}{\text{Number of new cases of the disease identified during the specified period}} \times 10^n$$

Death-to-case ratio = 10,000/50,000 × 1 = 0.2 or 20,000/100,000 × 100 = 20 per 100

Case-fatality Rate

The case-fatality rate is the proportion of persons with a particular condition (cases) who die from that condition. It is a measure of the severity of the condition (it represents the 'killing power' of a disease). Case-fatality rate is generally used in acute infectious diseases (food poisoning, cholera, measles). Case fatality is expressed in percentage.

The case-fatality rate is a proportion, so the numerator is restricted to deaths among people included in the denominator. The time periods for the numerator and the denominator do not need to be the same. The case-fatality rate is a proportion, not a true rate. As a result, some epidemiologists prefer the term case-fatality ratio.

Example: Case-fatality rates

In an epidemic of swine flu, 500 cases were identified. 50 patients died as a result of their infections. Calculate the case-fatality rate.

$$\text{Case-fatality rate} = \frac{\text{Number of cause-specific deaths among the incident cases}}{\text{Number of incident cases}} \times 100$$

Case-fatality rate = (50/500) × 100 = 10%

Proportionate mortality

Proportionate mortality describes the proportion of deaths in a specified population over a period of time attributable to different causes. Each cause is expressed as a percentage of all deaths, and the sum of the causes must add to 100%. These proportions are not mortality rates, because the denominator is all deaths rather than the population in which the deaths occurred.

Sometimes, particularly in occupational epidemiology, proportionate mortality is used to compare deaths in a population of interest (say, a workplace) with the proportionate mortality in the broader population. This comparison of two proportionate mortalities is called a proportionate mortality ratio, or PMR. A PMR greater than 1.0 indicates that a particular cause accounts for a greater proportion of deaths in the population of interest than you might expect.

For example, construction workers may be more likely to die of injuries than the general population. However, PMRs can be misleading, because they are not based on mortality rates. A low cause-specific mortality rate in the population of interest can elevate the proportionate mortalities for all of the other causes, because they must add up to 100%. Those workers with a high injury-related proportionate mortality very likely have lower proportionate mortalities for chronic or disabling conditions that keep people out of the work-force. In other words, people who work are more likely to be healthier than the population as a whole—this is known as the **healthy worker effect**.

Survival Rate

Survival is proportion of cases that do not die in a given interval after diagnosis (and is equal to 1 fatality). The survival time is defined as the time that elapsed between diagnosis and death. Computation of survival depends upon follow-up of diagnosed patients for deaths or withdrawal from observation. There are two related approaches to the estimation of survival: The Kaplan-Meier and actuarial, or life-table, methods.

Kaplan and Meier is particularly useful when exact survival times are available, since smooth estimates of survival as a function of time since diagnosis can be obtained.

The actuarial method requires a life-table with survival times grouped usually into intervals that permit the calculation of the cumulative probability of survival at time (t_i) from the conditional probabilities of survival during consecutive intervals of follow-up time up to and including t_i (Cutler and Ederer 1958; Ederer *et al.*, 1961). Information from all cases is used in the estimation of survival, including those withdrawn due their follow-up ending owing to closure of study, and those who are lost to follow-up before the termination.

In both cases follow-up is censored before the time of the outcome event, usually the death of the patient. **'Observed survival'** is influenced not only by mortality from the disease of interest, but also by deaths from other causes. If these deaths can be identified, they can be treated as withdrawals, and the **'corrected survival'** (also referred to as **'net**

survival') calculated. Alternatively, allowance for deaths due to causes other than the disease under study is made by calculation of **'relative survival'** (Ederer *et al.*, 1961).

MEASURES OF DISABILITY

Disability is the umbrella term for impairments, activity limitations and participation restrictions, referring to the negative aspects of the interaction between an individual (with a health condition) and that individual's contextual factors (environmental and personal factors).[9]

Information on disability is an important component of health information, as it shows how well an individual is able to function in general areas of life. Along with traditional indicators of a population's health status, such as mortality and morbidity rates, disability has become important in measuring disease burden, in evaluating the effectiveness of health interventions and in planning health policy.[10]

Global Burden of Disability

There are over 1 billion people with disabilities (PWD) in the world. This corresponds to about 15% of the world's population. Disability is more common among women, older people and children and adults who are poor. PWDs face wide-spread barriers in accessing services in healthcare (including rehabilitation), education, transport and employment.

South-east Asia Region Situation

Of the WHO regions, the South-east Asia region has the second highest prevalence rate of moderate disability (16%) and the third highest prevalence rate of severe disability (2.9%). Both percentages are assumed to be underestimated as most South-east Asia region countries used an impairment-based definition rather than the ICF definition, except Indonesia and Thailand.

Defining and measuring disability, however, has been challenging. The World Health Organization (WHO) has tried to address the problem by establishing an international classification scheme known as the international classification of functioning, disability and health (ICF).

The conceptual framework of the ICF captures an individual's level of functioning in six major life domains (Flowchart 7.1—(i) cognition (understanding and communication); (ii) mobility (ability to move and get around); (iii) self-care (ability to attend to personal hygiene, dressing and eating, and to live alone); (iv) getting along (ability to interact with other people); (v) life activities (ability to carry-out responsibilities at home, work and school); (vi) participation in society (ability to engage in community, civil and recreational activities).[11,12]

Flowchart 7.1: The ICF model

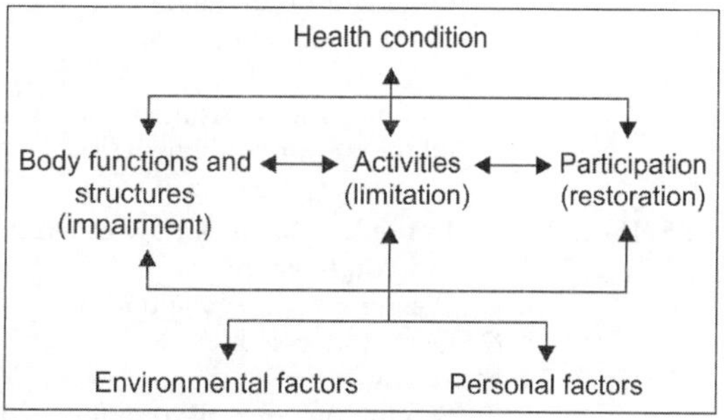

Measurement of Disability[13,14]

In World Health Organization Disability Assessment Schedule 2.0 (WHODAS 2.0) all domains were developed from a comprehensive set of ICF items and made to correspond directly with ICFs 'activity and participation' dimension (Table 7.13), which is applicable to any health condition. For all six domains, the WHODAS 2.0 provides a profile and a summary measure of functioning and disability that is reliable and applicable across cultures in adult populations.

Tables 7.14 and 7.15 depict prevalence in SEA region (2001–2010) and impairment ranking, respectively.

Table 7.13: World Health Organization Disability Assessment Schedule 2.0, 36 items over six domains with the corresponding international classification of functioning, disability and health (ICF) codes*[14,15]

Domain	*Domain question*	*ICF code*
1: Cognition	**In the last 30 days, how much difficulty did you have in:**	
1.1	Concentrating on doing something for 10 minutes	d160 Focusing attention; b140 attention functions; d110-d129 Purposeful sensory experiences
1.2	Remembering to do important things	b144 Memory functions
1.3	Analysing and finding solutions to problems in day-to-day life	d175 Solving problems; d130-d159 Basic learning
1.4	Learning a new task, for examole, learning how to get to a new place	d1551 Acquiring complex skills
1.5	Generally understanding what people say	d310 Communicating with—receiving—spoken messages
1.6	Starting and maintaining a conversation	d3500 Starting a conversation; d3501 Sustaining a conversation
2: Mobility	**In the last 30 days, how much difficulty did you have in:**	
2.1	Standing for long periods such as 30 minutes	d4154 Maintaining a standing position
2.2	Standing up from sitting down	d4104 Standing
2.3	Moving around inside your home	d4600 Moving around within the home
2.4	Getting out of your home	d4602 Moving around outside the home and other buildings
2.5	Walking a long distance such as a kilometre (or equlvalent)	d4501 Walking long distances
3: Self-care	**In the last 30 days, how much difficulty did you have in:**	
3.1	Washing your whole body	d5101 Washing whole body
3.2	Getting dressed	d540 Dressing
3.3	Eating	d550 Eating
3.4	Staying by yourself for a few days	d510-d650 Combination of multiple self-care and domestic life tasks
4: Getting along	**In the last 30 days, how much difficulty did you have in:**	
4.1	Dealing with people you do not know	d730 Relating with strangers and domestic life tasks;
4.2	Maintaining a friendship	d7500 Informal relationships with friends
4.3	Getting along with people who are close to you	d760 Family relationships; d770 Intimate relationship; d750 Informal social relationships;
4.4	Making new friends	d7500 Informal relationships with friends; d7200 Forming relationships;
4.5	Sexual activities	d7702 Sexual relationships
5: Life activities	**In the last 30 days, how much difficulty did you have in:**	
5.1	Taking care of your household responsibilites	d06 Domestic life

(Contd.)

Table 7.13: World Health Organization Disability Assessment Schedule 2.0, 36 items over six domains with the corresponding international classification of functioning, disability and health (ICF) codes*[14,15] *(Contd.)*

Domain	*Domain question*	*ICF code*
5.2	Doing most important household tasks well	d640 Doing housework; d210 Undertaking a single task; d220 Undertaking multiple tasks
5.3	Getting all the household work done that you needed to do	d640 Doing housework; d210 Undertaking a single task; d220 Undertaking multiple tasks
5.4	Getting your household work done as quickly as needed	d640 Doing household; d210 Undertaking a single task; d220 Undertaking multiple tasks
5.5	Your day-to-day work/school tasks well	d850 Remunerative employment; d830 Higher education; d825 Vocational training; d820 School education
5.6	Doing your most important work/school tasks well	d850 Remunerative employment; d830 Higher education; d825 Vocational training; d820 School education; d210 Undertaking a single task; d220 Undertaking multiple tasks
5.7	Getting done all the work that you needed to do	d850 Remunerative employment; d830 Higher education; d825 Vocational training; d820 School education d210 Undertaking a single task; d220 Undertaking multiple tasks
5.8	Getting your work done as quickly as needed	d850 Remunerative employment; d830 Higher education; d825 Vocational training; d820 School education; d210 Undertaking a single task; d220 Undertaking multiple tasks
6: Participation	**How much of a problem do you have:**	
6.1	Joining community activities	d910 Community life
6.2	Because of barriers or hindrances in the world	d9 Community, social and civic life
6.3	Living with dignity	d940 Human rights
6.4	From time spent on health condition	Not applicable (impact question)
6.5	Feeling emotionally affected	b152 Emotional functions
6.6	Because health is a drain on your financial resources	d8700 Personal economic resources
6.7	With your family facing difficulties due to your health	Not applicable (impact question)
6.8	Doing things for relaxation or pleasure by yourself	d920 Recreation and leisure

* The WHO DAS 2.0 also includes two preliminary sections that ask about demographic variables and general health. These sections are to be used if the WHO DAS 2.0 is used alone, but may be dropped or modified if WHO DAS 2.0 is used in conjunction with other instruments that already collect such information. A final optional section asks about the attributes and impact of identified problems.

Table 7.14: Estimated prevalence of disability in South-east Asia region countries during 2001–2010[16]

Country	*%*	*Year*
Bangladesh[a]	5.6	2005
Bhutan[a]	3.4	2005
Democratic People's Republic of Korea[b]	3.4	2007
India[c]	2.1	2001
Indonesia[a]	21.3	2006
Maldives[d]	4.7	2010
Myanmar[e]	2.4	2009
Nepal[a]	1.6	2001
Sri Lanka[a]	2.0	2001
Thailand[a]	2.9	2007
Timor-Leste[a]	1.5	2006

* The figures are estimated from the available data from country census or other surveys of different time periods.

Sources: [a]*World report on disability;* [b]*Disabled in Korea 2007;* [c]Census of India Reports 2001; [d]Human Rights Commission 2010; [e]Union of Myanmar 2009.

Table 7.15: Ranking of impairment/disability based on prevalence in Soutih-east Asia region countries*[16]

Country	*Rank 1 impairment*	*Rank 2 impairment*	*Rank 3 impairment*	*Rank 4 impairment*
Bhutan	Speech and hearing	Visual impairment	Mobility	Intellectual disability
Democratic People's Republic of Korea	Mobility disability	Visual impairment	Speech and hearing	Intellectual disability
India	Visual disability	Mobility impairment	Speech and hearing	Intellectual disability
Indonesia	Mobility disability	Speech and hearing	Visual impairment	Intellectual disability
Maldives	Mobility disability	Speech and hearing	Intellectual disability	Visual impairment
Myanmar	Mobility disability	Visual impairment	Speech and hearing	Intellectual disability
Nepal	Mobility disability	Speech and hearing	Visual impairment	Intellectual disability
Sri Lanka	Mobility disability	Speech and hearing	Visual impairment	Intellectual disability
Thailand	Mobility disability	Speech and hearing	Visual impairment	Intellectual disability
Timor-Leste	Visual impairment	Mobility impairment	Speech and hearing	Intellectual disability

* Information from Bangladesh is not available.

Source: Situation analysis of community-based rehabilitation in the South-east Asia region, WHO, New Delhi, 2012.

Approaches to Measurement[10–16]

Approaches to measuring disability vary across countries and influence the results. Operational measures of disability vary according to the purpose and application of the data, the conception of disability, the aspects of disability examined—impairments, activity limitations, participation restrictions, related health conditions, environmental factors—the definitions, question design, reporting sources, data collection methods, and expectations of functioning. Information on health and disability can come from a variety of sources requiring different data collection methods.

Prevalence estimates can be done by national survey and census but data cannot be compared directly with the World Health Survey or global burden of disease estimates, because there is no consistent approach across countries to disability definitions and survey questions.

The ICF can inform the data collection process across these various sources and methods, and the manner in which it is used differs accordingly. In clinical settings, the relevance of the ICF may be more apparent given the long history of implementing major coding systems (such as ICD). However, the ICF can also be used to inform population-based data collections.

Until recently, those interested in understanding functioning and disability in a population context were faced with two major challenges—(1) deciding upon an acceptable conceptualization and definition of disability; and (2) choosing an instrument designed to measure disability that effectively operationalized that definition in the population of interest. Historically available instruments produced data lacking in reliability or validity.

In the past, many low-income countries reported disability prevalence rates well under 5%, far below the rates observed in some high-income countries, commonly over 10%, some over 20%. What has been lacking is a standardized approach to the measurement of functioning and disability that would allow for the collection of valid data for use within countries as well as for international comparisons of disability statistics.

The ICF provides a framework for the definition and operationalization of disability in surveys and censuses. The World Report on Disability (WHO and WB 2011) makes specific recommendations to enhance the availability and quality of data on disability. These include the adoption of the ICF as a framework for the development of questions on disability, improved comparability of data, the development of appropriate tools (both quantitative and qualitative methodologies) to improve and expand data collection on disability, and the collection of national population census data.

SUMMARY MEASURES OF POPULATION HEALTH (SMPH)[17-19]

Regular assessment of population health is a key component of public health policy development. So far, we have seen indicators of morbidity, mortality and health states. These are useful for planning, evaluating, etc. However, if these different indicators are to be used for making comparisons of health status between 200 countries, a vast array of indicators would need to be generated and their interpretation would become extremely challenging. It would become even more unwieldy if a large number of diseases are being compared over time, across population groups, or else before and after some intervention. Summary measures of population health are measures that combine information on mortality and non-fatal health outcomes to represent the health of a particular population as a single number (Field and Gold 1998). Such 'summary figures' are called 'summary measures of population health' (SMPH).

Uses of SMPH

1. **Comparing the health of one population to the health of another population.** Such comparisons are essential to evaluate the performance of different health systems. Comparisons allow decision-makers to focus their attention on those health systems with the worst performance. In addition, they also provide the possibility of analyzing the key contributors to differences in health between populations.
2. **Comparing the health of the same population at different points in time.** Monitoring changes in health status over time is essential for the evaluation of health system performance and progress towards stated goals for a given society.

3. **Identifying and quantifying overall health inequalities within populations.**
4. **Providing appropriate and balanced attention to the effects of non-fatal health outcomes on overall population health.** In the absence of summary measures, conditions that cause decrements in function but not mortality tend to be neglected relative to conditions that primarily cause mortality.
5. **Informing debates on priorities for health service delivery and planning.** When a summary measure is combined with information on the contributions of different causes of disease and injury or risk factors to the total, such information should be a critical input to debates on the identification of a short-list of national health priorities that will consume the attention of senior managers in public health agencies and government leaders.
6. **Informing debates on priorities for research and development in the health sector.** The relative contributions of different diseases, injuries and risk factors to the total summary measure is also a major input to debate on priorities for research and development investment (World Health Organization 1996).
7. **Improving professional training curricula in public health.**
8. Analyzing the benefits of health interventions for use in cost-effectiveness analyses.

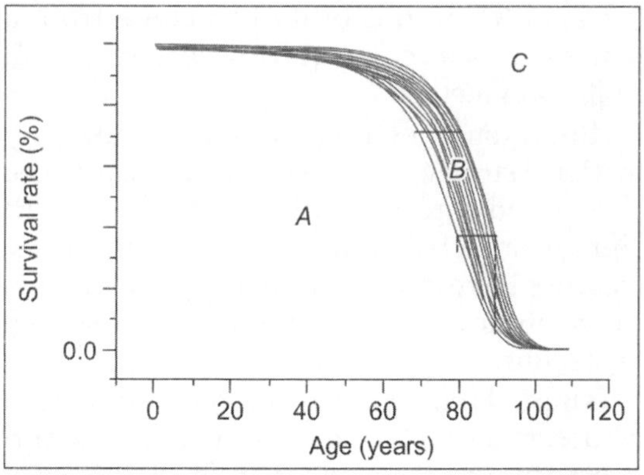

Fig. 7.5(a): Adapted from Murray CJL and Lopez AD Legend: *A* = time lived in optimal health, *B* = time lived in suboptimal health, *C* = time lost due to mortality.

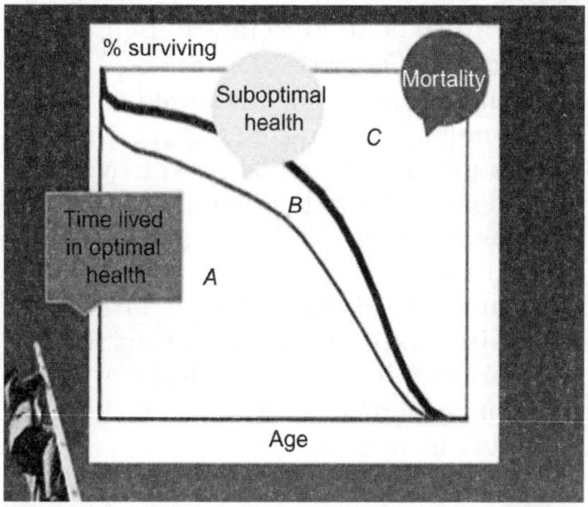

Fig. 7.5(a): The survivor curve. (*Source:* https://www.slide share.net/vicksy02/measuring-burden-of-disease

Types of SMPH

Broadly, there are two categories of SMPH based on simple survivorship curve (Fig. 7.5):

Health expectancies: Health expectancies measure years of life gained or years of improved quality of life. In this group of measures, among others, following measures are classified:

- Active life expectancy (ALE),
- Disability-free life expectancy (DFLE),
- Disability-adjusted life expectancy (DALE),
- Health-adjusted life expectancy (HALE),
- Quality-adjusted life expectancy (QALE).

Health gaps: Health gaps measure lost years of full health in comparison with some 'ideal' health status or accepted standard. In this group of measures among others, following measures (indicators) are classified:

- Potential years of life lost (PYLL),
- Healthy years of life lost (HYLL),
- Quality-adjusted life years (QALY),
- Disability-adjusted life years (DALY).

Both approaches use time and multiply number of years lived (or, not lived in case of premature death) by the 'quality' of those years. The process of adjustment of the years of healthy life lived is called 'quality adjustment' (expressed as QALYs), and the process of adjustment of the years of healthy life lost is called 'disability adjustment' (expressed as DALYs). It means that QALYs represent a gain which should be maximized, and DALYs represent a loss which should be minimized. In the QALY approach the quality is weighted (sometimes called 'utility', as it is the case of cost-utility analyses) on a scale from 1 indicating perfect health and the highest quality of life, to 0 indicating no quality of life and is synonymous to death. In the DALY approach, the scale goes in opposite way—a disability weighted zero indicates perfect health (no disability), and weighted 1 indicates death. The disability weighting is the most difficult and controversial part of the DALY approach.

There are two lines (upper and lower) and three areas (*A*, *B* and *C*). The upper line is the survivorship curve from a hypothetical life table population. The lower curve is a hypothetical curve of survivors to each 'age x' in optimal health. Area *A* represents time lived in optimal health, area *B* time lived in suboptimal health, and area *C* time lost due to mortality.

Total life expectancy at birth: LE = $A + B$, where, LE = total life expectancy at birth, A = time lived in optimal health, B = time lived in suboptimal health.

Health expectancies are population indicators that estimate the average time that a person could expect to live in a defined state of health.

Health expectancy (HE): HE = $A + f(B)$, where, HE = health expectancy, A = time lived in optimal health, B = time lived in suboptimal health and $f(B)$ = function that assigns weights to years lived in suboptimal health (optimal health has a weight of 1).

Health gaps measure the difference between actual population health and some specified standard or goal. HG = $C + g(B)$ where, HG = health gap, B = time lived in suboptimal health, C = time lost due to mortality (premature death) and $f(B)$ = function that assigns weights to health states lived during time B, but where a weight of 1 equals to time lived in a health state equivalent to death.

Health expectancy is often called **active life expectancy (ALE),** when activities of daily living (ADL) and instrumental activities of daily living (IADL) are used as measures of health status. Specifically, ALE measures health in terms of functional ability, not disease status.

Health expectancy is a generic term typically referring to the average number of years an individual can expect to live in a given health state (Mathers, Robine and Wikins, 1994). An attractive feature of HE is that it combines the fundamental dimensions of health (mortality, morbidity and disability) into a summary indicator to provide infor mation on the length of life and the health fulness of life. It shares other important properties with life expectancy (LE) such as independence from the age structure of the population and its measurement in expected years of life (Nusselder and Looman, 2004). The concept of HE resulted from a broadening in the conceptualization of health from a metric (which uses length of life as a measure of health status) to a quality of life perspective.

Health-adjusted Life Expectancy

Health-adjusted life expectancy (HALE) is a measure of population health that takes into account mortality and morbidity. It adjusts overall life expectancy by the amount of time lived in less than perfect health. This is calculated by subtracting from the life expectancy a figure which is the number of years lived with disability multiplied by a weighting to represent the effect of the disability (Fig. 7.6).

Disability-free Life Expectancy or Sullivan's Index

Disability-free life expectancy (DFLE) is basically an extension of the well-known concept of life expectancy. Life expectancy shows the number of years that a person of a particular age can expect to live considering current mortality, that is, the age- and sex-specific mortality rates. If additionally the share of

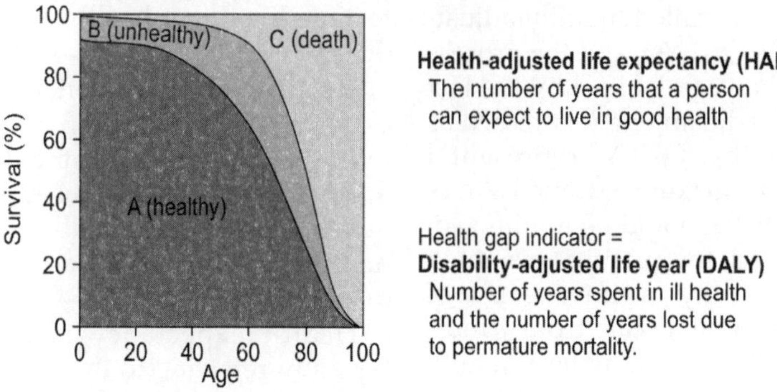

A = time lived in good health
C = time lost due to premature mortality
Life expectancy = A + B
Health expectancy indicators (e.g. healthy life expectancy and HALE) = A + f(B)
Health gaps indicators (e.g. DALYs) = C + g(B)

Fig 7.6: Health-adjusted life years

population in a healthy or unhealthy condition in different age groups is considered, we can determine the number of healthy life years, as a way to quality life expectancy estimates.

The main reason for the popularity of the Sullivan method is its simplicity and the fact that it does not require many input data. Only the following data by 5-year sex-age groups are needed.

- Mean annual population,
- Number of deaths (to estimate death rate),
- Proportion of disability-free persons in the given age group.

Quality-adjusted Life Year

The quality-adjusted life year (QALY) was introduced in 1976 to provide a guiding principle for selecting among alternative tertiary healthcare interventions. The idea was to develop a single measure of quality of life in order to compare expected outcomes for a disease from different interventions; a measure that valued possible health states for their quality of life as well as their duration (Table 7.16).

The central notion behind the QALY is that a year of life spent in one health state may be preferred to a year spent in another. It is a generic measure that sums time spent in different health states using weights for each health state on a scale of 0.00 (dead) to 1.00 (perfectly healthy), i.e. the arithmetic product of duration of life and a measure of quality of life (health state weight) (Table 7.16). So, 5 years of perfect health = 5 QALYs, while 2 years in a state measured as 0.5 of perfect health followed by 3 years of perfect health = 4 QALYs.

Years of Potential Life Lost (YPLL)

Rationale for use years of life are lost (YLL) take into account the age at which deaths occur by giving greater weight to deaths at younger age and lower weight to deaths at older age. The years of life lost (percentage of total) indicator measures the YLL due to a cause as a proportion of the total YLL lost in the population due to premature mortality. Years of potential life lost (YPLL) is one measure of the impact of premature mortality on a population.

Definition

YLL are calculated from the number of deaths multiplied by a standard life expectancy at the age at which death occurs. The standard life expectancy used for YLL at each age is the same for deaths in all regions of the world and is the same as that used for the calculation of disability adjusted life years (DALY).

Table 7.16: Variables and formula for disability adjusted life years (DALYs) and basic formulation for quality-adjusted life years (QALYs)

S.No.	*Particulars*	*Unit*
1.	Years of potential life lost due to death before expectation of life had the disease not occurred	(YLL) Year
2.	Years lost due to disability multiplied by disability weight years	(YLD) Year
3.	Number of deaths	(N) Number
4.	Number of incident cases	(I) Number
5.	Life expectation or duration of disability	(DW) Number
6.	Discount rate	(r) %
7.	Age-weighting correction constant	(0.1658) = C
8.	Parameter for age-weighting function	(0.04) = b
9.	Age at onset of disease	(a) = years
10.	Parameter for setting age-weighting	(K) = 1 or 0

DALY = YLL + YLD, where YLL = N Ce(ra)/(+ r)2 [e(+ r) (L + a) [–(+ r) (L + a)–1] – e(+ r) a [–(r) a–1]], (YLD = I DW {K Ce(ra)/(+ r) 2 [e(+ r)(L + a) [–(+ r)(L + a)–1] – e (+ r)a [–(r)a–1]] + (1–K) (L/r) (1– e rL)}

QALYs (basic formulation) QALY = Life years lived (duration) × Quality of life (health state) indicator. These would be based on a number of different quality of life scales.[2]

Additionally 3% time discounting and non-uniform age weights which give less weight to years lived at young and older ages were used as for the DALY. With non-uniform age weights and 3% discounting, a death in infancy corresponds to 33 YLL, and deaths at ages 5 to 20 to around 36 YLL.

Calculations

YPLL is calculated as the sum of the differences between a predetermined end-point and the ages of death for those who died before that end-point. The two most commonly used end-points are age 65 years and average life expectancy.

The use of YPLL is affected by this calculation, which implies a value system in which more weight is given to a death when it occurs at an earlier age. Thus, deaths at older ages are 'devalued.' However, the YPLL before age 65 ($YPLL_{65}$), places much more emphasis on deaths at early ages than does YPLL based on remaining life expectancy (YPLLLE). In 2000, the remaining life expectancy was 21.6 years for a 60-year-old, 11.3 years for a 70- year-old, and 8.6 for an 80-year-old. $YPLL_{65}$ is based on the fewer than 30% of deaths that occur among persons younger than 65. In contrast, YPLL for life expectancy (YPLLLE) is based on deaths among persons of all ages, so it more closely resembles crude mortality rates.

YPLL rates can be used to compare YPLL among populations of different sizes. Because different populations may also have different age distributions, YPLL rates are usually age-adjusted to eliminate the effect of differing age distributions.

Method for Calculating YPLL from a Line Listing

Step 1. Decide on end-point (65 years, average life expectancy, or other).

Step 2. Exclude records of all persons who died at or after the end-point.

Step 3. For each person who died before the end-point, calculate that person's YPLL by subtracting the age at death from the end-point. ($YPLL_{individual}$ = end-point – age at death)

Step 4. Sum the individual YPLLs (YPLL = Σ $YPLL_{individual}$)

Method for Calculating YPLL from a Frequency

Step 1. Ensure that age groups break at the identified end-point (e.g. 65 years). Eliminate all age groups older than the end-point.
Step 2. For each age group younger than the end-point, identify the mid-point of the age group, where mid-point = age group's youngest age in years + oldest age + 1÷ 2.
Step 3. For each age group younger than the end-point, identify that age group's YPLL by subtracting the mid-point from the end-point.
Step 4. Calculate age-specific YPLL by multiplying the age group's YPLL times the number of persons in that age group.
Step 5. Sum the age-specific YPLLs.

The **YPLL rate** represents years of potential life lost per 1,000 population below the end-point age, such as 65 years. YPLL rates should be used to compare premature mortality in different populations, because YPLL does not take into account differences in population sizes. The formula for a YPLL rate is as follows:

$$\text{YPLL} = \frac{\text{Years of potential life lost}}{\text{Population under age of 65 years}} \times 10^n$$

Disability-adjusted Life Years (DALYs)[20]

The DALY is a summary measure, which combines time lost through premature death and time lived in states of less than optimal health, loosely referred to as 'disability'. The DALY is a generalization of the well-known potential years of life lost measure (PYLLs) to include lost good health. One DALY can be thought of as one lost year of 'healthy' life and the measured disease burden is the gap between a population's health status and that of a normative reference population. DALYs for a specific cause are calculated as the sum of the YLLs from that cause and the YLDs for people living in states of less than good health resulting from the specific cause:

DALY (c,s,a,t) = YLL (c,s,a,t) + YLD (c,s,a,t)
for given cause (c), age (a), sex (s) and year (t)

The YLLs for a cause are essentially calculated as the number of cause-specific deaths multiplied by a loss function specifying the years lost for deaths as a function of the age at which death occurs.

The basic formula for YLLs is the following for a given cause (c), age (a), sex (s) and year (t).

$$\text{YLL}(c,s,a,t) = N(c,s,a,t) \times L(s,a)$$

where, N (c,s,a,t) is the number of deaths due to the cause (c) for the given age (a) and sex (s) in year (t), and L (s,a) is a standard loss function specifying years of life lost for a death at age (a) for sex (s).

One DALY is one lost year of 'healthy' life and the measured disease burden is the gap between a population's current health status and that of an ideal situation, where everyone lives into old age, free of disability. The normative reference population has a life expectancy at birth of 82.5 years for females and 80.0 years for males.

Time-discounting and non-uniform age weights, which give less weight to years lived at young and older ages, are used in calculating standard DALYs as reported in recent WHO World Health Reports. With age weights and time discounting, a death in infancy corresponds to 33 DALYs, and deaths from ages 5 to 20 to around 36 DALYs. Thus a disease burden of 3300 DALYs in a population would be the equivalent of 100 infant deaths or to approximately 5500 persons aged 50 years living one year with blindness (disability weighting = 0.6).

DALYs were designed to guide World Bank investment policies for health and to inform global priority setting for health research and international health programs.

Analysis of DALYs due to a variety of causes and risk factors has given new perspectives on the relative importance of different areas of disease prevention.

Physical Quality of Life Index[21,22]

Physical quality of life index (PQLI) was developed by famous economist Morris David in 1979 for 23 developed and developing countries. Morris David used the following three indicators to prepare a composite index known as physical quality of life index—1. life expectancy rate at 1 year of age (LER), 2. infant mortality rate (IMR), and 3. basic literacy rate (BLR). This index combines three measures into a single indicator. Each of the three components is marked on a scale of 0 (absolutely hopeless state) to 100 (absolutely best state). An average of the three components, with equal weight to each is calculated, which again would range from 0 to 100. PQLI has been often used in making international comparisons.

$$PQLI = LER + IMR + BLR \div 3$$

Example: Suppose, the LER for India is rated as 75, the IMR is rated as 40 and BLR is rated as 65, then the PQLI will be 60. [(75 + 40 + 65)/3]

Advantages of PQLI (smart code: AHEAD)

1. Aspect of welfare has been considered
2. Helps the government for analysis
3. Easy to compare
4. Also Considers Distribution
5. Data required is easily available

Limitations of PQLI (smart code: MAN)

1. Many other factors have been ignored
2. All factors have been given equal importance
3. Not a proper measure of economic development

Life Tables[23]

One important method of assessing the health of a population is to ask how long people can expect to live. Life expectancy, usually reported at birth, although it can be applied to other ages as well, is a commonly used summary measure that can also be used to compare across countries. Life expectancy is calculated using life tables.

A life table is a table which shows, for a person at each age, what the probability is of them dying before their next birthday. From this starting point, a number of statistics can be derived and are also included in the table:

- The probability of surviving any particular year of age
- The remaining life expectancy for people at each age
- The proportion of the original birth cohort still alive.

Life tables are usually constructed separately for men and for women because of their substantially different mortality rates. The Office of National Statistics is one organization which produces life tables.

Construction of Life Tables

Age-specific mortality rates are applied to a notional population, typically of 100,000 (an example is the European Standard population). Starting at birth, the probability of dying in each period is applied to the number of people surviving to enter that period, so that the initial figure slowly reduces to zero.

The different elements required for a life table include (using standard notations).

Ix	Number of survivors at age x
nqx	Probability of dying between age x and x + n
nDx	Number of deaths between age x and x + n
nLx	Number of person years lived between age x and x + n
Tx	Total number of person years lived after age x
ex	Life expectancy at age x

This sort of life table is based on current age-specific death rates for each age or age band used and are called 'period life tables' and are the most frequently used type. In contrast, actual life expectancy of a particular birth cohort can only be calculated when everyone in this cohort is dead. This is called a 'cohort life table' and requires data over many years to prepare just a single complete cohort life table.

Strength and Weaknesses

- Summary measure of mortality providing an overall picture of mortality, allowing countries and regions to be compared.
- Hypothetical measure that has the potential to be misunderstood by general public/ media.

It does not say much about who is still alive, and their quality of life; for example, how many years are lived with disability before dying. This has led to attempts to bring together morbidity and mortality, with measures such as Health-Adjusted life expectancy and disability adjusted life.

Other characteristics can also be used to distinguish different risk factors for life expectancy, such as smoking-status, occupation, socio-economic class, and others. More complex analyses for assessing cancer survival, that involve comparisons between two populations or a population at two points in time can also be undertaken.

MEASURES OF FERTILITY INCLUDING NATALITY (BIRTH)

Fertility is important to public health, population change, and the quality of human life. The role it plays in determining the size, composition, and growth of populations is a powerful factor governing the course of population change. In addition, fertility change influences the health of women, their offspring, their families, and, therefore, public health practice.

Fertility, in its most specific sense, refers to the actual birth of living offspring. Natality is often used synonymously for fertility. Additionally, the capacity to bear children is termed fecundity, and the probability of conceiving in a given month is called fecundability. Natural fertility describes the level of fertility found in populations that use neither contraception (temporary or permanent) nor induced abortion.

Table 7.17: Commonly used measures of fertility including natality (birth)[24,25]

Measure	*Numerator*	*Denominator*	*10^n*	*Formula*
Crude birth rate	Number of live births during a specified time interval	Mid-interval population (mid-year population)	1,000	$\frac{\text{No. of live births during a specified time interval}}{\text{Mid-year population}} \times 1000$
Crude fertility rate (general fertility rate)	Number of live births during a specified time interval	Number of women ages 15–44 years at mid-interval	1,000	$\frac{\text{No. of live births during a specified time interval}}{\text{Number of women ages 15–44 years at mid-interval}} \times 1000$
Age-specific fertility rate	Number of live births born to woman of a given age or age group	Mid-year female population of the same age or age group during the same year	1,000	$\frac{\text{No. of live births born to woman of a given age or age group}}{\text{Mid-year female population of the same age or age group during the same year}} \times 1000$
Crude rate of natural increase	Number of live births minus number of deaths during a specified time interval	Mid-interval population (mid-year population)	1,000	$\frac{\text{No. of live births minus number of deaths during a specified time interval}}{\text{Mid-year population}} \times 1000$
Low-birth weight ratio	Number of live births <2,500 grams during a specified time interval	Number of live births during the same time interval	100	$\frac{\text{No. of live births <2,500 grams during a specified time interval}}{\text{Number of live births during the same time interval}} \times 100$
Child–women ratio	Number of children 0–4 years of age	Females of child-bearing age	10,000	$\frac{\text{No. of children 0–4 years of age}}{\text{Females of child-bearing age}} \times 1000$
Adolescent fertility rate	Number of births to women aged 15–19 years	Number of women aged 15–19 years at mid-interval	1,000	$\frac{\text{No. of births to women aged 15–19 years}}{\text{Number of women aged 15–19 years at mid-interval}} \times 1000$

Natality measures are population-based measures of birth. These measures are used primarily by persons working in the field of maternal and child health (Table 7.17).

Crude birth rate (CBR) is the number of live births for a specified geographic area (nation, state, county, etc.) during a specified period (usually a calendar year) divided by the total population (usually mid-year) for that area and multiplied by 1,000. **India's** crude birth rate (CBR) during 2013 was 21.4 per 1000 mid year population.

The reason the CBR is 'crude' because the total population is represented in the denominator, similar to the crude death rate, e.g. the 'population at risk' of giving birth to a live neonate is poorly represented by the total population. As a result, the CBR is affected by the demographic distribution of the population in the denominator, especially by sex and age, but also by race or ethnicity category and other demographic characteristics.

Example: Calculation of CBR

CBR = Number of live births ÷ Mid-year population × 1,000

In a state, there were 180,000 live births in calendar year 2010 and 12,300,000 estimated population in calendar year 2010.

(180,000 ÷ 12,300,000) × 1,000 = 14.6 live births per 1,000 population in 2010

Crude marriage rate (CMR) is a gross measure of the level of the relative frequency of marriages in an area for a given year. It expresses additions, by the formal means of legal marriage, being made to the married segment of the total population. This refers to the number of marriages per 1,000 mid-year population.

General fertility rate (GFR): It is defined as number of live births in a given area during a year per 1000 mid-year population of females in the reproductive age groups (15 to 44 years) in that area, during that year. While GFR is definitely an improvement over CBR, comparisons between two populations based on GFR may not be accurate because the populations structure of ladies within the category of 15 to 45 years age may be quite different between the two populations (for example, one population may have much higher proportion of females aged 15 to 30 years, while the other population may have higher proportion of females aged 30 to 45 years). Secondly, the GFR does not allow for identifying the 'high risk' age group of females, as far as conception is concerned, so that family planning activities can be directed towards such high risk groups. This difficulty is overcome by computing the age-specific fertility rates (ASFR).

Total fertility rate (TFR)[26,27] refers to the number of births a woman would have if (a) she lived from age 15 to age 50 and (b) she experienced throughout her reproductive life exactly the ASFRs observed for the year in question. India's TFR was 2.1 in 2016. (SRS2016)

Seven ASFRs are normally calculated, one for each 5-year age group (15–19, 20–24, 25–29, 30–34, 35– 39, 40–44 and 45–49 years). Single-year rates can also be computed. Assuming that ASFRs have been computed for each 5-year age group and are expressed per 1000 women, the total fertility rate per woman can be computed as follows:

TFR (per woman) = ASFRs × 5 ÷ 1000, Numerator: Sum of the ASFRs × 5, denominator: 1000

Age-specific fertility rate (ASFR) refers to the number of live births born to woman of a given age or age group (prevailing age-specific fertility rates from age 15 to 49 years) by the mid-year female population of the same age or age group during the same year. ASFRs are often expressed per 1000 women. The age-specific fertility rate (ASFR) is derived as follows:

ASFR = Births in year to women aged 'X' ÷ No. of women aged 'X' at mid-year

Use of TFR and ASFR

The TFR is probably the most commonly used demographic indicator. It is closely associated with contraceptive prevalence and other indicators of reproductive health such as the maternal mortality ratio. It is a useful indicator of population momentum and a good proxy measure for the success (or failure) of family planning services. The TFR may also be used as a measure of poor physical reproductive health, since high parity (>5 births) represents a high risk of maternal morbidity and mortality. The main strength of the TFR is that it is a single summary measure that is independent of age structure, unlike the general fertility rate that only partially controls for age structure and the crude birth rate that does not do so at all. It is thus useful for international comparisons and for monitoring trends over time. It should be emphasized, however, that the TFR is a hypothetical measure of completed fertility; in cases of rapid fertility transition its value is primarily illustrative. As mentioned above, disaggregation of the ASFRs is useful in reflecting the age pattern of fertility, especially in high-risk groups such as adolescents and older women. TFRs are not useful in gauging the direct impact or success of family planning programmes. Family planning programmes can reduce total fertility only by reducing unintended as opposed to intended fertility. Nevertheless, there is strong empirical evidence that high contraceptive prevalence is associated with a low TFR and that increasing contraceptive prevalence is related to lowering the TFR.[28]

Adolescent fertility rate refers to annual number of births to women aged 15–19 years per 1000 women in that age group.

Very young adolescents are more likely to experience complications during pregnancy and childbirth than adult women and are at greater risk of maternal-related death. The infants of adolescent mothers are at higher risk of mortality and morbidity. The measure does not indicate the full dimensions of teen pregnancy as only live births are included in the numerator. Stillbirths and spontaneous or induced abortions are not reflected. The adolescent fertility rate (births per 1000 women aged 15–19 years in 2012), was highest in the WHO African region (116) and in low-income countries (112) compared with a global average of 50.

The value for adolescent fertility rate (births per 1,000 women ages 15–19) in India was 77.00 as of 2011. Over the past 14 years this indicator reached a maximum value of 116.10 in 1997 and a minimum value of 77.00 in 2011.

Gross reproductive rate (GRR): This is a measure of the average number of female live births that would occur to a female newborn, growing up and passing her entire reproductive age, if the current fertility rate were to apply. The GFR assumes that these women will not die before completing their child-bearing age, which is more of a hypothetical assumption and this drawback is overcome through compilation of net reproductive rate (NRR). The GRR is thus equivalent to TFR for female children only.[24]

Net reproduction rate (NRR): The average number of daughters a hypothetical cohort of women would have at the end of their reproductive period if they were subject during their whole lives to the fertility rates and the mortality rates of a given period. It is expressed as number of surviving daughters per woman. India's NRR in 2010 was 1.09.[24]

NRR is always lower than GRR, because it takes into account the fact that some women will die before entering and completing their child-bearing years. Correspondingly NRR will be less than half the magnitude of the TFR.

Replacement level fertility is said to have been reached when NRR = 1.0 – Surviving women in the hypothetical cohort have exactly enough daughters (on average) to replace themselves in the population. At this time GRR >1 and TFR >2. (Roughly, this is when couple have an average of two children.) When NRR = 1.00, it does not imply: CBR = CDR, population growth rate = 0.[24]

Relationship between Reproduction Measures and Population Growth

Population momentum is the propensity for a population to grow for many years after

Example: Calculating TFR and NRR

Suppose that in a country one-third of all females born die in infancy, one-third die at age 30, and one-third live to age 60. Women bear one child at age 25, one child at age 28, one child at age 32, and one child at age 35. One-half of children are girls.

a. Compute the total fertility rate and the net rate of reproduction.
b. Suppose that mortality is reduced so that there is no infant mortality. Half of all women die at age 30 and half at age 60. Compute the net rate of reproduction.
c. Suppose now that age-specific fertility changes, so that women have (on average) one-half child at ages 25, 28, 32, and 35. Compute the total fertility rate and the net rate of reproduction.

Answer

a. The total fertility rate (TFR) is the number of children that a woman can expect to have during her child-bearing years conditional on the probability of living through those years and had the given age-specific fertility at each age. In this country, the child-bearing years are 25–35. So, the TFR will be

   TFR = (1 child) × (Probability of reaching age 25) + (1 child) × (Probability of reaching age 28) + (1 child)* (Probability of reaching age 32) + (1 child) × (Probability of reaching age 35)

   Substituting in the given information, we get TFR = (1) × (2/3) + (1) × (2/3) + (1) × (1/3) + (1) × (1/3) = 2

   The net rate of reproduction (NRR) is fraction of kids that will be girls, which in this case is half.

   NRR = (2) × (1/2) = 1
b. Now women will live with certainty till age 30. So, the previous expression for TFR is

   TFR = (1) + (1) + (1/2) + (1/2) = 3 and NRR = 1.5
c. Now women have half as many kids at each age. Keeping the same assumptions from part (b), the TFR and NRR would simply be half of what they were in the previous part: TFR = 1.5 and NRR = 0.75

fertility declines to reach the replacement level of the 'two-child family'. (TFR ~2.2 and NRR = 1.0). This population momentum during the fertility transition is a function of young age structure of the population due to high levels of fertility in the past.

Low Birth Weight Ratio[29]

The percentage of live born babies who weigh less than 2500 g.

Numerator: Number of live born babies who weigh less than 2500 g × 100

Denominator: Total number of live births

Birth weight is the first weight of the infant obtained after birth. For live births, birth weight should preferably be measured within the first hour of life before significant post-natal weight loss has occurred, with measurement accuracy of at least 10 g, and a correct reading technique. While statistical tabulations include 500 g groupings for birth weight, weights should not be recorded in those groupings but to the degree of accuracy to which it is measured.

- **Low birth weight (LBW):** Less than 2500 g (up to and including 2499 g).
- **Very low birth weight:** Less than 1500 g (up to and including 1499 g).
- **Extremely low birth weight:** Less than 1000 g (up to and including 999 g).

The definitions of low, very low and extremely low birth weight do not constitute mutually exclusive categories. Below the set limits they are all-inclusive and therefore, overlap (i.e. 'low' includes 'very low' and 'extremely low', while 'very low' includes 'extremely low').

Use of Low Birth Weight Ratio

Although duration of pregnancy is the most important determinant of weight at birth, many other factors contribute. The rate of LBW is a rough summary measure of many factors, including maternal nutrition (during childhood, adolescence, pre-pregnancy and pregnancy), lifestyle (e.g. alcohol, tobacco and drug use) and other exposures in pregnancy (e.g. infectious diseases and altitude).

LBW is strongly associated with a range of adverse health outcomes, such as perinatal mortality and morbidity, infant mortality, disability and disease in later life, but is not necessarily part of the cause.

The main strength of LBW data is that they are relatively easy to measure. LBW is a strong predictor of an individual baby's survival. The lower the birth weight, the higher the risk of death. Groups with lower mean birth weights show higher infant mortality rates. Examples are twins and infants of mothers with lower socio-economic status.

HEALTH GOALS AND INDICATORS

With the goal of good health in mind,
think of an indicator as
"...a measure that helps quantify the
achievement of a goal."

— Mark Friedman

Goal is an ambitious commitment to address a single challenge. These are general guidelines that explain what you want to achieve. They are usually long term and represent global visions such as 'protect public health and safety.'

Target is a specific, measurable and time-bound outcome (result) that directly contributes to achievement of a goal.

Objectives define strategies or implementation steps to attain the identified goals. Unlike goals, objectives are specific, measurable, and have a defined completion date. They are more specific and outline the 'who, what, when, where, and how' of reaching the goals.

Indicator is a metric used to measure progress towards a target; generally based on available or established data. Example is mentioned in Table 7.18.

An indicator is something that points to an issue or condition. Its purpose is to show you how well a system is working. An indicator is something that helps you understand where you are, which way you are going and how far you are from where you want to be. A good indicator alerts you to a problem before it gets too bad and helps you recognize what needs to be done to fix the problem.

Health-related Millennium Development Goals[30]

In September 2000, world leaders at the United Nations Millennium Summit recognized a collective responsibility to work toward "a more peaceful, prosperous and just world" (UN, 2000). The MDGs reaffirmed this vision and launched an ambitious global partnership for development, setting specific targets to be met by 2015 and using numerical indicators to measure progress (Table 7.19).

By 2015, the world will have met some of the MDGs' key targets, such as halving the poverty rate, and will get close to completing primary education for all children; but achieving the health goals looks difficult and Africa lags behind, despite the substantial progress it has made since 2000. Overall, the MDGs have been remarkably successful in focusing attention and mobilizing

Table 7.18: Health goals and indicators

Goal	*Target*	*Indicator*
Achieve universal primary education	Ensure that, by 2030, children everywhere, boys and girls alike, will be able to complete a full course of primary schooling	• Net enrollment ratio in primary education • Literacy rate of 15–24-year-olds
Reduce child mortality	Eradicate under-five mortality	• Infant mortality rate • Under-five mortality rate

Table 7.19: Global and regional progress towards the achievement of the health-related MDGs[30]

	Target	Global	AFR	AMR	SEAR	EUR	EMR	WPR
Target 1.C: Halve, between 1990 and 2015, the proportion of people who suffer from hunger								
% reduction in proportion of underweight children under 5 years of age, 1990–2013	50	40	27	60	43	86	36	79
Target 4.A: Reduce by two-thirds, between 1990 and 2015, the under-five mortality rate								
% reduction in under-five mortality rate, 1990–2013	67	49	49	64	60	63	46	71
Measles immunisation coverage among 1-year-olds[a] (%), 2013	90	84	74	92	78	95	78	97
Target 5.A: Reduce by three-quarters, between 1990 and 2015, the maternal mortality rate								
% reduction in maternal mortality ratio, 1990–2013	75	45	49	37	64	59	50	60
Births attended by skilled health personnel[b] (%), 2007–2014	90	74	51	96	68	98	67	96
Target 5.B: Achieve, by 2015, universal access to reproduction health								
Antenatal care coverage (%)—at least one visit 2007–2014	100	83	77	96	77	—	78	95
Unmet need for family planning (%), 2012	0	12	24	9	13	10	18	6
Target 6.A: Have halted by 2015 and begun to reverse the spread of HIV/AIDS								
% reduction in HIV incidence, 2001–2013	>0	46	59	24	45	20	<–50	21
Target 6.C: Have halted by 2015 and begun to reverse the incidence of malaria and other major diseases								
% reduction in incidence of malaria[a], 2000–2013	75	30	34	76	49	100	39	69
% reduction in mortality rate of tuberculosis (among HIV-negative people)[a], 1990–2013	50	45	40	69	54	11	15	74
Target 7.C: Halve, by 2015, the proportion of the population without sustainable access to safe drinking-water and basic sanitation								
% reduction in proportion of population without access to improved drinking-water sources, 1990–2012	50	54	32	60	70	60	13	76
% reduction in proportion of population without access to improved sanitation, 1990–2012	50	32	8	40	27	22	32	53

[a] Target tablished via resolutions of the World Health Assembly or agreed upon by WHO multi-lateral partnerhips.
[b] Target set by the International Conference on Population and Development.

Met or on tract   Substantial progress   No or limited progress   ⊟ Data not available or not applicable

resources to address the major gaps in human development.

The outcome/progress of health-related MDGs are given in the Table 7.19 and depicted in different colours bases on the following categories.

Met or on track—indicates that the relative target reduction has already been met or will be achieved by 2015, should the trends observed since 1990 continue. In the case of absolute targets, the criterion used is that the latest observed data are within 5 percentage points of the target value.

Substantial progress—indicates that for relative target reductions the latest observed data are at least half-way to achieving the target. For the absolute coverage targets, indicates that the difference between the latest observed data and the target is no more than half the gap between the target and the global baseline (after rounding to the nearest 5% this leads to the following cutoff values: (a) Measles immunization coverage among 1-year-olds—80%; (b) births attended by skilled health personnel—75%; (c) antenatal care coverage: At least one visit—80%; and (d) unmet need for family planning—10%) but greater than 5 percentage points.

No or limited progress—indicates that latest observed data are not yet half-way to achieving the relative target reduction. For the absolute coverage targets, indicates that the difference between the latest observed data and the target is more than half of the gap between the target and the global baseline. SEAR countries progress towards achieving MDGs are mentioned in Tables 7.20 and 7.21.

The indicators used in this report have been included on the basis of their relevance to global public health, on data availability and quality, and on the reliability and comparability of the resulting estimates (Table 7.22). Taken together, these indicators provide a comprehensive summary of the current status of national health and health systems in the following nine areas (Table 7.23).

1. Life expectancy and mortality,
2. Cause-specific mortality and morbidity,

Table 7.20: South-east Asia region countries progress towards the achievement of the health-related MDGs (Target 4A and 5A, B)

	Target 4.A: Reduce by two-thirds, between 1990 and 2015, the under-five mortality rate		*Target 5.A: Reduce by three-quarters, between 1990 and 2015, the maternal mortality ratio*		*Target 5.B: Achieve, by 2015, universal access to reproductive health*	
Target	**67**	**90**	**75**	**90**	**100**	**0**
Bangladesh	72	93	69	44	59	14
Bhutan	73	94	87	58	74	12
DPR Korea	37	99	–2	100	100	15
India	**58**	**74**	**66**	**67**	**75**	**21**
Indonesia	65	84	56	83	96	11
Maldives	89	99	93	99	99	29
Myanmar	53	86	66	78	83	—
Nepal	72	88	76	36	58	28
Sri Lanka	52	99	41	99	99	7
Thailand	65	99	38	100	98	7
Timor-Leste	68	70	78	21	84	32

Table 7.21: South-east Asia region countries progress towards the achievement of the health-related MDGs (Target 6A, C and 7C)

	Target 6.A: *Have halted by 2015 and begun to reverse the spread of HIV/AIDS*	*Target 6.C:* *Have halted by 2015 and begun to reverse the incidence of malaria and other major diseases*	*Target 7.C:* *Halve by 2015, the proportion of the population without sustainable access to safe drinking water and basic sanitation*	
	% reduction in HIV incidence, 2001–2013	*% reduction in mortality rate of tuberculosis (among HIV negative people), 1990–2013*	*% reduction in proportion of population without access to improved drinking-water sources, 1990–2012*	*% reduction in proportion of population without access to improved sanitation, 1990–2012*
Target	**>0**	**50**	**50**	**50**
Bangladesh	—	36	53	36
Bhutan	—	96	—	—
DPR Korea	—	75	< –50	62
India	**57**	**50**	**77**	**22**
Indonesia	< –50	64	50	37
Maldives	—	92	86	97
Myanmar	75	68	68	51
Nepal	86	67	65	33
Sri Lanka	< –50	22	81	75
Thialand	68	37	71	61
Timor-Leste	—	—	36	3

3. Selected infectious diseases,
4. Health service coverage
5. Risk factors,
6. Health systems,
7. Health expenditure,
8. Health inequities,
9. Demographic and socio-economic statistics.

An overarching health indicator for the post-2015—way forward (candidate indicators) ***also see under SMPH***[34]

A health goal—'ensure healthy lives and promote well-being for all at all ages'.

The following sections briefly summarize definitions, relevance, methods, data sources and pros and cons for four potential candidate indicators—life expectancy at birth, premature mortality (deaths below age 70), and healthy life expectancy (population survey based or burden of disease based).

An overarching health outcome indicator should meet the following criteria.

- Understandable and relevant to the health goal and development outcomes, and reasonably easy to communicate to the general public.

Table 7.22: The selection criteria for ideal indicators[31]

Criterion	*Explanation*
Scientifically robust	An indicator must be a valid, specific, sensitive and reliable reflection of that which it purports to measure.
Valid	An indicator must actually measure the issue or factor it is supposed to measure
Reliable	An indicator must give the same value if its measurement were repeated in the same way on the same population and at almost the same time.
Sensitive	An indicator must be able to reveal important changes in the factor of interest.
Specific	An indicator must reflect only changes in the issue or factor under consideration.
Useful	At national level, an indicator must be able to act as a 'marker of progress' towards improved reproductive health status, either as a direct or proxy measure of impact or as a measure of progress towards specified process goals. Since computation of national-level indicators usually requires aggregation of data collected at a local level, the data should also be useful locally, i.e. follow-on action should be immediately apparent
Representative	An indicator must adequately encompass all the issues or population groups it is expected to cover. For national-level indicators the group of interest is the population as a whole, including minority groups and adolescents.
Understandable	An indicator must be simple to define and its value must be easy to interpret in terms of reproductive health status.
Accessible	The data required should be available or relatively easy to acquire by feasible data collection methods that have been validated in field trials.
Ethical	An indicator must be seen to comply with basic human rights and must require only data that are consistent with the morals, beliefs or values of the local population.

- Measurable for most countries using data available at national level for recent time periods.
- Allows the setting of meaningful and potentially attainable targets that are motivating for policy makers and communicators.
- Universal, flexible, and allow for country adaptation.

An overarching health outcome indicator not only measures the performance of the health sector but is also closely linked to other development processes, as health is closely linked to the economic, social and environmental factors.

The following four **potential candidate indicators:** Life expectancy at birth, premature mortality (deaths below age 70), and healthy life expectancy (population survey based or burden of disease based) are briefed.

Life Expectancy At Birth[35]

Brief definition: The average number of years that a newborn could expect to live, if he or she were to pass through life subject to the age-specific death rates of a given period.

Relevance to sustainable development health goal: Life expectancy at birth is a summary indicator of mortality conditions and, by proxy, of health conditions. It summarizes mortality risks and trends across all age groups, including older people. Measurement of life expectancy at birth also allows reporting of life expectancy at other ages to track health improvements for specific age groups in populations.

Methods of calculation: Calculation of life expectancy at birth is based on age-specific death rates for a particular calendar period and methods are well known and

Table 7.23: Area-wise list of core health indicators[32,33]

S.No.	*Areas*	*Indicators*
1.	Life expectancy and mortality	• Life expectancy at birth (years) • Life expectancy at age 60 (years) • Healthy life expectancy at birth (years) • Neonatal mortality rate (per 1000 live births) • Infant mortality rate (probability of dying by age 1 per 1000 live births) • Under-five mortality rate (probability of dying by age 5 per 1000 live births) • Adult mortality rate (probability of dying between 15 and 60 years of age per 1000 population)
2.	Cause-specific mortality and morbidity	• Age-standardized mortality rates by cause (per 100,000 population) • Years of life lost (per 100,000 population) • Number of deaths among children aged <5 years (000s) • Distribution of causes of death among children aged <5 years (%) • Maternal mortality ratio (per 100,000 live births) • Cause-specific mortality rate (per 100,000 population) • Incidence rate (per 100,000 population per year) • Prevalence (per 100,000 population)
3.	Selected infectious diseases	• Cholera, diphtheria, human African trypanosomiasis • Japanese encephalitis, leishmaniasis, leprosy, malaria, measles • Meningitis, mumps, pertussis, poliomyelitis, congenital rubella syndrome • Rubella, neonatal tetanus, total tetanus, tuberculosis, yellow fever
4.	Health service coverage	• Unmet need for family planning (%) • Contraceptive prevalence (%) • Antenatal care coverage (%) • Births attended by skilled health personnel (%) • Births by caesarean section (%) • Neonates protected at birth against neonatal tetanus (%) • Immunization coverage among 1-year-olds (%) • Children aged 6–59 months who received vitamin A supplementation (%) • Children aged <5 years with ARI symptoms taken to a health facility (%) • Children aged <5 years with suspected pneumonia receiving antibiotics (%) • Children aged <5 years with diarrhoea receiving ORT (ORS and/or RHF) (%) • Children aged <5 years sleeping under insecticide-treated nets (%) • Children aged <5 years with fever who received treatment with any antimalarial (%) • Pregnant women with HIV receiving antiretrovirals to prevent MTCT (%) • Antiretroviral therapy coverage among people eligible for treatment (%) • Case-detection rate for all forms of tuberculosis (%) • Treatment-success rate for new tuberculosis cases (%)
5.	Risk factors	• Population using improved drinking-water sources (%) • Population using improved sanitation (%) • Population using solid fuels (%) • Infants exclusively breastfed for the first 6 months of life (%) • Children aged <5 years who are wasted (%) • Children aged <5 years who are stunted (%) • Children aged <5 years who are underweight (%) • Children aged <5 years who are overweight (%) • Prevalence of anaemia among women aged 15–49 years (%) • Prevalence of raised fasting blood glucose among adults aged ≥18 years (%) • Prevalence of raised blood pressure among adults aged ≥18 years (%)

(Contd.)

Table 7.23: Area-wise list of core health indicators[32,33] *(Contd.)*

S.No.	*Areas*	*Indicators*
		• Adults aged ≥18 years who are obese (%) • Alcohol per capita consumption (≥15 years) (litres of pure alcohol) • Prevalence of smoking any tobacco product among adults aged ≥15 years (%) • Prevalence of current tobacco use among adolescents aged 13–15 years (%) • Prevalence of condom use by adults aged 15–49 years during higher-risk sex (%) • Population aged 15–24 years with comprehensive correct knowledge of HIV/AIDS (%)
6.	Health systems	**Health workforce** • Density of physicians per 10,000 population • Density of nursing and midwifery personnel per 10,000 population • Density of dentistry personnel per 10,000 population • Density of pharmaceutical personnel per 10,000 population • Density of psychiatrists per 10,000 population **Infrastructure and technologies** • Hospitals (per 100,000 population) • Psychiatric beds (per million population) • Computed tomography units (per million population) • Radiotherapy units (per million population) • Mammography units (per million females aged 50–69 years) **Essential medicines** • Median availability of selected generic medicines in public and private sectors (%) • Median consumer price ratio of selected generic medicines in public and private sectors
7.	Health expenditure	**Health expenditure ratios** • Total expenditure on health as a percentage of gross domestic product • General government expenditure on health as a percentage of total expenditure on health • Private expenditure on health as a percentage of total expenditure on health • General government expenditure on health as a percentage of total government expenditure • External resources for health as a percentage of total expenditure on health • Social security expenditure on health as a percentage of general government **Expenditure on health** • Out-of-pocket expenditure as a percentage of private expenditure on health • Private prepaid plans as a percentage of private expenditure on health • Per capita health expenditures • Per capita total expenditure on health at average exchange rate (US$) • Per capita total expenditure on health (PPP int. $) • Per capita government expenditure on health at average exchange rate (US$) • Per capita government expenditure on health (PPP int. $)
8.	Health inequities	• Contraceptive prevalence—modern methods (%) • Antenatal care coverage—at least four visits (%) • Births attended by skilled health personnel (%) • DTP3 immunization coverage among 1-year-olds (%) • Children aged <5 years who are stunted (%) • Under-five mortality rate (probability of dying by age 5 per 1000 live births)

(Contd.)

Table 7.23: Area-wise list of core health indicators *(Contd.)*

S.No.	*Areas*	*Indicators*
9.	Demographic and socio-economic statistics	• Total population (000s) • Median age of population (years) • Population aged <15 years (%) • Population aged >60 years (%) • Annual population growth rate (%) • Population living in urban areas (%) • Civil registration coverage (%) of births and cause of death • Crude birth rate (per 1000 population) • Crude death rate (per 1000 population) • Total fertility rate (per woman) • Adolescent fertility rate (per 1000 girls aged 15–19 years) • Literacy rate among adults aged ≥15 years (%) • Net primary school enrolment rate (%) • Gross national income per capita (PPP int. $) • Population living on <$1 (PPP int. $) a day (%) • Cellular phone subscribers (per 100 population)

standardized (Preston *et al.*, 2001). The death rates are commonly tabulated for ages 0 to 1 year, 1 to 5 years, and for 5-year-age groups for ages 5 and above.

Life expectancy may be calculated separately for males and females, or for both sexes combined, and can also be presented for particular ages after birth. Life expectancy inequalities can also be calculated for population groups, (e.g. region of residence, or socio-economic status as defined by individual or area-level indicators in available data source).

Advantages: Calculation methods are well defined and non-controversial. The indicator is well-understood, widely used and reported. Regularly updated national data is available for almost half of countries, and there is now substantial global momentum to improve civil registration and vital statistics, including death registration data, in countries without reasonable national coverage at present. There are reasonably acceptable methods to estimate child mortality and adult mortality from other sources, though regularity of data availability and time delays remain a problem, as does the problems of assessing levels of under-reporting.

Disadvantages: Does not directly address non-fatal health outcomes, disability, etc. except through the proxy of mortality risks. For many countries with relatively high life expectancies at present, plausible targets will not involve large increases in life expectancy. Aiming for a 4-year increase in life expectancy at birth may not excite policy makers as much as reducing a death rate by 75%.

Premature Mortality

Brief definition: The total number of deaths that occur before age 70 years.

Relevance to sustainable development health goal: Targeting overall mortality before age 70 ignores no modifiable cause of death, nor causes of disability that also cause substantial numbers of deaths. 40% fewer premature deaths would be important in all countries, but implies very different priorities in different populations.

Methods of calculation: Calculation of premature mortality requires only age-specific death rates and population numbers for broad age groups for a particular calendar period and the method is extremely simple. Premature mortality requires less detailed data for its calculation than does life expectancy at birth. Premature mortality may be calculated separately for males and females, or for both sexes combined, and can also be disaggregated for broad age groups, (e.g. under 5, under 50, 50–69). Premature mortality inequalities can also be calculated for population groups (e.g. region of residence, or socio-economic status as defined by individual or area-level indicators in available data source).

Advantage: Simple to calculate and understand, allows nesting of specific subtargets for priority areas of health, and for country-specific priority setting.

This indicator would facilitate quantification of the target-setting process, based on analysis of mortality trends by age as well as by disease category. The proposed targets focus on premature mortality and avoid more complex metrics that are much harder to measure and track over time. Norheim *et al.* stress the importance of countries adapting the targets to their own circumstances. According to the author's detailed analyses, achieving these targets would result in a halving of deaths under age 50 years, avoiding a third of the NCD deaths in people aged 50–69 years, and, overall, result in avoidance of 40% of deaths under age 70 years by 2030.

Disadvantage: The indicator appears to exclude older people, and as for life expectancy measures, does not include non-fatal health/disability. In reality, concerted action to reduce non-communicable disease deaths in the ages 30–69 years will inevitably also help to reduce NCD death rates for people aged 70 years and over; however communication around this issue would require special attention.

Healthy Life Expectancy (HLE)[34] at Birth

Brief definition: The average equivalent number of years of full health that a newborn could expect to live, if he or she were to pass through life subject to the age-specific death rates and average age-specific levels of health states for a given period.

Relevance to sustainable development health goal: Healthy life expectancy (HLE) provides a summary of overall health conditions for a population, which are in turn an integral part of development. While communicable diseases such as HIV/AIDS, tuberculosis and malaria continue to cause substantial loss of health and mortality in developing countries, particularly African countries, non-communicable diseases and injuries are responsible for more than half of all lost years of healthy life in developing as well as developed countries. HLE thus provides a more complete picture of the impact of morbidity and mortality on populations, than simple life expectancy alone.

Methods of calculation: Sullivan's method is generally used to combine life table data with estimates of proportion of years lived in each life table age range which are 'healthy years'.

There are three main classes of method/data used:

a. Dichotomous classification into healthy/non-healthy, based usually on self-report of disability and functioning limitations, either in a module of questions or in response to a single global question such as "How is your health? Excellent/Good/Fair/Poor/Bad"
b. Use of survey data on functioning in a set of health domains together with a health state valuation function which enables summation across health states into a single 'equivalent healthy years'. Examples of survey modules of this type include SF-36, EQ-5D, HUI and the WHODAS and SAGE instruments. Examples of health state valuation functions include the EQ-5D values, the HUI valuation function and the WHO World Health Surveys valuation function.
c. Use of global burden of disease analyses estimating YLD for a comprehensive set of diseases and injuries to prepare age–sex-specific average YLD per capita, interpreted as the equivalent healthy proportion of years lived at that age group.

Advantage: It captures mortality risk and health states in a way that clearly covers both. Apart from life tables, the other inputs are derived directly from population-represen tative surveys using straightforward and relatively simple methods (though methods for deriving prevalence of health states from survey questions may vary greatly in complexity).

Disadvantage: Self-report data generally will have issues of comparability across countries, particularly if extended from high income to developing countries. There is some controversy around the use of health state valuations to summarize across various states of health. The monitoring of such an indicator at international level will require repeated population surveys, using a common survey instrument.

Health-adjusted Life Expectancy (HALE)[34] at Birth

Brief definition: The average equivalent number of years of full health that a newborn could expect to live, if he or she were to pass through life subject to the age-specific death rates and average age-specific levels of health states for a given period.

Relevance to sustainable development health goal: Health-adjusted life expectancy (HALE) provides a summary of overall health conditions for a population, which are in turn an integral part of development. While communicable diseases such as HIV/AIDS, tuberculosis and malaria continue to cause substantial loss of health and mortality in developing countries, particularly African countries, non-communicable diseases and injuries are responsible for more than half of all lost years of healthy life in developing as well as developed countries. HALE thus provides a more complete picture of the impact of morbidity and mortality on populations, than simple life expectancy alone.

Methods of calculation: Sullivan's method is generally used to combine life table data with estimates of proportion of years lived in each life table age range which are 'healthy years'.

This section describes HALE indicators based on use of global burden of disease analyses which estimate YLD for a comprehensive set of diseases and injuries to prepare age–sex-specific average YLD per capita, interpreted as the equivalent healthy proportion of years lived at that age group.

Alternate methods using population survey data to directly estimate prevalence of health states were described above in Section 3 (Healthy Life Expectancy).

Methods have been developed drawing on estimated cause-specific health state prevalence from burden of disease analysis using the disability adjusted life year (or DALY) (Salomon *et al.*, 2012). This approach requires relatively complex analyses and is data-demanding. A number of issues remain to be resolved around methods for dealing with comorbidity in the DALY-based approach.

Advantage: It captures mortality risk and health states in a way that clearly reflects all major health outcomes. The calculation methods of the GBD approach ensure reasonable cross-country comparability.

Disadvantage: It requires information on the prevalence of over 1000 health states. Since these data are not regularly collected for most countries, it can only be calculated by imputing prevalences based on relatively sparse population-representative studies. To date, empirical data required for comorbidity adjustments is not available and it is likely that simplifying assumptions will need to continue to be made for the foreseeable future.

Indicators of Overall Development

The human development index (HDI) is an index combining normalized measures of life expectancy, literacy, educational attainment and GDP per capita for countries, worldwide. It is claimed as a standard means of measuring human development, according to the United Nations Development Program (UNDP). The HDI combines three basic dimensions, viz. Life expectancy at birth, as an index of population health and longevity; secondly, knowledge and education, as measured by the adult literacy rate (with two-thirds weighting) and the combined primary, secondary and tertiary gross enrollment ratio (with one-third weighting) and, thirdly, the standard of living, as measured by the natural logarithm of gross domestic product (GDP) per capita at purchasing power parity (PPP) in US Dollars. The human development index (HDI) thus represents the average of these three general indices as shown in Table 7.24.

The HDI is finally calculated as (L+E+G)/3. An index of below 0.5 indicates poor development, while an index of 0.8 and above indicates good development of a country. Reviews in 2007 indicate that India, with an index of approximately 0.6 is progressing but has still a long way to go. Countries like Norway, Canada and Japan have been often taking the first place.

MEASURES OF HEALTHCARE SERVICE DELIVERY

These are indicators which either measure the 'availability' (as, doctor–population ratio, population served by each health centre, population–hospital bed ratio); or, 'expenditure on healthcare' (as, percentage of national budget earmarked for health sector, average finances spent per person on healthcare); or, 'health coverage' (e.g. percentage of children fully immunized, deliveries conducted by trained birth attendants, % of cases of pulmonary TB brought under ATT, % of houses that were adequately sprayed with an insecticide, etc.); or 'accessibility' (e.g. mean distance in kilometers required to be travelled in a village to reach the health centre); or, 'utilization' (e.g. % of women who availed of cervical cancer screening camp out of those who were eligible); or, finally, the 'policy' (e.g. availability of a stated health policy and enunciated targets).

INTRODUCTION

Strengthening service delivery is crucial to the achievement of the health-related millennium development goals (MDGs), which include the delivery of interventions to reduce child mortality, maternal mortality and the burden of HIV/AIDS, tuberculosis and malaria. Service provision or delivery is an immediate output of the inputs into the health system, such as the health workforce, procurement and supplies, and financing. Increased inputs should lead to improved service delivery and enhanced access to services. Ensuring availability of health services that meet a minimum quality standard and securing access to them are key functions of a health system.[35]

Some concepts that have frequently been used to measure health services remain extremely relevant and are part of the key characteristics. For example, terms such as access, availability, utilization and coverage have often been used interchangeably to reveal whether people are receiving the services they need.[36,37]

Access is a broad term with varied dimensions: The comprehensive measurement of access requires a systematic assessment of the physical, economic, and socio-psychological aspects of people's ability to make use of health services.

Availability is an aspect of *comprehensiveness* and refers to the physical presence or delivery of services that meet a minimum standard.

Table 7.24: Calculation of human development indices

Index	*Measure*	*Minimum value*	*Maximum value*	*Formula*
Longevity	Life expectancy (LE) at birth	25 years	85 years	L = LE–25/60
Education	Liyeracy rate (LR)	0%	100%	E = 2LR + CGER/3
	Combined gross enrollment ration (CGER)	0%	100%	
GDP	GDP per capita (PPP)	100 USD	40,000 USD	E = log GDP_{pc}-2/260206

Utilization is often defined as the quantity of healthcare services used. *Coverage* of interventions is defined as the proportion of people who receive a specific intervention or service among those who need it.

Key Characteristics of Good Service Delivery in a Health System[38]

Good service delivery is a vital element of any health system. Service delivery is **a fundamental input to population health status,** along with other factors, including social determinants of health. The precise organization and content of health services will differ from one country to another, but in any well-functioning health system, the network of service delivery should have the following ***key characteristics.***

1. **Comprehensiveness:** A **comprehensive range** of health services is provided, appropriate to the needs of the target population, including **preventative, curative, palliative** and **rehabilitative** services and **health promotion** activities.
2. **Accessibility:** Services are directly and permanently accessible with no undue barriers of cost, language, culture, or geography. Health services are **close to the people, with a routine point of entry to the service network at primary care level** (not at the specialist or hospital level). Services may be provided in the home, the community, the workplace, or health facilities as appropriate.
3. **Coverage:** Service delivery is designed so that all people in a **defined target population** are covered, i.e. the sick and the healthy, all income groups and all social groups.
4. **Continuity:** Service delivery is organized to provide an individual with **continuity of care across the network of services, health conditions, levels of care, and over the life-cycle.**
5. **Quality:** Health services are of high quality, i.e. they are **effective, safe, centred on the patient's needs** and given in a **timely** fashion.
6. **Person-centredness:** Services are **organized around the person, not the disease** or the financing. Users perceive health services to be responsive and acceptable to them. There is **participation** from the target population in service delivery design and assessment. People are partners in their own healthcare.
7. **Coordination: Local area health service networks are actively coordinated,** across types of provider, types of care, levels of service delivery, and for both routine and emergency preparedness. The patient's primary care provider facilitates the route through the needed services, and works in collaboration with other levels and types of provider. Coordination also takes place with other sectors (e.g. social services) and partners (e.g. community organizations).
8. **Accountability and efficiency:** Health services are **well managed** so as to achieve the core elements described above with a **minimum wastage** of resources. Managers are allocated the necessary authority to achieve planned objectives and held **accountable for overall performance and results.** Assessment includes appropriate mechanisms for the participation of the target population and civil society.

Service delivery monitoring has immediate relevance for the management of health services, which distinguishes this area from other health systems building blocks. Shortage of medicines, uneven distribution of health services, and the poor availability of equipment or guidelines must all be taken into account as part of basic service management.

The measurement strategies and indicators for monitoring as well as the 'inputs', 'processes' and 'outputs' to the health system as they relate to the service delivery building block.

Source of Data

Multiple sources of data on health service delivery are required including routine facility reporting systems, health facility assessments (both facility censuses and surveys), and other special studies as no single method provides all the information to assess service delivery.

Service Delivery Monitoring System

Data from routine health facility reporting systems need to be supplemented with data from health facility assessments. The topics included in these assessments will vary over time and the questionnaire should use a modular approach selected on the basis of current priorities and needs. In addition, data generated through facility assessments should be complemented or cross-checked with data from other sources, such as the databases of health workers, infrastructures, equipment and procurement, that are often available in various departments of the ministries of health. This can serve as a complementary or benchmarking material for data on service delivery generated through the routine HMIS.

Core Indicators[35,38,39]

Countries have often defined their own set of performance measures in the area of service delivery. The challenge is to devise a set of sensitive and specific indicators that can easily be collected at all facilities at relatively little cost, and with the possibility of becoming part of regular facility reporting systems.

The indicators listed below can be grouped into those that reflect *general service availability, general service readiness, and service-specific availability and readiness* (Box 7.4).

GENERAL SERVICE AVAILABILITY

General Service availability refers to the physical presence of delivery of services that meet a minimum standard. Availability comprises health infrastructure (**facilities and beds per 10,000 population**), the **health workforce per 10 000 population** and aspects of service utilization (**inpatient/outpatient visits per 10,000 population**).

Box 7.4

1. **General service availability**
   - Number and distribution of health facilities per 10,000 population
   - Number and distribution of inpatient beds per 10,000 population
   - Number of outpatient department visits per 10,000 population per year
2. **General service readiness**
   - General service readiness score for health facilities
3. **Service-specific availability**
   - Proportion of health facilities offering specific services
   - Number and distribution of health facilities offering specific services per 10,000 population
4. **Service-specific readiness**
   - Specific-services readiness score for health facilities

Number and Distribution of Health Facilities Per 10,000 Population

Definition

The number of health facilities available relative to the total population for the same geographical area.

Numerator: The number of health facilities, i.e. all public and private health facilities, defined as a static facility (a designated building) in which general health services are offered. It does not include mobile service delivery points and non-formal services, such as traditional healers.

Denominator: The total population for the same geographical area.

Matching Dimensions

Distribution implies urban–rural differences and could also include differences between regions or provinces, or sometimes between districts. Since the population size of districts tends to be small, comparisons of densities between districts have to be made cautiously.

Additional information can be presented based on the managing authority of health facilities—public, private not-for-profit (including faith based), private for profit, etc.

Number and Distribution of Inpatient Beds Per 10,000 Population

Definition

The number of inpatient beds available relative to the total population for the same geographical area.

Numerator: The number of inpatient beds. This includes total hospital beds (for long-term and acute care), maternity beds and pediatric beds, but not delivery beds. Public and private sectors are included.

Denominator: The total population for the same geographical area.

Matching Dimensions

Distribution implies urban–rural differences and could also include differences between regions or provinces, or sometimes between districts.

Additional information about beds can be presented based on the managing authority of health facilities—public, private not-for-profit (including faith based), private for profit, and other (such as parastatals).

Data on maternity beds can also be used to calculate the density of maternal beds per 1000 pregnant women per year.

True indicators of access need to measure the proportion of the population living within a specified travel time and/or distance from a health facility. Access is sometimes measured through household surveys which rely on respondent judgement or on basic spatial analysis of catchment areas around specified facilities. However, the latter is subject to weaknesses. For example, designing catchment areas around health facilities.

Number of Outpatient Department Visits Per 10,000 Population Per Year

The patient volumes at inpatient and outpatient facilities are not a coverage indicator because the population in need is not well defined. Low rates, however, are indicative of poor availability and quality of services. For example, several countries have demonstrated that outpatient department rates go up when constraints to using health services are removed, such as by bringing services closer to the people or reducing user fees. In contrast, once rates exceed an uncertain threshold the number of visits is no longer an indicator of the strength of the health services.

Definition

The number of outpatient visits to health facilities relative to the total population of the same geographical area.

Numerator: The number of visits to health facilities for ambulant care, not including immunization (can be divided into children under 5 years of age and aged 5 years and over).

Denominator: The total population for the same geographical area.

Matching Dimensions

Disaggregation by district or province/region can be presented.

Potential additional indicators of inpatient care and utilization include admission rates (number of new admissions per 10,000 population per year) and number of caesarean sections per 100 deliveries. Both indicators tend to vary considerably, however, with country practices and changes in admission or intervention policies. Very low rates tend to indicate that services are not available, but otherwise the statistics are difficult to interpret.

Two related indicators are:

1. Average length of stay: An indicator of quality and efficiency of health services.
2. Bed occupancy rate: An indicator of efficiency of services.

GENERAL SERVICE READINESS

Readiness is defined as the cumulative availability of components required to provide services. It comprises tracer items for the following major domains—infrastructure/ amenities, basic supplies/equipment including small surgery, standard precautions, laboratory tests, medicines and commodities.

General Service Readiness Score for Health Facilities

Estimation of general service readiness is derived from data on availability and functioning of tracer items in the facility on the day of assessment. These items are grouped in five domains, i.e. basic amenities, basic equipment, standard precautions for prevention of infections, laboratory, medicines and commodities.

Definition

Cumulative availability of components required in health facilities to provide general services, expressed as percentage. The overall score is the unweighted average of domain scores. Each domain score represents the average number of items present and functioning in the health facilities, expressed as a percentage of the total number of items in that domain.

Matching Dimensions

Scores for the different domains of general service readiness should be presented separately. All scores can be presented by district and by ownership of facilities.

Hospitals provide a wide range of services and an expanded version of the questionnaire should be administered during facility assessment, or regular reporting.

SERVICE-SPECIFIC AVAILABILITY

Service-specific availability refers to whether or not a specific service is offered. Availability is captured by the proportion of services offering a specific service and the density of the facilities offering the service per 10,000 population.

Specific services may include family planning, antenatal care, safe delivery, child health, HIV/AIDS, tuberculosis, malaria, chronic conditions and small surgery.

Proportion of Health Facilities Offering Specific Services/Number and Distribution of Health Facilities Offering Specific Services Per 10,000 Population

Definition

Proportion of health facilities ready to provide key services: The number of facilities that offer specific services relative to the total number of facilities.

Number and distribution of health facilities ready to provide key services per 10,000 population: The number of facilities that offer specific services relative to the total population in the same geographical area.

Numerator: The number of facilities in which a specific service is offered.

Denominator: The total number of facilities (to obtain the proportion), or, the total population for the same geographical area (to compute the density).

Matching Dimensions

Distribution implies urban–rural differences and could also include differences between regions or provinces, or sometimes between districts.

SERVICE-SPECIFIC READINESS

Service-specific readiness refers to the capacity of health facilities to provide a specific service, measured through the presence of tracer items that include trained staff, guidelines, equipment/supplies, diagnostic capacity, medicines and commodities. The main challenge is to develop a concise set of items for each domain so that all programs can be monitored through a single data collection mechanism.

Service-specific Readiness Score for Health Facilities

Definition

Cumulative availability of components required in health facilities to deliver specific services, expressed as percentage. The overall score for a specific service is the unweighted average of number of items present and functioning, expressed as a percentage of the total number of items in that service.

Matching Dimensions

Scores for the different domains of general service readiness should be presented separately. All scores can be presented by district and by ownership of facilities.

Hospitals provide a wide range of services and an expanded version of the questionnaire should be administered during facility assessment, or regular reporting.

Service Quality

Assessing quality of care can be difficult because it can cover both the complex processes of evaluating, diagnosing and treating a patient as well as the outcomes of that treatment for the patient. In most definitions, quality of care is seen to be multidimensional—care is said to be of high quality if it is effective, safe, centered on the patient's needs and given in a timely fashion (Table 7.25).

Matching Dimensions

Scores for the different domains of general service readiness should be presented separately. All scores can be presented by district and by ownership of facilities.

Hospitals provide a wide range of services and an expanded version of the questionnaire should be administered during facility assessment, or regular reporting.

Table 7.25: Some indicators for consideration in assessing healthcare quality[35]

Dimension of care	*Indicators*
Effectiveness	• Case-fatality rates for specific diseases • Hospital admission rate for asthma • Percentage of sick child visits during which health worker counselled mother on nutrition • Percentage of women aged 40 years and over who reported a mammogram within the past 2 years • Percentage of women who received prenatal care in the first trimester
Safety	• Percentage of providers who know hand hygiene guidelines • Birth trauma rate in neonate per 1000 live births • Percentage of adults whose provider asks about other prescribed medication
Patient centeredness	• Percentage of adults with recent health visit who stated their provider always listened to what they had to say • Percentage of adults with recent health visit who stated their provider explained things clearly • Percentage of adults with recent health visit who stated their provider showed respect to them
Timeliness	• Percentage of persons who state they have a usual source of care • Percentage of emergency department visits where patients left without being seen • For heart attack patients, median time to thrombolytic therapy or percutaneous transluminal coronary angioplasty (PTCA)

MEASURING THE TRANSMISSIBILITY OF INFECTIONS

Ingenuity, knowledge, and organization alter but cannot cancel humanity's vulnerability to invasion by parasitic forms of life. Infectious disease which antedated the emergence of humankind will last as long as humanity itself, and will surely remain, as it has been hitherto, one of the fundamental parameters and determinants of human history.

— *William H. McNeill, 1976*

Synonyms: Contagious, communicable, transmittable, transmissible, transferable, conveyable, spreadable, spreading.

INTRODUCTION

To understand transmissibility/infectiousness of infections, it is necessary to refresh our knowledge of chain/factors of transmission of a diseases and modes of diseases transmission. A brief account of the same is given below.

Chain of transmission: Six major factors can be identified—the infectious agent, the reservoir, the route/portal of exit, the mode of transmission, the route/portal of entry and the susceptible host (Figs 7.7 and 7.8).[40]

Infectious agents are organisms capable of producing in-apparent infection or clinically manifest disease and include bacteria, rickettsia, chlamydiae, fungi, parasites, viruses, and prions. Infectious disease may also be due to the toxic product of an infectious agent, such as the toxin produced by *Clostridium botulinum* causing classical botulism.

Agents can be described by their ability to cause disease (pathogenicity) as well as their ability to cause serious disease (virulence). The pathogenicity of an infectious agent is the

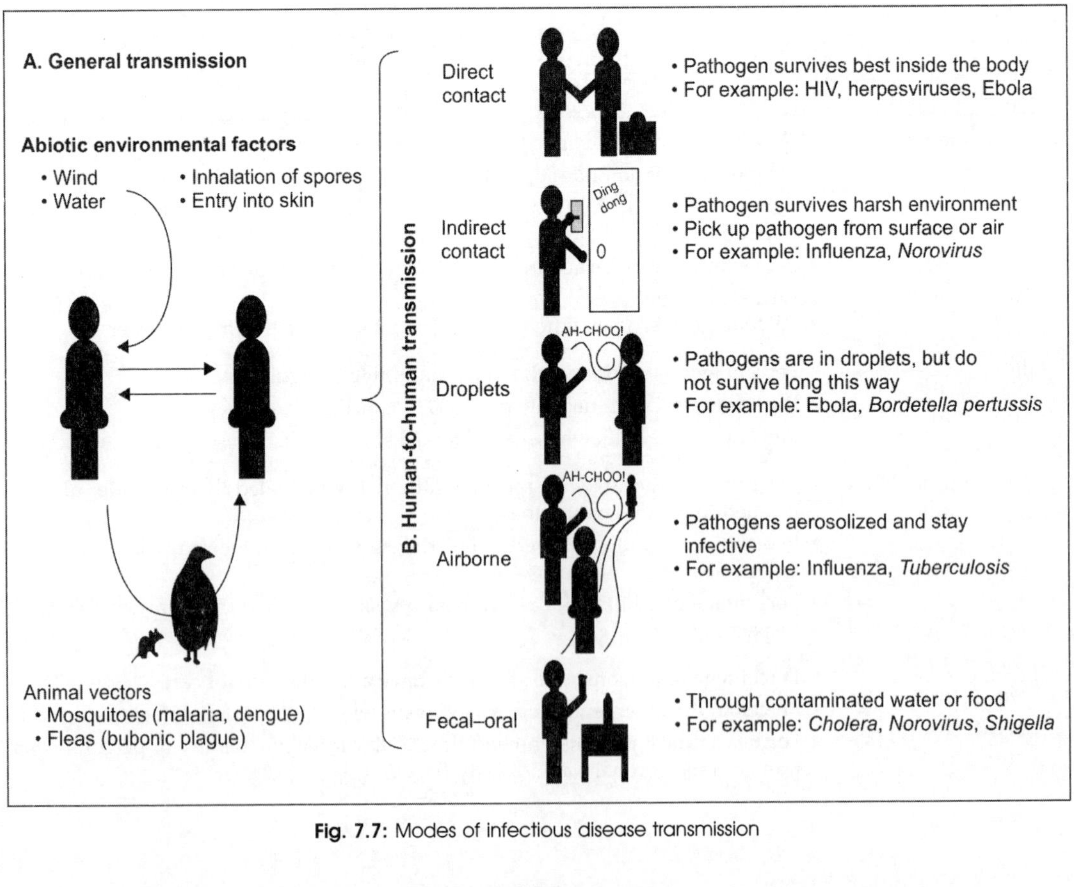

Fig. 7.7: Modes of infectious disease transmission

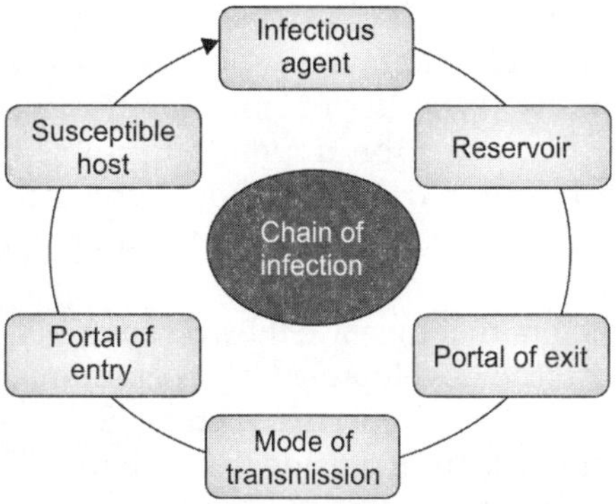

Fig. 7.8: Chain of transmission

extent to which clinically manifest disease is produced in an infected population and is measured by the ratio of the number of persons developing clinical illness to the total number infected. The **virulence** of an infectious agent is the extent to which severe disease is produced in a population with clinically manifest disease. It is the ratio of the number of persons with severe and fatal disease to the total number of persons with disease.

The infective dose of an infectious agent is the number of organisms needed to cause an infection. The infective dose may vary depending upon the route of transmission and host susceptibility.

A **reservoir** of an infectious agent is any person, other living organism, or inanimate material in which the infectious agent normally lives and grows. Many infectious agents can survive in different organisms, or on non-living objects, or in the environment. Some can only persist and multiply inside human beings, whereas others can survive in other animals, or for example in soil or water. The place where the infectious agent is normally present before infecting a new human is called a **reservoir**. Without reservoirs, infectious agents could not survive and hence could not be transmitted to other people. Humans and animals which serve as reservoirs for infectious agents are known as **infected hosts**, e.g. people infected with HIV and *Mycobacterium tuberculosis*; these infectious agents persist and multiply in the infected hosts and can be directly transmitted to new hosts.

A **portal of exit** is the site from where microorganisms leave the host to enter another host and cause disease/infection. For example, a microorganism may leave the reservoir through the nose or mouth when someone sneezes or coughs, or in faeces.

The routes of exit from the respiratory tract are the nose and the mouth. Some infectious agents get out of the infected host in droplets expelled during coughing, sneezing, spitting or talking, and then get transmitted to others. For example, people with tuberculosis in their lungs usually have a persistent cough; *Mycobacterium tuberculosis* uses this as its route of exit.[40–42]

Modes of transmission are the movement or the transmission of pathogens from a reservoir to a susceptible host. Once a pathogen has exited the reservoir, it needs a mode of transmission to the host through a portal of entry. Transmission can be by direct or indirect contact or through airborne transmission.

Direct contact is person-to-person transmission of pathogens through touching, biting, kissing, or sexual intercourse. Microorganisms can also be expelled from the body by coughing, sneezing or talking. The organisms travel in droplets over less than 1 meter in distance and are inhaled by a susceptible host.

Direct modes of transmission can occur in two main ways:

- **Person-to-person:** The infectious agent is spread by direct contact between people through touching, biting, kissing, sexual intercourse or direct projection of respiratory droplets into another person's nose or mouth during coughing, sneezing or talking. A familiar example is the transmission of HIV from an infected person to others through sexual intercourse.
- **Trans-placental transmission:** This refers to the transmission of an infectious agent from a pregnant woman to her fetus through the placenta. An example is mother-to-child transmission (MTCT) of HIV.

Indirect contact includes both vehicle-borne and vector-borne contact. A vehicle is an inanimate go-between, an intermediary between the portal of exit from the reservoir and the portal of entry to the host. Inanimate objects such as handkerchiefs and tissues, soiled laundry, and surgical instruments and dressings are common vehicles that can trans.

Indirect transmission has three subtypes:

- **Airborne transmission:** The infectious agent may be transmitted in dried secretions from the respiratory tract, which can remain suspended in the air for some time. For example, the infectious agent causing tuberculosis can enter a new host through airborne transmission.
- **Vehicle-borne transmission:** A **vehicle** is any non-living substance or object that can be contaminated by an infectious agent, which then transmits it to a new host. **Contamination** refers to the presence of an infectious agent in or on the vehicle.
- **Vector-borne transmission:** A **vector** is an organism, usually an *Arthropod,* which transmits an infectious agent to a new host. Arthropods which act as vectors include houseflies, mosquitoes, lice and ticks.

A **portal of entry** is the site through which microorganisms enter the susceptible host and cause disease/infection. Infectious agents enter the body through various portals, including the mucous membranes, the skin, the respiratory and the gastrointestinal tracts. Pathogens often enter the body of the host through the same route they exited the reservoir; for example, airborne pathogens from one person's sneeze can enter through the nose of another person.

The skin normally serves as a barrier to infection. However, any break in the skin invites the entrance of pathogens, such as tubes placed in body cavities (catheters) or punctures produced by invasive procedures (needles, IV).

The host (also called the susceptible host) is the human body—someone who is at the risk of infection. Infections do not necessarily occur when pathogens enter the body of the person whose immune system is functioning normally. Whether or not a pathogen will result in infection depends upon several factors related to the host (the person exposed), the pathogen itself, and the environment.

Factors that increase the susceptibility of a host to the development of a communicable disease are called **risk factors**. Some risk factors arise from outside the individual—for example, poor personal hygiene, or poor control of reservoirs of infection in the environment. Factors such as these increase the exposure of susceptible hosts to infectious agents, which makes the disease more likely to develop.

Pathogenicity, or the capacity to cause disease, is a relatively rare quality among microbes. It requires the attributes of transmissibility or communicability from one host or reservoir to a fresh host, survival in the new host, infectivity or the ability to breach the new host's defenses, and virulence, a variable that is multifactorial and denotes the capacity of a pathogen to harm the host.

Or pathogenicity is defined as the absolute ability of an infectious agent to cause disease/damage in a host—an infectious agent is either pathogenic or not.

MEASURE OF TRANSMISSIBILITY[42–45]

Epidemiology of infectious diseases, epidemic theory in particular, has played a significant role in understanding of the threshold phenomenon in spread of the infectious disease.

Threshold effects are always present in infectious diseases epidemiology, e.g. direct person-to-person infection transmission can only take off and lead to epidemic, if the density of susceptible population exceeds certain critical value. Herd immunity, a consequence of threshold behaviour, can be used to control the spread of the infection.

Among various threshold parameters arising in epidemic theory perhaps the most useful is the basic reproduction number, usually denoted as R_0.

Basic Reproduction Rate (R_0)[42]

The basic reproduction rate (R_0) is used to measure the transmission potential of a disease (the reproduction number is to forecast future incidence was estimated from the case-count data.).

The basic reproduction number, R_0, is defined as the expected number of secondary cases produced by a single (typical) infection in a completely susceptible population. It is important to note that R_0 is a dimensionless number and not a rate, which would have units of time.

Some authors incorrectly call R_0 the 'basic reproductive rate.'

We can use the fact that R_0 is a dimensionless number to help us in calculating it.

$R_0 \propto$ (Infection/contact) × (Contact/time) × (Time/infection)

$$R_0 = t \times c \times d$$

where, '*t*' is the transmissibility (i.e. probability of infection given to contact between a susceptible and infected individual), '*c*' is the average rate of contact between susceptible and infected individuals, and '*d*' is the duration of infectiousness.

R_0 excludes new cases produced by the secondary cases, etc.

The basic reproductive rate is affected by several factors:

- The duration of infectiousness
- The rate of contacts in the host population
- The probability of infection being transmitted during contact

Infectious Period

Some diseases are contagious for longer periods than others. For example, according to the Centers for Disease Control and Prevention (CDC), adults with the flu are typically contagious for up to 8 days, while children can be contagious for up to 2 weeks. The longer the infectious period of a disease, the more likely an infected person is to spread the disease to other people. A long period of infectiousness will contribute to a higher R_0 value.[44]

Contact Rate

If a person who is infected with a contagious disease comes into contact with many people who are not infected or vaccinated, the disease will spread more quickly. If that person remains at home, in a hospital, or otherwise quarantined while they are contagious, the disease will spread more slowly. A high contact rate will contribute to a higher R_0 value.[44]

Mode of Transmission

The diseases that spread most quickly and easily are the ones that can travel through the air, such as the flu or measles. Physical contact with an infected person is not necessary for the transmission of such conditions. You can catch the flu from breathing near someone who has the flu, even if you never touch them.[44]

In contrast, diseases that are transmitted through bodily fluids, such as Ebola or HIV, are not as easy to catch or spread. This is because you need to come into contact with infected blood, saliva, or other bodily fluids to contract them. Airborne illnesses tend to have a higher R_0 value than those spread through contact.

If $R_0 > 1$:	Then each primary case produces more than 1 secondary case and will lead to **epidemic.**
If $R_0 < 1$:	Then each primary case does not produce enough cases to replace itself, there will not be any disease.
If $R_0 = 1$:	Then each primary case replaces itself and disease will continue to persist as endemic.

For example, if the R_0 for chickenpox in a population is 20, then we would expect it to spread rapidly because each new case of chickenpox would produce 20 new secondary cases.

Effective Reproductive Rate (R)[44,45]

In many circumstances not all contacts will be susceptible to infection. That is, some contacts will be immune, for example, due to prior infection which has conferred life-long immunity, or as a result of previous immunization. Therefore, not all contacts will become infected and the average number of secondary cases per infectious case will decrease. This is measured by the effective reproductive rate (R) (Figs 7.9 to 7.11).

A population will rarely be totally susceptible to an infection in the real world. The effective reproductive rate (R) estimates the average number of secondary cases per infectious case in a population made up of both susceptible and non-susceptible hosts. It can be thought of as the number of secondary infections produced by a typical infective.

$$R = R_0 x$$

It is the basic reproductive rate discounted by the fraction of the host population that is susceptible (x).

For example, if R_0 for Nipah is 10 in a population where 50% of the population is immune, the effective reproductive rate for Nipah is $10 \times 0.5 = 5$. Therefore, under these circumstances a single case of Nipah would produce an average of 5 new secondary cases. To successfully eliminate a disease from a population, R needs to be maintained.

Herd Immunity (HI)[44–46]

Herd immunity occurs when a significant proportion of the population (or the herds) have been vaccinated, and this provides protection for unprotected individuals. The larger the number of people who are vaccinated in a population, the lower the likelihood that a susceptible (unvaccinated)

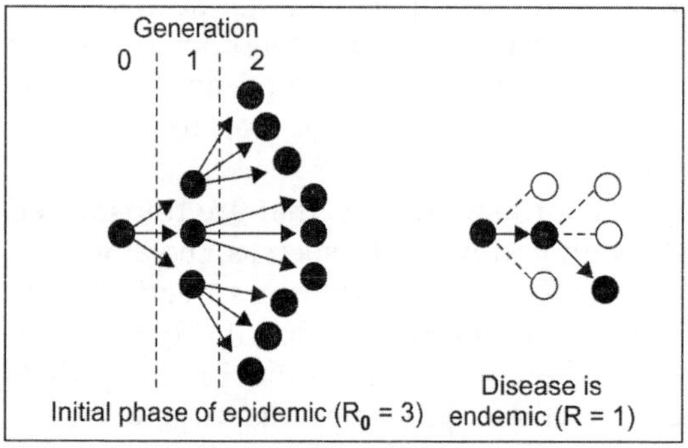

Fig. 7.9: Transmission in epidemic

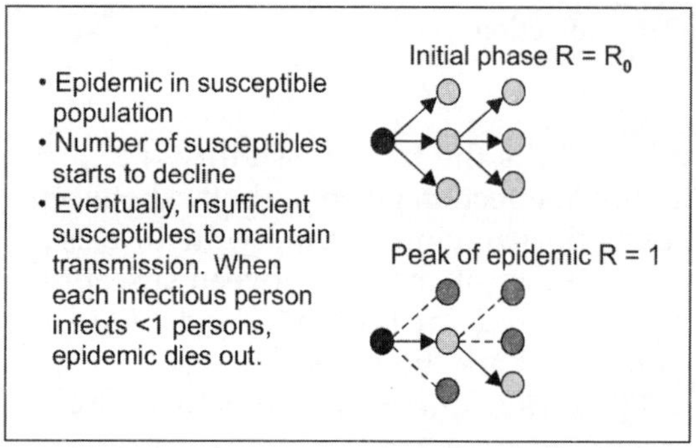

Fig. 7.10: Effective reproduction number R

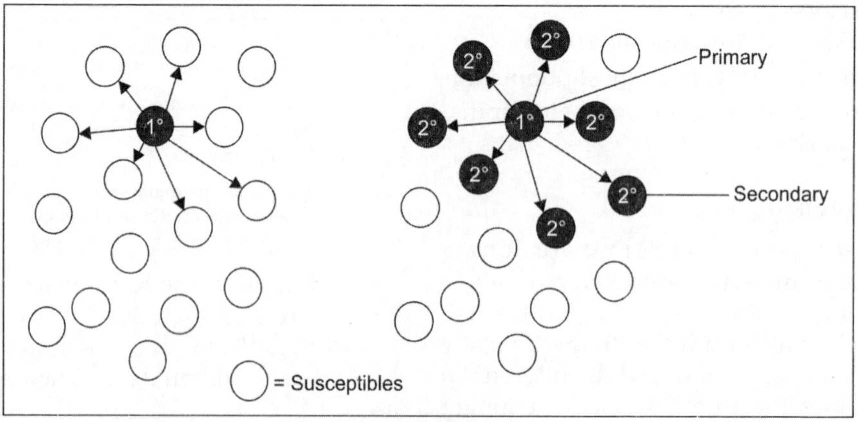

Fig. 7.11: Concept of R_0

person will come into contact with the infection. It is more difficult for diseases to spread between individuals if large numbers are already immune, and the chain of infection is broken.

The herd immunity threshold is the proportion of a population that needs to be immune in order for an infectious disease to become stable in that community. If this is reached, for example due to immunization, then each case leads to a single new case and the infection will become stable within the population. That is R = 1.

If the threshold is surpassed, then R

$$HIT = R_0 - 1 \div R_0 \text{ or } 1 - 1 \div R_0$$

- If some fraction of population is protected (p), then the remainder (1–p) is not directly protected.
- Pathogen will not be able to persist in the unprotected portion of the population if is now less than 1.
- Conversely, the infectious disease will only persist if the number of secondary cases in the susceptible population is at least equal to $1R_0$ (Fig. 7.12).

This is an important measure used in infectious disease control and immunization and eradication programs.

Relationship of R_0 and Herd Immunity

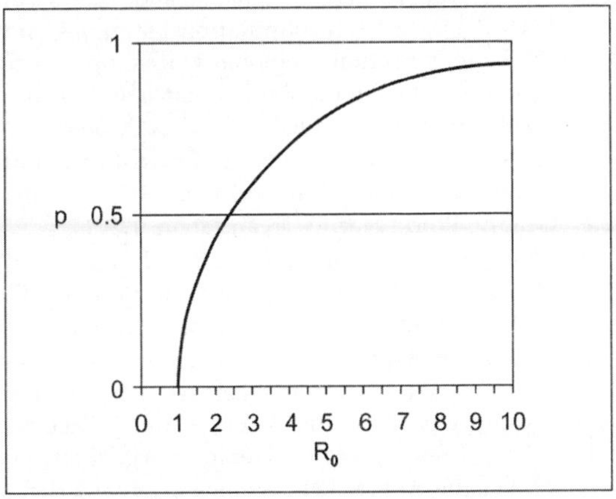

Fig. 7.12: Relationship of R_0 and herd immunity

Secondary Attack Rate (SAR)

Secondary attack rate (SAR) is used in the study of the spread of infectious diseases in small communities.

- Only for person–person transmission
- SAR = The proportion of those exposed to the primary case that develop disease as a result of the exposure

Depends On

- Closeness of contact, e.g. first Ebola outbreak SAR = 27% for close family
- Type of contact, e.g. for HIV—sharing needles > sexual contact, e.g. for Ebola—extensive contact with body fluid > skin contact
- Stage of illness, e.g. Ebola more infectious (higher viral load) as disease progresses

R_0 and SAR

R_0—average number of secondary cases per case in a totally susceptible population

SAR—proportion of those exposed to the primary case that develop disease as a result of the exposure in a particular situation

R_0 = SAR (household) × no. of contacts (household) + SAR (other family) × no. of contacts (other family) + S AR (community) × No. of contacts (community) + etc.

References

1. Principles of epidemiology in public health practice: An introduction to applied epidemiology and biostatistics, Ch. 3, (3rd edn.). Self study Course SS1000, published by US department of health and human services, Centers for Disease Control and Prevention (CDC), Office of Workforce and Career Development, Atlanta, GA 30333.
2. Epidemiological Research Methods, Stat 507 Ch. 2.2. Measures of disease frequency, dept. of statistics, HYPERLINK https://www.psu.edu/ The Pennsylvania State University, Source URL: HYPERLINK https://newonlinecourses. science. psu.edu/stat507/02/measures/https://online courses.science.psu.edu/stat507/02/measures
3. Rothman, Kenneth. Modern Epidemiology, Ch. 5 and pp 227–2290. Lilienfeld and Lilienfeld-Foundations of epidemiology, Measures of mortality, pp 71–80; Mausner & Kramer. Epidemiology: an introductory text, pp 338–44.

4. Gaffey WR. A critique of the standardized mortality ratio. J Occup Med 1976;18:157–60.
5. Victor J Schoenbach, Wayne D Rosamond. Understanding the fundamentals of epidemiology—an evolving text, Department of Epidemiology, School of Public Health, University of North Carolina at Chapel Hill, Fall 2000. pp 129–48.
6. Census India 2011.www.censusindia.gov.in
7. Omar R Ahmed, Cynthia Boschi-Pinto, Alan D Lopez, Christopher JL Murrey, Mie Inoue. Age standardization of rates: A new WHO standards, GPE discussion paper series: no. 31, EIP/GPE/EBD, WHO 2001.
8. Causes of deaths in India–2004–2006. HYPERLINK http://www.cghr.org/uploads/consolidated data/2004-6-final,pdf" www.cghr.org/uploads/consolidateddata/2004–6-final pdf. HYPERLINK http://www.censusindia.gov.in http://www.censusindia.gov.in
9. WHO. World report on disability. Geneva: WHO, 2011. http://www. who.int/disabilities/world_report/2011/ en/index.html-accessed 2013.
10. WHO. How to use the ICF: A practical manual for using the International Classification of Functioning, Disability and Health (ICF). Exposure draft for comment. October 2013. Geneva: WHO.
11. WHO. International classification of functioning and disability and health (ICF). Geneva: WHO–http://www.who.int/classifications/icf/en/index.html-accessed 21 May 2013.
12. WHO. International classification of functioning. disability and health. Geneva: WHO, 2001.
13. WHO. Ten facts on disability. Fact file. Geneva: WHO-http://www.who.int/features/factfiles/disability/facts/en/index.html-accessed 21 May 2013.
14. WHO. Disability report by the secretariat. Executive. Geneva: WHO, 2012. Document No. EB 132/10–30 November 2012.
15. WHO Regional Office for South-East Asia. Situation analysis of community based rehabilitation in the South East Asia. New Delhi: WHO-SEARO, 2012.
16. An overarching health indicator for the Post-2015 Development Agenda, Brief summary of some proposed candidate indicators Background paper for Expert Consultation 11–12 December 2014.
17. Paul J van der Maas. How summary measures of population health are affecting health agendas. Bulletin of the World Health Organization 2003;81 (5).
18. Christopher JL Murray Joshua A Salomon Colin Mathers. A Critical Examination of Summary Measures of Population Health https://www.who.int/healthinfo/paper02.pdf
19. Molla MT, Madans JH, Wagener DK, Crimmins EM. Summary measures of population health: Report of findings on methodologic and data issues. National Cancer for Health Statistics, Hyattsville, Maryland. 2003. https://www.cdc.gov/nchs/data/misc/pophealth.pdf
20. WHO, Health statistics and information systems, Disease burden and mortality estimates. https://www.who.int/healthinfo/global_burden_disease/en/
21. Physical Quantity of Life Index (PQLI): https://economicsconcepts.com/physical_quantity_of_life_index.htm
22. Morris MD. The Physical Quality of Life Index (PQLI). Dev Dig 1980;18(1):95–109. PubMed PMID: 12261723.
23. Life-tables and their demographic applications. https://www.healthknowledge.org.uk/public-health-textbook/health-information/3a-populations/life-tables-demographic-applications http://www.quantitativeskills.com/downloads/#Lifetable
24. HYPERLINK https://dhsprogram.com/Data/Guide-to-DHS-Statistics/Guide_to_DHS_Statistics_DHS-7.htm" Guide to DHS Statistics DHS-7 https://dhsprogram.com/Data/Guide-to-DHS-Statistics/index.htm#t=Current_Fertility.htm
25. Govt. of India, Estimates of fertility indicators - Census of India. Ch. 3, www.censusindia.gov.in›7. Ch. 3, Fertility Indicators-2015.pdf
26. Censusindia.gov.in › vital_statistics › SRS_Report_2012 › 10_Chap_3_2012
27. Govt. of India, Fertility Indicators | data.gov.in https://data.gov.in/resources/fertility-indicators-major-states-2006-2011
28. Thomas Spoorenberg. Evaluation and Analysis of Fertility Data (ppt). Population Estimates and Projections Section. Regional workshop on the Production of Population Estimates and Demographic Indicators Addis Ababa, 5–9 October.
29. ICD-10. International statistical classification of diseases and related health problems: 10th revision. Geneva, World Health Organization, 1992.
30. World Health Statistics 2015. Part-I, Health-related Millennium Development Goals. WHO Press, WHO, 20 Avenue Appia, 1211 Geneva 27, Switzerland.
31. WHO. 2006. Reproductive health indicators: guidelines for their generation, interpretation and analysis for global monitoring. Annexure 2. Page 63. WHO Press, World Health Organization, 20 Avenue Appia, 1211 Geneva 27, Switzerland https: //www.who.int/reproductivehealth/publications/monitoring/924156315x/en/

32. MoSP, GOI. Manual on health statistics in India. Central Statistical Office Ministry of Statistics and Programme Implementation Government of India New Delhi May, 2015 HYPERLINK http://Global Reference List of Core Health Indicators: Working Version 5, World Health Organization Geneva, 17 November 2014. www.who.int › healthinfo › country_monitoring_evaluation › GlobalRefL..."
33. Global Reference List of Core Health Indicators: Working Version 5, World Health Organization Geneva, 17 November 2014. www.who.int › healthinfo › country_monitoring_evaluation › GlobalRefL...
34. Indicator for the Post-2015 Development Agenda: Brief summary of some proposed candidate indicators, Background paper for Expert Consultation 11–12 Dec. 2014 https://www.who. int/health info/indicators/hsi_indicators_SDG_ Technical Meeting_December2015_BackgroundPaper.pdf
35. WHO. Toolkit on monitoring health systems streng thening. Service Delivery, 2008. HYPERLINK http://www.who.int › statistics › toolkit_hss › EN_ PDF accessed on 10 Sept. 2018 www.who.int › statistics › toolkit_hss › EN_PDF accessed on 10 Sept. 2018
36. Tanahashi T. Health services coverage and its evaluation. Bulletin of the World Health Organization 1978;56:295–303.
37. Shenghelia B, et al. Beyond access and utilization: defining and measuring health system coverage. In: Murray CJL, Evans DB, (Eds.). Health systems performance assessment: de7bates, methods and empiricism. Geneva, World Health Organization, 2003;221–235.
38. WHO. Health service delivery. https://www.who.int/healthinfo/systems/WHO_MBHSS_2010_section1_web.pdf accessed on 10 Sept. 2018
39. Service Availability Mapping (SAM) (assessment tool and country reports). Geneva, World Health Organization (http://www.who.int/healthinfo/systems/serviceavailabilitymapping/en/accessed 26 July 2018).
40. Communicable Diseases Module: 1. Basic Concepts in the Transmission of Communicable Diseases. http://www.open.edu/openlearncreate/mod/oucontent/view.php?id=84
41. Guide to monitoring and evaluating communicable disease surveillance and response systems, World Health Organization 2006; http://www.who.int/csr/resources/publications/surveillance/WHO_CDS_EPR_LYO_2006_2.pdf
42. Robert J. Kim-Farley, Global strategies for control of communicable diseases,Oxford Textbook of Public Health.
43. James Holland Jones, Notes On R0, Department of Anthropological Sciences, Building 360, Stanford, CA May 1, 2017, https://web.stanford.edu/~jhj1/teachingdocs/Jones-on-R0.pdf
44. Vanessa Bates Ramirez, HYPERLINK https://www.healthline.com/health/r-nought-repro duction-number" What Is R0? Gauging Contagious Infections, College of Medicine HYPERLINK https://www.healthline.com/medical-team University of Illinois-Chicago, June 24, 2016; https://www.healthline.com/health/r-nought-reproduction-number
45. Roberto Rigobon, Contagion: How to Measure It? URL: http://www.nber.org/chapters/c10638
46. Gao, Daozhou, "Transmission Dynamics of Some Epidemiological Patch Models" (2012). Open Access Dissertations. Paper 763.

Chapter
8

Epidemiological Study Designs: Descriptive Studies

Ram Chandra Goyal

Epidemiology is a scientific discipline with sound methods of scientific inquiry at its foundation.

According to **John M Last**, epidemiology is defined as "the **study** of the **distribution** and **determinants** of **health-related states or events** in **specified populations**, and the **application** of this study to the control of health problems".[1]

The core of the public health is epidemiology as it deals with quantitative discipline (disease frequency), causal reasoning (statistical association between an explanatory characteristic (exposure) and the outcome of interest (disease), generation and testing hypotheses in all scientific fields as biostatistics and informatics, with biologic, physics, ergonomics, economic, social, and behavioural sciences.

To summarize, epidemiology is the study (scientific, systematic, data-driven) of the distribution (**frequency, pattern**) and determinants (**causes, risk factors**) of health-related states and events (not just diseases) in specified populations (patient's community, group of individuals), and the application of (in public health) this study to the control of health problems.[2]

CLASSIFICATION OF EPIDEMIOLOGICAL STUDIES[3–8]

Classification depends on the nature of question to be addressed, whether one want to get an answer for their beliefs and ideas or magnitude of problem or prove the hypothesis.

A study design is a specific plan or protocol for conducting the study, which allows the investigator to translate the conceptual hypothesis into an operational one.

One of the challenging basic issues is in deciding the appropriate epidemiological study design for achieving the stated aim and objectives of the proposed research question.

It depends on the research question and hypotheses, resources and time available for the study, type of outcome of interest, type of exposure of interest and ethics.

Although there are endless ways of classifying epidemiological study designs, commonly used study designs are as follows:

A. **Classification based on nature of the enquiry**
   - **Explorative:** It lays emphasis on discovery of ideas and insights. It is also called formulative designs.
   - **Descriptive:** It describes the characteristics of an individual or a group or situation.

- **Diagnostic:** This type of study determines the frequency with which something occurs (disease/event) or its association with something else factor(s).
- **Experimental:** These designs try to prove the causal influence of one variable on another variable.

B. Classification based on taxonomy (Table 8.1 and Fig. 8.1).

Table 8.1: Classification based on observation and intervention

Type of study	*Alternate name*	*Unit of study*
A. Observational studies (non-experimental)		
Descriptive studies:		
Case report, case series		Individuals
Ecological	Co-relational	Populations
Cross-sectional (single sample from large population without comparison)	Prevalence	Individuals
Analytical studies		
Cross-sectional (single sample from large population with comparison)	Prevalence	Individuals
Case control	Case reference	Individuals
Cohort	Follow-up/longitudinal	Individuals
B. Experimental/intervention studies		
Randomized controlled studies	Clinical trial	Patients
Field trial		Healthy person
Community trial	Community intervention studies	Communities

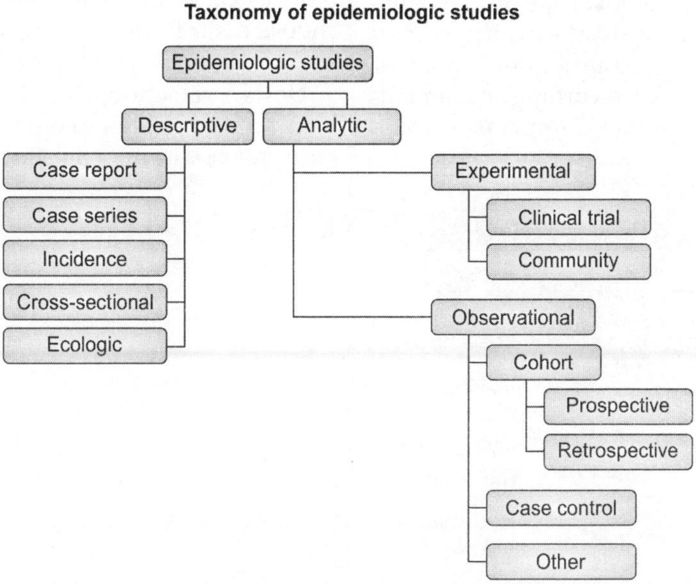

Fig. 8.1: Classification based on observation and intervention

C. Classification based on type of research

Quantitative

- Observational—studies that do not involve any intervention or experiment—descriptive, analytical and experimental
- Experimental—studies that entail manipulation of the study factor (exposure) and randomization of subjects to treatment (exposure) groups

OR

- Preliminary (case reports, case series)
- Basic [cross-sectional, case control, cohort (prospective, retrospective)]
- Hybrid (two or more of the above, nested case control within cohort, etc.)
- Incomplete (ecological, PMR, etc.)
- Others (repeated, case cross-over, migrant, twin, etc.)

Qualitative

- Case study/comparative study/sample survey/panel survey
- Experiment/interventional
- Participant observation

In qualitative research sources of data collection/elicitation are participatory inquiry, systematic observations, participant observation (fieldwork), interviews (individual/family/group), questionnaires, focus group, film, AV recording, documents and text and researcher's impressions and reactions.

Table 8.3: Relative ability of different study designs to prove causation

Type of study design	*Ability to prove causation*
Ecological	Weak
Cross-sectional	Weak
Case control	Moderate
Cohort	Moderate
Randomized controlled trials	Strong

A good study design must fulfill the following criteria.

- *Objectivity*—methods used for collection of data and scoring of responses should be objective.
- *Reliability*—it is the consistency throughout a series of measurements.
- *Validity*—the method/equipment should measure what it is supposed to measure.
- *Generalisability*—should provide information regarding generalisability of the findings of the present study to parent population.

Selection of study designs also depends on the purpose and ability of the study designs to prove the causation of the disease/event. We must choose a study design which can prove the causal relationship (Tables 8.2, 8.3 and 8.5).

Design selection, decision algorism and hierarchy of epidemiological study designs are mentioned in Table 8.4 and shown in Fig. 8.2.

Table 8.2: Epidemiological studies and their reasoning

Type of study	*Reasoning*
Ecological	Descriptive; association on group level may be used for development of general hypothesis
Cross-sectional	Descriptive; association on group level may be used for development of specific hypothesis
Case control	Increases prevalence of risk factor among diseases may indicate a causal relationship
Cohort	Increases risk of disease among exposed indicates a causal relationship
Intervention/experimental	Modification (reduction) of the incidence rate of disease confirms a causal relationship.

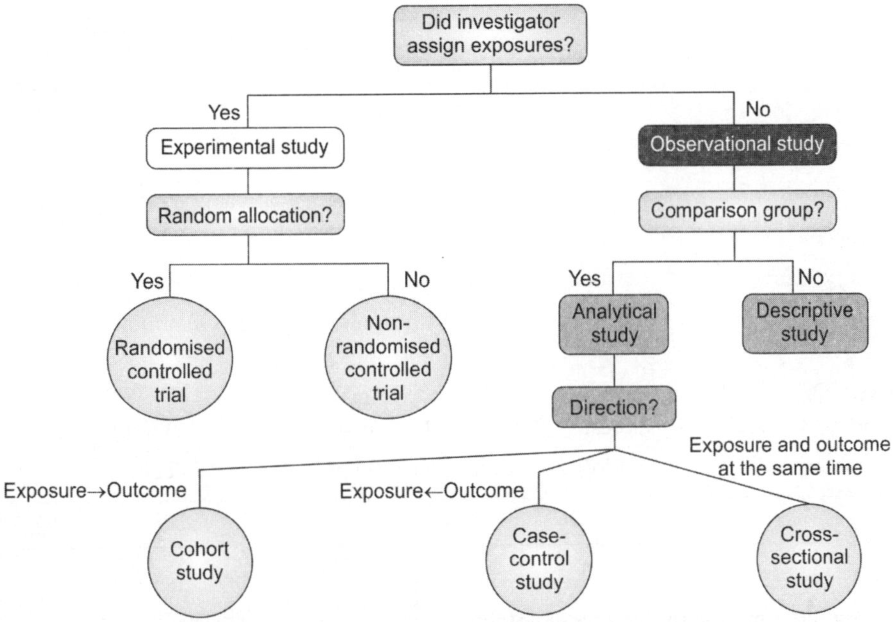

Fig. 8.2: Decision algorism for choosing a study design

Table 8.4: The hierarchy of epidemiological study designs

Descriptive study designs:	
Case report	Single case
Case series	Collection of similar cases
Correlational	Population based study—using secondary data
Cross-sectional (descriptive)	Single sample from larger population—no comparison
Analytical study designs:	
Cross-sectional (analytical)	Single sample from larger population—compares two or more groups in the sample
Case control	Compares risk factors between diseased (cases) and non-diseased (controls) groups
Cohort	Compares outcomes between groups exposed and non-exposed to a risk factor for a disease
Interventional study:	
Clinical trial	Investigator allots the subjects to different groups—intervention versus non-intervention

DESCRIPTIVE STUDIES

The descriptive epidemiology is concerned with "describing the characteristics of the occurrence or distribution of diseases or health-related states and events within a population."

Descriptive patterns of disease occurrence often lead to the generation of hypotheses about disease causation.

To describe descriptive epidemiology three basic questions can be asked:

- Who is getting the disease? or person distribution.
- Where is it occurring? or place distribution.
- When is the disease occurring? or time distribution.

Table 8.5: Purpose and appropriateness of epidemiological study design

Basis	*Cohort*	*Case control*	*Cross-sectional*
Rare condition	Impracticable	Bias is more	Not appropriate
To determine a precise risk	Best	Only estimates are possible	Output is only prevalence and not incidence
To determine whether exposure preceded disease	Best	Not appropriate	Not appropriate
Administrative purpose	Not appropriate	Not appropriate	Best
If attrition a serious problem	Not appropriate	Attrition is minimal	Attrition may occur before the study
If selective survival is a problem	Best	Not appropriate	Not appropriate
If all factors are not known	Best	Not appropriate	Not appropriate
Time and money	Most expensive	Least expensive	In between

The 5W's of descriptive epidemiology:
- What = health issue of concern
- Who = person
- Where = place
- When = time
- Why/how = causes, risk factors, modes of transmission

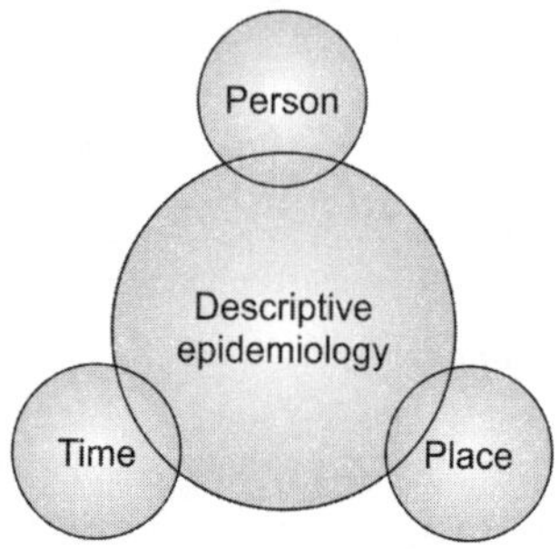

These three questions serve as the basis for a descriptive investigation and these three features, i.e. person, place and time are used to track the occurrence of a disease (Table 8.6).

Person Distribution

One of the basic tenets of epidemiology is that diseases do not occur at random and all persons in a population are not equally likely

Table 8.6: Descriptive epidemiology (person, place and time characteristics)

Person (some personal characteristics)		*Place*	*Time*
Age	Physical parameters like height, weight, BP, etc.	Villages, town, cities, institutions	Duration
Gender, ethnicity, religion	Biochemical parameters like lipid profile, blood sugar, LFT, KFT, etc.	Urban, rural, tribal, reachable/unreachable	Hours, day,
Marital status	Habits, hobbies	Region, state, country	Week, month
Occupation, education	Birth order, family size	Climatic zones	Year, season
Social class, income	Addictions, use of medication, etc.	—	—

to develop a particular condition due to the differences in their exposure and susceptibility to causal/risk factors. The personal characteristics which can be examined in relation to disease occurrence can be grouped as inherent characteristics of people (e.g. age, sex, race), biologic characteristics (immune status), acquired characteristics (marital status), activities (occupation, leisure activities, use of medications/tobacco/drugs), lifestyle, behavioural factors or the conditions under which they live (socio-economic status, access to medical care), etc. Age and sex are two most commonly person's attribute used in all kind of studies/data set. There are many more personal characteristics which as impact on spectrum of health and disease. Some of the commonly used characteristics are described below.

Age

It has been noticed that occurrence of various diseases are at various stages of life. It is strongly related to disease as certain diseases are more common in certain age groups than in others, e.g. mumps, measles, chickenpox in childhood (unvaccinated children), injuries, violence, substance use in adolescence, injuries, cancer in middle age and atherosclerosis, arthritis, Alzheimer in old age. As age increases the immunity decreases and susceptibility increases. Apart from this number of factors that also vary with age like opportunity for exposure, latency or incubation period of the disease, and physiologic response to the causative factor (Figs 8.3 and 8.4).

Bar diagram: A total of 100 patients were treated for breast cancer in the 4 years period. Mean age of patients was 51 years (standard deviation = 10.48). Minimum age was 28 years and the maximum was 80 years and median age was 49 years. Number of patients 50 years and below 50 years of age was 60. Out of 60 patients 19 (31.6%) were 40 and below 40 years of age. The age distribution showed two peaks at 41–50 years and 51–60 years with 42 and 24 patients, respectively in both the age groups. Number of patients in age groups 21–30, 31–40, 41–50, 51–60, 61–70 and 71–80 were 1, 18, 42, 24, 11 and 4, respectively (Fig. 8.5).[10]

Pie diagram: A study conducted in Maharashtra in 2012 showed 30% of the patients who were admitted due to respiratory infection belonged to the paediatric group, which was found to be the most vulnerable to infections as compared with other age groups. The patients of adolescence group (6–20 years) were 11%, whereas the middle aged groups (21–40 years) comprised 34% (Fig. 8.6).[10]

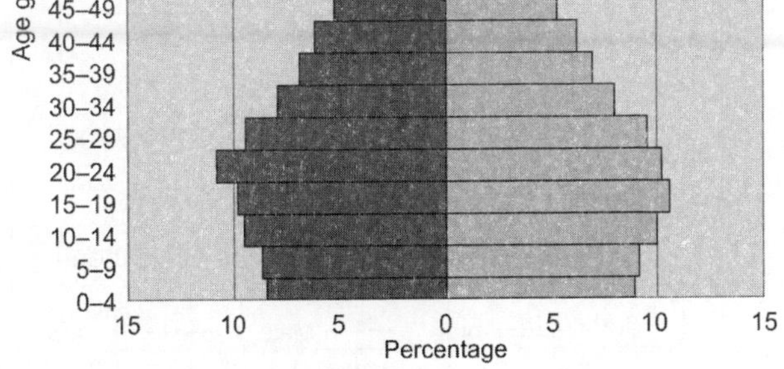

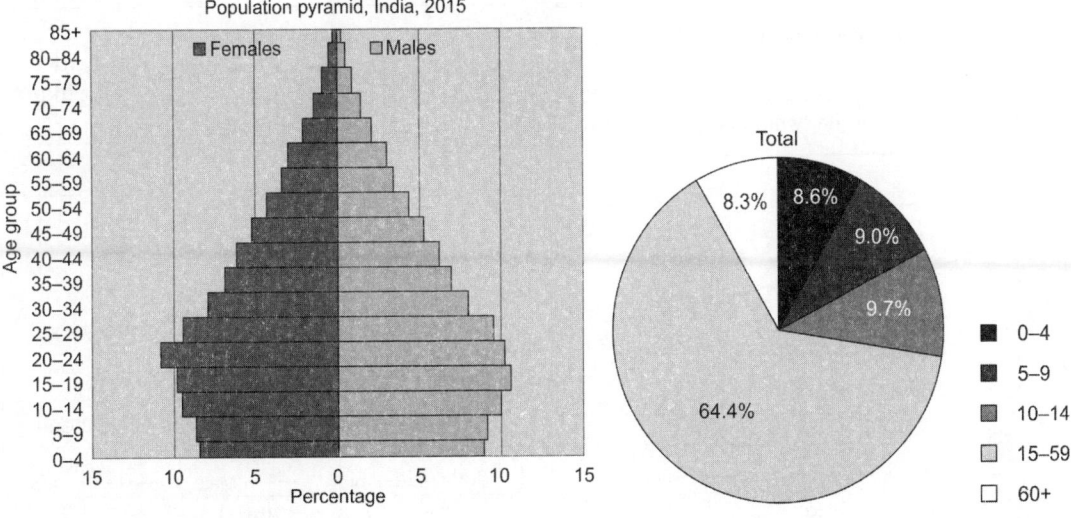

Fig. 8.3: Age pyramid of populationin India[3]

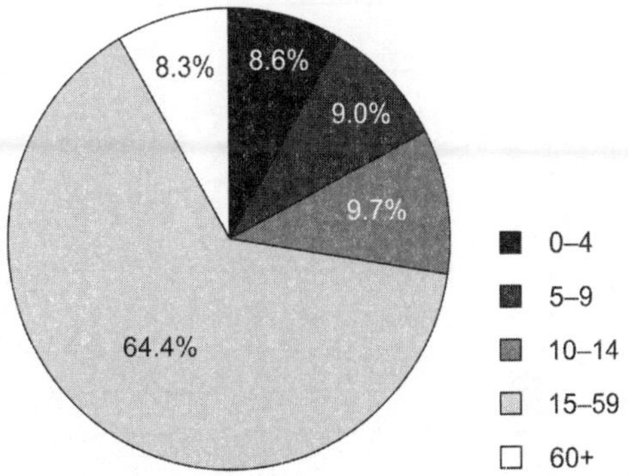

Fig. 8.4: Distribution of population in India[9]

Gender (Sex)

Mortality rates from several common causes of death, such as ischaemic heart disease, malignant neoplasms, and HIV-AIDS (in Western countries), have sex ratios substantially greater than one. The disparity is due to socio-cultural, behavioural practices and lifestyle of men and women. Other factors like environmental exposures, genetic predisposition, endogenous factors, such as the sex hormones, may contribute to differences in risk between the sexes.

Some diseases are more common in women than men, e.g. chronic diseases such as diabetes, hyperthyroidism, obesity, etc. and some others such as lung cancer and coronary heart disease are more common in men than women. Following graphs (Figs 8.7a and b) and Table 8.7 show the difference in male and female mortality in India.

Table 8.7: Prevalence of metabolic syndrome and components in urban Asian Indians

Variable	*Male*	*Female*
High WC	18.4	29.3
Low LDL	4.7	68
High TG	43.1	36.8
High FBG	39.2	31.9
High BP	45.1	40.6
Metabolic syndrome	17.6	44.2

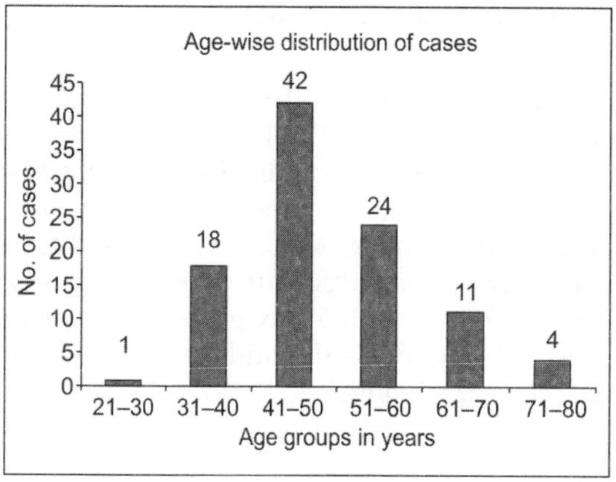

Fig. 8.5: Bar diagram

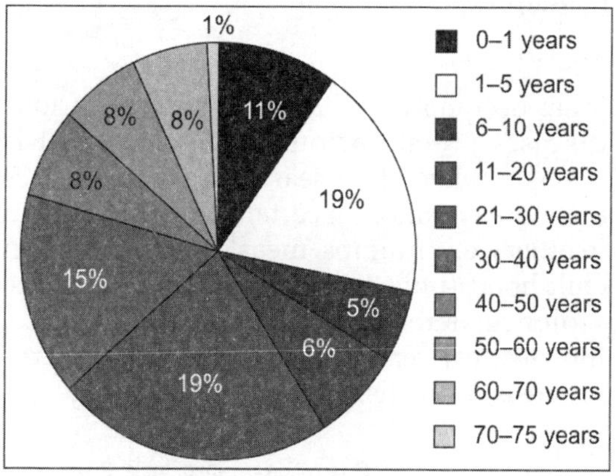

Fig. 8.6: Pie diagram

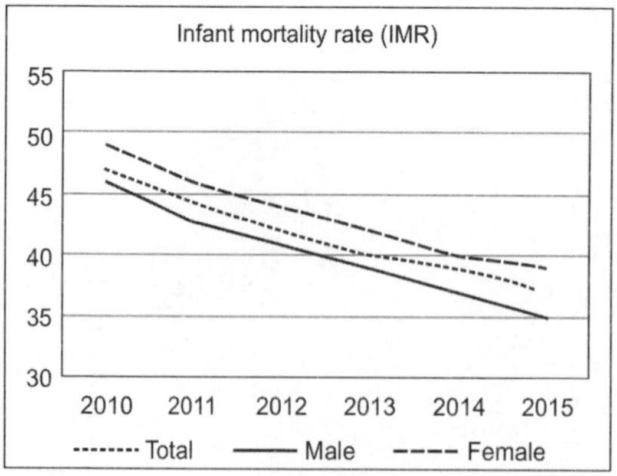

(a)

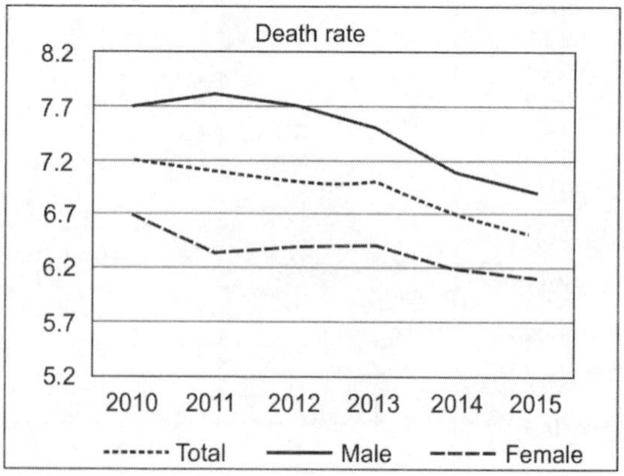

(b)

Figs 8.7: (a) IMR and (b) death rate

Marital Status

Although the true nature of the association between marriage and ill-health is not certain, however, it has been found that mortality rates are lower for married males and females than for the unmarried of the same age and sex. It may be due to the differences in life-styles and behavioural factors. On the other hand, it may be a risk factor for certain conditions such as cancer cervix is long been studies and found to have positive association. Table 8.8. shows age at first marriage and carcinoma.[11]

Ethnicity (Race)[11,12]

Studies within multi-ethnic societies are more valuable than international comparisons, if the primary variable of interest is ethnicity or racial group, since at least some of the environmental differences present in international comparisons are reduced or eliminated.

There are differences in disease occurrence between racial and ethnic sub-groups in the population, e.g. coronary heart disease, hypertension, cancer, sickle-cell anemia, etc. These differences may be due to genetic or environmental factors and thus a stimulus for further epidemiological studies.

The most fruitful approach using routine data sources is through the study of migrants, that attempt to separate the 'genetic' and 'environmental' components of differences by studying disease risk in a given migrant population in comparison with that in the host population (similar environment, different genetics) and in the population living in place of origin (similar genetics, different environment).

Table 8.9 showed that several population-based studies based on predominantly white European populations have found the prevalence of PAD to be between 6% and 18% over the age of 55 years. The prevalence rises with age and has been found to be approximately 20% in people over 70 years of age 12 and up to 60% in the over 85 age group. There has, however, been very little research into the prevalence of PAD in non-Caucasian populations, although previous population-based studies have shown variations in the prevalence of this disease amongst different ethnic groups (Table 8.9 and Fig. 8.8).

Occupation

There are various types of occupations ranging from simple writing work (sedentary) to farm workers/blacksmith (heavy workers), but everyone gets one or the other occupational hazard. Several determinants,

Table 8.8: Age at first marriage and carcinoma

Age (year)	*No. of women*	*Cases of invasive carcinoma*	*Cases of carcinoma in-situ*
<15	764	9	7
15–19	14,261	73	105
20–24	13,950	42	57
25–29	4,985	5	18
30–34	1,474	2	2
35 and over	877	1	3
Unknown	2,565	9	7
Never married	2,628	2	3
Totals	**41,504**	**143**	**202**

(Christofherson WM and Parker JE. Relation of Cervical Cancer to Early Marriage and Childbearing *N Engl J Med* 1965; Vol. 273, no. 5)

Table 8.9: Examples of population-based studies investigating PAD in different ethnic groups[13]

Study	*Country*	*Race/ethnic group studied*	*Sample size*	*Age*	*PAD prevalence* (%)
Fowkes *et al.*	UK	European	1592	55–74	18.3
Meijer *et al.*	Netherlands	European	6450	>55	19.1
Fabsitz *et al.*	US	Native American Indians	4549	45–74	5.3
Premalatha *et al.*	South India	Indian	631	>20	3.2
Diehm *et al.*	Germany	European African–American Non-hispanic white	6821	⩾65	18
Selvin and Erlinger	US	Hispanic African–American Non-hispanic white	2174	>40	4.3 (AA:7.9; NHW:4.4; H:3.0)
Collins *et al.*	US	Hispanic African–American Non-hispanic white	403	>55	16.6 (AA22.8; NHW:13.2; H:13.7)
McDermott *et al.*	US	Hispanic Chinese	6560	45–84	3.7 M (NHW:2.7; Ch:1.1; AA7.1;H:3; F (NHW:3.5; Ch:2.2; AA:6.1; H:1.7)
Criqui *et al.*	US	African–American Non-hispanic white Hispanic Asian	2343	29–91	4.4 (AA:7.8; NHW:4.9; H:1.8; As:1.4)
Allison *et al.*	US	African–American Non-Hispanic white Hispanic Chinese	6653	45–85	4.3 (AA:7.2; NHW:3.6; H:2.4; Ch:2)
He *et al.*	China	Chinese	2334	⩾60	19.8
Al-Sheikh *et al.*	Saudi Arabia	Arabic	471	⩾45	11.7
Garofolo *et al.*	Brazil	Japanese	1008	⩾30	20.4
Sritara *et al.*	Thailand	Thai	2305	52–73	5.2
Carbayo *et al.*	Spain	European	784	⩾40	10.5
Sigvant *et al.*	Sweden	European	5080	60–90	18
Kumar *et al.*	South Africa	Black African	542	>50	29.3

PAD defined as ABPI <0.9. All studies include males and females. AA: African American; H: Hispanic; NHW: Non-Hispanic White; Ch: Chinese; As: Asian

Source: Bennett PC, Silverman S, Gill PS, Lip GYH. Ethnicity and peripheral artery disease, QJM: An International Journal of Medicine, 2009;102(1):3–16, https://doi.org/10.1093/qjmed/hcn140

including risk factors at workplace (e.g. working hours, salary, workplace policies, health promotion and protection provisions of employment and working conditions, etc.) leading to accidents, musculo-skeletal diseases, respiratory diseases, hearing loss, circulatory diseases, stress-related disorders, communicable diseases, cancers and other conditions.[14]

The major occupational diseases/morbidity of concern in India are silicosis, musculo-skeletal injuries, coal workers' pneumoconiosis, chronic obstructive lung diseases, asbestosis, byssinosis, pesticide poisoning and noise-induced hearing loss.

It has an important bearing on the health status as the occupation may alter the habit pattern of employees, e.g. sleep, alcohol,

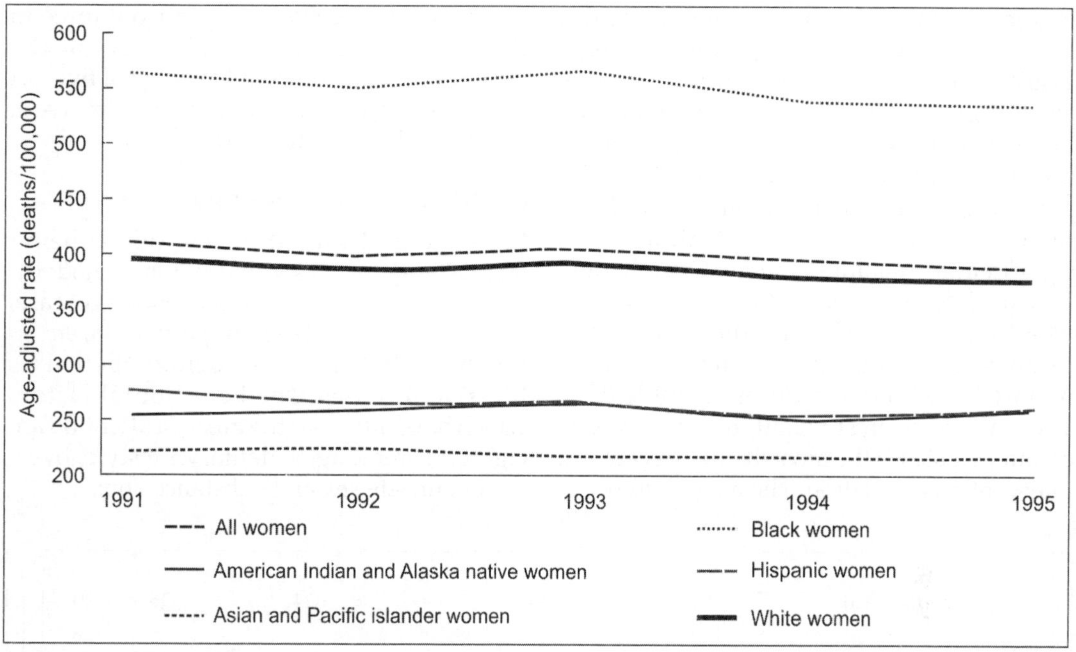

Fig. 8.8: Trends in heart disease mortality among women 35 years of age and older, by race and ethnicity, 1991–1995

smoking, drug addiction, night shifts, etc. It is obvious that persons working in a particular occupation may be exposed to particular types of risks, e.g. workers in coal mines are more likely to suffer from silicosis whereas those in sedentary occupations have more risk of suffering from heart disease.

Apart from the above, workers are also exposed to long working hours, poor and adverse working environment and inadequate coverage of health leads to minor and major mental disorders.

Socio-economic Status (SES)

There are many factors included in SES such as occupation, income, educational, housing, purchasing power, access to health services and social standing play an important role in health and disease. Sometimes, only family income is considered for classifying the SES, e.g. BG Prasad classification, Parikh's classification, etc. in India.

WHO regions and World Bank income categories: WHO Member States are grouped into low and middle-income countries (LMIC) by WHO region (the 6 WHO regions are used), separating out high-income countries within each of these regions into a 7th group.

World Bank income groups—WHO Member States are grouped into 4 income groups (low, lower-middle, upper-middle, and high) based on the World Bank list of analytical income classification of economies for the fiscal year, which is based on the Atlas gross national income per capita estimates.

Epidemiological studies have shown that health and diseases are not equally distributed in social classes. Individuals in the upper social classes have longer life expectancy and better health and nutritional status than those in the lower social classes. Certain diseases like coronary heart disease, hypertension and diabetes have shown a higher prevalence in upper classes than in the lower classes. However social classification varies from country to country and may have different meanings for different persons.

It is clear that in low- and lower-middle-income countries large gaps persist in basic maternal, child and environmental health services coverage. These gaps are not evenly distributed across population groups (Figs 8.9 and 8.10). Whereas 39% of mother–child pairs in these countries received at least six of the seven basic interventions, 4% of mother–child pairs received no interventions at all. When the data are stratified by wealth quintile, significant inequalities emerge. Overall, only 17% of those in households in the poorest wealth quintile (Q1) in their countries received at least six basic interventions as opposed to 74% in the richest quintile (Q5). Those in the poorest wealth quintile in each country were also the most likely to receive no interventions at all (9%). The mean number of interventions received ranged from three in the poorest wealth quintile to six in the wealthiest, with an overall average of five out of the seven interventions being received. (WHO health statistics, 2018).[15]

Lifestyle and Human Behaviour

Lifestyle and human behaviour is being increasingly seen as a risk factor in modern-day diseases such as coronary heart disease, cancer, obesity, diabetes, hypertension, etc. so much so that these are being labelled as lifestyle diseases. The behavioural factors which have attracted the greatest attention are cigarette smoking, sedentary lifestyle, over-eating, unsafe sex and substance abuse.

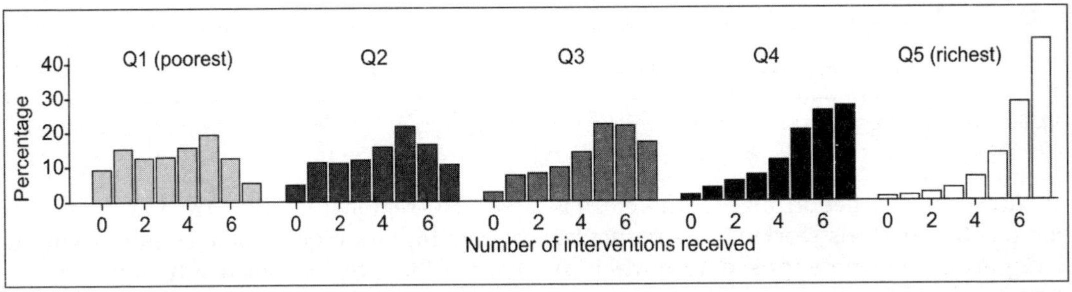

Fig. 8.9: Proportion of mother-child pairs in low- and lower-middle-income countries, by wealth quintile and number of basic interventions received (out of seven), 2005–2015[15]

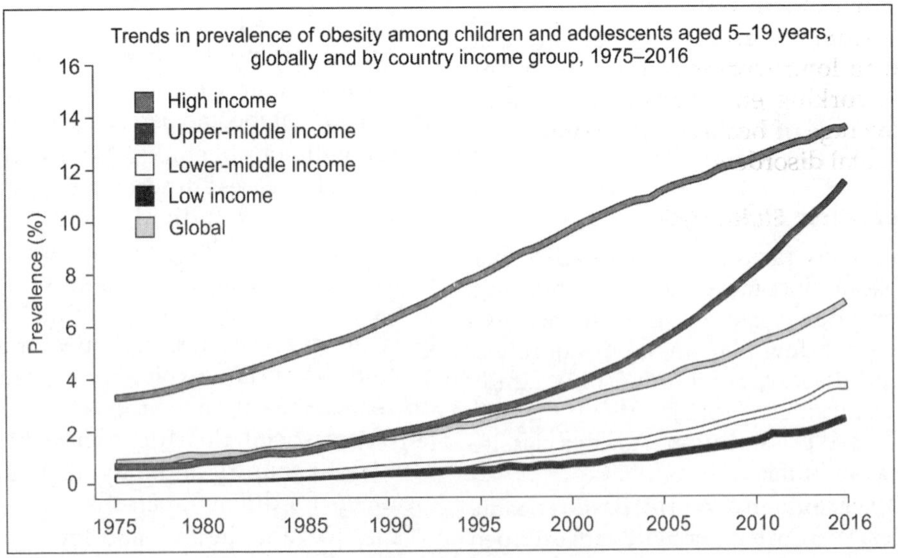

Fig. 8.10: Trend in prevalence of obesity

PLACE DISTRIBUTION (GEOGRAPHICAL COMPARISONS)

Health and diseases vary from place to place and study of geographical distribution and its determinants can provide clues about the causes of the disease. The study of place distribution is not only limited to place of residence but to any geographic location relevant to disease occurrence. For example, place of diagnosis or report, birthplace, workplace, school, district, hospital unit, or recent travel destinations, village, district, region or state or nations. These variations may be classified as following.

International Variations

The international variations are seen due to differences in culture, lifestyle, behaviour, dietary pattern, genetic composition, environment, access to healthcare, etc. As we know, infectious diseases, malnutrition and diarrheal diseases are more common in developing countries than developed world and vice-versa for non-communicable diseases.

There is a marked difference between the incidences of different cancers in different parts of the world. The cancer of stomach is very common in Japan but unusual in the United States. There are also international variations in the incidence of breast cancer and esophageal cancer as well as in the occurrence of cardiovascular diseases.

The variation may be appreciated from the trend of prevalence of obesity among boys and girls from Fig. 8.11.[15]

In 2016, 132,121 cholera cases and 2420 deaths were reported to WHO from 38 countries, including 47 imported cases reported in 9 countries (Fig. 8.12).

National Variations

Disease frequency can be different between different regions and states within a country or national boundaries. This information can be used to set priorities for health services and resource allocation.

The bar diagram (Figs 8.13 and 8.14) showed that percentage share of population in the selected age groups (below 5 years of age) for bigger States/UTs by residence and sex. At the national level, 7.3% population in urban areas constitutes below 5 years of age as against 9.2% for rural area. Sex differences in the share of child population are negligible both in rural and urban areas. The difference in the share of male child population to female child is maximum (about 1% higher) in rural areas of Delhi, Kerala and Uttarakhand. The

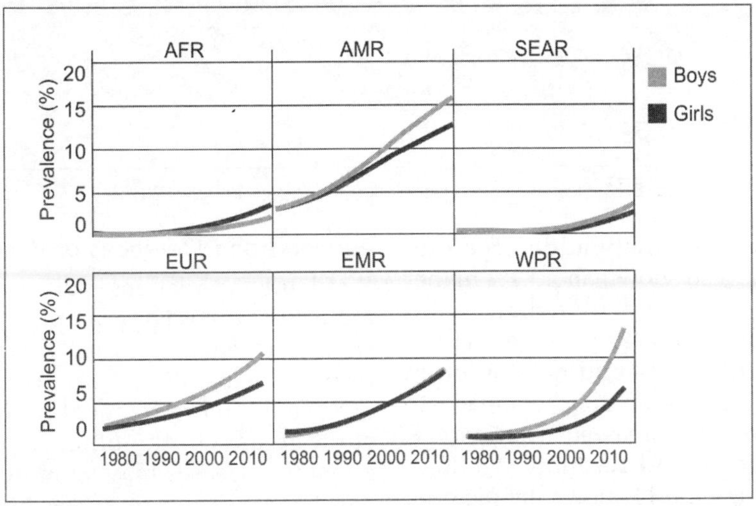

Fig. 8.11: Trends in prevalence of obesity among boys and girls aged 5–19 years, by WHO region, 1975–2016

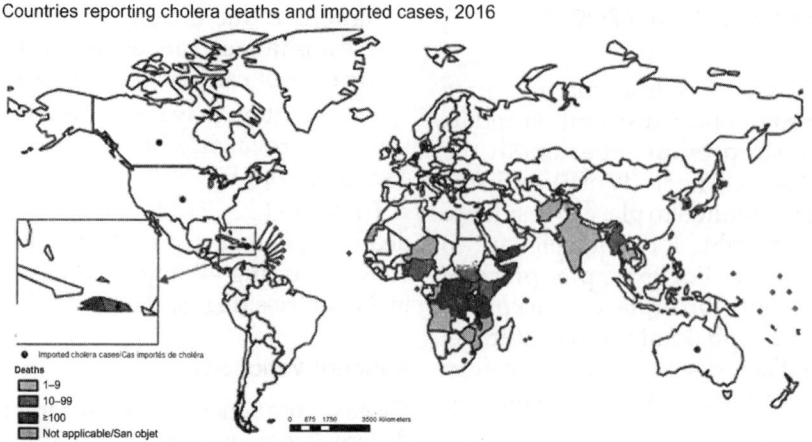

Fig. 8.12: Cholera reported figures in 2016.
Source: http://gamapserver.who.int/mapLibrary/Files/Maps/Global_Cholera(WER)_2016.png

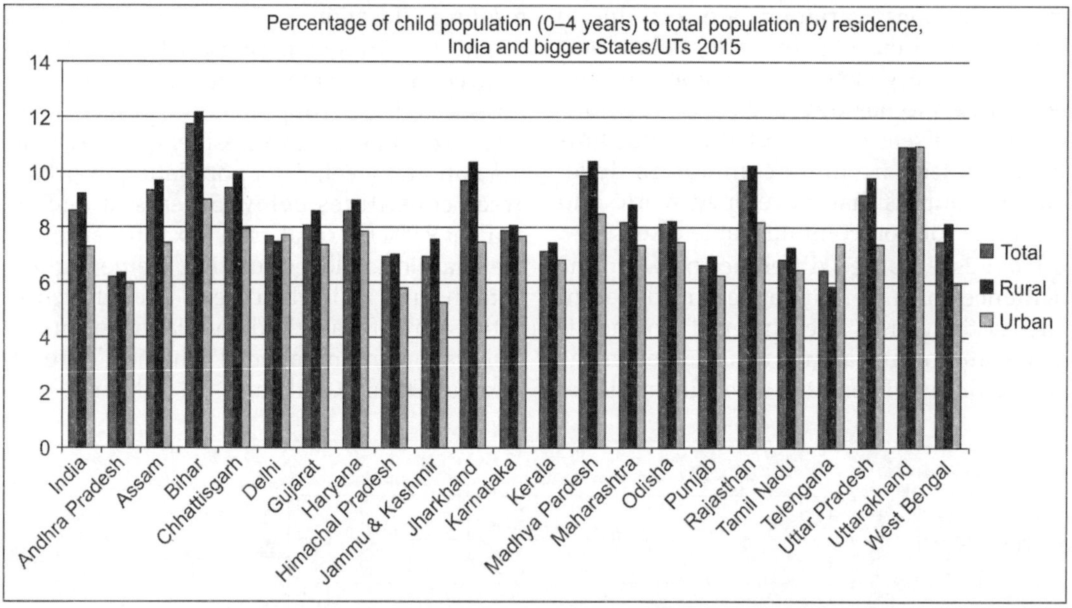

Fig. 8.13: State-wise child population (0–4 years) in India, 2015[16]

urban areas of the newly added State of Telangana have also shown about 1% higher difference in the male to female child population share. Among the bigger States/ UTs, the percentage of child population in rural areas varies from 5.9 in Telangana to 12.2 in Bihar. In urban areas, such variation is from 5.3 in Jammu and Kashmir to 11.0 in Uttarakhand. Figure 8.14 shows the pictorial presentation of percentage of child population for bigger states/UTs.[16]

Ruralñurban Differences or Variations

Rural–urban variations in disease distribution are well known. For example, chronic bronchitis, accidents, lung cancer, cardio-vascular disease, mental illness and drug dependence are usually more frequent in urban than in rural areas. On the other hand, skin and zoonotic diseases may be more common in rural than in urban areas. Birth rate and death rates in India are higher in rural than in urban areas. These variations may be due to

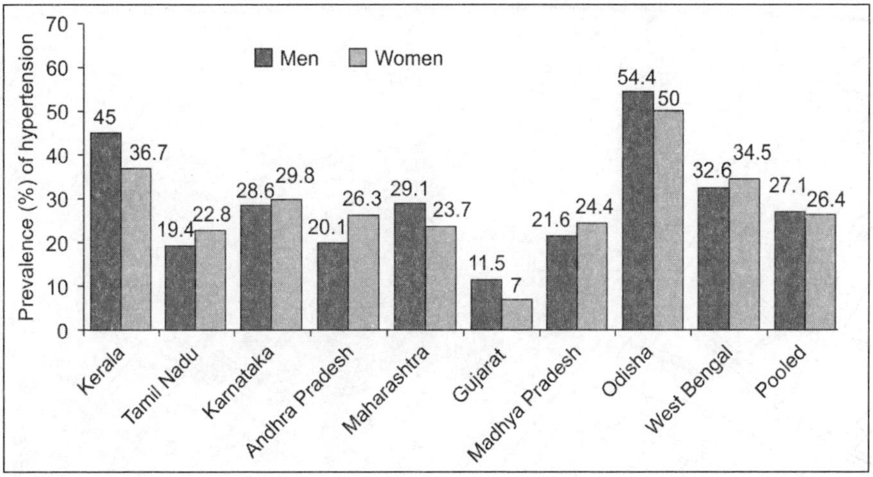

Fig. 8.14: Age-adjusted state-wise prevalence of hypertension among tribal men and women aged ≥20 yr in 9 states of India[16]

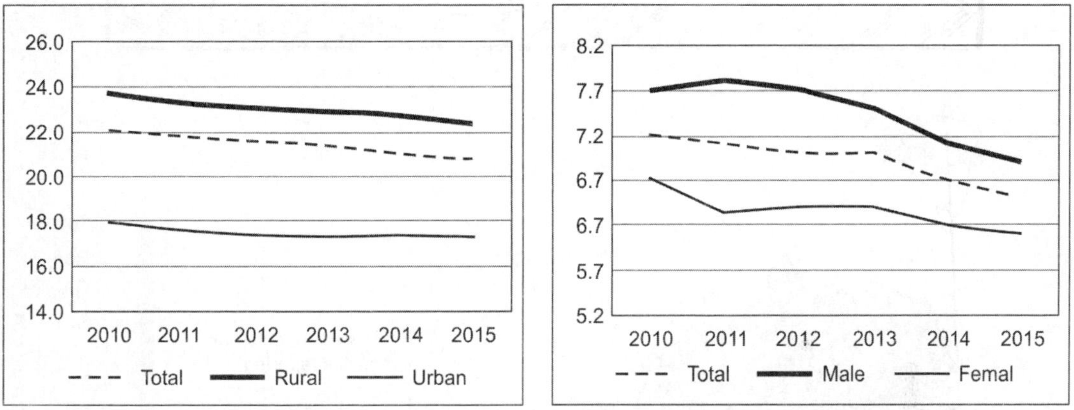

(a) **(b)**

Figs 8.15: (a) Birth rate and (b) death rate

differences in population density, social class, levels of education, sanitation, etc. (Figs 8.15 and 8.16).

Local Distributions or Variations

Inner and outer city variations in disease frequency are well known. These variations are best studied with the aid of 'spot maps' or 'shaded maps' which show at a glance area of high or low frequency. For example, John Snow in his classic investigation of cholera epidemic in London in 1854, by studying local variations, was able to hypothesize that cholera was a water-borne disease, long before the birth of bacteriology (Fig. 8.17).

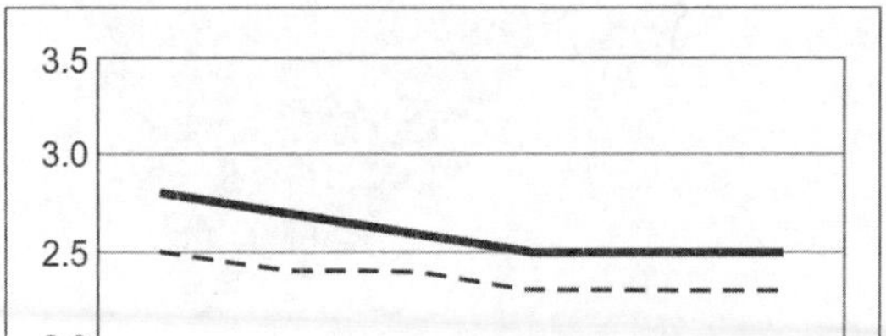

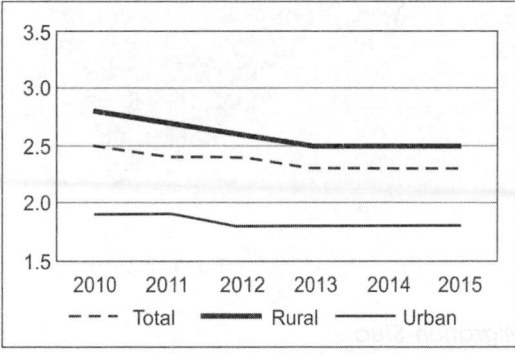

Fig. 8.16: Total fertility rate

Local distribution of measles can be seen in a district starts from a small village in district Almora in India (Fig. 8.17).

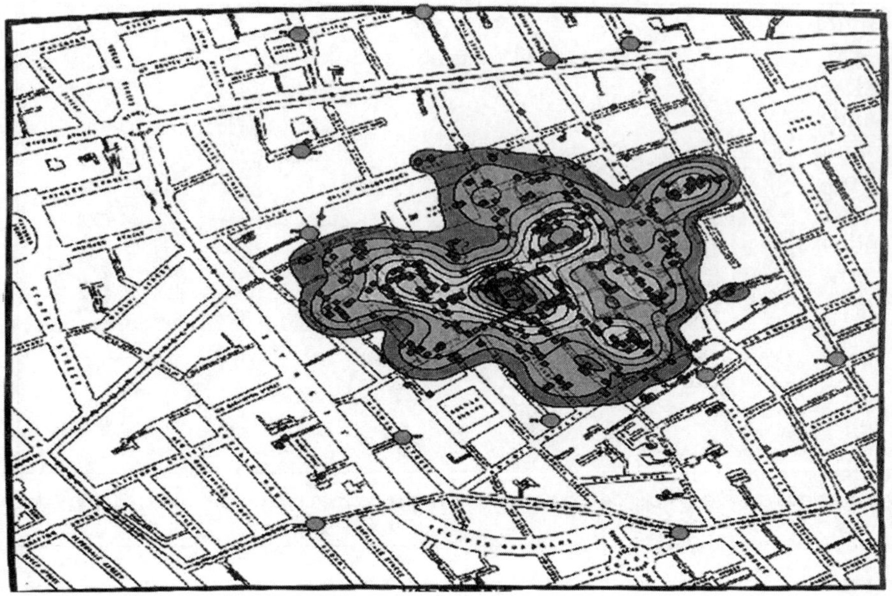

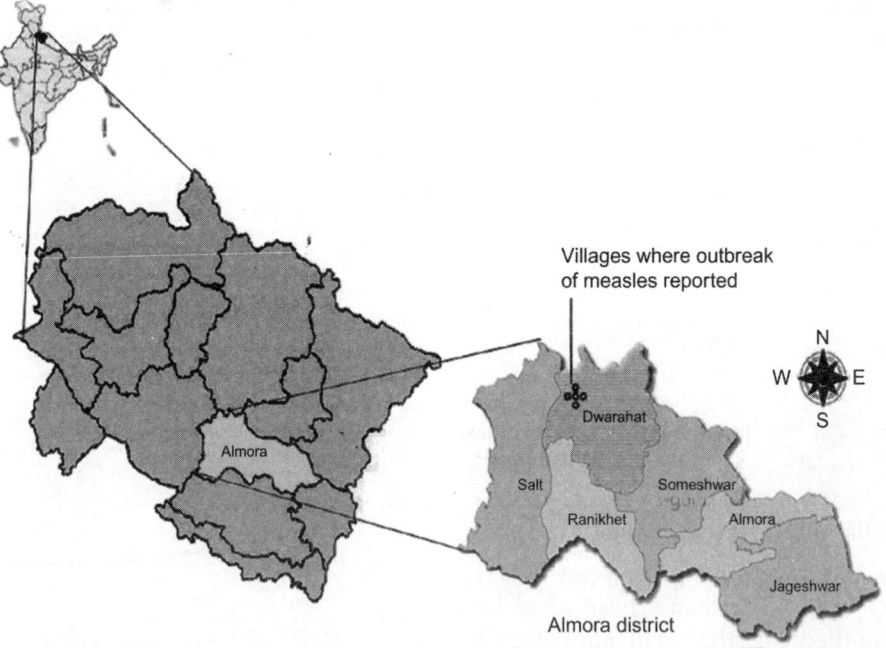

Fig. 8.17: Distribution of measles in district Almora[17]

Migration Studies

One of the useful techniques in descriptive epidemiology is the examination of the effects of migration on the rate of disease occurrence. These studies can help to clarify whether a disease of unknown cause is determined either by genetic inheritance or by environmental factors. Migration from a high-risk population to a low-risk population should not affect the occurrence of a geneticallydetermined disease among the migrants. On the other hand, migration from a high-risk population to a low-risk population should result in a reduction in the occurrence of an environmentally-determined disease. In other words, migration reduces the chances of exposure to the environmental risk factors and hence the occurrence of disease should come down. A demographic and mobility process approach to these considerations is presented in Table 8.10.

The epidemiological analysis of illnesses and disease in migrants is most commonly approached in one of two ways in receiving countries. The first is to consider the health issue of concern in terms of the status at the time of migration, while the second is to study the evolution of the health characteristic over time. The reference population for the first analytical approach is normally the host or receiving population, while the reference group for the second approach can be either the host population or a comparison cohort at the migrants' place of origin.

Age-specific prevalence of the diseases among males with a history of migration and non-migrants. Diabetes, hypertension, and cardiac complaints are more prevalent among those with duration of migration of over 5 years when compared with those with no history of migration (Table 8.11). The age-specific increase in prevalence is substantially higher

Table 8.10: The impact of different health environments and the phases of population mobility[18]

Occurrence	*Examples*	*Consequence at destination*
Pre-departure existing medical condition	• Prevalence of endemic disease • Level of development • Access to care • Availability of care	Arriving population displays health indicators of origin: • Differing incidence and prevalence of illness • Differences in awareness of and use of health-care services • Preventive • Promotional • Diagnostic • Therapeutic
Health impacts during migration	• Trauma (physical-psychosocial) • Deprivation • Violence • Exposure • Injury	Some populations display greater prevalence of illness resulting from torture, trauma, abuse and exposure • Refugees • Refugee claimants or asylum seekers • Trafficked/smuggled migrants
Health impacts arising after arrival	Administrative/legal limits • Poverty • Language culture • Occupational risks	Awareness of and use of healthcare services in migrant populations may be limited by immigration status, poverty, language and culture Working conditions may be associated with health risks: • Migrant agricultural labor • Commercial sex workers • Illegal workers • Trafficked migrants
Health consequences of return travel	Health environment at origin may have changed—health systems improvements or declines Children born to foreign-born parents have no exposure to risks present at origin	Population making return journeys to place of origin (particularly children born at new destination) may be at increased risk of disease or illness: 'Visiting friends and relative' travellers – Locally born children of foreign-born parents

among migrants for diabetes and hypertension though the trend is unmistakable even for cardiac diseases. The same trend is seen for women aged 30–69 (Fig. 8.18).

A study conducted by Ebrahim S *et al.* showed that obesity prevalence (BMI 0.25 kg/m^2) was greatest in urban women (53.5%, 95% CI 50.5–56.5) and lowest in rural men (18.0%, 95% CI 17.0–21.0), with migrants in an intermediate position. The age, occupation, and factory adjusted odds of obesity were between 3- and 4-fold greater in migrant than rural men and women.[20]

Time Distribution or Time Trends

Health and diseases are dynamic and never constant, therefore, occurrence of diseases- and health-related events are ever changing with time. By observing and describing the time trends, we can know as to which diseases are increasing or decreasing, measure effectiveness of prevention and control program, the efficacy of treatment regimes, lead to the formulation of etiological hypotheses as well as their explanations, and help to formulate guidelines for prevention and control of diseases.

The pattern of disease frequency may be described by the time scale of its occurrence such as by the hour, day, week, month, year(s).

Time trends are usually displayed with a two-dimensional graph. The vertical or *y*-axis usually shows the event/disease number or rate. The horizontal or *x*-axis shows the time periods. It is depicted as graphs (line, bar, histogram).

Three types of time trends or fluctuations (increase or decrease) have been identified:

A. Short-term fluctuations or epidemic changes.

B. Periodic fluctuations or trends.

C. Long-term or secular trends or fluctuations.

SHORT-TERM FLUCTUATIONS OR EPIDEMIC CHANGES*

The best known short-term fluctuation in the occurrence of a disease is an epidemic which is "a rapid and remarkable increase in the incidence of a disease over the endemic rate". The endemic rate is described as "the usual rate of occurrence for a disease in a population". The variations of a short-term fluctuation of an epidemic are:

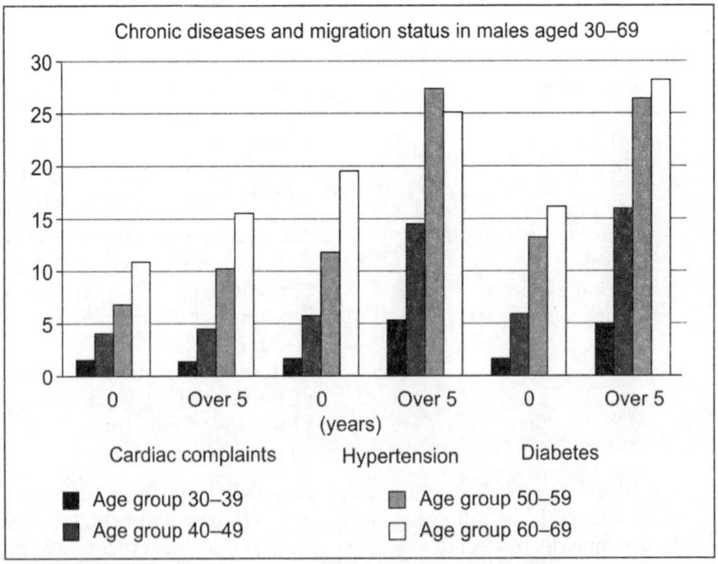

Fig. 8.18: Chronic diseases and migration status in males aged 30–69 years[19]

*Short-term fluctuations or epidemic changes are discussed in detail in Chapters 3 and 6.

Table 8.11: Odds ratios (95% CI) for the risk of disease in a sibling compared to a rural sibling, adjusted for occupation, age, age group, and factory with an individual-specific random effect of sib-pair[20]

Risk factors	*Men*					*Women*				
	Urban	*Migrants*	*Rural*	*p for trend**	*Text Urban = Migrant*	*Urban*	*Migrants*	*Rural*	*p for trend**	*Text Urban = Migrant*
Hypertension	1.76 (1.37–2.27)	1.67 (1.31–2.12)	1	<0.0001	0.67	1.55 (1.13–2.12)	1.22 (0.90–1.65)	1	0.005	0.08
Obese	3.83 (2.95–4.98)	3.12 (2.44–3.98)	1	<0.0001	0.08	4.89 (3.56–6.72)	3.86 (2.88–5.19)	1	<0.0001	0.05
Underweight	0.21 (0.14–0.31)	0.10 (0.06–0.16)	1	<0.0001	0.002	0.23 (0.14–0.38)	0.18 (0.11–0.31)	1	<0.0001	0.37
Diabetic	2.43 (1.72–3.43)	2.15 (1.55–3.00)	1	<0.0001	0.42	2.96 (1.69–5.17)	2.68 (1.59–4.52)	1	0.0001	0.64
Fasting blood glucose >7 mmol/L	2.33 (1.46–3.73)	2.38 (1.51–3.76)	1	0.0006	0.92	2.38 (1.18–4.80)	2.26 (1.13–4.51)	1	0.02	0.83
Regular alcohol	1.42 (1.08–1.88)	1.38 (1.05–1.73)	1	0.007	0.70	0.31 (0.11–0.86)	0.63 (0.28–1.42)	1	0.02	0.15
Current smoker	0.82 (0.66–1.03)	0.61 (0.49–0.75)	1	0.03	0.01	0.28 (0.09–0.89)	0.66 (0.27–1.63)	1	0.02	0.11
Physically inactive	2.00 (1.66–2.41)	1.62 (1.33–1.97)	1	<0.0001	0.02	1.14 (0.87–1.50)	1.20 (0.92–1.57)	1	0.41	0.65

* Test for trend on the log-odds scale
doi:10.1371/journal.pmed.1000268.t003

i. **A common source epidemic which may be a single-exposure (point-source) epidemic,** e.g. an epidemic of food poisoning or a continuous (repeated) exposure epidemic, e.g. from a well of contaminated water (Figs 8.19a and c).

ii. **Propagated epidemics,** e.g. epidemics of hepatitis A, polio, cholera, which usually result from person to person transmission of an infectious agent (Figs 8.19b and d).

PERIODIC FLUCTUATIONS OR TRENDS

These are of two types:

i. **Seasonal fluctuations or trends:** There are variations of various diseases in different seasons. These may be related to environmental factors like temperature, humidity, rainfall and life-cycles of vectors, etc. It is well known that measles and varicella (chickenpox) are more common in spring whereas upper respiratory tract infections

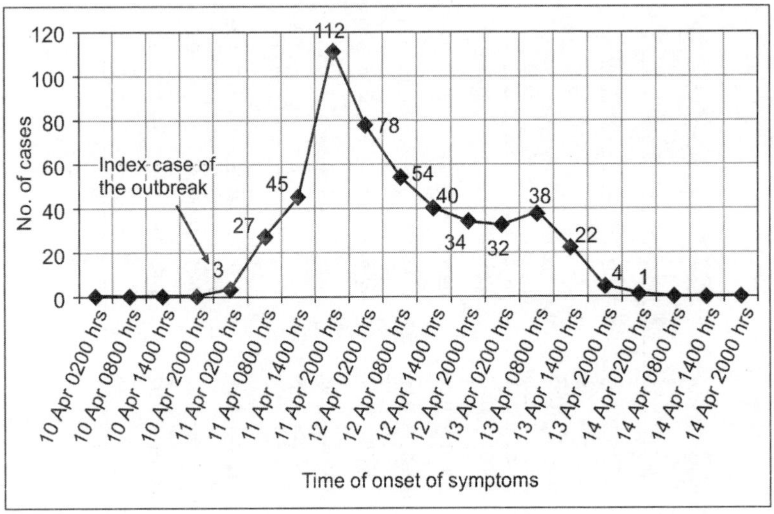

Fig. 8.19a: Common source epidemic[21]

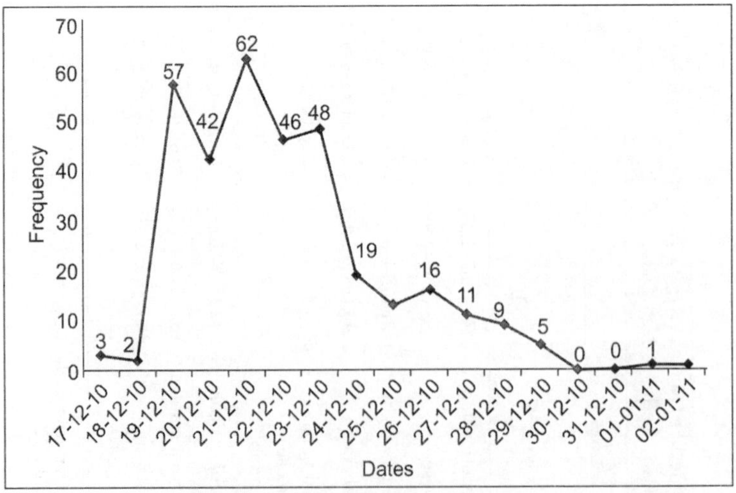

Fig. 8.19b: Propagated epidemics[22]

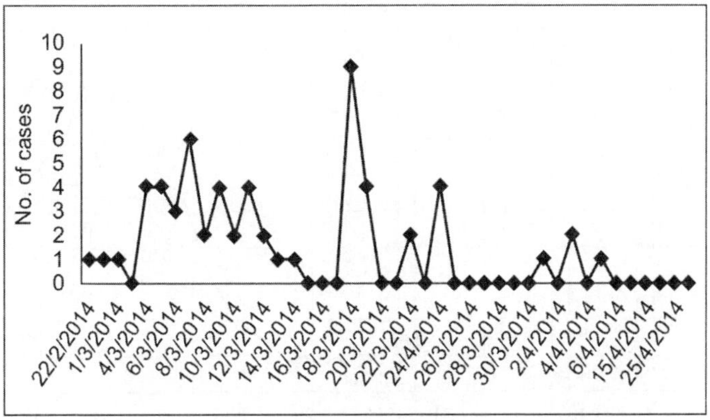

Fig. 8.19c: Trend of measles cases during outbreak[23]

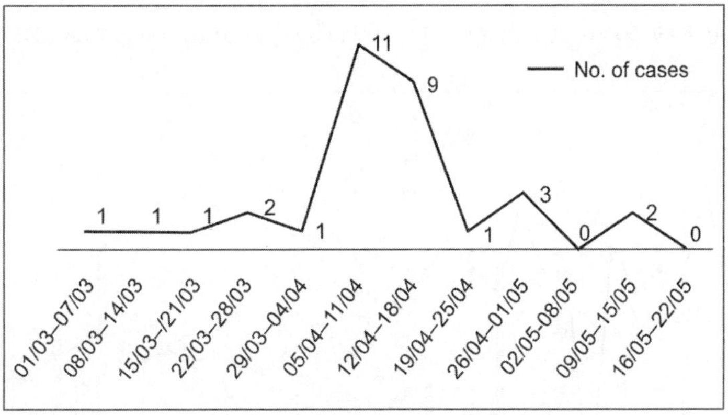

Fig. 8.19d: Epidemic curve (all cases)[21]

are more common in winter and mosquito-borne diseases (malaria, dengue) and gastro-enteritis are more during summer and rainy seasons (Fig. 8.20). Some non-infectious diseases may also exhibit seasonal variations, e.g. drowning, sun-stroke, hay-fever and snake-bite, etc.

ii. **Cyclic trends or fluctuations:** Some diseases occur in cycles spread over short periods of time which may be days, weeks, months or years. For example, in the pre-vaccination era, epidemics of measles occurred every 2–3 years and rubella (German measles) every 6–9 years. It was due to naturally occurring variations in herd-immunity. Influenza pandemics are known to occur every 7–10 years due to antigenic variations. Some non-infectious conditions may also show cyclic trends, e.g. automobile accidents are more on the week-ends and at hours of the day. The knowledge of cyclic trend is useful for the communities to defend themselves by taking preventive and control measures (examples are shown in Figs 8.21 and 8.22).

LONG-TERM OR SECULAR TRENDS OR FLUCTUATIONS

Secular trends (Figs 8.23a to f) are the changes that occur in the frequency of a disease (a progressive increase or decrease) over a long period of time, i.e. several years or decades. Examples include non-infectious diseases like coronary heart disease (CHD), lung cancer and diabetes, which have shown a consistent upward trend during the last six decades and infectious diseases like typhoid, cholera, diphtheria and polio, which have shown a

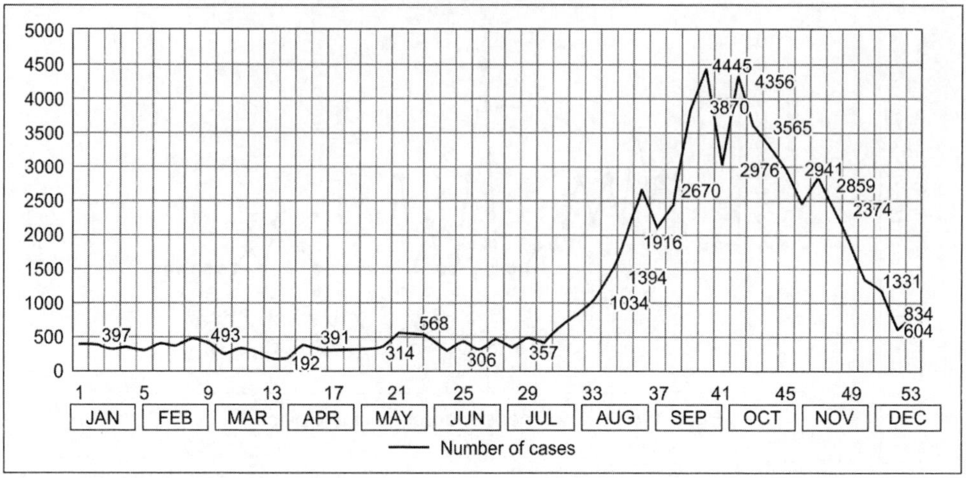

Fig. 8.20: Seasonal distribution of propable dengue cases in Rajasthan 2015[24]

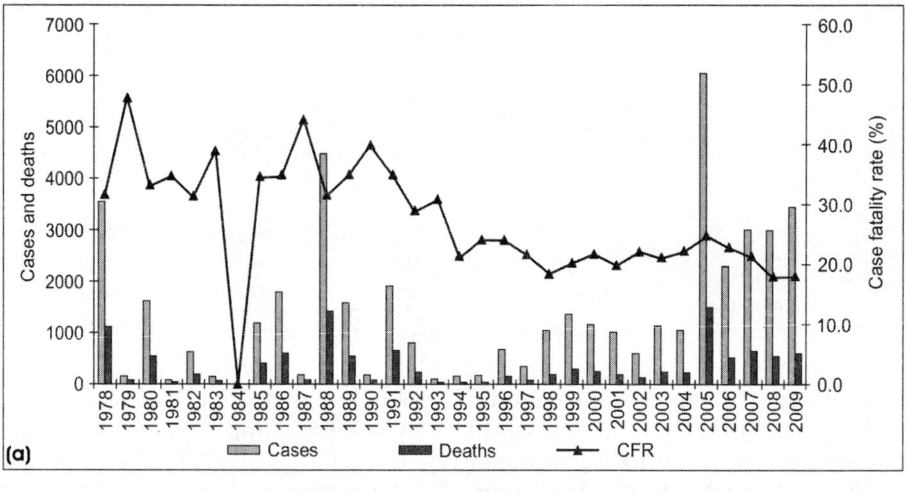

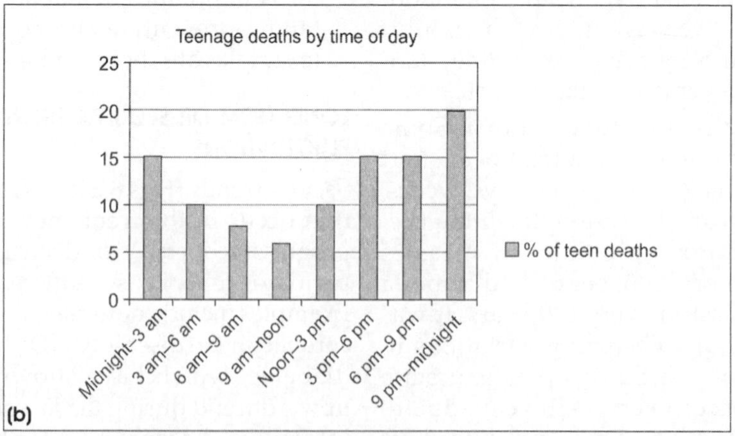

Figs 8.21a and b: Teenage deaths by time of day[25]

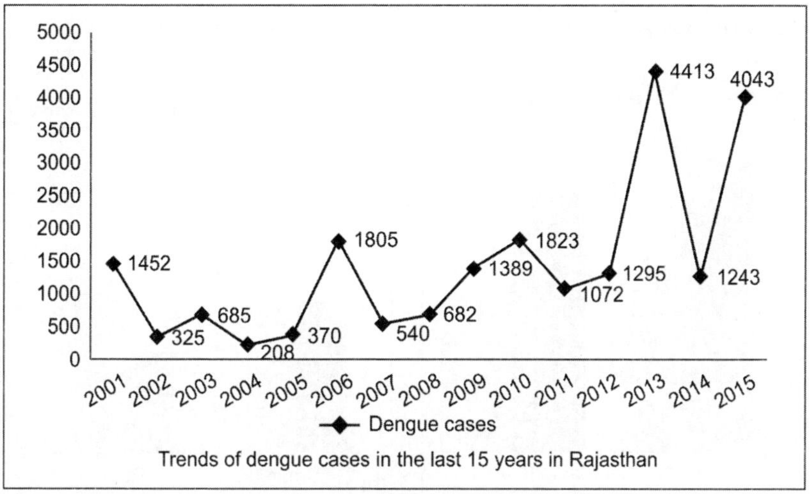

Fig. 8.22: Trends of dengue cases[24]

downward trend or decline. Following charts of NFHS-4 survey conducted by Government of India shows the trends of various key indicators from NFHS-1 in 1992–93 till NFHS-4 in 2015–16.[26,27]

TYPES OF DESCRIPTIVE STUDIES

A descriptive study involves describing the characteristics of a particular situation, event or case. Descriptive studies can be carried out on:

(i) **Individual** (small) level—individual-level data include case reports, case series, and cross-sectional studies.

(ii) **Aggregate** (larger) scale—aggregate-level data include city, district, or country.

Ecological studies are aggregate descriptive studies. It always describes the event in time, place and person. The descriptive study can answer the research question by asking what, when, where, who, and how for an event.

Individual (Small) Level Descriptive Studies

Case Reports[29,30]

Descriptive case reports describe in-depth the characteristics of one or a limited number of 'cases'. The case report is a presentation of a newer normal (to be proved)/abnormal finding or outcome which, otherwise, would not be present. A case may be, for example, a patient, a health centre, or a village. Such a study can provide quite useful insight into a problem. Case studies are common in social sciences, management sciences, and clinical medicine. For example, in clinical medicine the characteristics of a hitherto unrecognized illness may be documented as a case study. This is often the first step toward building up a clinical picture of that illness.

It is generally limited to presuming the association between the risk factor/a variable and the disease/outcome. Another example may be of an adverse (or beneficial) side-effect of a new drug, which may not have been documented before.

Case report—advantages

- Case reports can help to identify new clinical issues and may lead to development of hypotheses. However, they are normally regarded as low level evidence as the observations may be subject to bias.
- Report rare events—provide source for further research about disease frequency, risk, prognosis and treatment.

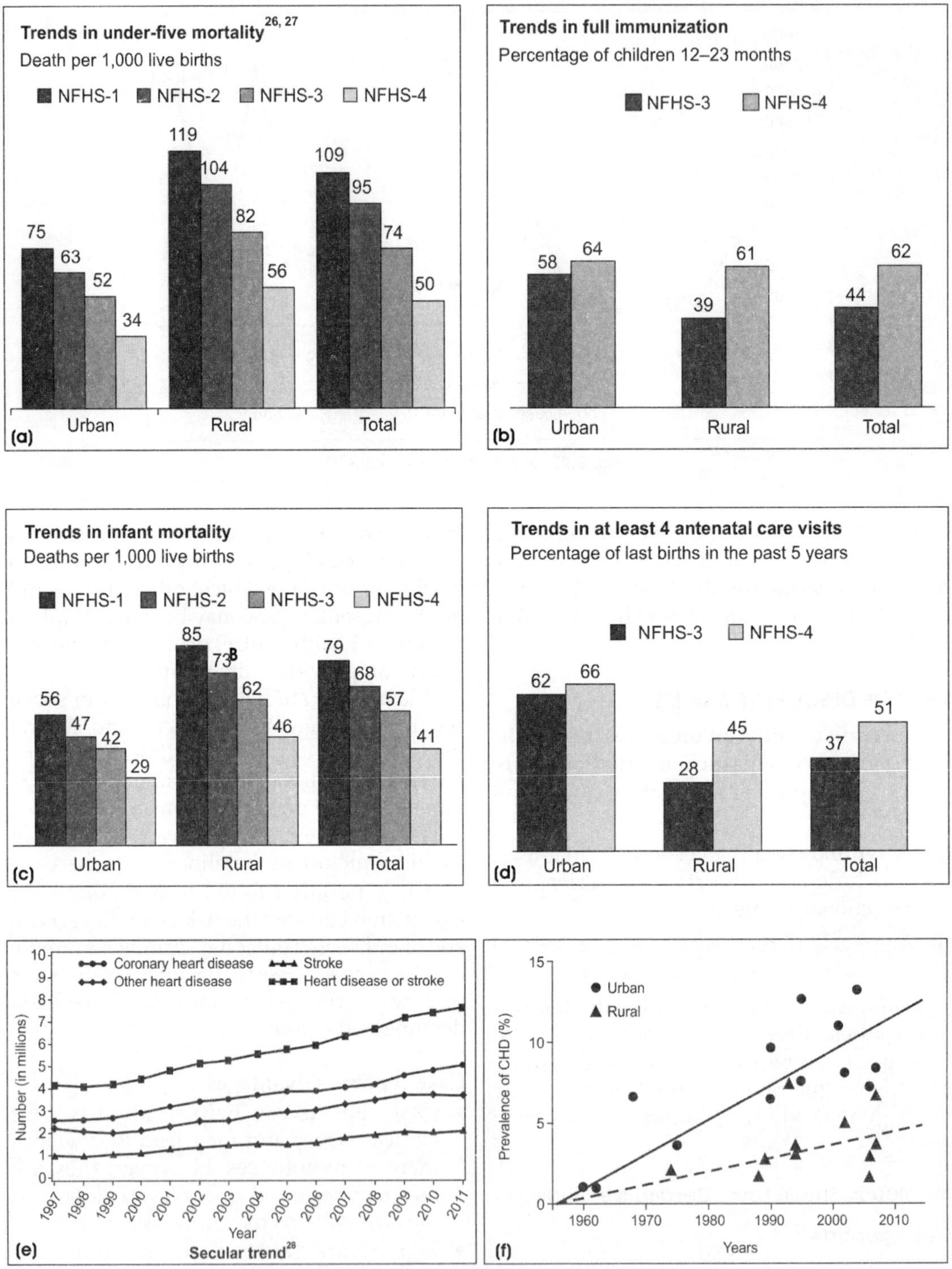

Figs 8.23a to f: Trends of various key indicators[26–28]

- Describe the management of a condition through history, clinical findings, laboratory studies, or treatment.
- Describes the side effects and complications of drug treatments.
- Easy and inexpensive to conduct in clinical settings

Case report—disadvantages:

- Susceptible to chance
- The absence of a comparison group means that case reports can only generate a hypothesis about an exposure outcome relationship.
- No conclusions can generally be drawn about an exposure-outcome relationship.

Case report series: Objective and brief report of a clinical characteristic or outcome from a group of clinical subjects. Generalization is not possible due to biased selection or un representativeness of subjects, lack of control group, etc.[30,31]

Case series—advantages

- Informs first cases of an emerging new condition or disease.
- Provide the first clues for formulating hypotheses.
- Easy and inexpensive

Case series—disadvantages

- Patient's selection may be biased.
- It may be unclear whether the confluence of findings is merely a chance occurrence or is truly characteristic of a new disease or syndrome.
- Case series studies have no comparison group and only be used to generate hypotheses about the relationship between an exposure and an outcome.

However, if one wishes to test whether the findings pertain to a larger population, a more extensive, cross-sectional survey has to be designed.

CROSS-SECTIONAL STUDIES

Cross-sectional study is also known as instantaneous study or prevalence study **or simultaneous study.**

A cross-sectional study is observational and the investigator has no control over the exposure of interest (e.g. smoking, alcohol intake, diet). The purpose of the study to find-out characteristics of the population at one point of time (sometimes referred as 'snap shot' study). It measures range of variables on an individual basis and the same time measuring outcome of interest. There is no comparison group and it estimates the prevalence.

This methodology can be used to assess the burden of disease or health needs of a population, and helps in the planning and allocation of health resources.

Example of variables that may be studied in cross-sectional studies:

- *Physical characteristics* of people, materials or the environment, as in prevalence surveys of tuberculosis, leprosy, HIV, etc.
- Evaluation coverage of immunization, latrines, etc.
- *Socio-economic characteristics* of people such as their age, education, marital status, number of children and income.
- The *behaviour* or practices of people and the *knowledge, attitudes, beliefs, opinions* which may help to explain that behaviour (KAP studies), or *events* that occurred in the population.

Types of Cross-sectional Study

Descriptive

A cross-sectional study may be purely descriptive and used to assess the frequency and distribution of a particular disease in a defined population, e.g. school survey for refractive errors or obesity, dental caries survey, etc.

Analytical

Analytical cross-sectional studies may also be used to investigate the association between a assumed risk factor and a health outcome. However, this type of study is limited in its ability to draw valid conclusions about any association or possible causality because the presence of risk factors and outcomes are measured simultaneously. It may therefore be difficult to work out whether the disease or the exposure came first or vice versa. It is a retrospective study and hence there is risk of recall bias.

Census is an example of cross-sectional surveys. A cross-sectional survey may be repeated in order to measure changes over time in the characteristics that were studied. The surveys may be very **large**, with hundreds or even thousands of study units. In these cases only a **limited number of variables** will usually be included, in order to avoid problems with analysis and report writing. If cross-sectional surveys are **smaller** they can be **more complex**. They may include all the elements just mentioned. Small surveys can reveal interesting associations between certain variables, such as between having tuberculosis and socio-economic status, sex, and ways of coping.

Steps in Conduction Cross-sectional Studies

Cross-sectional studies are used to estimate the prevalence of diseases or the prevalence of exposure to risk factors or both. The following steps have to be completed.

i. **Define target population:** Usually defined by age, sex and place of residence.
ii. **Decide sample size and Draw sample:** This requires a population register maintained by the district authorizes or Pachayatiraj institutions (PRI) in India.
iii. **Decide standard case definition:** Define fixed criteria by which the condition is identified.
iv. **Complete case ascertainment:** Apply the case definition to the sample, obtaining a high response rate.
v. **Analyze data and share:** Estimate the prevalence rate.
vi. **Dissemination of information**

Merits

- Short duration
- Relatively inexpensive
- Subject dropout not a problem
- Can study several outcomes
- Better control over subject selection and measurements.
- Good pre-study for a cohort study

Demerits

- Does not address sequence of events (weaker proof of causality)
- Increased bias potential
- Needs large sample size for uncommon diseases
- Does not give information about incidence or true relative risk.

Problems and Issues with Cross-sectional Designs

- **Choosing a representative sample:** It is difficult to include all sections of society from all geographical areas with all variables under consideration. A cross-sectional study should be representative of whole the population.
- **Sample size:** The sample size should be sufficiently large enough to estimate the prevalence of the conditions of interest with adequate precision. The large sample in the study will have minimal chances of bias and also provide better results.
- **Data collection:** Primary or secondary data may be used for this type of design. Specific inclusion and exclusion criteria should be established before the start of the study. The standardization of questionnaire, interview tools and other methods are to be finalized for its validity along with pilot study before actual conduct of survey.
- **Impending bias in cross-sectional studies:** Could occur at any stage of study such as sampling bias; recall bias, non-response bias, etc.

Analysis of Cross-sectional Studies[32]

Following measurements can be done from a cross-sectional study.

Mean, median, odds ratio, prevalence (point prevalence and period prevalence), and chi-squared test (for analytical study) can be done.

$$\text{Prevalence} = \frac{\text{No. of cases in defined population at one point in time}}{\text{No. of persons in defined population at same point in time}}$$

ECOLOGICAL STUDIES[33,34]

An ecological or aggregate study focuses on the comparison of groups, rather than individuals as individual-level data are missing on the joint distribution of at least two and perhaps all variables within each group; in this sense, an ecologic study is an incomplete design.

Characteristic of ecological studies:

- *The exposure* and *outcome* are measured on *populations/groups*, rather than on individuals.
- The pre-existing sources of information/data are used to find out outcome (morbidity, disability, fertility or mortality trend).
- Exposure is expressed as population mean, median, proportion, etc. based on observations from individuals within the group.
- Ecological studies can be used to generate (or test) aetiological hypotheses, and to evaluate interventions at the population level.

TYPES OF ECOLOGICAL STUDIES

In an ecological study design, the planned unit of analysis is the group. Ecologic designs may be classified on two dimensions—the method of grouping and the method of exposure measurement (an ecologic design is called exploratory, if the primary exposure of potential interest is not measured and analytic if the primary exposure variable is measured and included in the analysis) (Table 8.12).

Advantages of Ecological Studies

- Quick and less expensive (using already available information)
- Used to investigate differences between populations
- Useful for generating hypotheses
- Can be used to study group specific effects (smoking ban in workplace)
- Helps in analyzing impact of the programs
- Simplicity of analysis and presentation

Disadvantages of Ecological Studies

- *Ecological fallacy*—population level observation may not match at the individual level due to heterogeneity of exposure level and/or covariate levels within groups and between the groups.
- Cannot control for confounding factors
- Ecologic analysis poses major problems of interpretation when making ecologic inferences and especially when making biologic inferences (due to ecologic bias)
- Data on exposure and outcomes may have been recorded differently between countries or regions leading to biased results.
- Geographical comparisons may suffer from migration of populations between groups over the period of the study which may dilute the difference between groups.
- Reliance upon existing published statistics may limit the types of exposure-outcome relationships that can be investigated in an ecological study.
- The crude 'population level' data used in ecological studies renders them unsuitable for detecting subtle or complicated

Table 8.12: Types of ecological studies

Based on the unit of observation	*Based on the method of exposure measurement in ecological study*	
By time (time trend design)	Exploratory	Analytical/aetiological
By place (multiple group design)	Exploratory	Analytical/aetiological
By person	Exploratory	Analytical/aetiological
By combination of time, person and place (mixed design)	Exploratory	Analytical/aetiological

relationships between exposures and outcomes.

- Due to the many limitations of ecological studies they provide us with relatively weak evidence about 'cause and effect' relationships between exposure and outcomes.

Sources of Data in Descriptive Studies

They are of two broad types:

1. Primary data or systems based on populations, containing data collected through personal interviews or examinations.
2. Secondary/systems based on records, containing data collected from vital and medical records. They include:
   - Census data, or population registers (SRS, NASSO, etc.)
   - Vital statistics (especially death certificate data)
   - Disease registers (e.g. cancer, diabetes), recording new cases of specific diseases in defined populations
   - Notification systems (e.g. Dengue, cholera, polio, Japanese encephalitis, HIV/AIDS, etc.)
   - Hospital activity statistics, especially on admissions/discharges from hospital, Diagnostics records
   - Primary care contacts
   - Community surveys (e.g. those carried out by the NFHS and ICMR).

References

1. Last JM, editor. Dictionary of epidemiology. 4th ed. New York: Oxford University Press; 2001. p. 61.
2. Global Health–health protection. https://www.cdc.gov/globalhealth/healthprotection/fetp/training_modules/19/desc-and-analytic-studies_ppt_final_09252013.pdf License: CC BY-NC-SA 3.0 IGO.
3. Kenneth J. Rothman and Sander Greenland. Types of Epidemiologic Studies http://www.med.mcgill. ca/epidemiology/hanley/bios601/RothmanGreen land 98/RothmanGreenland05TypesEpi Studies.pdf
4. RothmanJ,GreenlandS.Modernepidemiology. Secondedition.Lippincott-RavenPublishers,1998.
5. Principles of Epidemiology in Public Health Practice, Third Edition, published by U.S. DEPARTMENT OF HEALTH AND HUMAN SERVICES. Centers for Disease Control and Prevention (CDC),Office of Workforce and Career Development, Atlanta, GA 30333https://www. cdc.gov/ophss/csels/dsepd/ss1978/ss1978.pdf
6. Wolfgang Ahrens and Iris Pigeot. Handbook of epidemiology. Published by Springer-Verlag Berlin Heidelberg 2005.
7. Visanou HANSANA. Epidemiological study designs. https://www.gfmer.ch/Activites_ internationales_Fr/Laos/PDF/Epidemiologic_study_designs_Hansana_Laos_2009.pdf
8. Omair Aamir. Selecting the appropriate study design for your research: Descriptive study designs. Journal of Health Specialties 2015;3:153. 10.4103/1658-600X.159892.https://sph.unc.edu/files/2015/07/nciph_ERIC8.pdf
9. Govt. of India, Ministry of Home Affairs. Census 2011. Downloaded from http://www.censusindia.gov.in/2011-common/census_data.html.
10. Chavan RD Kothari ST, Zunjarrao K, Chaowdhary AS. Surveillance of acute respiratory infections in Mumbai during 2011–12. Indian j Med Microbiol (serial online) 2015 (cited 2018 Aug 8;33:43–50 Available from: http://www.ijmm.org/text.asp?2015/33/1/43/148376
11. Christofherson WM, Parker JE. Relation of Cervical Cancer to Early Marriage and Childbearing N Engl J Med 1965;273(5):235–39, doi:10.1056/NEJM196507292730502
12. Dev V, Adak T, Singh OP, Nanda N, Baidya BK. Malaria transmission in Tripura: Diseases distribution and determinants. India J Med Res (serial online) 2015, (cited 2018 Aug8);142(Suppl S1):12–22. Available at http://HYPERLINK "http://www.ijmr.org.in/text.aps?2045/142/7/12/176597" www.ijmr.org.in/text.aps?2045/142/7/12/176597.
13. Bennett PC, Silverman S, Gill PS, Lip GYH. Ethnicity and peripheral artery disease, QJM: An International Journal of Medicine 2009;102(1):3–16, https://doi.org/10.1093/qjmed/hcn140
14. A Dharanipriya, S Ganesh Kumar. Prevalence and pattern of occupational injuries at workplace among welders in coastal south India. Indian Journal of Occupational and Environmental Medicine 2014;18(3):135–39 DOI: 10.4103/0019-5278.146911
15. World health statistics 2018: Monitoring health for the SDGs, sustainable development goals. Geneva: World Health Organization; 2018.
16. Laxmaiah A, Meshram II, Arlappa N, Balakrishna N, Rao KM, Reddy CG, Ravindranath M, Kumar S, Kumar H, Brahmam G. Socio-economic and demographic determinants of hypertension and knowledge, practices and risk behaviour of tribals in India. Indian J Med Res 2015;141:697–708.

17. Hashmi S, Singh AK, Rawat V, Kumar M, Mehra A K, Singh RK. Measles outbreak investigation in Dwarahat block of District Almora, Uttarakhand. Indian J Med Microbiol 2015;33:406-9
18. Gushulak BD, MacPherson DW. The basic principles of migration health: Population mobility and gaps in disease prevalence. Emerging Themes in Epidemiology 2006;3:3. http://doi.org/10.1186/1742-7622-3-3
19. Safraj Shahul Hameed, Vellapallil Raman Kutty, Krishnapillai Vijayakumar, Ajayan Kamalasanan, "Migration Status and Prevalence of Chronic Diseases in Kerala State, India," International Journal of Chronic Diseases, vol. 2013, Article ID 431818, 6 pages, 2013. https://doi.org/10.1155/2013/431818.
20. Ebrahim S, Kinra S, Bowen L, Andersen E, Ben-Shlomo Y, Lyngdoh T. ... for the Indian Migration Study group Membership of the Indian Migration Study group is provided in the Acknowledgments. (2010). The Effect of Rural-to-Urban Migration on Obesity and Diabetes in India: A Cross-Sectional Study. PLoS Medicine, 7(4), e1000268. http://doi.org/10.1371/journal.pmed.100026
21. Kumar MK, Bhaskar V, Ray S. Food poisoning outbreak in a training establishment: A retrospective cohort study. J Mar Med Soc 2017;19:28–33
22. Shah HD, Shah VP, Desai AN. An epidemic outbreak of Vibrio Cholerae El Tor 01 serotype ogawa biotype in a Lalpur town, Jamnagar, India. J Postgrad Med 2012;58:14–8.
23. Bajaj S, Bobdey P, Singh N. Measles outbreak in adults: A changing epidemiological pattern. Med J DY Patil Univ 2017;10:447–52.
24. Rathore M, Kashyap A, Kapoor P. Journey of dengue in Rajasthan in the last 15 years (2001–2015) with special reference to 2015. Indian J Health Sci Biomed Res 2017;10:3–8.
25. Kumari R, Joshi PL. A review of Japanese encephalitis in Uttar Pradesh, India. WHO South-East Asia J Public Health 2012;1:374–95.
26. International Institute for Population Sciences (IIPS) and ICF. 2017.
27. National Family Health Survey (NFHS-4), 2015-16: India. Mumbai: IIPS.
28. Tan ST, et al. Coronary heart disease in Indian Asians. HYPERLINK "https://www.ncbi.nlm.nih.gov/pubmed/25054115"Glob Cardiol Sci Pract. 2014 Jan 29;2014(1):13-23. doi: 10.5339/gcsp.2014.4. e-Collection 2014.
29. Sayre JW, Toklu HZ, Ye F, et al. (August 07, 2017) Case Reports, Case Series – From Clinical Practice to Evidence-Based Medicine in Graduate Medical Education. Cureus 9(8): e1546. DOI 10.7759/cureus.1546
30. Case Reports, Case Series–from Clinical... available from: https://www.researchgate.net/publication/318971117_Case_Reports_Case_Series_-_From_Clinical_Practice_to_Evidence Based_Medicine_in_Graduate_Medical_Education [accessed Aug 11 2018].
31. Chan K, Bhandari M. (2011). Three-minute critical appraisal of a case series article. Indian Journal of Orthopaedics, 45(2), 103–104. http://doi.org/10.4103/0019-5413.77126
32. Health Knowledge, Epidemiology. Available from: http://www.healthknowledge.org.uk/e-learning/epidemiology
33. Hart J. On Ecological Studies: A Short Communication. Dose-Response. 2011;9(4):497–501. doi:10.2203/dose-response.10-046.Hart.
34. Morgenstern Hal. Ecologic Studies In Epidemiology: Concepts, Principles, and Methods .Annu. Rev. Public Health 1995;16:61–81.

Chapter

9

Case-Control Study

Pradeep Kumar and Ram Chandra Goyal

"Judging from the manner in which the subject is usually handled, the study of the etiology of diseases is generally undertaken with great levity, even by men of high acquirement. Some slight general knowledge, supported by a little more or a little less common sense, is quite sufficient to fit its possessor for the discovery of the causes of disease, in other words, to qualify him for the most complicated problem within the whole range of pathology."

— PCA Louis (Louis 1844: 487)

The case-control study is an observational analytical study because no intervention is made to alter the course of the disease. Although, it is simple and cost-effective but less powerful than cohort and experimental studies. Case control studies are also known as 'retrospective studies' and 'case-referent studies.' This is one of the methods for testing the hypotheses.

INTRODUCTION

Historical Background

The following time-line (Table 9.1) tries to trace the origins and early development of the case-control study, focusing on its evolution in the 19th and early 20th century. A number of clinical investigations, and several sociological studies, in the first half of this century can be described as case-control studies, the most fully developed of which was Janet Lane-Claypon's 1926 study of breast cancer.[1,2]

Definition

A study that compares persons with a disease or outcome of interest (cases) and people without disease or outcome (controls). It retrospectively determine the exposure to the risk factor of interest from both the groups of individuals (cases and controls) to determine the relationship between the risk factor and the disease.

The case group represents the 'observed' level of exposure, and control group the 'expected level' of exposure. Differences in exposure between the two groups indicate that the disease is associated with the exposure or not.

Components of the Case-control Study

The case-control study has basically six essential components, i.e. three each elements and practices (Fig. 9.1).[3]

These elements include three inter-related underlying concepts:

Table 9.1: Timeline of development of case-control study	
Year	*Investigator and their studies*
1843	William August Guy's investigation of occupation in relation to pulmonary consumption was the first case-control study quoted by (Lilienfeld and Lilienfeld, 1979).
1862	James Paget (of Paget's diseases) studied but authored by WM Baker, entitled 'Statistics of cancer' (Baker 1862).
1884	Louis prefigured the case control approach by considering the hereditary predisposition to phthisis.
1885	John Snow's observations on cholera further investigated by Whitehead concluded that "among those attacked, the ratio of pump water drinkers to non-drinkers of the same water is 80 to 20, whilst among those who escaped disease, the ratio of pump water drinkers to non-drinkers of the same 57 to 279". This gives an odds ratio of 19.6 for pump water use and cholera ($p < 0.001$).
1920	Broders discovered an association between pipe smoking and lip cancer.
1920	Goldberger and Sydenstricker work on case control on pellagra and its deficiency.
1926	Janet Lane-Claypon, who selected matched hospital controls, investigated the relationship between reproductive experience and female breast cancer.
1928	Lombard and Doering study which was related to pipe smoking to oral cancer.
1939	Franz Müller conducted a case-control study on smoking and lung cancer in Germany.
1947	Schrek and Lenowitz—a US medical case-control study of penile carcinoma and circumcision.
1949 and 1950	Record and McKeown's case-control study of risk factors including folic acid deficiency for congenital malformations of the nervous system in Birmingham.
1950	Levin *et al.*, 1950; Wynder and Graham, 1950; Doll and Hill, 1950, studies on association between cigarette smoking and lung cancer generated enormous interest in case control, methodology.
1950 and 1952	The landmark study of Doll and Hill inspired future generations of epidemiologists to use this methodology. It remains to this day a model for the design and conduct of case-control studies, with excellent suggestions on how to reduce or eliminate selection, interview and recall bias.
1953	Aird *et al.* discovered the association between gastric cancer and the ABO blood groups.
1970	Mac Mahon *et al.* found the association between late first pregnancy and breast cancer.
1971	Herbst *et al.* studied association between diethylstilbestrol and vaginal adenocarcinoma.
1975	Ziel and Finkle; Smith *et al.*—treatment of menopausal women with exogenous estrogens similarly increased the risk of endometrial cancer.
1975	Prince *et al.*—liver cancer and hepatitis B carrier status
1977	Tuyns *et al.*—synergistic effects of alcohol and tobacco consumption on esophageal cancer.
1981	Kehrberg *et al.* able to found use of tampon causes toxic-shock syndrome.
1987	Hurwitz *et al.* found association between aspirin and Reyes syndrome.
1991	Martin *et al.* confirmed the association between L-tryptophan and eosinophilia-myalgia.
	Since last 7 decades a number of case-control studies have been conducted specially after Doll and Hill study on smoking and lung cancer.

1. The idea of the case, that is, those disease entities are specific, and are likely to have one or more specific causes.
2. An interest in disease aetiology and prevention.
3. A focus on individual, as opposed to group, aetiologies.
4. A history taking from patients/cases with disease under study.
5. Grouping individual cases together into series (case series/case cohort).
6. Making comparisons of the differences between groups to calculate **average** risk at the level of the individual.

In case-control study, we measure the proportion of cases and controls who were exposed or nor to a risk factor(s).[4] The following Table 9.2 depicts the scheme of the study.[5]

Situations Needed to Conduct Case-control Studies (Fig. 9.1)

1. To study rare disease or outcome.
2. The disease or outcome has a long induction and latent period (i.e. a long time between exposure and the eventual causal manifestation of disease).
3. No or limited evidence for causation and association in early stages of finding an aetiology of diseases under study.
4. Exposure data is difficult or expensive to obtain.
5. To the study dynamic population.

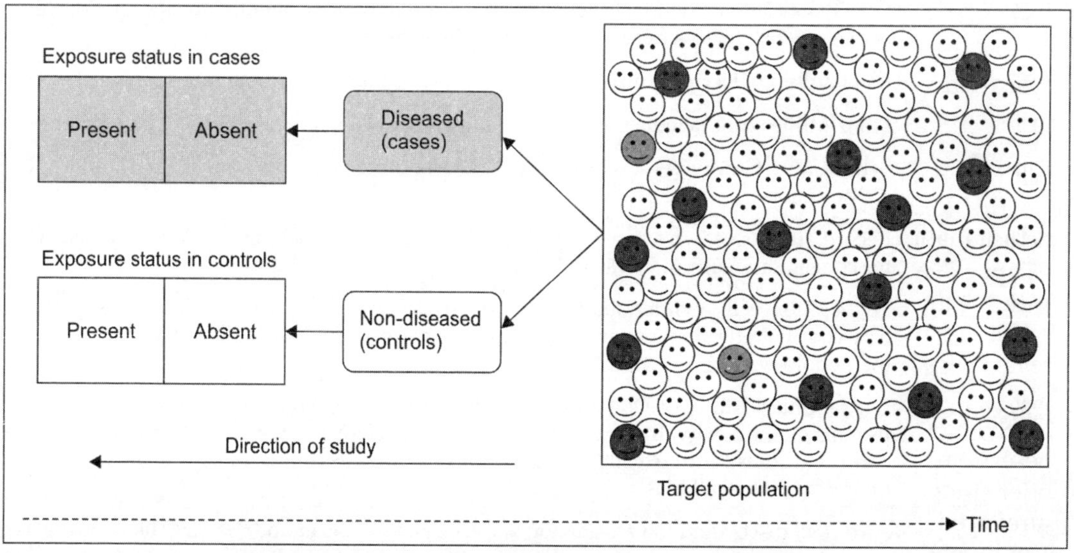

Fig. 9.1: Schematic presentation of case-control study design

Table 9.2: Case-control study design

Past exposure	*Cases (with disease)*	*Control (without disease)*
Present	A	B
Absent	C	D
Total	A + C	B + D
Proportion who were exposed	A/A + C	B/B + D
Proportion who were not exposed	B/A + C	B/B + D

If exposure is associated with disease, then proportion of the cases who were exposed, A/A + C, to be greater than the proportion of the controls who were exposed, B/B + D.

6. Availability of limited resources to conduct study to find out multiple potential risk factors.

Types of Case-control Studies

Various types of case control studies are shown in Fig. 9.2.

Selection of Study Subjects (cases and controls)

The cases and control study should start with the clearly defined hypothesis, identifying the target population and sample population to be decided.

Selection of Cases

Definition of Cases

In the case-control design, investigator should ensure that all true cases in a given population have chance to be included in the study. This requires a standard definition of the disease/ health problems being studied. They should also fulfill the diagnostic and eligibility (inclusion and exclusion) criteria.

Types of cases (to include in case-control studies)—there are two types of cases may be used in case-control studies, i.e. incident or prevalent cases.

Incident Cases

These are newly diagnosed cases of a disease under study during a defined time period. It is preferred over prevalent cases especially for chronic conditions due to:

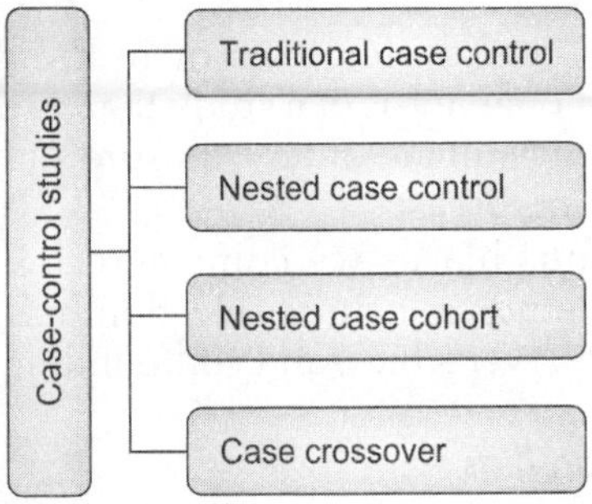

Fig. 9.2: Types of case-control studies

- High motivation
- The recall of past exposure(s) may be more accurate
- Diagnostic criterion among the cases is more consistent
- It avoids complicating factors related to selection of longer duration
- The temporal sequence of exposure and disease is easier to assess among incident cases.

However, it is sometimes impossible to have an adequate sample size if only recent cases are enrolled.

Prevalent Cases

It comprises individuals who have had the outcome (old and new cases) under investigation for some time. Recall bias is much higher than incident cases as it may be more difficult to ensure adequate reporting of events related to a time before the development of disease.

Sources of Cases

Typical sources for cases include:

- Public and private hospital patients (selection should be from multiple hospitals)
- Patients visiting at medical practitioners/ nursing homes
- Disease registries (e.g. cancer, diabetes, stroke, mental retardation, etc.).
- Data of notifiable diseases/surveillance systems.
- Cross-sectional surveys

Selection of Controls[6]

In principle, the controls should be selected from the same risk population from where cases are selected, but it may not be possible all the time. Therefore, Wacholder *et al.* have suggested three aspects that must be considered in the selection of controls, which may reduce selection bias, confounding and information bias:

1. The study base—the comparison group ('controls') should be representative of the source population that produced the cases.

2. The confounding elimination—the 'controls' must be sampled in a way that is independent of the exposure, meaning that their selection should not be more (or less) likely if they have the exposure of interest.
3. The comparable accuracy

Sources of Controls[3,5,6]

Drawing Controls from General Population

Selecting controls from general population is the best choice if one assure the following.

- Surety of the same study base population in the two groups of comparison;
- The establishment of precise criteria of exclusion similar to cases and
- The possibility of generalization to the base of the distribution of exposures.

Hospital or Clinic Controls

This is the most frequently used method for selection of controls due to assumption that all patients admitted in the hospital are from the same population base that generate the cases as well as controls and that the quality of information would be good as that of cases.

As we know, the hospital per se does not have defined catchment area, so the cases and controls may be entirely different. In order to reduce this selection bias, controls are recruited from the cases' friends or relatives, which usually represent the same population.

Neighborhood Controls

Mainly in population-based studies, controls may be selected from neighborhood as they are more cooperative, belongs to similar social class and easily accessible. They are usually chosen non-randomly within a geographical set what may lead to an independence of the selection process and the exposure. The use of neighborhood controls may lead to 'over-matching' on the study exposure if the exposure is related to residence.

Friend Controls

This seems to be an attractive alternative for case-control study in terms of resources and logistics aspects. They can be selected from a list of friends or associates obtained from the case. As the case and friend control will have similar socio-economic status, the biases due to social class are reduced.They can also lead to overmatching regarding factors that depends on lifestyle and occupational exposures.

Sometimes, however, it may be useful to select a spouse or sibling control; a sibling may provide some control over genetic differences between cases and controls.

Size of Control Group

The size of the control group may be determined by circumstances, resources, or power of study. For example, the number of eligible controls—sometimes is a limiting factor. At other times, time and resources may limit the number of controls that can be enrolled. However, when the size of the population from which the cases arose is large and resources are adequate, power calculations can be performed to determine the optimal number of controls needed to identify an important association.

Most case-control studies use a control-to-case ratio of either 1:1, 2:1, or 3:1. In general, little power is gained with control-to-case ratios in excess of 3:1 or 4:1. While uncommon, the number of eligible and enrolled cases can exceed the number of eligible or available controls. Since 80% of maximum efficiency can thus be obtained with 4:1, it is often inadvisable to seek a higher ratio.

Bias in Case-control Study[5–7]

Bias is "any systemic error in the design, conduct or analysis of a study that results in a mistaken estimate of an exposure's effect on the risk of disease."

Various biases we come across in case-control studies include selection bias, recall bias, observer's bias, and confounding bias.

Selection Bias

Selection bias may occur when those individuals selected as controls are unrepresentative of the population that produced the cases, i.e. cases and controls should then be selected from the same identifiable group. Ideally all cases in a defined population would be included, but if only a sample is used they should be truly representative of all cases arising in the population. The controls too should then be selected to be representative of this population.

Berkesonian bias is a bias introduced in hospital based case-control studies, due to varying rates of hospital admissions. As the potential for selection bias is likely to be less of a problem in population-based case-control studies, neighborhood controls may be a preferable choice when using cases from a hospital or clinic setting.

Some other that may contribute to selection bias are as follows:

Patient dies before interview: When cases are ascertained through a population-based disease registry, a significant interval of time may elapse between initial diagnosis and notification to the registry. Some patients whose disease course is rapidly fatal may therefore not be interviewed in person, but are either excluded from the study or represented by a proxy interview subject to increased measurement error. This selection factor may affect both cases *and* controls in hospital-based studies.

Subject: The most common reason for selection bias in case-control studies is refusal of the subject to participate, either actively by refusing to sign a consent form or passively by failure to provide history or agreeing for laboratory examination.

Recall bias: Due to very nature, the case-control study is retrospective, therefore the recall bias is the major potential problem in case control studies. Ernst Wynder, a well-known epidemiologist, also called it 'rumination bias.'

Recall bias occurs at the level of study subjects, as the information about cause is either generated by asking the subjects or from the records. This occurs when study subjects, are unable to recall correctly the exposure which may have occurred long ago. This inability to recall correctly (recall bias) may occur in both cases and controls and in either case will influence the observations and will influence the results. This recall bias can be **differential** (more in case of either the case or control) or **non-differential** (equally prevalent in both cases and controls). It may be noted that the non-differential recall bias is also damaging and can lead to spurious conclusion, but the differential recall bias is even more damaging.

Observer's bias: The problem of bias is not confined only to the subjects but can occur at the level of observers as well. Here the investigator, if knows about the status of the subject that whether he/she is a case or control, as per his/her convictions may made an extra effort to dig out the information of exposure or conversely may ignore the information provided. In order to deal with the observer's bias, same sort of questionnaire should be used or the same amount of efforts be made to get the information about the exposure. Use of available records to get the history of exposure is better than relying on the recall of study subjects or the efforts of observers to dig out the information. Still better if the investigator is blinded or is unaware of the fact that whether he/she is dealing with a case or a control (blinding).

Confounding bias: Confounding factor is the one which independently influences both factor and disease under study and its distribution is also unequal among cases and controls. This is also dealt by the adequate matching of cases and the controls. Matching is done to ensure the compliance of a basic principle of epidemiology that the only the alkies shall be compared. In other words, apples should be compared only with the apples and oranges with oranges only. Under no situation, apples be compared with oranges or vice versa. Let us take the classical example of smoking and lung cancer. We all know that age in itself is a determinant of any cancer including lung cancer and it may happen that cases have higher age than controls. In this case, apart from smoking (under study), we are not sure that whether the age is also not contributing to the incidence of lung cancer. So, to ward off the effect of age, it is advised to match the age of cases and controls; each control should have identical or comparable (± 1or 2 years). Also, when we select the controls from the relatives of cases, we automatically match many environmental characteristics which are logically common for all members of same family.

Examples

Influence of Recall Bias on the Interpretation

1. True situation

Group	*Exposure present*	*Exposure absent*	*Total*	*OR*
Cases	400	100	500	16
Controls	100	400	500	

2. Non-differential recall bias (20%): Both cases and controls under report exposure by 20%

Group	*Exposure present*	*Exposure absent*	*Total*	*OR*
Cases	320	180	500	9.3
Controls	80	420	500	

3. Non-differential recall bias (10%): Both cases and controls under report exposure by 10%

Group	*Exposure present*	*Exposure absent*	*Total*	*OR*
Cases	360	140	500	11.7
Controls	90	410	500	

4. Differential recall bias cases and controls under report exposure by 20% and 10%, respectively

Group	*Exposure present*	*Exposure absent*	*Total*	*OR*
Cases	320	180	500	8.1
Controls	90	410	500	

Hybrid Studies[8]

Nested case control and case-cohort designs are the most common approaches for reducing the costs of exposure assessment in prospective epidemiologic studies. Exposure data in these designs are obtained on a subset of the full cohort. Nested case control designs (or equivalently, incidence density sampling designs) include all cases and a pre-specified number of controls randomly chosen from the risk set at each failure time. Case-cohort designs include all cases and one randomly selected sub-cohort from the risk set at baseline.

Nested Case-control Study[3,4,7]

A nested case-control study is a type of case-control study that draws its cases and controls from a pre-existed cohort population (ongoing cohort study) that has been followed for a period of time (Fig. 9.3).

This cohort, at its inception or during the course of follow-up, has had exposure information. The investigator identifies cases of disease that occurred in the cohort during the course of follow-up period. The investigator also identifies disease-free individuals within the cohort to serve as controls. Using previously collected data and obtaining additional measurements of exposures from available subjects. The investigator analyses and compares the exposure frequencies in cases and controls as in traditional case-control study with the calculation of odds ratios.

The nested case-control study is considered as a strong observational study, comparable to its parent cohort study in the likelihood of an unbiased association between an exposure and an outcome.

Advantages of Nested Case-control Studies

- Relatively cheap and easy to conduct.
- Data related to exposure and confounding have often already been collected.

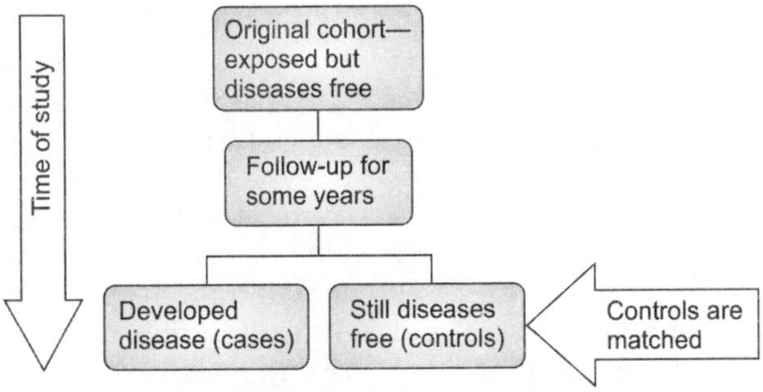

Fig. 9.3: Nested case-control study

- Can utilise the baseline data on exposure and confounding collected before the onset of disease, which reduces the potential for recall bias and uncertainty regarding the temporal sequence between exposure and disease onset.
- As cases and controls drawn from the same cohort, it decreases the likelihood of selection bias.

Disadvantages of Nested Case-control Studies

- Causal inference is still limited.
- Not all relevant risk factor/exposure data may have been recorded.
- Data may not have been recorded in the same way, or with the same accuracy and consistency, over time.
- Recall bias may persist if some data are collected retrospectively.
- Non-diseased persons from whom the controls are selected may not be fully representative of the original cohort due to loss to follow-up or death.

Case-cohort Study

This study design is a kind of hybrid between case control and cohort methodologies.

A case-cohort study compares a series of cases to a sub-cohort (control); the sub-cohort is randomly selected from the defined cohort (original cohort) with which the study began. This subset of the full cohort is called the sub-cohort and represents the entire cohort. These controls are not individually matched to each case, it is possible to study different diseases (different sets of cases) in the same case-cohort study using the same cohort for controls. It selects only incident cases for their case groups as it is a prospective study. But since the sub-cohort is selected at the beginning of follow-up, some of its members may develop the disease during follow-up.The case-cohort study design seeks to improve efficiency by making a sub-cohort its focus, rather than the entire cohort (Fig. 9.4).

Case-crossover Study

Case-crossover studies are another type of case-control studies (Fig. 9.5). Thses studies

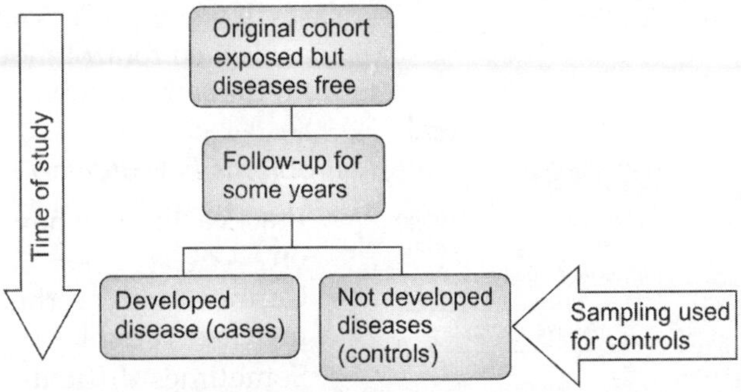

Fig. 9.4: Nested case-cohort study

also have a backward logical and retrospective temporal direction. The investigation begins with the identification of a series of cases and exposure is retrospectively assessed. In contrast to case-control studies, case-crossover studies use the same individuals as cases and controls. A case-crossover study assesses the frequency of exposure in the cases immediately before the onset of disease, and compares this to another time when the same people did not develop the disease. If an exposure precipitates disease, that exposure should occur more frequently during the interval before the onset of disease than during some other interval when disease did not occur.This design is generally used to study outcomes that rapidly, and typically temporarily, follow exposure because the comparisons occur within individuals, individual characteristics that don't change over time and might contribute to the outcome are 'matched' and cannot, therefore, act as confounders of the exposure-disease relationship.

Matching[7]

Matching is defined as the process of selecting the controls so that they are similar to the cases. The goal of the matching is to compare 'like with like'. The characteristics most correctly specified for matching are those that are potential confounders of the exposure-diseases associations of interest. By matching cases and control such variables like age, race, sex, socio-economic status, and occupation will help to interpret the results correctly.

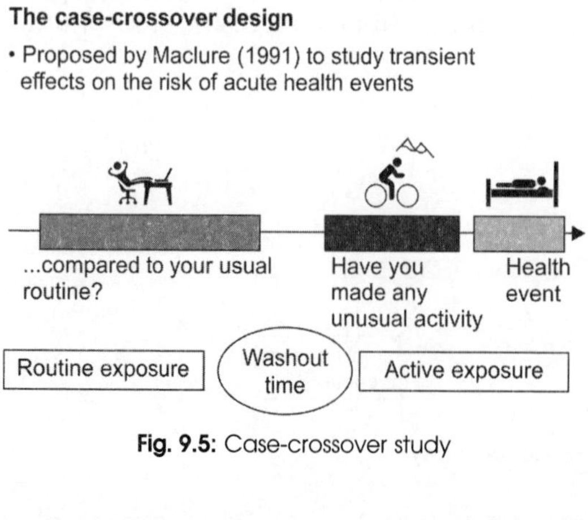
The case-crossover design
• Proposed by Maclure (1991) to study transient effects on the risk of acute health events
...compared to your usual routine?
Have you made any unusual activity
Health event
Routine exposure
Washout time
Active exposure

Fig. 9.5: Case-crossover study

While matching it should be borne in mind that the suspected aetiological factor or the variable we wish to measure should not be matched, because by matching, its aetiological role is eliminated in that study. The cases and controls will then become automatically alike with respect to that factor. It should be noted that if matching is overdone, it may be difficult to find controls. Further with excess zeal in matching, there may be a tendency to reduce the odds ratio.

Matching is of two types:
1. Individual matching and
2. Group matching.

Individual Matching or Pair Matching

Pair matching is the selection of one or more controls for each case who have the same or similar specified characteristics as that case. Although the term pair matching implies one case and one control, the term may also refer to two, three, or more, or even a variable number of controls matched to each case. Suppose we select case of 50 years male from a hospital suffering from lung cancer, then we must choose a 50 years old male from the same hospital who is not suffering from lung cancer, he might have some other diseases say diabetes or cataract.

Group Matching or Frequency Matching

Frequency matching, also called category matching or group matching, is an alternative to pair matching. Frequency matching involves the selection of controls in proportion to the distribution of certain characteristics of the cases. If we select 50% females as cases from a schools then control should also be 50% males from the same school.

Problems in Matching

- Practical limit on how many you can match on
- Cannot analyse the association for the matched variables
- Sometimes difficult, expensive (requires large number of cases and controls)

- Over-matching (matched by factors strongly related to the exposure which is the main interest.)

Analysis in Case-control Studies

For an unmatched case-control study, the data look like this (Table 9.3):

- odds of = number of cases with the exposure = A
- exposure (cases) number of cases without the exposure = C
- odds of = number of controls with the exposure = B
- exposure (controls) number of controls without the exposure = D
- odds ratio = odds of exposure (cases) = AD
- odds of exposure (controls) = BC

a. **Exposure rates** = A/A + C (among cases) and B/B + D (among controls), it is depicted as percentages (%)

b. **Risk estimation:** The estimation of disease risk associated with exposure is obtained by an index known as 'relative risk' (RR) or 'risk ratio', which is defined as the ratio between the incidence of disease among exposed persons and incidence among non-exposed.

Relative risk (RR) = Incidence among exposed/incidence among non-exposed

True relative risk can only be calculated in cohort study as in case control, true incidence is not there.

c. The **odds ratio** is the measure of association for a case-control study. It tells us how much higher the odds of exposure is among cases of a disease compared with controls.

The odds ratio compares the **odds of exposure** to the factor of interest **among cases** to the odds of exposure to the factor **among controls**. (The **odds** is the probability that an event will happen divided by the probability that it won't happen.)

An odds ratio:

- **Close to 1.0** means that the odds of exposure among cases is the same as the odds of exposure among controls. The exposure is not associated with the disease.
- **Greater than 1.0** means that the odds of exposure among cases is greater than the odds of exposure among controls. The exposure may be a risk factor for the disease.
- **Less than 1.0** means that the odds of exposure among cases is lower than the odds of exposure among controls. The exposure may be protective against the disease.

Hypothetical Example (Table 9.4)

An outbreak of cholera was detected among residents of Bhilai, India. In a case-control study, investigators found that 30 of 40 case patients and five of 60 controls drank contaminated water. Inserting these numbers into the 2 × 2 table:

Exposure among cases = A/A + C = 30/40 = 0.75, i.e. 75% and

Exposure among controls = B/B + D = 0.08, i.e. = 8%

Table 9.3: Hypothetical example—obesity and high fat diet (case-control study)

Age group	*No. of cases selected*	*No. of control selected—unmatched*	*No. of control selected—unmatched*
5–10 years	50	30	50
11–15 years	30	20	30
16–20 years	30	80	30
21–25 years	60	70	60
26–30 years	80	50	80
	250	**250**	**250**

Table 9.4: Case-control study design

Drank contaminated water	*Cholera cases*	*Control (no cholera)*	*Total*
Yes	A = 30	B = 5	A + B = 35
No	C = 10	D = 55	C + D = 65
Total	**A + C = 40**	**B + D = 60**	**A + B + C + D = 100**

Odds ratio (OR) = AD/BC = 30 × 55/5 × 10 = 33

Interpretation: The odds of exposure to contaminated water was over 33 times higher among cases than controls, means there is a definite association between contaminated water and cholera.

Relative risk (RR) = Incidence among exposed/incidence among non-exposed

RR = A/A + B ÷ C/C + D = 30/35 ÷ 10/65 = 5.73

Differences between case-control and cohort studies are given in Chapter 10.

References

1. Nigel Paneth, Ezra Susser, Mervyn Susser. Series: History of epidemiology—origins and early development of the case-control study: part 1, Early evolution. 2002 pp 282–88.
2. Nigel Paneth, Ezra Susser, Mervyn Susser Series: History of epidemiology—origins and early development of the case-control study: part 2, The case-control study from Lane-Claypon to 1950. 2002, pp 259–265.
3. Wallace/Maxcy-Rosenau-Last, Public Health and Preventive Medicine, 15th edn., Ch 3. Epidemiology and public health. The McGraw-Hill Companies, Inc. doi: 10.1036/0071441980.
4. Kumar R, Khan AM, Chatterjee P. Types of observational studies in medical research. Astrocyte 2014;1:154–9.
5. Gordis, Leon (author) 1934. Epidemiology. Ch 10 Leon Gordis 5th edn. Saunders, an imprint of Elsevier Inc. 1996.
6. Sao Paulo. Selection of subjects in case-controls studies. Med J 1995;113(2 Supl.) http://dx.doi.org/10.1590/S1516-31801995000700024
7. Gregg Michael. Field epidemiology (Ed.), Oxford University Press, Inc.198 Madison Avenue, New York, 10016. 3rd edn. 2008.
8. Ahrens Wolfgang, Pigeot Iris (Eds). Handbook of Epidemiology, *Norman E. Breslow (author)*. Case-control studies. Ch 1.6, page 287. https://publichealthdentistryindia.files.wordpress.com/.../wolfgang ahrens, irispigeot.

Chapter

10

Cohort Studies: 'Master Craftmen' of Medical Research

Badrinarayan Mishra

Box 10.1: Learning objectives

This chapter will enable the reader:

- To learn the importance of cohort studies and the pivotal role they play in medical research.
- To distinguish between the various types of cohort designs including open, fixed and closed cohort and retrospective, prospective, ambi-directional and special cohort designs.
- To describe the key features in conducting cohort studies including the selection of exposed and unexposed populations, the sources of information on exposures, outcomes and other key variables, approaches to follow-ups, calculating person time and data analysis.
- To understand ethical concerns and expense management in cohort studies.
- To compare and contrast between cohort studies and RCT, case-control and cross-sectional studies.
- To understand important cohort studies conducted across the globe.
- To describe the strengths and limitations of cohort studies

Box 10.2: Cohort study highlights

1. This is the best study to ascertain both the incidence and natural history of disease.
2. This answers the chicken–egg question; which often frustrates cross-sectional and case-control studies.
3. Here temporal association between putative cause and outcome is usually clear.
4. It is useful in investigation of multiple outcomes that might arise out of single exposure.
5. Assessment of many outcomes is a positive attribute of cohort study.
6. Cohort study can test hypothesis or generate hypothesis. Examining the planned primary or secondary association is called hypothesis conformation. Looking (reporting) at other outcome measured is called hypothesis generation.
7. There is limited ethical concern which is common to non-experimental research—since the investigator does not assign exposure.
8. Cohort study allows calculation of incidence rates, absolute risk, relative risks, and attributable risk.
9. Other outcome measures of interest are cumulative incidence analysis by Poisson regression and time to event or survival analysis by Kaplan Meier method and proportional hazard model.

HISTORICAL OVERVIEW

A perfect cuisine has a royal history. Of all cuisines in medical research 'cohort study' the 'Cullen Queen' has a vibrant one. It dates back to ancient Rome. The mighty Roman Army was known for its 'legions' and 'cohorts'. A 'legion' was a major unit in Roman army and ten 'cohorts' coming together constituted one 'legion' (Fig. 10.1). 'Cohors' in Latin means a group of soldiers and 'one cohort' constituted of 300–600 soldiers.[1, 2]

Once a cohort was formed, no new soldiers were added to it. Thus, the recruited soldiers

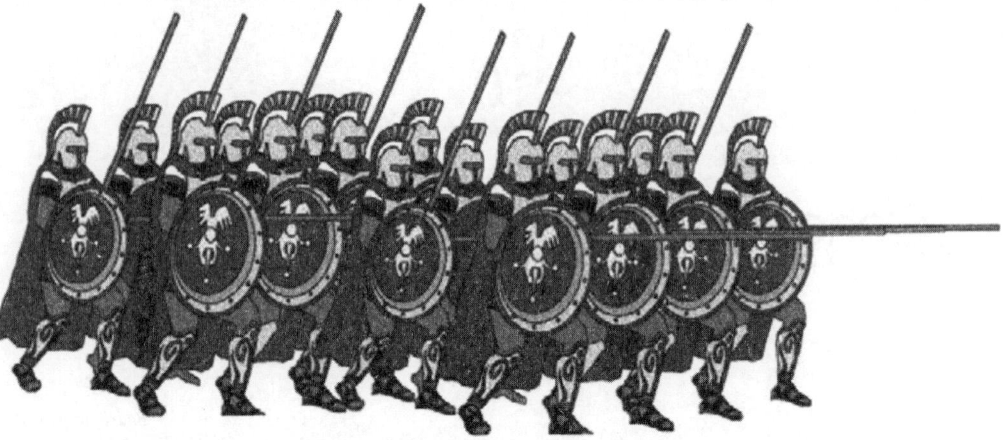

Fig. 10.1: A cohort in Roman army *(courtesy: The Lancet Publishing groups)*

remained in the same cohort for the duration of their service—a classic example of 'fixed cohort'. Attrition occurred mainly through death. This 'militarized cohort' of yester years formed the basis of the popular 'medical cohort' of today. In medicine, the word cohort is used to describe any designated group of persons who are followed over a period of time; or to describe a group of individuals with a common characteristic or experience, i.e. a birth cohort, marriage cohort, occupational cohort, etc. Cohort study in medicine describes an epidemiological investigation that follows such groups with common characteristics in respect to exposure so as to measure outcomes that may arise out of it.

The credit of medicalization of cohort goes to Wade Hampton Frost; the leading American epidemiologist of early 20th century. Frost compared the trends with age in the sex-specific incidence of tuberculosis in groups of men and women born at different dates. Such groups were called cohorts by Frost. The use of this technique found mention in a paper entitled "The age selection of mortality from tuberculosis in successive decades" published in 1939.[3]

INTRODUCTION

It is rightly said "you can observe a lot by just watching".[4] The watchfulness in medical research is epitomized by cohort study, which effectively combines descriptive and analytical research designs. Thus cohort study is considered as an observational research with strong analytical power which can assess causal association in terms of temporality of event occurrence and it has all the goodness of interventional control design. Though it comes next to randomized control trails (RCTs) in the evidence hierarchy pyramid (Fig. 10.2) in its ability to synthesize quality research evidence, but the commonness and feasibility of its conduction specially in community and public health research puts it ahead of RCTs. On many occasions it is the only possible interventional design that can be conducted due to ethical and other restrictions on RCTs. Furthermore, its population-based design has better generability and external validity than RCTs. Thus it will not be out of place to rate cohort study as the best study available in most conditions and more so in public health scenario where deliberate intervention by introduction of new agents of change is mostly unconceivable and aptly unethical.

Basic Concepts of Cohort Study

In its simplest form; a cohort study follows-up two or more groups from exposure to outcome and compares the experience of a group exposed to some factor with another group not exposed to it. If the former group

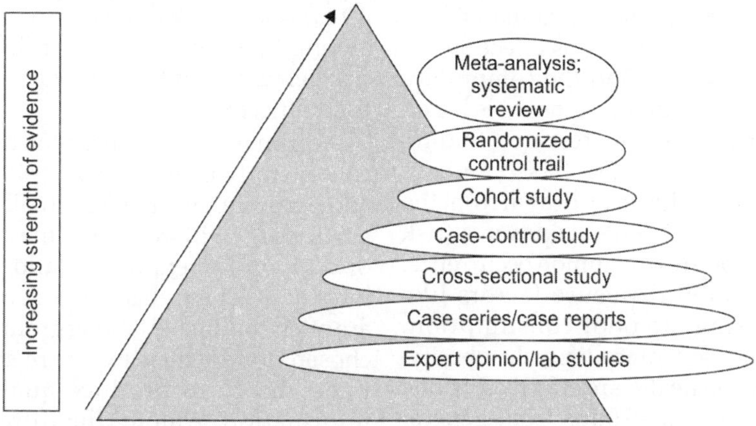

Fig. 10.2: Evidence-based ladder/pyramid for interpretation of medical research

has a higher or lower frequency of an outcome than the unexposed, then an association between exposure and outcome is evident. The defining characteristic of all cohort studies is that they track people forward in time from exposure to outcome. Researchers doing this kind of study must, therefore, go forward in time from the present or go back in time to choose their cohorts (Fig. 10.3). Either way, a cohort study moves in the same direction, although gathering data might not.

Principle of Cohort Study

Only a technically well designed cohort can produce a valid and generalized result. So, the selections of exposure and comparison groups should be scientific and mutually complementing. Analysis and interpretation of synthesized information must follow research or deal. Thus the success of a cohort study depends on selection of exposure group, finding a suitable comparison to exposed population, drafting a suitable cohort design and finally analyzing and interpreting the results in a valid manner. These four principles are discussed one-by-one in the following sections.

Exposure Groups in Cohort Study

The first step in starting a cohort study lies in identifying an exposure and selecting an exposure group. Exposure status of an event is determined by results of previous observational and analytical studies. This exposure or risk factor may be harmful or protective in nature. For example, in case of administration of vaccines to a defined population; which when considered as exposure has protective

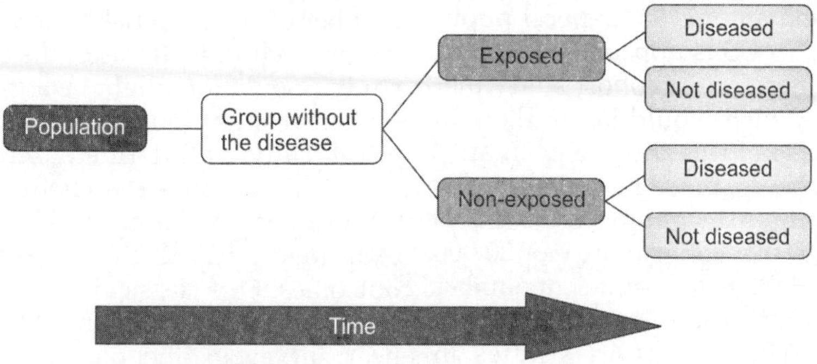

Fig. 10.3: Basic design of cohort study

effect and exposure to nuclear radiation to a group of people has deleterious effect on the health of the individual and the community alike. While finding out an exposure is based on knowledge from previous research, finding out an exposure group is based on the population at risk. This can be drawn from the general population when the exposures (risk factors) in question are of common occurrence. Studies of common exposure factors like cigarette smoking, alcohol consumption, tobacco chewing, sedentary lifestyle, obesity, etc. and its effect on health are effectively done by selecting 'exposure groups from general population'.

But, there are instances where the exposures with proven health effects are rare in general population; for example, exposure to alanine dye and its outcome in the form of bladder and skin cancer. In this scenario, though the exposure to alanine in general population is very rare but we can find out special occupational groups where the working population has unusual high exposure to this dye stuff. Thus the workers in dye industries using alanine qualify to be a special exposure cohort. Hence, even though an outcome may be extremely rare in a general population, it may be sufficiently common in a special exposure group so as to allow for collection of adequate number of cases for conduction of epidemiological study. The advantage of 'special exposure cohort' is that it permits the evaluation of rare outcomes that would otherwise require a prohibitively large number of individuals from general population. For example, the annual incidence rate of mesothelioma among the general population of males in US is approximately 8.42 per million.[5] Therefore, a cohort study that included 20,000 men would be unlikely to identify any case of this disease even after 5 years of follow-up. Since mesothelioma is relatively common in people exposed to asbestos, however a cohort study of 20,000 such workers might yield a sufficient number of cases to explore various exposure disease relationships. Though cohort studies in general are not optimal for the evaluation of rare diseases, but if the occurrence is not rare among those exposed, i.e. if the attributable risk percentage is high, a cohort design can be used efficiently.

A primary requirement for the validity of cohort study is the ability to obtain complete and accurate information on all participants, particularly with respect to the ascertainment of data on the exposures and outcomes of interest. Keeping this in mind, cohort studies are often conducted among groups specifically chosen not for their exposure status, but for their ability to produce quality relevant information. Among the different groups preferred for cohort studies are members of certain professions, such as doctors or nurses, workers of different occupations or entire company, union members, prepaid medical care plan holders, veterans, student alumni, etc. Each of these groups offers some logistic advantage to the investigators, ranging from annually updated addresses, to a mechanism of periodic follow-up, to the provision of complete medical and employment records. These groups are termed as 'special convenient groups', which are in a position to generate quality data from their well maintained records. Since the groups were not selected because of unusually high level of specific exposures, these populations are most usually studied when the exposures of interest are common or the groups are very large.

Thus the choice of a particular group to serve as a study population for any given cohort is related to both the hypothesis under investigation and specific features of the design. For example, in order to investigate a number of common risk factors for relatively common chronic diseases, the best choice of study population might be a general cohort, drawn from a geographically and demographically well defined area who can be surveyed to establish baseline exposure status with respect to a number of factors and then examined periodically to ascertain future outcomes. One classic design of this type of prospective cohort design is the Framingham heart survey. In other places for events of rare occurrence a special exposure group like industrial workers in solvent (alanine) factories can be studied by retrospective cohort design for evaluation of cancer risk.

To sum it up; exposed population can be drawn from general population for common exposure (risk factors) or from different occupational groups where there is a chance of unusual high exposure or from special population groups which generate quality information and are ideal for long follow-up (Fig. 10.4 and Table 10.1).

Comparison Groups in Cohort Study

The second principle for success of cohort study stresses on selection of a valid comparison group. A comparison group in cohort studies constitutes of group of individuals who are similar to the cohort population in respect to all other variables except the exposure (risk factor) under study. Thus they constitute the non-exposure group which is closest to the exposed cohort in other aspects. The data of these two groups are compared with each other to determine the presence or absence of causality.

Idealistically speaking the perfect comparison is 'comparing the same individual for a risk factor with himself'. This theoretical concept is known as 'counterfactual idea'; where the ideal comparison group consists of exactly the same individuals in the exposed group had they not been exposed. As it is impossible for the same individual to be exposed and unexposed to a risk factor simultaneously it becomes mandatory to select different groups of individuals as

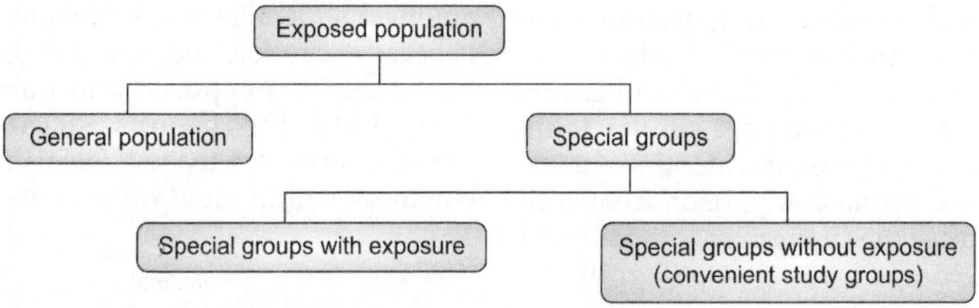

Fig. 10.4: Selection of exposed group

Table 10.1: Exposure groups in cohort studies

Types of exposure group	*Strength*	*Weakness*
General population	• Suitable for common exposures • Study of multiple exposures and its outcomes • Generability of study results	• Loss to follow-up is common and can reduce validity • May be difficult to assemble • Unsuitable for rare exposures
Special groups		
1. Special groups with exposure	• Suitable for rare and single or limited exposures • Easy to constitute • Good source for information • Low rate of loss to follow-up	• Generability is limited • Losses of subjects before defining cohort • Suffers from 'health workers effect'
2. Special groups without exposure or convenient study group	• Suitable for common exposure • Study of multiple exposures • Easy to constitute • Low rate of loss to follow-up • Good source for quality and comparable information	• Generability is limited • Suffers from 'health workers effect' • Requires large number of participants

comparison groups who are either not exposed to the risk factor under investigation or has comparatively less exposure to the factor in question. So in the selection of comparison groups an effort is made to select the group which is as close to the exposed cohort as possible baring the risk factor. For example, as in 'the British doctors cohort' study the comparison group was doctors who were non-smokers and the study cohort constitutes doctors who were smokers. The effects of cigarette smoking like lung cancer, cardiovascular diseases, bronchitis, and other respiratory problems of these two groups of doctors were compared.

Classification of Comparison Groups

Depending on their source of origin, we have two major comparison groups. They are 'internal' and 'external comparisons'. The external one is further divided into groups selected from general population and groups from another cohort who are similar to the study cohort baring the exposure (risk factor). A variant to external comparison frequently used to increase the strength of comparability is 'multiple comparisons' group (Fig. 10.5).

Internal Comparison Group

This is also known as 'General population group'. Here a single general cohort is chosen for study purpose and its member then classified to study cohort and comparison cohort based on exposure status (Fig. 10.6). For example, in Doll and Hill cohort study of British physicians with respect to cigarette smoking and lung cancer, the study cohort was all doctors who smoked cigarette and the internal comparison group was all doctors who were non-smokers. Both these groups were derived from a single selected cohort of British physicians irrespective of their smoking status. Similarly, in the famous Framingham heart study; baseline levels of blood cholesterol, systolic and diastolic BP was determined for all selected participants. Then they were divided into quintiles of exposures based on these baseline values. The rates of coronary heart diseases within these groups were compared for risk evaluation.

Internal comparison groups are the best amongst all available comparison options. It is because the selected cohort is divided into two groups as exposed and non-exposed. Thus both the groups share common parameters except the risk factor. This design enhances validity and often considered as a

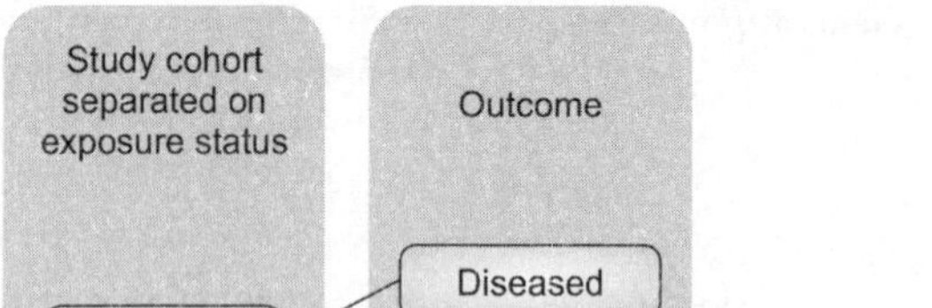

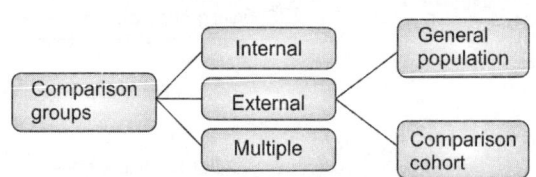

Fig. 10.5: Classification of comparison groups

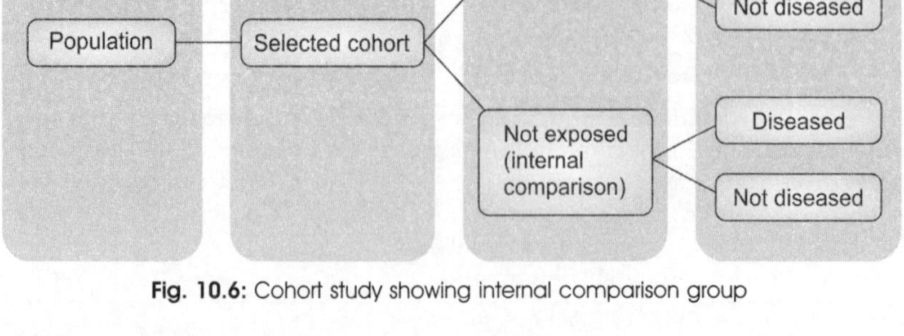

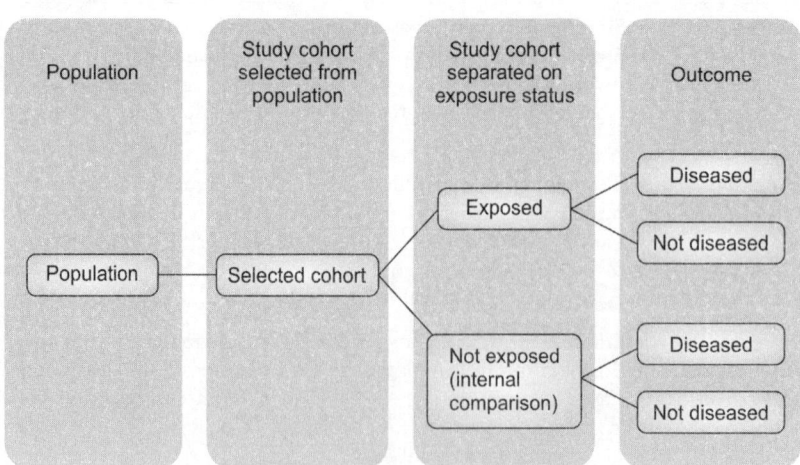

Fig. 10.6: Cohort study showing internal comparison group

variant of 'non-randomized control trial design' (NRCT); where the exposure (risk) factor equivocates the experimental intervention of NRCT.

If a suitable internal comparison group is not available, then the investigators look for the alternate ones. They are 'external comparison groups' derived from general population or other related cohorts known as 'comparison cohorts'. Another way of satisfying the need is by employing 'multiple comparison groups' if the available single external options are not satisfactory.

External Comparison Group

For studies involving 'special exposure groups' like workers in different occupational settings it is difficult to gather an internal comparison group. Firstly, it is because all the members working in the occupational setup are exposed to the risk factor under study though may be at varying degrees. So getting a reliably unexposed comparison is not possible. Secondly, even an attempt at gathering an internal comparison may look possible by defining the quantum of exposure to different working classes; still it becomes difficult to get a comparison group which is close to the study cohort in other characters. For example, in an oil refinery where manual labourers are allowed to handle most of the toxic materials, the level of exposure to labourers may be exceptionally high in comparison to other office workers like executives (blue collar workers) and desk clerks thereby making them comparable with respect to the exposure. But in most occasions the comparability stops here. Because socio-economic and other demographic characters of on field workers (labourers) and other office workers differ in most industrial settings. Most of the labourers are men, younger in age and from low socio-economic background, whereas majority of desk clerks are women and blue collar executives are from higher economic strata. Thus, adopting an internal comparison strategy may not succeed in assembling adequate numbers for valid comparison.

Thus, begins the search for a comparison group without exposure from external sources like the general population or another comparable cohort which is not exposed to the risk factor under investigation. So, we look for external comparison group from general population or other comparable cohorts (Fig. 10.7).

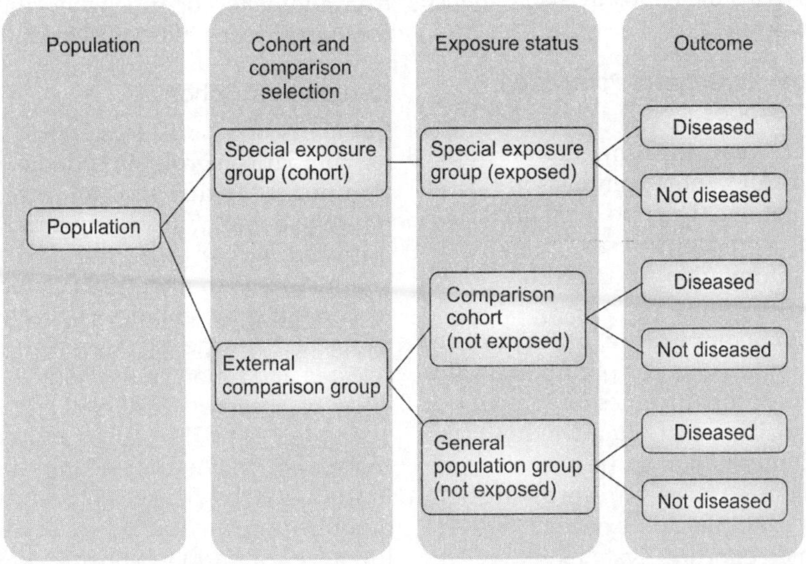

Fig. 10.7: Cohort study showing external comparison group—an example of multiple comparison groups

General Population Comparison Groups

Most 'special exposure cohorts' are too small for the derivation of reliable age, sex, and cause specific rates. Thus, the observed number of cases or outcomes arising out of study cohort is compared with the expected number which is generated from or available at general population level. Here pre-existing available data on disease occurrence and death in a population becomes the basis of comparison. For example, comparisons with population rates are possible only for outcomes for which these rates are available such as mortality, cancer incidences, or other events for which special data can be obtained. In most countries such data are available in the form of death certificates, cancer registry, etc. Good quality internationally comparable data are also compiled and maintained by world health organization.

Drawing a well matched 'population comparison group' is no small challenge. The comparison group should be as close to the study cohort as possible. Therefore, besides general items like age, sex, socio-economic status, etc.; other relevant issues should be considered. For example the importance of geographical similarity, ethnicity, etc. cannot be ignored as increased comparability of study groups sans the exposure will enhance the study quality.

Disadvantages of General Population Comparison Groups

Applying information from general population groups for cohort comparison has its inherent limitations. The two most important ones which need mention are 'paucity of comparable information' and 'health workers effect'.

Paucity of comparable information: Naturally comparisons for population rates are possible only for outcomes for which such rates are available. Most often we don't find the required information in the formats available or the required formats (records) are non-existent. For example, non-existence of event recording and reporting systems like cancer registry or immunization registry or their token existence in most developing and under developed countries severely jeopardizes their use. Similarly, non-adherence to ICD codes for reporting morbidity and mortality by concern reporting agencies severely limits their applicability.

Health workers effect: Employment of workers in occupational set-ups follows set norms. The prime objective of these set norms is to choose healthy work force which will contribute to increased production. The unhealthy ones are either not employed or removed from working population with suitable compensations. Thus, the study cohorts from occupational sectors enjoy better health in comparison to the general population. General population on other hand consists of both ill and healthy subject. The rates of death and diseases among a working population are usually lower than those of the general population, even if a noxious agent is present that elevates certain disease rates. This inappropriateness of comparability forms the basis of 'health worker effect'. Enjoyment of average better general health of working population incorporates an element of bias to cohort studies when an occupational study cohort is compared with general population. This is coined as 'health worker effect'. This can be countered by employing a comparison group from another occupation where the groups are comparable sans the exposure under study.

Comparison Cohort

Comparison cohorts are adopted as an external comparison group in order to eliminate or minimize 'health worker effect' and to improve demographic comparability thereby minimizing confounding and improving validity. Here another cohort which is similar in demographic characteristics to the study cohort except the exposure in question are selected and followed over time for comparability of observed exposure effects. In most occasions both the study and comparison cohorts are drawn from the same industry like in the study by Seltser and Starwell, where mortality rate in radiologists due to sustained low level radiation exposure is evaluate by comparing them with a cohort of unexposed colleagues like ophthalmologists, otolaryngologist and internists who didn't have the exposure.[6] Here all study participants were from the same industry, i.e. healthcare providers. In other instances occupational groups form different industries may be recruited. As in a study involving 'asbestos processing and lung cancer' workers from asbestos industry were compared with workers from cotton textile industry. In these two types of industries workers engage in same types of tasks and share many socioeconomic characteristics baring the exposure factor, i.e. exposure to asbestos fibres.

Multiple Comparison Groups

Multiple comparison policy is adopted when no single external group appears sufficiently similar to exposure group so as to provide assurance about the validity of comparison. Under such circumstances, it is assumed that if similar association is observed for a number of different comparison groups, then the association can be validated. This has warranted the use of multiple comparisons in cohort studies. Here for example one group can be from general population and other from a comparison cohort. One of the historic examples of multiple comparisons is the study of mesothelioma in asbestos workers in US.[7] Here, in addition to comparison with textile workers, mortality rates were also compared with that of the general US white male population. It was found that asbestos workers had excess mortality from all causes; like lung cancer and other respiratory diseases, hypertensive heart diseases, etc. relative to both cotton textile workers and general population. Thus, the mortality experience of asbestos workers was not only greater than of the general population but also substantially higher than that of a group of workers engaged in similar work but without asbestos in their environment. The consistency of the result of these two comparisons enhanced the belief in the existence of true increases in disease risk. This approach can also be adopted when we have no definite comparison group which is clearly superior to others under consideration.

The strengths and weaknesses of comparison groups are summarized in Table 10.2.

Designing of Cohort Studies

The third step in conduction of cohort study is to select a correct cohort design which will

Table 10.2: Comparison groups in cohort studies

Types of comparison group	*Strength*	*Weakness*
Internal	• Most comparable to exposed group • Preferred first choice • Yields valid result	• May be difficult to identify • May not be possible to draft one in all occasions
External		
General population	• Accessible • Stable data	• Lack of comparability with exposed group • Result may suffer from healthy worker effect. • Data on key variables may be missing.
Comparison cohort	• Fairly comparable • Minimizes health workers effect	• Results are often difficult to interpret because comparison cohort often has other exposures.
Multiple comparison groups	• Good comparability • Method of choice among external groups when no suitable general population or comparison cohorts are available.	• Difficult to conduct • Expensive

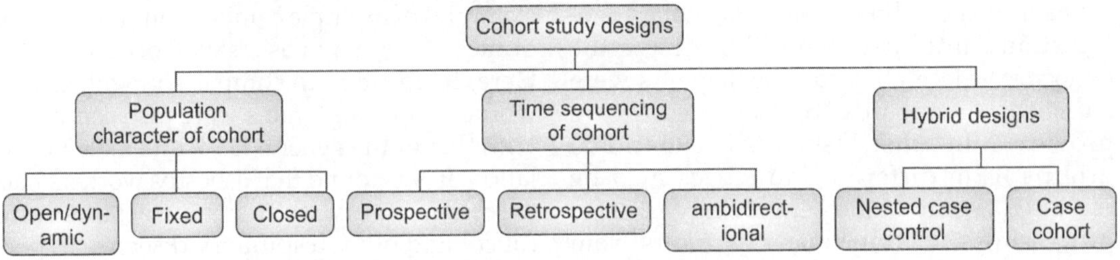

Fig. 10.8: Cohort study designs

suitably answer the research hypothesis. Here we have handful of options to bail us out. What is of outmost importance is to find the right one. Let us examine the options, their strengths and limitations. On broader term, we can have two types of cohort depending on population character and time sequencing. Though these two are not mutually exclusive still we prefer to start the discussion under these categories for sound interpretation (Fig. 10.8).

Cohort Based on Population Character

Here the population dynamics of study subjects becomes the basis of cohort classification. We can have open, closed or fixed cohort depending on recruitment and follow-up strategy of study participants.

Open Cohort

Here the study subjects are recruited at the start of the study and also at different points when they become eligible to enter. They are then followed up over certain predefined time period. This predefined time may be either the end of the study time or the occurrence of the event of interest, whichever is earlier. Thus, for example if the study duration for a proposed cohort designed to study the association of leukaemia with radiation exposure is 10 years, then logically all participants enrolled for the study, i.e. both study subjects and comparison groups should be followed over 10 years from the time of recruitment. But, if someone develops the proposed outcome, i.e. leukaemia at the end of 5 years, then the follow-up for that participant ends there. Thus, we have an openness element for follow-up. Similarly, a person may terminate his association with the study due to varied reason. These are issues like migration, death, voluntary discontinuation, etc. In other instances, persons may be allowed to join the study as soon as they become eligible for enrolment. For example, a subject becomes eligible for a cohort study for occupation related exposure only at the end of completion of 10 years of service, the time considered as cut off for exposure criteria. Thus, persons are added to study cohort at different time on qualifying exposure criteria, hence we have openness in approach for enrolment or entry to study group. So, studies where there designs are adopted are called open cohorts.

Fixed Cohort

This design involves enrolling participants at a fixed point in time and following them over. For example, in the study of infamous and inhuman atomic exposure to the residents of the twin towns of Hiroshima and Nagasaki of Japan during World War 2, those present in these cities at the time of bombing qualified to be considered as study subject from the fixed episode.[8] Though the entry point is fixed the exit is variable, as the subjects were assessed for the occurrence of outcome, i.e. leukaemia. Thus, a closed cohort has its origin from an irrevocable event and this cohort doesn't gain members in contrast to open cohort. But losses may occur as in line of open cohort design.

Closed Cohort

The key features of this design are that the subjects enter the study as they do for fixed cohort and there is no loss to follow-up. All subjects enter the study after an irrevocable event and all participants are followed up till the end point without losing a subject. Thus, all subjects have the same maximum observation time and no subject become unobservable. These assumptions are very restrictive and rarely satisfied in practice. For example, in a case of food poisoning after a dinner party all members those attained the dinner becomes eligible for study. They are followed-up to a logical end point, i.e. longest incubation period for the poisoning in question assuming no loss to follow-up as the duration of study is likely to be short and the poisoning non-fatal and most invitees are from a population which is assessable.

Cohort Based on Time Sequencing

The second classification is based on time sequencing of cohort. Time sequencing means the time of assembling the study population. Thus, if the population is assembled on present time and followed up thereafter to future to establish outcomes, it is called a prospective cohort. On contrary, if the study cohort is assembled back in time and followed up till date when the outcome of interest has already occurred, it is called a retrospective cohort. A combination of these two is called an ambidirectional one. The decision to adopt a prospective, retrospective or ambidirectional study depends on the research question, practical constraints such as time and money, and the availability of suitable study populations and records (Table 10.3).

Prospective Cohort (synonymsóconcurrent cohort, longitudinal cohort, panel study)

A prospective study watches for outcomes, such as the development of a disease, during the study period and relates this to other factors such as suspected risk or protection factor(s). The study usually involves taking a cohort of subjects and watching them over a predefined period which in most cases is a long one, running into years and even decades. The outcome of interest should be of common occurrence; otherwise, the number of outcomes observed will be too small to be statistically meaningful. All efforts should be made to avoid sources of bias such as the loss of individuals to follow-up during the study. Prospective studies usually have fewer potential sources of bias and confounding than retrospective studies.

For example, an investigator who wants to study the epidemic of multiple births stemming from assisted reproductive technologies could begin a cohort study now.[9] Women exposed to these technologies and a similar group who conceived naturally could be tracked forward through their pregnancies to monitor the frequency of multiple births thereby making the study concurrent or prospective in nature.

As pointed out, earlier cohort classified on basis of population character and timing of event occurrence and recording are not mutually exclusive. In a prospective cohort, we can follow an open population, fixed population or closed population. Here also we can adopt any of the control selection

Table 10.3: Characteristic of population-based cohort study

Type of population studied	*Defined by*	*Follow-up*	*Appropriate measure of disease frequency*
Open or dynamic	Changeable characteristic	• Members come and go • Losses may occur	Incidence rate
Fixed	Irrevocable event	• Does not gain members • Losses may occur	Incidence rate
Closed	Irrevocable event	• Does not gain members • No loss occurs	Cumulative incidence

procedures discussed previously like, internal comparison, external comparison or multiple comparisons. The selection of exposure groups can be based on from general population, at risk population or special population groups. Prospective cohort design incorporates the original concept of an ideal cohort study. For example, in the classic Framingham heart study, open cohorts of adult residents from the city were prospectively followed over many years. The risk or exposure status was determined by baseline parameters at entry point and exposed, and comparison groups were selected on the percentile score of entry point biomarkers, thus adopting an internal comparison method.

The cohort study of the infamous atomic bombing in Hiroshima and Nagasaki followed a fixed cohort of exposed population prospectively over years to determine the effect of radiation on health and the result was compared with the unexposed population by adopting an external comparison policy and with population having different levels of exposure by adopting an internal comparison method.

Strengths and limitation of prospective cohort studies: Most idealistic study design amongst all cohort studies is the prospective one. But it is not without flaws. Like any other design, it has its own inheriting strengths and limitations. The ascertainment of exposure criteria, collection of base data in the form of baseline information and biological and other samples, selection and follow-up of study subjects and data recording in accordance with study objectives are its strong point. They help in establishing causal association of events of interest by study of temporality of events occurrence, dose response nature of exposures and outcomes and minimizing bias. The major limitations are the long duration of follow-up, cost and losses to follow-ups (Table 10.4).

Retrospective Cohort (synonymsóhistorical cohort, non-concurrent prospective study, database research)

Retrospective cohort once considered as the second option or junior sibling in cohort design to prospective cohort is gaining popularity in recent years. This study was traditionally used to ascertain exposure and outcome relationship for suspected industrial exposures after its occurrence, thereby lending support to the risk hypothesis. Thus, all relevant events, i.e. cause and effects have already occurred when the study is initiated.

For example, a hypothetical retro-cohorts design begun in 2010 to study the outcomes of lipid lowering medication on recent MI survivors from the city of Mumbai. Here

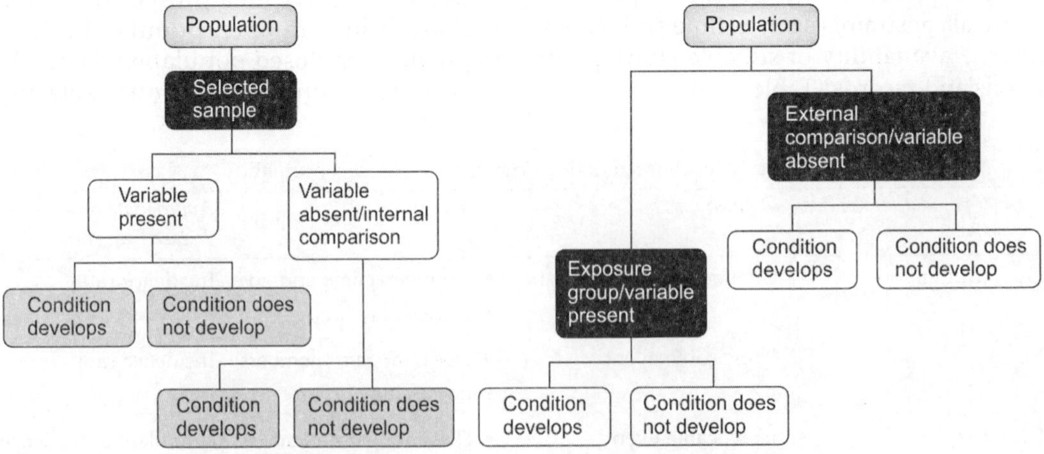

Fig. 10.9: Flow diagrams of cohort with internal and external comparison

Table 10.4: Strengths and limitation of prospective cohort studies

Strengths	*Limitations*
• Can establish time order	• Loss to follow-up
• Can obtain incidence rate	• Misclassification of disease or exposure status
• Can study more than one disease or outcome	• In case of large numbers of subjects or long follow-up it leads to more cost or logistic challenges
• Minimizes bias in ascertainment of exposure status	• Hard to study rare diseases
• Efficient for rare exposure	• Changes over time in staffs or methods
• No control, so no bias in control selection	

exposure group was selected from medical records and included those who received lipid lowering medication, and the comparison group comprised individuals who didn't receive it immediately after the event (MI). These groups were assembled over 2001 to 2006. The outcomes in their immediate 6-month time period following acute MI was recorded from medical records and data analyzed.

Conventionally, in a retro-cohort study (Fig. 10.10) exposure and comparison groups are assembled from records like employment register as it once existed in past and the select subjects followed-up from that time till date for the occurrence of an event or outcome of interest. The follow-up is done by collecting information from data sources like, treatment records, death certificates, information from surviving persons regarding the event of interest or information from other reliable sources. The key to success depends on three factors. First one is to have access to appropriate historical records or documents that will allow the investigators to identify the subjects and their exposure status. Secondly, a valid outcome assessment will require access to documents like death certificates, disease registries, and medical records. Third and the last but no way the least one is about

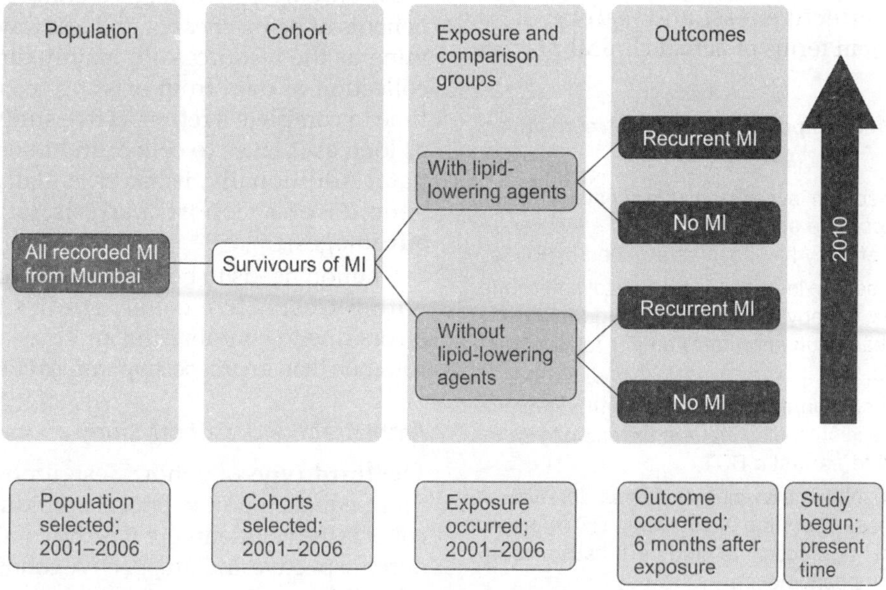

Fig. 10.10: Retro-cohorts design

blinding the investigators to outcomes till the group assignment is complete. In fact, it is not legitimate for the investigators to search the data base for the outcomes until they have completed the assignment process; even though these outcomes have already occurred by the time the investigation is begun as is the case in retrospective cohort studies.

Over-dependency of the study design on medical and other data base has sown the seed for its most recent synonyms 'database research'. In recent years application of computer and medical software in healthcare delivery has transformed medical research. This has made available quality medical records on ongoing medical care and other health-related issues. The recent retro-cohort studies are increasingly using this information to study the outcome of therapies, their effectiveness and safety. Thus, they can often complement the information that can be obtained from randomized control trials (RCTs). Therefore, information from RCTs and information based on collection of data in course of clinical practice can be used together to provide a future picture that cannot be obtained from either one alone. Hence, on present day scenario retrospective cohort studies are providing important information on the effectiveness and safety of the treatment in terms of actual clinical practice.

Box 10.3: Important uses of retrospective cohort studies

1. Are useful in investigating the impact of therapy in a practice setting to establish effectiveness after efficacy has been established by RCTs.
2. Are useful in investigating issues of safety after a new therapy has been approved for clinical use based on short term and/or relative short RCTs.
3. Are useful in investigating potential improvements in outcomes that are expected to be too small to warrant a RCT.
4. Are useful in providing evidences for 'altering the case alters the effect' when RCTs are not ethical or practical to study this causal contributory phenomenon.

Prospective versus Retrospective Cohort Study

It is important to understand that the methodology of prospective and retrospective cohort studies is fundamentally the same. In both instances exposure and comparison groups are established and then they are followed over in time. But the major differences lie in timing of events, collection of data, costs involved and validity of results. In case of a retrospective cohort study, the investigator basically collects data from past records and does not follow patients up as is the case with a prospective study. Based on available recorded information two groups are established as exposed versus non-exposed and these groups are followed up in the ensuing time period. So, in retrospective cohort study all the events like exposure, latent period, and subsequent development of disease or outcome have already occurred in the past. We merely collect the data now and try to establish the risk of disease development in the event of established exposure. On the other hand, prospective cohort study is conducted by starting with two groups at the current point, and following them up in future for occurrence of disease or event of interest.

Obviously retrospective cohort has the benefits of being cheaper and less time consuming as the resources are mainly directed at collection of data from existing records and time to complete a retrospective study is only as long as it takes to collect and interpret the data. Additionally, it has essentially all the benefits of a cohort analysis (statistical advantages).

Caution needs to be exercised in particular with retrospective cohort studies because errors due to confounding and bias are more common than in prospective studies (Table 10.5).

Ambidirectional Cohort Study

The **third type** of cohort design possible in time sequencing of events is ambidirectional cohort study. Essentially it is the combination of retrospective and prospective cohort design adopted to study the short-term and long-

Table 10.5: Prospective *vs.* retrospective cohort

Distinguishing parameter	*Prospective cohort*	*Retrospective cohort*
Direction/follow-up	Futuristic	Posthoc
Cost	Costlier	Less costly
Duration	Long	Short
Latency of disease	Ideally short	Long
Loss to follow-up	Common	Uncommon
Availability and quality of data	Good	Was poor, but has improved in recent years due to better record keeping
Confounding and bias	Errors due to confounding and bias are less common	Errors due to confounding and bias are more common
Importance of scientific question	More valid interpretation of data	Validity of interpreted information lower in quality

term effects of an exposure in the same cohort. As the name implies, data collection goes in both directions. Here exposure is recorded from past records as in case of retrospective cohort and groups are followed. The follow-up continues into future to measure the outcomes.

For example, let us hypothesize that assisted reproductive technology may lead to multiple births, birth defects and ovarian cancer. So, the investigator might, therefore, starts with a cohort who has adopted assisted reproductive technology in past and look back through records for multiple births and birth defects. Through, this retrospective component, he can study the short-term effects of exposure, i.e. birth-related outcomes. These women can then be followed up into the future for ovarian cancer occurrence as a prospective cohort.

We mentioned at the start of discussion on study designs that though the designs are discussed under separate heads, in fact, they are not water-tight compartments. An open cohort can be studied prospectively, and ambidirectionally. For example, as mentioned in the hypothetical study of 'assisted reproductive technology may lead to multiple

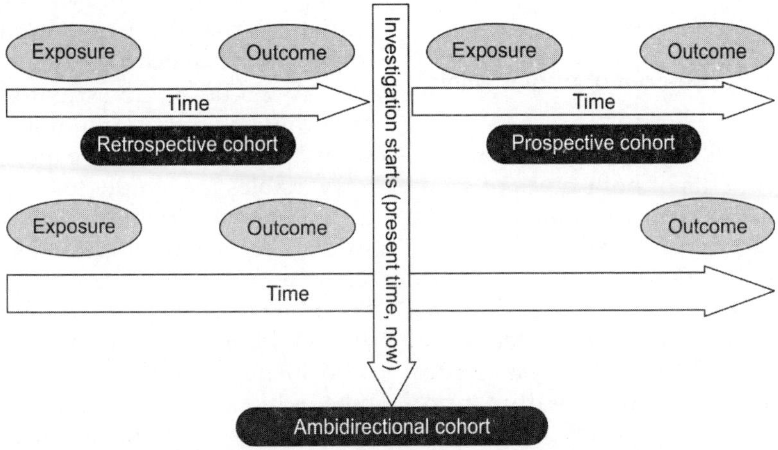

Fig. 10.11: Time sequensing of different cohort study designs

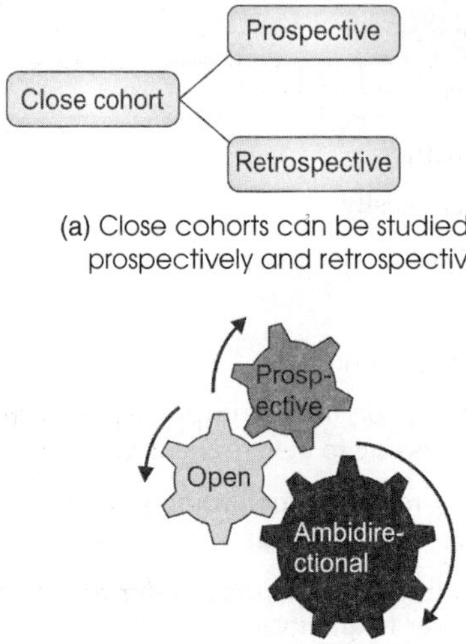

(a) Close cohorts can be studied both prospectively and retrospectively.

(b) A prospective cohort can be open in nature, and studied ambidirectionally. An ambidirectional study can engage open cohort and be forward looking.

Figs 10.12: Diagrams explaining interplay of different cohort study designs

births, birth defects and ovarian cancer' above. Birth defects can be studied by retro-cohort design and cancer incidences by prospective continuation of the same study in future. Similarly a closed cohort can be studied retrospectively and prospectively as was the case for alanine dye industry workers and Hiroshima and Nagasaki nuclear bombing, respectively. A fixed cohort can be studied prospectively as the case is in most non-fatal food poisonings. This concept is presented in Figs 10.12a and b.

Hybrid Designs: Case-control Studies within a Cohort

In recent years lots of thinking has gone into cash-on the benefits of both types of study design possibly by ways of combining at least some elements of them whenever possible. This synthetic end result is called a 'hybrid cohort', where a case-control study is initiated within a cohort study. Here selection of participants is carried out using a case control approach, which takes place within a pre-defined cohort. The case group consists of all or a sample of individuals with the outcome occurring in the defined cohort over a specified follow-up period. The control groups can be selected either from individuals at risk at the time each case occurs or from the baseline cohort. Based on these selection criteria for control, we have two types of hybrid cohorts—one where the controls are selected from at risk population each time a case occurs is called 'nested case control study' and the other where the controls are randomly selected from the baseline cohort for the cases those occurs during the follow-up of the original cohort is called 'case cohort study'.

Nested Case-control Study

Here controls are a random sample of individuals remaining in the cohort at the time each case occurs. This sampling approach is known as 'incidence density sampling' or 'risk set' sampling, where cases are compared with a subset (a sample) of the 'risk set' that is the cohort members who are at risk (that could become a case) at the time when each case occurs. Therefore, a case occurring latter in the follow-up is eligible to be controlled for earlier cases, as a control which is selected early in the study could later develop the disease and can become a case in the course of the same study. By this incidence density sampling technique cases and controls are matched on calendar time and length of follow. This is equivalent of matching cases and controls on duration of follow-up in a standard case control study, thus permitting us to use straightforward statistical analysis like standard multiple regression for matched and survival data.

Why would an investigator carve out a case-control study in the midst of a cohort study? It is because some exposure or predictor variables are simply too expensive to be determine on everyone in a concurrent cohort study. Let us assume a sophisticated blood test as a prototype. A clever way to skirt the financial obstacle is to do a cohort study that will yield sufficient number of cases. All participants entering the cohort study have a tube of blood drawn at enrolment; serum is frozen and stored until the study's conclusion. All those in the cohort study who develop the outcome of interest now become the cases for the nested study. The investigator then chooses a random sample from all participants who did not develop the outcome (controls). Next, the blood test is done on serum from only the cases and selected controls, not the whole group of exposed and unexposed study population. In this way, the laboratory cost is minimised while assuring that the exposure, i.e. a positive laboratory test, was present before development of the outcome.

For example, a nested case-control study examined the potential relation between body concentrations of organochlorines and non-Hodgkin's lymphoma. The blood samples were obtained on entry to a large cohort study started in Maryland, USA, in 1974. Blood samples were eventually analysed for only 74 individuals with lymphoma and 147 controls.[10] Thus, instead of measuring organochlorine concentrations of the entire cohort of 25,802, the investigators incurred this laboratory expense for less than 1% of the cohort. In view of the increased availability of banked blood specimens around the world, this type of research design is getting popular.

Controls are selected at each time a case occurs—(incidence density sampling) from at risk groups (Fig. 10.13).

Case-cohort Studies

Here controls are selected as a random sample of the total cohort at base line for cases as they occur during the follow-up of the cohort under study. This chosen subset of study cohort is called a 'sub-cohort'. Some cases that develop during the follow-up might also be a part of the control group of sub-cohort.

The added advantages of case cohort design over nested case control design is that one sample of baseline cohort (sub-cohort) can serve as control group for different sets of cases (or diseases) occurring in the same cohort. Whereas nested case control design needs separate control groups for each disease type or set of cases or outcome variables.

For example, in arthrosclerosis risk in community (ARIC) cohort studies by Dekker *et al.* a cohort of 15,800 men and women aged 45–64 years were assembled over 1986–1989 and followed-up prospectively for 6 years to study heart rate variability as a risk factor for the outcomes.[11] This cohort reported 443 deaths from all cause, 140 deaths from CV risk, 173 cancer deaths, and 345 incident coronary heart diseases (CHD). As a comparison group for all four case groups, 900 baseline cohort participants were identified and heart rate variability measured in ECG records for 900 controls and all the four case groups. A nested case control design would have asked for a separate control for each group of cases, i.e. four control groups in case of one.

If the same study was designed for a prospective cohort analysis then elaborate and time consuming coding of ECG for all

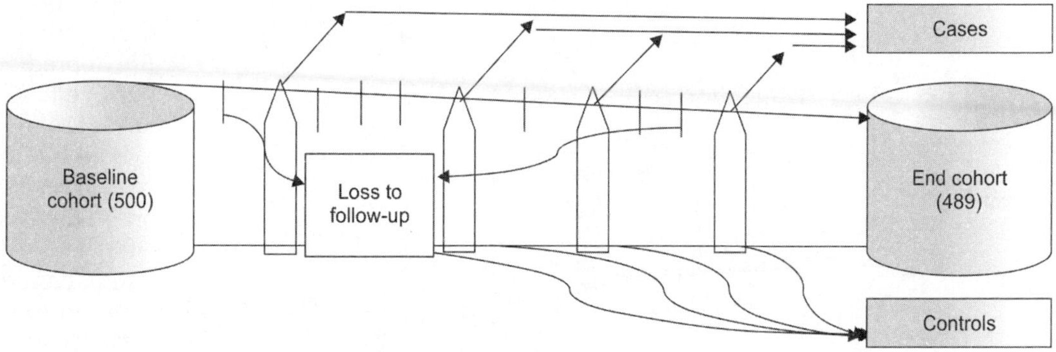

Fig. 10.13: Nested case control study

cohort participants (15,800) should have been done in place of only 900 controls and four groups of cases.

Another practical advantage of case cohort design is that the baseline control sample is the representative of source population. Thus, risk factors distribution and prevalence rates needed for population attributable risk estimation can be obtained.

Controls are selected from baseline cohort for the number of cases (Fig. 10.14).

Advantages of hybrid designs:

1. These are fundamentally efficient when additional information that was not obtained or measured for the whole cohort is needed. For example, in a concurrent cohort study serum samples were obtained at recruitment stage from study participants and stored in freezer. After a sufficient number of cases have occurred during follow-up the frozen samples of cases and controls can be analyzed. This reduces the cost and preserves samples for future use.
2. These types of studies eliminate recall bias as data are collected before the development of any disease. For example, data like interview, blood samples, etc. are collected at the beginning of study at baseline.
3. If abnormalities in biological values are found, it is more likely that these findings represent risk factors or other pre-morbid conditions than the manifestation of early subclinical diseases because the specimens were collected years before the development of clinical diseases or event outcome. When such abnormalities are found in traditional case control studies we do not know whether they preceded the disease or were a result of the disease.
4. Such studies are often more economical to conduct.
5. Finally in both nested case control and case cohort studies cases and controls are derived from the same original cohort. So, there is likely to be greater comparability between the cases and the controls than one might ordinarily find in traditional case control study.
6. Here, we also have advantages of methodological soundness of cohort design like restricting detection bias and the efficiency of the case-control approach.

These designs have received considerable attention in recent years. The availability of increasing numbers of well designed and established large prospective cohort studies and newer methodological and analytical advances are set to borden their scope further.

Analysis of Cohort Studies

This is the final frontier in cohort study. All the hard work encored in cohort study will be futile if the collected data doesn't fulfil 'research order'. By research order, it is meant that the source of data, follow-up of subjects, recording of events and analysis of information are done as per the demand of cohort research protocol. Let us take these issues one by one in that sequence.

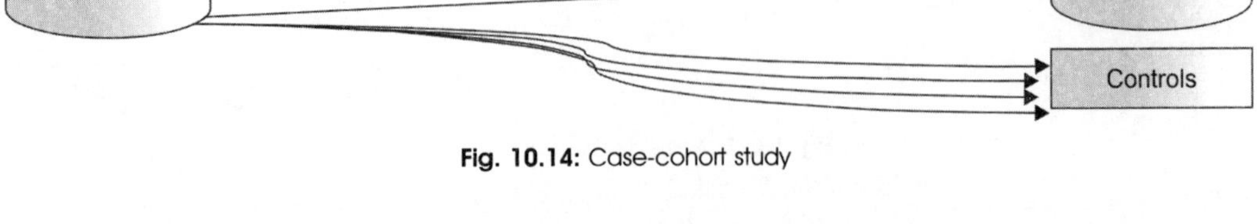

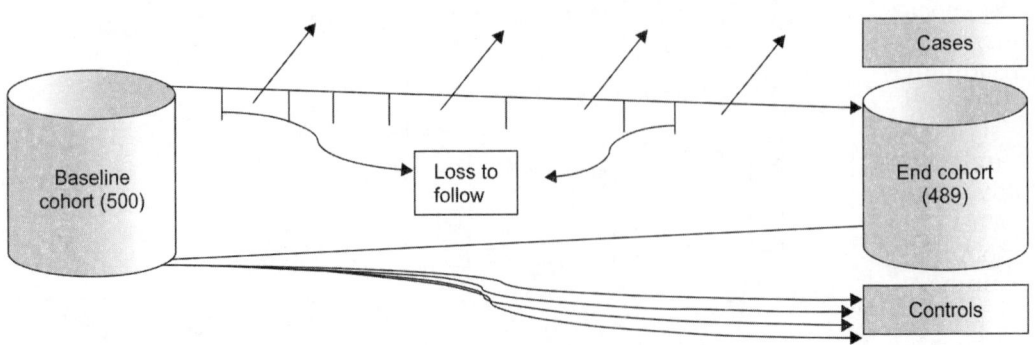

Fig. 10.14: Case-cohort study

Sources of Data

The success of cohort study depends on information on exposures, outcomes, and other key variables. These information are usually provided by medical and employment records, interviews, direct physical examinations, laboratory tests, biological specimens, and environmental monitoring.[12] Some of these sources are pre-existing, and others are designed specifically for the study purpose. Because each type of source has advantages and disadvantages, investigators often use several sources to piece together all of the necessary information thereby improving data quality.

Healthcare records are used to describe a participant's exposure history in studies of possible adverse health effects stemming from medical procedures. The advantages of these records include low expense and a high level of accuracy and details regarding a disease and its treatment. Their main disadvantage is that information on many other key characteristics, apart from basic demographic characteristics is often missing.

Employment records are used to identify individuals for studies of occupational exposures. Typical employment record data includes job title, department of work, years of employment, and basic demographic characteristics. Like medical records, they usually lack details on exposures and other important variables.

Because existing records such as healthcare and employment records often have limitations, many studies are based on data collected specifically for the investigation. These include interviews, physical examinations, and laboratory tests. Interviews and self-administered questionnaires are particularly useful for obtaining information on lifestyle characteristics such as use of cigarettes or alcohol, which are not consistently found in records.

Whatever the source of information, it is important to use comparable procedures for obtaining information on the exposed and unexposed groups. Biased results may occur if different sources and procedures are used. Thus, all resources used for one group must be used for the other. In addition, it is a good idea to mask investigators to the exposure status of a subject so that they make unbiased decisions when assessing the outcomes. Standard outcome definitions are also recommended to guarantee both accuracy and comparability.

Follow-up of Subjects and Recording of Events

Success of medical research is heavily dependent on completeness of recorded information. This includes following up selected participants till the completion of study and obtaining the required data from them or their records as the case may be. If there occurs loss of study subjects or incomplete recording of events of interest then the study results will be biased.

'Loss to Follow-up' in Cohort Design

In all cohort design like prospective, retrospective or ambidirectional, the ascertainment of outcome involves tracing or following all study participants from the point of exposure to the future, in order to determine whether they develop the disease of interest or not. Failure to obtain such informations on every subject, or for that matter on a greater proportion of individuals in either the exposed and non-exposed groups, can be a major source of bias that could render the results of a cohort study uninterpretable. If this happens before defining the cohort as in retrospective cohorts, the results may be internally valid, but their general applicability will be compromised. On the other hand if this loss occurs after defining the cohort as the case is in prospective cohort studies, the validity of study is affected (Fig. 10.15).

Loss before Defining Cohort

On many occasions, it may not be possible to realize the health effects of a particular exposure until many years have lapsed. This may be due to unavailability of facilities to detect the outcome at warranted time or very long latency of the disease condition. In such a scenario which is no way less commonly encounter, the ideal study option is retro-

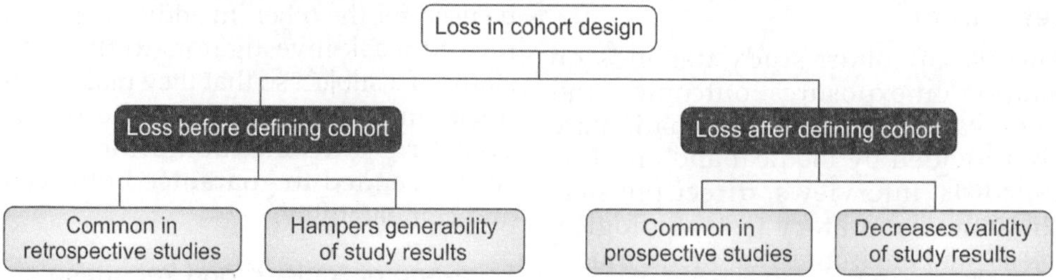

Fig. 10.15: Types of 'loss to follow-up' in cohort studies and their interpretations

spective cohort analysis. But collection of information on exposed group may be severely limited due to unavailability of valid records or late ascertainment of outcome. For example, Wada *et al.* conducted a cohort study in 1965 for respiratory cancer deaths among former employees of mustard gas factory workers which were in operation from 1929 to 1945.[13] With great difficulty a list of 2620 employees was assembled from the total 5000. So, we had a loss close to 50% before starting the study. Again causes of death could not be ascertained before 1952, thereby restricting the observation period from 1952 to 1976. Thus, they missed out those deaths which occurred before 1952, thereby leading to losses of those cases. Ultimately, this study only included a portion of exposed person.

Non-participation in Cohort Study

Another way of recording losses prior to defining cohorts is by way of non-participation. Out of the eligible candidates, only a select few participates in the study with vigour and commitment. Virtually, in every cohort study only a proportion of those, who are eligible to participate actually agree to do so. For example, in the Framingham heart study, 4469 (69%) out of 6507 eligible persons actually underwent the first examination.

Those who agree to participate may differ in a number of ways from non-participants. Non-participants are more likely to have lesser motivation, poorer attitude towards health and diseases and harbour more amounts of risks.[14]

Thus, losses occurring before the definition of cohort may limit generalibility of the study result. Negative findings would not exclude the possibility that excess illness occurred prior to the definition of the cohort or among persons not included in the cohort. However, such losses do not affect the validity of the findings in the cohort itself.

Loss after Defining Cohort

Here loss to follow-up occurs either when the participant no longer wishes to take part or when he or she cannot be located. Minimizing these losses are crucial for two reasons. First, losses to follow-up effectively decrease the sample size and reduce the ability of the study to detect an association. Second, those who are lost to follow-up may differ in important ways from those, who are successfully traced. Of particular concern is that lost individuals are more likely to have developed the disease under study. If lost individuals are more or less likely to be from the exposed group than those who are successfully traced, the study results may suffer from a form of bias known as 'information bias'. These types of loss are commonly encountered in prospective studies and decreases validity of study results.

Retention Strategy

Before looking into the modalities involved in preventing losses to follow-up, it will be prudent to analyze important issues that leads to this event. First and foremost in the list is the length of required period of follow-up, or the interval that elapses between definition of exposure status and ascertainment of outcome. Outcomes that have a short latency period measuring unto days or weeks, as in cases of acute illnesses like food poisoning, or measuring up to months, as in cases of congenital malformations or spontaneous abortions, require far shorter periods of observations than chronic diseases with latency period lasting many years or even decades, such as cancer or coronary heart diseases. In general, the longer the observation period, the more difficult it will be to achieve complete follow-up. Because people are more like to move, change job, change their names, or lose touch with the study organization.

The next in line are 'issues of the subjects'. If the subjects are ill motivated, moribund due to elements other than condition in study, and less committed then they may add on to the list of 'increased loss to follow-up'. Lack of study feedback to the participants may be another hinderent.

The last one is 'issues of investigators'. An unsympathetic investigator can turn the participants away. Investigators unwilling to share the study progress with the participants can compound the problem further.

A loss to follow-up in excess to 10% of study population can severely jeopardize its result thus making high retention critical to the success of a cohort study, investigators have developed many methods to maximize retention and trace study participants. For prospective cohort studies, strategies include collection of information such as full name, social security number, and date of birth that help locate participants as the study progresses. In addition, regular contact is recommended for participants in prospective studies. These contacts might involve requests for up-to-date outcome information or news letters describing the study's progress and findings.[15] The best strategy to use when participants do not initially respond is to send additional mailings.

When participants are truly lost to follow-up, investigators employ a number of strategies. These include sending letters to the last known address with 'address correction requested'; checking telephone directories, directory assistance, newly available internet resources, vital statistics records, driver's license rosters, voter registration records; and contacting relatives, friends, and physicians identified at baseline.

So, it is seen that people are more likely to continue active participation in longitudinal studies when they believe that the research is important, and that they are making a valuable contribution, are receiving regular feedback, and are treated with courtesy and respect by researchers. Observational human exposure studies sometimes involve substantial burdens of time and effort. Over long periods, this level of burden can reduce retention. It may be necessary to develop novel methods that reduce participant time and effort or to focus the study design so that fewer study procedures are implemented at any time point. Because the time needed to analyze samples, verify results, and perform data analyses can be long, it may be difficult to provide timely feedback to participants in observational human exposure studies. Researchers might consider including simple measures that can provide immediate and useful information of value to participants to encourage continued participation. Effective use of these strategies will reduce the need for higher cost and encourage retention.

Censoring

Two inherent design drawbacks of cohort studies are the unusual length of follow-up especially in concurrent or prospective study and the population dynamics of the study participants. So holding on to the group participants till the logical study end points is not achievable for all. Participants may leave the study for reasons unrelated to its outcome. This can be due to death from causes outside the study exposure, end of follow-up arising from migration or switching of job, termination of follow-up by the investigators due to exhaustion of funding, disenrollment from health plan, dropout, etc. When such an event occurs it becomes necessary to put a stop to the contribution made by such participants to the study or else the results will be fallacious. So, censoring in cohort study means putting an end to follow-up of study participants who discontinue the study before the occurrence of its final outcome. It is also known as incomplete observation of event of interest. Depending on the nature of dropout, we have

Table 10.6: Minimizing loss to follow-up[15] (designing clinical research by Stephen B Halley)

During enrolment

(A) Exclude those

- Who are likely to be lost
- Planning to move
- Uncertainty about willingness to return
- Suffering from ill health or fatal diseases unrelated to research question

(B) Obtain information to allow future tracking

- Address, telephone numbers, e-mail
- Social security/health numbers
- Name, address, telephone numbers, e mail of one or two close friends or relatives who do not live with the subject
- Name, address, telephone numbers, e mail of physicians

During follow-ups—periodic contact with subject to collect information, provide results, express care, etc.

- By telephone at weekends and evening hours
- Request forwarding address from postal services
- Seek address through other public sources, i.e. telephone directory, national health services, etc.
- For fellows covered by Medicare collect data about hospital discharge
- Determine vital status from state health department

At all time

- Treat study subjects with appreciation, kindness and respect.
- Helping them to understand the research question, so they will want to join as partner in making the study successful.

Source: Stephen B Hulley, Steven R Cummings, Warren S Browner, MPH, Deborah G Grad, Thomas B Newman. Designing Clinical Research (4th edn): ISBN-10:1608318044; ISBN-13:9781608318049. Publisher: LWW

different types of censoring. They are administrative censoring, censoring due to loss to follow-up, and right censoring.

Administrative censoring means the follow up of study participants is ended by the investigator either due to exhaustion of fund or end of the stipulated duration. These persons who are at risk but didn't develop the study outcome may develop it at a later date. ***Censoring due to loos to follow-up*** is the most common prototype. Here a person who is not contributing to the study anymore is censored. The reasons for his discontinuation is mostly personal like, death from causes outside the study exposure, end of follow-up arising from migration or switching of job, disenrollment from health plan, dropout, etc. this type of censoring is also called ***right censoring.***

Once the person becomes untraceable he or she is removed from the study and the number of time (years) they stayed in the study before dropping out is only considered in calculating the person time or person years, the most common denominator employed in cohort analysis.

Concept of Time in Cohort Analysis

Cohort study is the only observational analytical study where participants are followed over time to observe the occurrence of events of interest. This nature puts cohort much ahead of other descriptive studies. The timing of events during the follow-up period helps in establishing causality. So, it is important to understand the concept of time in relation to cohort studies.

Calendar Time

Recording of events in the study population as and when they occur is called calendar time of events. All observations in cohort studies are recorded in calendar time at data collection stage. Thereafter, they are suitably compiled to estimate person time and survival time for data exploration and evidence synthesis.

Person Time

An inherent drawback of cohort studies is loss to follow-up especially in open and fixed cohorts. Here, retaining all participating individuals for a long period of time in the ambit of study period is difficult. Nevertheless, the contributions made by the subjects for whatever period they stayed under observation can not be sidelined. The investigators have to consider all possible contributions lend by the participants in order to strengthen the data pool. So, the participants are followed up to the censoring point and the total time period the cohort population stayed under observation is calculated as person time. Thus, this measurement combines both the number of persons and time (days, months, years, etc.), over which they were observed. For example, the number of person year for two people each of whom is observed for 5 years is 10 person years, so also is the result for 10 people each of whom is observed for 1 year, i.e. 10 person years. The number of person years can be added together and then the number of events calculated per number of person years observed. For example a useful way of expressing mortality is in terms of numbers of death divided by the person years over which a group is observed.

Person-time calculation is most useful in identifying exposures and their different outcomes in terms of absolute numbers. It describes heterogeneities in the incidence of the disease where the individuals in the groups have certain fixed characteristics like age between 50–60 years, smoking 1–2 packs of cigarettes or having a particular genetic mutation, etc. It is also used for evaluating exposures for chronic diseases and conditions for which the point of origin of exposure is considered unimportant.

Survival Time

Its use started in survival analysis literature, where the study end point was referred as 'death' and the length of follow-up for a given object as the 'survival time'. Thus, when we speak of a subject surviving to the end of the study we mean that, for this individual, the end point of interest did not occur or the person survived the exposure. This old terminology is retained to present day irrespective of whether the study has a mortality end point or not.

The nature of cohort study provides the temporal structure necessary to associate a particular exposure with a subsequent event of interest. Documentation of time sequences of exposures and events generates data upon which the course of event development can be modelled. Such data provides flexibility to define the study outcomes according to the amount of time elapsed between exposure and event. The time at which the exposure first occurred placing the individual at risk for event development is called the origin. The use of time to event outcome requires that variable be anchored at the origin, resulting in the characterization of the event incidence across the time since origin. Thus, the incidence of events from 5 to 7 years past origin will be handled differently in data analysis from 9 to 11 years even though both time periods record equal spans, i.e. 2 person years. Here the calendar time observations are shifted to a common starting point to facilitate data analysis. The total duration of observation as observed in calendar time stays unaltered.

For example, in Fig. 10.16a, an open cohort study is presented which involves 8 subjects who are designed to be followed up for a maximum observation period of 8 years.[16] They are divided into two groups based on their exposure status. The first four enrolments belong to exposure group and the last four to comparison group. The horizontal axis represents calendar time. The line of each subject, which is referred as follow-up line stretches between the calendar time points that the individual was under observation. A solid dot indicates that the subject died, and a circle means that the subject is censored. So subject one entered after 6 months of recruitment was followed for 5 years and exited the study by virtue of his death at 5 and ½ years. Subject two entered after 3 years and 2 months from the beginning of recruitment but

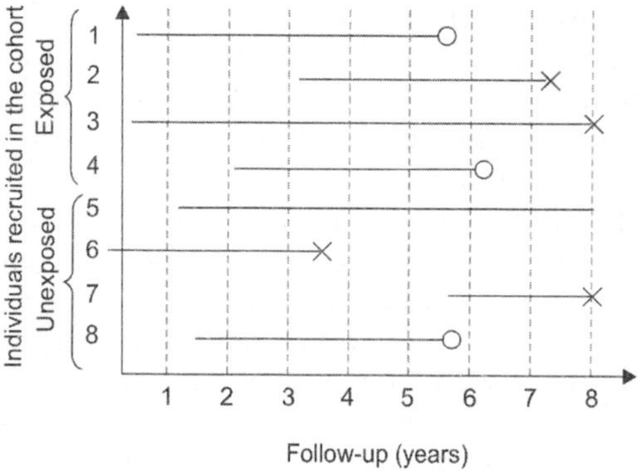

Fig. 10.16a: Calendar time

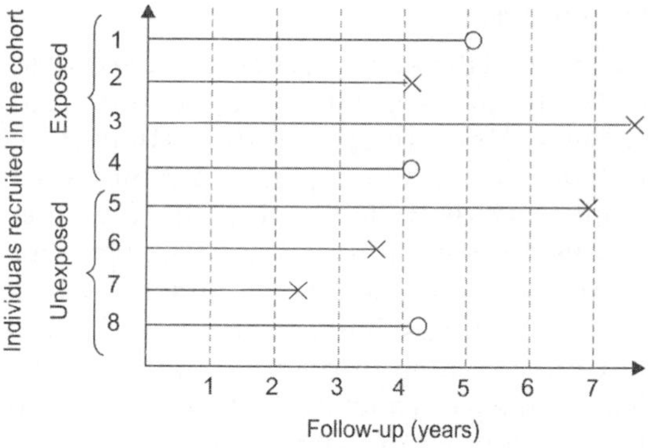

Fig. 10.16b: Survival time

* Example of calendar time in open cohort study (timing of occurrence of events is recorded as and when they occurred).
* Example of survival time (the timing of event is shifted to a common point for easy interpretation and analysis).
* As persons were followed-up over different time periods ranging from years to months and days, then the ideal denominator that can be drafted out of these types of observation is 'person time', i.e. the actual time the person was in study either in exposure or comparison group.

dropped out after 4 years of follow-up. Subject 3 was enrolled at the 6-month point, was followed till the end and exited the study alive. Subject 4 entered the study after 2 years of recruitment, and died out of the event of interest after 4 years. Similarly, in the comparison group; subject 5 entered the study after 1 year and made an exist at the stipulated end point alive. Subject 6 was enrolled at the starting of the study and died after 3½ years. Subject 7 entered the study after 5½ years and completed the study without experiencing the outcome. The last subject entered the study after 1½ year and met the outcome after 4 years of follow-up.

In Fig. 10.16b, the same cohort is represented to highlight the concept of survival time. Here, all follow-up lines are given the same starting point. Note that now the horizontal axis is levelled as survival time.

The difference between person time and survival time is mentioned in Table 10.7.

Table 10.7: Difference between person time and survival time[16]

Person time	*Survival time/time to event*
Based on person year (time) calculation	Based on survival time calculation
Measures strength of association	Measures temporality of association
Estimates absolute risk or incidence density	Estimates relative risk or relative hazard/relative time
Origin of event ill-defined	Origin of event well defined
Primary objective is to identify the exposures	Primary objective is to study dose response effect of exposure
Useful for analysis of trend and change in incidence of disease over calendar time by Poisson regression methods	Quantify how the hazard is modified by the exposure and estimates to what extent exposures shortens or extends disease-free time
Measures whether exposure results in outcome or not.	Observes whether the observed outcome differs in any way over the observed time.

Concept of Risk and Risk Estimations

Measurement of association and causality between exposure and outcome is done by estimation of any, some or all of these. They are risk, rates and odds which are used in one or other form for evaluation of occurrence of events in studied cohort population.

Risk in its simplest form represents finding out the Proportion of people who develop the disease over a specified period of time or it is the average probability that an event (disease) will occur given a particular exposure. It is calculated as

Risk = Number of sick people/total population

For example, if 1000 people are observed for 5 years and 42 out of them became sick whereas 958 stayed healthy, then risk = 42/1000 = 0.042. It can also be expressed in percentage.

Rates are another measure of occurrence of event. The common one employed in cohort studies is estimation of incidence rate. Here rate means proportion of people who develop the disease (event) during the total amount of observation time.

Rate = Number of sick people/total amount of time people are observed (total time at risk)

For example, in estimating the incidence of type 1 diabetes mellitus (T1DM) in Norwegian children 1,382,602 children were observed for 15 years out of which 1,382,547 never became sick, 55 developed type 1 diabetes and the total observation period for all was estimated to 8,184,994 person-years. Hence the rate of T1DM in Norwegian children was found out to be; rate (incidence) = 55/8 184 994 = 0.067 per 1000 person-years.[17]

Odds estimation is the third parameter of event measurement. This can be estimation of odds ratio as commonly done for case-control study or relative risk as in cohort studies. Thus, event (disease) odds is calculated as

Odds = Probability of disease/probability of not disease = Probability of disease/1 – probability of disease = risk/1 – risk.

Let us built our further discussion on these basic understanding. As mentioned previously persons are said to be at risk, if they do not have the disease of interest, but are capable of developing the disease within a specified time frame. Hence, risk means the probability of occurrence of an event in an individual within a pre-stipulated time period. For example, if an individual manifests illness or succumb to an event, or recovers from one within a prefixed time period, then he is referred to be at risk to the event or factor. This factor in question is known as risk factor. So a risk factor is an exposure which can be harmful or protective. The amount of the effect of risk associated with risk factors is estimated by risk estimation. Risk estimation of an event is of paramount importance in public health. The estimated risk in both exposed and comparison population becomes the basis for prediction of outcome measures directed at risk elimination.

For example, lung cancer is caused by exposure to smoking, asbestos, radiation or some chemical products; a classic example of multiple exposure. In this scenario, an individual, a physician or a public health policy maker would like to know that; if smoking is eliminated, what would happen to the incidence of lung cancer? Would smokers' risk of lung cancer disappear, if they stopped smoking? If not, then what amount of risk could be reduced by implementing such a major? These questions can also be asked in relation to other factors mentioned above. Especially for public health decision-making purposes, it is valuable to be able to answer these questions. Public health experts would like to know not only the impact of elimination of exposure on those who are exposed, but also the impact of elimination of exposure on the entire population, i.e. both exposed and unexposed. It helps them answer the following questions.

1. What amount of the risk of developing a disease is attributable to a particular exposure?

2. By what percent would the risk of developing disease be reduced if the exposure were eliminated?

The answer to these questions lies in estimation of different rates and ratio like incidence rate, relative risks, attributable risks, etc.

Incidence rate (synonyms—incidence density, hazard rate, and mortality rate)— though unit risk and incidence rates are considered interchangeable, but strictly speaking, risk denotes the rate of new cases in a fixed interval of time, whereas incidence rate (or incidence) denotes the rate of new cases per unit time. It is a measure of disease frequency that assesses the force of morbidity, or the probability of developing a disease in a given period of time. This is the most precise estimate of the impact of exposure in a population. It is calculated by dividing the number of new cases during the given period (usually 1 year) by total person time of observation over the same period.

$$\text{Incidence rate} = \left\{ \begin{array}{l} \text{New cases of disease/total} \\ \text{person time of observation} \end{array} \right.$$

The denominator presents the sum of each individual's time at risk or the sum of the time that each person remained under observation and free from the disease of interest. This allows the researcher to account for those who dropped out of the study and no longer contribute to person-year calculation.

Advantages of incidence rates: It denotes average rate at which disease develops in a population. It calculates the actual rate of event occurrence with units of time. There is no need of a closed population as it accounts for differing rates of follow-up.

Cumulative incidence: This differs from incidence rate calculation with respect to the denominator. Instead of person time the denominator considers only numbers of persons at risk. So, logically this calculation is applicable for closed cohort where losses to follow-up do not occur.

$$\begin{array}{l}\text{Cumulative} \\ \text{incidence}\end{array} = \left\{ \begin{array}{l} \text{No. of new cases of disease} \\ \text{during a period of time/No.} \\ \text{persons at risk of developing the} \\ \text{disease during same time period} \end{array} \right.$$

This also measures the probability of event occurrence and estimates risk like incidence rate but for a closed population.

Estimation of Risk

Conventionally, in a cohort study persons are followed up from the point of exposure till the occurrence of outcome of interest. The association of risk factor or exposure with the event of interest and prediction of outcome modifications that can be achieved by controlling the exposure in question are measured by different risk estimates. These are—absolute risk, relative risk, and attributable risk.

Absolute Risk (AR)

It is the estimation of the probability that an individual will experience the specified outcome during a specified period. It lies in the range 0 to 1, or is expressed as a percentage.

Absolute Risk Increase (ARI)

It is the absolute difference in risk between the exposed and comparison groups in a cohort. It is used when the risk in the experimental group exceeds the risk in the control group, and is calculated by subtracting the AR in the control group from the AR in the experimental group. This figure does not give any idea of the proportional increase between the two groups—for this, estimation of relative risk is needed.

Absolute Risk Reduction (ARR)

This refers to absolute difference in risk between the exposed and comparison groups in a cohort. It is used when the risk in the comparison group exceeds the risk in the exposed group, and is calculated by subtracting these absolute risks (ARs). This figure also does not give any idea of the proportional reduction between the two groups—for this, relative risk (RR) is needed.

Relative Risk (risk ratio)

The relative risk is a measure of association between a disease or condition and a factor

Table 10.8: Cumulative incidence vs. incidence rate[17]

Parameters	*Cumulative incidence*		*Incidence rate*	
	Follow-up complete	Follow-up incomplete	Individual data	Group data
Numerator	Number of cases	Classical life table	Number of cases	Number of cases
Denominator	Initial population	Kaplan Meier	Person time	Average population
Population	Can be measured only in closed population		Accounts for differing rates of follow-up so do not need closed population	
Units	Proportion with no units (unitless)		Actual rate with units of time (time $^{-1}$)	
Range	0 to 1		0 to infinity	
Estimates	Probability of developing disease		Average rate at which disease develops in a population	
Measures	Measure of risk		Measure of risk	
Synonyms	Proportion probability		Incidence density	

* No time unit whatsoever is attached to cumulative incidence (0–1; probability) which must be always specified like cumulative probability for the initial 3 years of follow-up.

under study. It is calculated by dividing the incidence rate among those exposed to the factor by the incidence rate among those not exposed to the factor. So we define relative risk as the absolute risk in the exposed group divided by the AR in the comparison group or the risk ratio as the ratio of two risks, i.e. between exposed *vs.* unexposed (exposed/unexposed).

From a 2 × 2 table of a cohort study, the relative risk could also be calculated as follows:

	Event develops	*Event does not develop*	*Total*
Exposed	*a*	*b*	*a* + *b*
Non-exposed	*c*	*d*	*c* + *d*
Total	*a* + *c*	*b* + *d*	*a* + *b* + *c* + *d*

Probability of incident in the exposed = *a*/*a* + *b*.
Probability of incident in the unexposed = *c*/*c* + *d*.
The risk ratio (RR) being the ratio of two risks, usually exposed/unexposed = [*a*/*a* + *b*]/[*c*/*c* + *d*].

The RR is a measure of the relationship between the incidence in the exposed and that in the non-exposed. RR = 1 means that the incidence in the exposed is the same as that in the non-exposed, and so there is no association between exposure and disease. RR >1 denotes a larger incidence in the exposed than in the non-exposed, thus exposure to the factor seems to increase the probability of developing the disease. RR <1 denotes a smaller incidence in the exposed as compared to the non-exposed, thus exposure to the factor seems to decrease the probability of developing the disease or is protective in nature.

So we can summarize that RR denotes the number of times more likely (RR >1) or less likely (RR <1) an event is to happen in one group compared with another. It is the ratio of the absolute risk for each group. It is analogous to the odds ratio (OR) when events are rare.

Relative Risk Increase (RRI)

The proportional increase in risk between exposed and comparison groups in a cohort.

Relative Risk Reduction (RRR)

The proportional reduction in risk between exposed and comparison groups in a cohort. It is a complement of the relative risk (1-RR).

Hazard Ratio (HR)

This is broadly equivalent to relative risk. It is useful when the risk is not constant with

Box 10.4: Relative risk (risk ratio)

Actually, this in actuality is estimated as a ratio of disease incidence among exposed to disease incidence among non-exposed. It is interpreted as follows—

- Quantifies magnitude of the association between exposure and disease
- Varies from 0 to infinity
- RR = 1: No association
- RR >1: Exposure is a risk factor for disease; increases risk for disease
- RR <1: Exposure decreases the risk for disease or protective in nature

Example:

- RR = 2.0 can be interpreted as twofold increase in risk
- RR = 0.7 can be interpreted as 30% decrease in risk

respect to time. It uses information collected at different times. The term is typically used in the context of survival over time type of data. If the HR is 0.5 then the relative risk of dying in one group is half the risk of dying in the other group. If HR is recorded in the original paper then we prefer these reports rather than calculating RR, because HRs takes account of more data, where relative risk measure the strength of association, which is a major consideration in deriving causal inferences, it does not answer how much of the disease that occurs can be attributed to a certain exposure? In order to find an answer to this we need to know and calculate attributable risk.

Attributable Risk (synonyms—risk ratio, incidence rate ratio)

The attributable risk is the excess of event due to the exposure to a specific condition. This answers to how much of the disease that occurs can be attributed to a certain exposure. AR is defined as the amount or proportion of disease incidence or risk that can be attributed to a specific exposure. For example, how much of lung cancer risk experienced by smokers can be attributes to smoking? The attributable risk is in many ways more important in clinical practice and public health because it answers the question that how much of disease we can prevent by eliminating exposure? In order to understand this, we must know the background risk, exposure attributable risk and population attributable risk.

Background Risk

The risk of the disease is not zero even in nonexposed population. Every person shares the background risk regardless of whether or not he or she has had the specific exposure in question. If we want to know how much of the total risk in exposed persons is due to the exposure, we should subtract the background risk from the total risk; because the risk in non-exposed person is equal to background risk.

Attributable risk has four measures. They are—exposure attributable risk, exposure attributable risk percent (AR%), population attributable risk and population attributable risk percent (PAR%).

Exposure attributable risk (AR)—it is the portion of the incidence of an event in the exposed population that is due to the exposure. It is the incidence of a disease in the exposed that would be eliminated if exposure were eliminated. The AR is calculated by subtracting the incidence in the unexposed from the incidence in the exposed.

Exposure attributable risk percent (AR%)—it is the percent of the incidence of a disease in the exposed that is due to the exposure. It is the proportion of the incidence of a disease in the exposed that would be eliminated if exposure were eliminated. The AR% is calculated by dividing the attributable risk by the incidence in the exposed and then multiplying the product by 100 to obtain a percentage.

Population attributable risk—the attributable risk for the total population is a valuable concept for the public health personnels. In the smoking and lung cancer study, the question addressed is what proportion of lung cancer in the total population can be attributed to smoking? If smoking were eliminated what proportion of the incidence of lung cancer in the total population (both smokers and non-smokers) would be prevented? This is answered by the population attributable risk. Thus, population attributable risk (PAR) is the portion of the incidence of a disease in the population (exposed and non-exposed) that is due to exposure. It is the incidence of a disease in the population that would be eliminated if exposure were eliminated.

The PAR is calculated by subtracting the incidence in the unexposed from the incidence in total population (exposed and unexposed).

Population attributable risk percent (PAR%) is the percent of the incidence of a disease in the population (exposed and non-exposed) that is due to exposure. It is the percent of the incidence of a disease *in the population* that would be eliminated if exposure were eliminated. The PAR% is calculated by dividing the population attributable risk by the incidence in the total population and then multiplying the product by 100 to obtain a percentage.

As we see attributable risk is a critical concept in virtually any area of public health and clinical practice, particularly in relation to questions regarding potentiality of preventive measures or success of intervention programmes.

Another application of PAR is in relation to holding industries and other public sector organization accountable for health-related responsibilities. One of the legal criteria used in finding a company or organization responsible for an environmental injury is if it has contributed to the injury by a quantum represented by greater than 50% of attributable risk. So, it can be suggested that an attributable risk of greater than 50% might represent a quantitative determinant of the legal definition of 'more like than not' in causing the effect.

Risk difference or difference in risk is also a measure of attributable risk which is calculated by subtracting the risk in unexposed from that of exposed (risk in exposed–risk in unexposed).

Relative Risk vs. Attributable Risk

The size of relative risk is a better index than attributable risk for establishing casual relationship. The more the relative risk the strong are the assumptions. If same exposure has different outcomes (smoking and ca lungs, chronic bronchitis, CV risk) relative risk is a better measure for assessment of causation and strength of association. Once the causality is established then attributable risk is a better predictor of success in intervention than relative risk.

Measures of RR and AR might give different impressions as to the importance of a particular exposure. If several factors those are aetiologically significant in the same disease are compared the same order of importance of the factors will be suggested whether RR or AR is examined. However, when the same exposure is assessed for several different manifestations this may not be the case? Thus, they may speak two different things. A high relative risk does not always mean an equally proportionate high attributable risk. For example, in male British physicians' cohort study for lung cancer and CHD mortality; the relative risk is much higher for lung cancer than CHD and the attributable risk much higher for CHD than lung cancer. This means if an effective smoking elimination program is initiated to eliminate smoking, then more CHD deaths will be prevented than lung cancer deaths. But the casual association of smoking with lung cancer is higher than to CHD as expressed by higher relative risk for lung cancer. Relative risk is valuable in aetiological studies of disease, whereas attributable risk has major application in clinical practice and public health. Relative risk and odds ratio are important as measures of the strength of association, which is an important consideration in deriving a causal inference. The attributable risk is a measure of how much of the disease risk is attributable to a certain exposure. Consequently, the attributable risk is useful in answering the question of how much of disease can be prevented if we have an effective means of eliminating the exposure in question. So the concept of relative risk and attributable risk are essential for understanding causation and the potential for prevention where one measures the strength of causation the other potential for prevention.

Reporting of Analysed Cohort Data

So far we have found out that the primary objective of the analysis of cohort study data is to compare the occurrence of outcomes like symptoms, disease, death and recovery in the exposed and unexposed groups. The occurrence of the outcome is usually measured using cumulative incidence or incidence rates, and the relationship between the exposure and outcome is quantified using absolute or relative difference between the risks or rates. The fundamental measure of disease outcome in a cohort study is the incidence rate. In fact, the type of incidence rate employed in a cohort study will determine the appropriate measure of association. If the cumulative incidence rate is used, the appropriate measure of association will be the relative risk or the risk difference. This is because these measures are calculated from the cumulative incidence rates in the exposed and unexposed groups. Similarly, if the person time incidence rate is used, the measure of association will be the rate ratio or the rate difference. This is because these measures are calculated from the person- time incidence rates in the exposed and unexposed groups. Since the two basic methods of analyzing cohort studies depend on the types of incidence rates used, they are discussed separately in the following two sections.

Reporting Based on Cumulative Incidence Rates

On the most basic level, cohort studies employing cumulative incidence rates can be analyzed using a standard 2 × 2 contingency table. When the results of a cohort study employing cumulative incidence rates are placed in a contingency table, it will be fairly simple to calculate measures of association based on risk. Unlike in case-control studies, in cohort studies cumulative incidence rates can be calculated directly from the data in the contingency table. This is possible because $a/(a + b)$ represents the actual proportion of cases that developed among the exposed group, and $c/(c + d)$ represents the actual proportion of cases that developed among the unexposed group. When multiplied by an appropriate rate base, these are the cumulative incidence rates in the exposed and unexposed groups. Thus, we can use them to calculate relative risk and risk difference. The statistical significance of the measure of association can be calculated using the chi-square test of independence. A 95% confidence interval for the relative risk can also be estimated.

Reporting Based on Time-to-event

For certain outcomes (including mortality), it may be particularly relevant to consider the time until the event occurs, rather than the incidence of the event. To give an absurd example, the incidence of death would be equal in all subgroups of a cohort study after two centuries had elapsed, regardless of any true association between exposure and risk. Even when the outcome is inevitable, refining estimates of risk by considering time to event usually results in increased statistical power compared with analyses that simply evaluate whether the event occurred.[18] Two commonly used approaches for analyzing time-to-event data include Kaplan-Meier analysis (which allows univariate comparison of survival times between groups) and Cox proportional hazards analysis (which allows both univariate and multivariate comparisons).

Survival Analysis (log-rank test; Kaplan-Meier survival curve)

Survival analysis is useful when lengths of follow-up vary substantially or when participants enter a study at different time.[8] The Kaplan-Meier method provides a more sophisticated expression of the risk of the outcome over time than does a simple dichotomous outcome. It can determine the probability of the outcome at any point in time. The log-rank test compares survival curves of different groups.[19]

Proportional Hazard Model (multivariate technique)

Another approach to different lengths of follow-up is the Cox proportional hazard model. It is a multivariate technique that has time-to-event such as illness as the dependent variable.[19] Coefficients from this model can be used to calculate the risk ratio (hazard ratio) of the outcome, after controlling for other covariates in the equation. The hazard ratio with 95% confidence limits is interpreted in the same way as a relative risk for dichotomous outcomes.[20]

In **multiple logistic regression,** we have 'yes–no' as dependant variables in contrast to time to event as is the case with Cox proportional hazard model. This method (logistic regression) yields an adjusted odds ratio that approximates the adjusted relative risk when disease incidence is rare (<10%), while adjusting for potential confounders.[21] It is also used to analyze the results of changes in biomarkers in a cohort study as a substitute to time-to-event analysis.

To sum it up depending on the nature of study design and follow-up of participants the cohort analysis can be based on cumulative incidence analysis, where the timing of event is in terms of absolute persons as the cases are in closed cohort or proportional mortality ratio (PMR). Or it can be based on person time analysis, where the exposure is calculated in terms of total time of exposure in participating persons within a predefined time, i.e. the study duration. These calculations are suited for open cohort, fixed cohort or standardized mortality ratio (SMR) studies.

Proportional mortality ratio (PMR) study—both PMR and SMR studies are a part of occupational epidemiology, where it is difficult to find a truly unexposed population as an internal comparison group.

PMR study design is used specially in industrial or occupational set-ups, where it is hard to find a population devoid of exposure. As internal comparison in terms of unexposed population is not feasible, the researchers look for external comparisons which are drawn from the general population. Death certificates are the source of information in PMR study. We collect data on age, cause of death, date, etc. from this certificate. The observed number of death due to a specific cause in the exposed group is compared with the expected number which is derived from the proportion of death resulting from that cause in the general population. The resulting PMR which is interpreted like a relative risk shows the relative importance of a specific cause of death in relation to all deaths.

For example, let us consider the PMR study involving pulp and paper-mill workers and US population.[22] Here, the study population consisted of members of United Paper Workers International Union who worked for at least 10 years in the industry and died from 1970 to 1984. Information on their year and date of birth, sex and race year of death and cause of death was collected from death certificates. For each cause of death

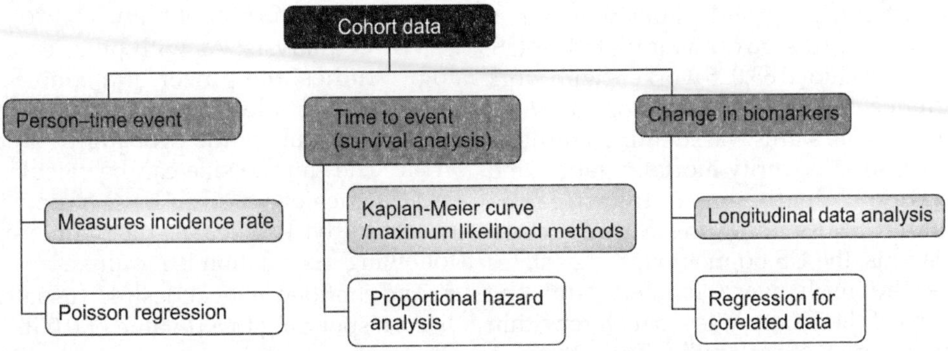

Fig. 10.17: Types of outcome and methods of analysis in cohort studies

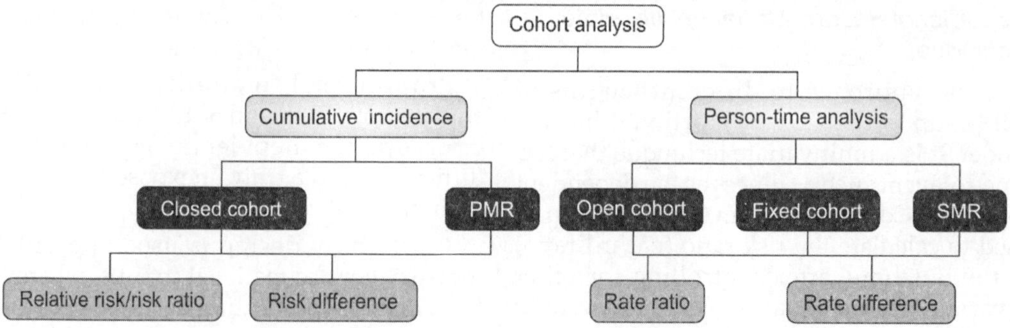

Fig. 10.18: Interpretation of reported information of cohort data

investigators compared the observed number of death to the expected number while controlling for sex, race, and age and calendar year of death from the general population. The study found a 31% increased risk of death from malignant neoplasm particularly cancer of lungs, lymphopoetic system and large intestine. A reduced risk of death was observed for cancer of stomach and pancreas. Death due to atherosclerotic causes did not record any deviation.

Standardized Mortality Ratio (SMR) Study

Here researchers require additional information to compare the mortality experience of the exposed group with that of the general population. It is because SMR compares the mortality rates of two groups whereas PMR compares the mortality proportions. Thus, information on person year of follow-up is needed among the study groups to calculate the expected number of deaths in SMR study.

For example, following reports of several PMR studies demonstrating an increased cancer risk in pulp and paper workers, a nationwide SMR study was initiated in US. This study included 63,025 workers with work experience of over 10 years from 51 mills across US. Vital status was identified through the mills, social security mortality tapes, and the national death index. Investigators calculated SMRs using three comparison populations, the US population, the 20 states where the mills were located, and the residents of the 330 counties that were within a 50 mile radius of each mill.[23] The latter two comparison population were used because their demographic characteristics were similar to those of the workers.

Total 7171 deaths occurred among cohort members by the end of 1991. Person time of follow-up was calculated for cohort members starting within 10 years after first employment and ending with the termination of study or death of participant. SMRs were calculated that adjusted for age, race, time and sex. It was observed that the overall mortality rate in pulp and paper-mill workers was significantly lower than that of the US population (SMR = 0.74) and the workers mortality rate was not elevated for any specific cause including that of malignancies (Table 10.9).

Improving Efficiency of Cohort Studies

Increase efficiency of cohort can be achieved by increasing its precision and validity. Improvement in precision is achieved by addressing issues concerning study size, whereas controlling of bias and confounding improves validity. These points are discussed under the headings of power analysis, effect modification and confounding control.

Power analysis: As with other epidemiologic studies, the power of a cohort study should be considered before it is initiated in order to minimize the probability of type II error. The sample size can be calculated in order to achieve a given level of power in a cohort study. To calculate the sample size the following information is required.[24]

- The confidence level desired (usually 95% corresponding to a p-value of 0.05).
- The level of power desired (usually between 80 and 95%).

Table 10.9: Proportional mortality ratio (PMR) *vs.* standardized mortality ratio (SMR)

PMR	*SMR*
Takes less time and usually retrospective	Lengthy in nature and usually prospective
Costs less money	More costly than PMR
Conducted first to find a risk and its association	Conducted to establish or diffuse the claims made by PMR studies
Suffers from health worker effect though to a lesser extent. Suffers from see-saw effect, i.e. deficit in one cause of death results in corresponding increase in other causes of death (as the total number of death in study population must equal the expected number of death derived from general population)	Suffers from health workers effect to a larger extent
	No see-saw effect
	Can establish causal association

- The ratio of unexposed subjects to exposed subjects.
- The expected frequency of the outcome in the unexposed group (usually estimated from previous research; 50% can be used if there is no estimate available, since it will maximize the sample size required).
- The smallest relative risk one would like to be able to detect, which should be based on practical significance.

It is important to remember that the power of a study decreases as the sample size decreases. Therefore, cohort studies that experience large losses to follow-up or have significant missing data may have markedly less power than that determined at the initiation of the study. In addition, some subgroup analyses may be based on substantially smaller sample sizes and will have significantly less power than that in the overall analysis as is the case with cohort studies based on cumulative incidence rates. Studies based on person time incidence rates should also consider the power of the study and potential confounding and effect modification.

Effect modification: Effect modification in cohort studies can be recognized by examining the stratum-specific relative risks in a manner similar to that for case-control studies. For example, if the relative risk in one stratum does not equal the relative risk in another stratum, and the difference is unlikely due to random variation, then effect modification is probable. This may be due to presence of confounders.

Bias and confounding: An internal valid epidemiological study measures what it is supposed to measure. There are distracters which can mislead or deviate the study results or inferences from 'truth' thereby rendering it unproductive. There are dozens of them, but the major ones are selection bias, information bias and confounders. These are major issues in any epidemiologic study design.

Selection bias: The essential feature of a cohort study is comparison of two groups for disease or exposure frequency. These groups should be the true representative of the population. When the representativeness of the population is compromised by selecting individuals from a particular group instead of general population; then effects estimated among subjects included in the study become different from the estimates obtainable from the targeted population. Thus, selection bias acts as a distracter to effects measured. It can result from procedures used to select subjects. Examples of selection bias are self-selection, health workers effect and diagnostic bias.

Information bias (misclassification): Unlike selection bias which occurs at the time of group selection or prior to it; information bias happens after group allocation at data collection phase. Information bias can occur whenever there are errors in classification of subjects. This can lead to error in collecting needed information from study groups. There are two types of misclassification based on its relationship with different study groups. They are differential and non-differential misclassification.

Differential misclassification occurs when classification errors in one group is independent of other group. For example, in study evaluating emphysema and cigarette smoking, smokers may be evaluated more stringently for emphysema by physicians than non-smokers because of the existing knowledge of their association. This practice may over-estimate emphysema incidence in smokers.[25] Other methods of recording differential misclassification are through recall bias, interviewer bias, non-response bias. Thus, differential misclassification can result in an information bias that exaggerate or underestimate an effect.

In **non-differential misclassification** the disease classification is incorrect for equal proportions of subjects in the compared groups. It is generally considered as a lesser threat to validity in comparison to differential misclassification as the bias introduced by it is always in a predictable direction, i.e. towards a null condition.

Confounding: The simplest description of confounding is mixing of effect. Here the estimate of effect of exposure of interest is distorted because it is mixed with the effect of an extraneous factor. This phenomenon is known as Simpsons' paradox.[26] This distortion introduced by the confounding factor can be large and lead to over-estimation or under-estimation of effect depending on the direction of association that the confounding factor has with the exposure and the disease. An extraneous factor to qualify as a confounder should met set criteria. This factor in question must be a risk factor for the disease, be associated with the exposure under study in the population from which the case are derived and must not be an intermediate step in the causal path between the exposure and the disease. Thus, confounders are some baseline characteristics that can significantly influence the development of the event, but who were not considered as similar parameter for the cohort at the entry stage.

Confounders can be identified by their epidemiological impact like age, differentiation of the tumour, myometrial invasion, etc. They can also be identified at univariate analysis by comparing the outcome in subset of patients presenting the characteristic or not and also in multivariate analysis.

Potential confounding in cohort studies can be controlled in the design stage by restriction or matching or in the analysis stage by stratification or multivariable methods.

Uniqueness of Cohort Design

Cohort studies bridges the gap between observational and experimental research. It imbibes methodological soundness from both categories. The prospective observational component gives it analytical power and natural intervention in the form of exposure factors endows upon the advantages of experimental designs. Thus, cohort studies like most controlled clinical trials can estimate the temporal relationships between exposure and outcomes. In fact, a clinical trial design is a special type of cohort study in which the study subjects are randomly assigned to different experimental groups. The role of randomization in clinical trials is to make the two groups comparable so that the effect of therapy can be determined. The difference between these study designs lies on the weight or validity of the conclusions regarding the potential causal relationships between exposure and disease, which is influenced by the inherent limitation of observational designs in controlling the problem of the potential confounding variables not identified by the investigators.

Advantages and disadvantages cohort studies: From our discussion so far, we are aware that cohort studies are a forte on its own. It has several subtypes with their inherent strengths and limitations. But on top of it cohort study as a unit has several advantages and disadvantages. These are presented in Table 10.10.

Managing Expense in Cohort Study

Follow-up studies are generally large enterprises. Lengthy studies of large population are

Box 10.5: Uniqueness of cohort studies

- Though observational in nature, it is prospective in character like experimental studies.
- It has amphibious character in the evolution of epidemiology and clinical research, i.e. it shares characters both of observational and experimental studies.
- Cohort studies and clinical trials are also called prospective studies in contrast to retrospective studies a term typically utilized for case-control studies.
- It is analytical in nature.
- It also harbours an interventional component. The intervention experienced here is natural intervention; like being a member of a family or intervention by choice like being a member of a particular occupation, or being associated with a particular habit.

expensive. Expenses running into millions of dollars even in excess to $100 millions are not uncommon. Most of the expenses are aimed at maintaining a continuous system for monitoring disease occurrence. Two bright examples are the special exposure group of Japanese exposed to nuclear bombing and the detailed medical and personal records of population of Framingham, Massachusetts.

There are various ways through which expenses incurred in cohort studies can be reduced. One of them is by using established existing systems for monitoring disease or event occurrence like cancer registry, immunization registry, etc. For example, the use of regional cancer registry to ascertain cancer occurrence among cohort members takes up the expenses needed for case ascertainment. Adopting an historical cohort design wherever feasible can reduce cost of the study in contrast to concurrent cohort selection and their follow-up. Substitution of control cohort by general population information like death certificate wherever applicable can save the cost that could have been incurred in following the control group. Adopting nested case control and case cohort desing during the course of a cohort study can also reduce the cost substantially.

Ethical Issues in Cohort Study

Research ethics has under gone a sea of change over the course of the 20th century. On present day respect for individual rights, their dignity, integrity, privacy, private life and personal autonomy has taken the centre stage. These rights are protected by the rule of informed consent and getting protocol clearance from institutional review board/Independent Ethics Committee (IRB/IEC), which in turn are guided by international agreements, such as the **Helsinki Declaration** and the **Council for International Organizations of Medical Sciences (CIOMS).**[27] Helsinki Declaration is the ethical standard for the International Committee of Medical Journal Editors. Here, the requirement states that "When reporting experiments on human subjects, authors

Table 10.10: Advantages and disadvantages of cohort studies in general

Advantages	*Disadvantages*
Can study time sequence of events (exposure precedes disease)	Costly
Ethical (exposure not assigned by investigators, occurs as a natural event)	Not appropriate for rare diseases
Can studied rare exposure	Low in validity (cross-over; differential misclassification of observed and exposure status, loss to follow-up affects validity
Can assessed multiple outcomes	Confounding possible
Not dependent on past records	Generalizability may be limited by non-response
Can determined exposure-specific incidence rates	Degree of accuracy of classification of exposure, confounders and disease status may not be precise
All types of outcomes (mild-to-severe) can be ascertained	

should indicate whether the procedures followed were in accordance with the ethical standards of the responsible committee on human experimentation (institutional and national) and with the Helsinki Declaration of 1975, as revised in 2000".[28] Indeed, the Helsinki Declaration applies to all types of medical research, including observational research. The other important international principles and rules concerning observational research is CIOMS. CIOMS in collaboration with the World Health Organization (WHO) has published International Ethical Guidelines for Biomedical Research Involving Human Subjects.[29] This document indicates that all research must benefit from both scientific and ethical expertise. It states that "all proposals to conduct research involving human subjects must be submitted for review of their scientific merit and ethical acceptability to one or more scientific review and ethical review committees. Ethical review committees may function at the institutional, local, regional, or national level, and in some cases at the international level. The ethical review committee is responsible for safeguarding the rights, safety, and well-being of the research subjects. Scientific review and ethical review cannot be separated—scientifically unsound research involving humans as subjects is ipso facto unethical in that it may expose them to risk or inconvenience to no purpose; even if there is no risk of injury. Wasting of subjects and researchers time in unproductive activities represents loss of valuable resource.

Normally, therefore, an ethical review committee considers both the scientific and the ethical aspects of proposed research. It must either carry out a proper scientific review or verify that a competent expert body has determined that the research is scientifically sound.

Examples

There are many famous examples of Cohort studies including the Framingham heart study, the UK study of doctors who smoke and survivors of the atomic bombing of Hiroshima and Nagasaki, Japan. Two of these the Framingham heart study and study on atomic bomb survivors of Hiroshima and Nagasaki are presented in a tabular format for the ready referral of readers (Table 10.11).

Table 10.11: Famous examples of cohort studies

Name of study	*Framingham study*	*Study of atomic bomb survivors*
Study aim	Incidence and risk factors for CVA and HTN	Incidence and risk for leukaemia and other cancers
Type of study	Concurrent	Special exposure group
Date	1949–current	1950—till the extinction of the cohort
Study population	Adult population in Framingham, WA, USA	Population from all age groups from Hiroshima and Nagasaki, Japan who survived the atomic bombing incident
Sample size	5126	120,128
Sex	Males and females	All gender groups
Age at baseline	30–62	All age groups
Active follow-up	Study variables every 2 years including physical examination, electrocardiogram, and laboratory examination	Study variables like occurrence of leukaemia based on dose as a function of distance, position and shielding.
Passive follow-up	Clinical records (in case of hospitalization); death certificates.	Clinical records, death certificates and Japanese family registration (Koseki) system.

Comparison of cohort and case-control study design: The two major observational research designs with analytical potential are case-control and cohort studies. Both of them have their strengths and limitations. A first-hand comparison of these methods will be appropriate before we windup the discussion (Table 10.12).[30]

Table 10.12: Difference between cohort and cace-control studies

Criteria	*Cohort studies*		*Case-control studies*
	Prospective	*Retrospective*	
Study group	Exposed person ($a + b$)	Exposed person ($a + b$)	Persons with disease (cases) ($a + c$)
Comparison group	Non-exposed persons ($c + d$)	Non-exposed persons ($c + d$)	Persons without diseases (controls) ($b + d$)
Outcome measurements	Incidence in the exposed ($a/b + c$) and incidence in the non-exposed ($c/c + d$)	Incidence in the exposed ($a/b + c$) and incidence in the non-exposed ($c/c + d$)	Proportion of cases exposed ($a/a + c$) and proportion of controls exposed ($b/b + d$)
Measures of risk	Absolute risk, relative risk, odds ratio, attributable risk	Absolute risk, relative risk, odds ratio, attributable risk	Odds ratio
Estimates	Incidence	Incidence	Prevalence
Temporal relationship between exposure and disease	Easy to establish	Sometimes hard to establish	Hard to establish
Multiple associations	Possible to study associations of an exposure with several diseases	Possible to study associations of an exposure with several diseases	Possible to study associations of a disease with several exposures or factors
Time required for the study	Generally long as there is need to follow-up the subjects	May be short	Relatively short
Cost of the study	Expensive	Less expensive than a prospective cohort	Relatively inexpensive
Population size needed	Relatively large	Relatively large	Relatively small
Potential bias	Assessment of outcome	Susceptible to bias both in assessment of exposure and outcome	Assessment of exposure
Best when	Exposure is rare; disease is frequent among exposed	Exposure is rare; disease is frequent among exposed	Disease is rare; exposure is frequent among the diseased
Problems	Selection of non-exposed comparison group often difficult; changes over time in criteria and methods	Selection of non-exposed comparison group often difficult; changes over time in criteria and methos	Selection of appropriate controls often difficult; incomplete information on exposure

Summary

Cohort studies in the original sense of the generation studies introduced by Andvord helped our understanding of the spread of tuberculosis and the aetiology of several cancers. The simplest cohort design is to obtain exposure data at baseline and follow-up individuals to obtain data when the event of interest occurs. There are two major types of cohort studies. They are prospective cohort studies and retrospective cohort studies. A distinguishing feature of both types of cohort studies vis-à-vis other major analytic an observational study is that the exposure status of the subjects is always assessed before their outcome status. Both prospective and retrospective cohort studies follow a cohort over time. In prospective designs the cohort is followed from the present into the future whereas in retrospective designs it is followed from some time in the past up to the present.[31]

Cohort studies in the modern time have established themselves as essential tools for epidemiological research. The nested case-control study and the use of biomarkers, which will in the course of time involve the techniques of molecular biology, provide us with powerful weapons for testing hypotheses about both the genetic and environmental causes of disease. In time to come cohort study in general and hybrid cohorts in particular are set to play even more important parts in the future of medical research than they have had in the past.[32]

Well-designed cohort studies have a number of advantages, including maintaining a clear temporal sequence between exposure and outcome, allowing direct calculation of incidence rates, allowing multiple outcomes to be assessed, providing an indication of incubation or latency periods for diseases, allowing uncommon exposures to be assessed, and precluding exposure suspicion bias. Disadvantages include potentially large sample size requirements, long follow-up periods, losses to follow-up, exposure and outcome misclassification, and diagnostic suspicion bias.[33]

A rewarding cohort design includes regularly schedule visits at which data on exposures are updated. The exposures can either be fixed over time like sex of the participants; change directly with time like age and calendar time of event occurrence; or do not change directly with time like biological markers. According to the scientific aims of a cohort study, disease occurrence can be measured as an event in person time, time to end point of interest, i.e. survival time, or change in a biomarker repeatedly measured at follow-up visits. So, analytical methods include survival analysis to handle censored observations due to incomplete observation of the development of events and longitudinal data analysis for the trajectory of markers of disease progression. Stratification, multivariate regression, and causal inference methods are key tools to accomplish comparability between exposed and unexposed groups. Identification of exposure and risk factors for disease provides a basis for prevention strategy. Data from cohort studies can be used to assess the effects of interventions by using data at individual level to determine individual effectiveness or by comparing occurrence of disease in the population when typically none or only a few are intervened to determine population effectiveness. It also quantifies the reduction of disease achieved by treating the subject of the population that needs therapy the most. By virtue of these cohort studies have established themselves as cornerstones of public health practice and policy.

Study Questions

1. Discuss the strengths and weakness of cohort studies.
2. Compare and contrast prospective and retrospective cohort studies.
3. Elaborate different types of bias encountered in cohort studies.
4. What are hybrid designs in cohort? Mention their advantages.
5. Different study designs have particular advantages and disadvantages. Contrast

the case-control and cohort designs with respect to the following factors.

a. Cost
b. Time required for completion of study
c. Efficiency (in terms of information per subject)
d. Design issues
e. Difficulty in obtaining information
f. Bias
g. What can they estimate?

References

1. Pickett JP, Exec Ed. The American Heritage Dictionary of the English Language; 4th edn. Boston, MA: Houghton Mifflin; 2000.
2. Grimes DA, Schulz KF. Cohort studies: Marching towards outcomes: The Lancet 2002;359:341. www.thelancet.com
3. Doll R. History of epidemiology; Cohort studies: history of the method. 46: 152, 2001.
4. Hyde J. Epidemiology/Biostatistics, Tufts Open Course Ware: Tufts University, Lecture 2008;2:1.
5. Ram WN, Lockey JE. Diffuse malignant mesothelioma: a review. West J Med 1982;137:548.
6. Matanoski GM, Seltzer R, Sartwell PE, et al. The current mortality rates of radiologist and other physician specialists: Specific causes of death. Am J Epidemiol 1975;101:199.
7. Enterline PE. Mortality among asbestos products workers in the United States. Ann NY Acad Sci 1965;32:154.
8. Shimizu Y, Kato H, Schull WJ. Studies of the mortality of A-bomb survivors. 9. Mortality, 1950–1985: Part 2. Cancer mortality based on the recently revised doses (DS86). Radiat Res 1990;121:120–41.
9. Fletcher RH, Fletcher SW, Wagner LA. Clinical epidemiology, risk; looking forward 2005;4(5):83.
10. Szklo M. Population-based Cohort Studies. Epidemiologic Reviews by the Johns Hopkins University School of Hygiene and Public Health 1998;20(1):2.4.
11. Szklo M, Nieto FJ. Measuring disease occurrence. Epidemiology beyond the basic 2007;2(2):69.
12. Aschengraw A, Seage III GR. Overview of Epidemiologic Study Designs. Essentials of epidemiology in public health 2007;5(7):142.
13. Wada S, Miyanishi M, Nishiomoto Y, et al. Mustard gas as a cause of respiratory neoplasia in man. Lancet 1 1968;1161–63.
14. Bergstrand R, Vedin A, Wilhelmsson C, et al. Bias due to non participation and heterogeneous subgroups in population survey. J Chron Dis 1983; 36:725.
15. Hunt JR, White E. Retaining and tracking cohort study members. Epidemiol Rev 1998;20:57–70.
16. Stefano P, Bottarelli Ezio. Survival analysis in epidemiology: A brief introduction. Ann Fac Medic Vet di Parma (Vol. XXVIII, 2008) pp 17–42.
17. Stefano P, Bottarelli Ezio. Poisson regression model in Epidemiology—An Introduction: Ann Fac Medic Vet di Parma, XXVI: 25–44: 2006.
18. Stene LC, Magnus P, Lie RT, Søvik O, et al. Birth weight and childhood onset type 1 diabetes: population based cohort study. BMJ 2001; 322(7291):889–92.
19. Thadhani R, Tonelli M. Cohort Studies: Marching Forward. Clin J Am Soc Nephrol 2006;1:1117–23.
20. Cox C, Chu H, Schneider M, et al. Parametric survival analysis and taxonomy of hazard functions for the generalized gamma distribution statistics in medicine 2007;26:4352–74.
21. Breslow NE, Day NE. The design and analysis of cohort studies. Statistical methods in cancer research II: 1987;132–39.
22. Zeger SL, Liang KY. An over view of methods for analysis of longidutinal data. Statistics in Medicine. 1992:11;1825–39.
23. Solet D, Zoloth SR, Sullivan C, et al. Patterns of mortality in pulp and paper workers. J Occup Med 1989;31:627–30.
24. Matanoski G, Kanchanaraksa S, Lee PSJ, Tao XG, et al. Industry wide study of mortality of pulp and paper mill workers. Am J Ind Med 1998;33:354–65.
25. Lilienfeld AM, Lilienfed DE. Fundamentals of epidemiology 2:1980. NY. Oxford University Press.
26. Greenland S. Response and follow up bias in cohort studies. Am J Epidemiol 1977;105:184–87.
27. Rothman KJ. A pictorial representation of confounding in epidemiological studies. J Chron Dis 1975;28:101–8.
28. Claudot FL, Alla F, Fresson J, Calvez T, Coudane H, et al. Ethics and observational studies in medical research: various rules in a common framework. International Journal of Epidemiology 2009; 38(4):1104–8.
29. International Committee of Medical Journal Editors. Uniform Requirements for Manuscripts Submitted to Biomedical Journals: Writing and Editing for Biomedical Publication. [Online]. February 2006. http://www.icmje.org/
30. Council for International Organizations of Medical Sciences (CIOMS). International Ethical Guidelines for Biomedical Research Involving Human Subjects. [Online]. 2002. [cited 2007 July 10]. http://www.cioms.ch/frame_guidelines_nov_2002.htm
31. Gordies L. A pause for review. Epidemiology 2009;4(13):225.
32. Schlesselman JJ. Case-control studies. New York. Oxford university press.1982.
33. Analytic study designs 131, rev. 8/1/00; w.sph unc. edu/courses/EPID168/

Chapter

11

Experimental Studies Including Clinical Trials

Paramita Sengupta

INTRODUCTION

Experimental studies (Fig. 11.1) are also known as intervention studies in which there is an attempt to change a variable in one or more groups of people. Experimental designs have been considered by many to be the gold standard design for evaluating effectiveness, but it may not always be ethical or feasible to randomly allocate people to a public health intervention.

True experimental designs are those where the researchers have complete control over the extraneous variables and can predict confidently that the observed effect on the dependable variable is only due to the manipulation of the independent variable. Experimental designs are called the gold standard.

True experimental designs have all three of the primary characteristics (i.e. manipulation, randomization, and control). They can be thought of as being most similar to a highly controlled laboratory experiment. As such, these designs have the most safeguards against sources of bias and therefore the greatest degree of overall scientific validity. Quasi-experimental designs are missing one or two of these elements. They have the element of manipulation or control but rarely randomization.

There are several types of true experimental designs and they are as shown in Fig. 11.1.

HISTORY

The *first unintentional clinical trial* was conducted by Ambroise Pare (1510–1590),[1] who had applied a digestive made up of egg yolk, rose oil and turpentine oil to the wounded victims of war, in place of the standard treatment of applying boiling oil, as it was in short supply, and he was successful.[2] A *planned trial* was conducted by James Lind, a Scottish surgeon in 1747, when he attributed a dietary cause to scurvy. Lind conducted a controlled, comparative trial on 12 patients suffering from scurvy on board a ship named *Salisbury*. The patients were given the same diet consisting of water gruel sweetened with

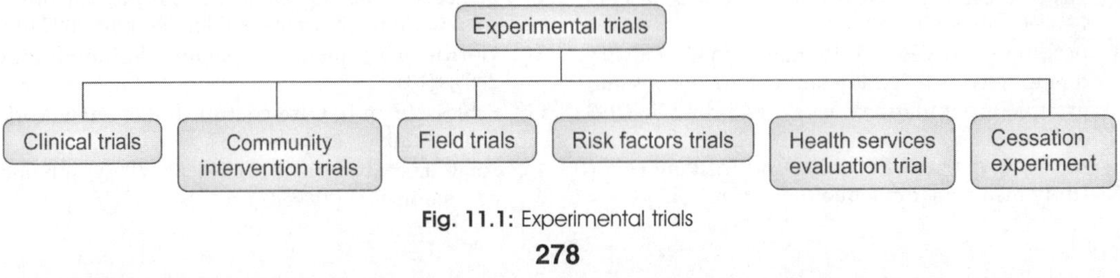

Fig. 11.1: Experimental trials

sugar in the morning; fresh mutton broth for dinner; puddings, boiled biscuit with sugar; and for supper barley, raisins, rice and currants, sago and wine. Two of these were given a quart of cyder a day, two others given 25 gutts of elixir vitriol, the third group was given 2 spoons of vinegar, the fourth group was put under a course of sea water, fifth group was given the bigness of a nutmeg, and the sixth had two oranges and one lemon. The patients who were given oranges and lemons showed remarkable change and were fit for duty within a week.

Sir RA Fisher first developed the concept of experimental randomization in 1925. JB Amberson and BT McMahon (1931) randomized patients by using a coin flip to see who received treatment for tuberculosis. Sir Austin Bradford Hill introduced the use of random numbers in the allocation of patients in the study of streptomycin and tuberculosis.

CLASSIFICATION OF RESEARCH DESIGNS BY DEGREE OF SCIENTIFIC RIGOR[3]

The research design classification system commonly used is 'classification by scientific rigor.' This system helps judge the validity of the results of the study, and categorizes the research designs based on levels of overall scientific integrity.

True Experimental (Table 11.1)

- Have all three design elements
- Are always prospective
- Have high scientific validity

Quasi-experimental

- Have one or two design elements
- Use manipulation or control
- Generally lack randomization
- Are generally prospective in nature
- Are moderate in scientific validity

Non-experimental

- Have one or none of the core design elements
- Lack manipulation and randomization
- May also lack control
- Are generally retrospective
- Have the lowest scientific validity

Clinical trials: Clinical trials are experiments that test hypothesis concerning the effects (favourable or unfavourable) of interventions on human subjects. The interventions can be on the effects of drugs, vaccines, treatments or devices. Clinical trials are used to determine whether new biomedical or behavioural interventions are safe, efficacious and effective. Clinical trials are done for the following.

- New drugs and new treatment of diseases
- New medical and healthcare technology
- New methods of primary prevention
- New programs for screening
- New ways of organizing and delivering health services
- New community health programs
- New behavioural intervention programs

DESIGN METHODS FOR CLINICAL TRIALS[4]

Traditional Designs for Clinical Trials

- Parallel group design
- Cross-over design
- Factorial design
- Add-on design
- Randomized withdrawal design
- Early escape design

Table 11.1: True experimental designs

Two arm	*Three arm*	*Follow-up*	*Factorial*	*Cross-over*
R O X O	R O X1 O	R O X O1 O2	R O X1 O	R O X1 O X2 O
R O C O	R O X2 O	R O C O1 O2	R O X2 O	R O X2 O X1 O
	R O C O		R O X1 X2 O	
			R O X2 X1 O	

Special Designs for Small Clinical Trials

- n-of-1 design
- Sequential design
- Decision analysis-based design
- Ranking and selection design
- Adaptive design
- Risk-based allocation design

Other Important RCT Designs

- Efficacy versus effectiveness
- Phase I, II, III, IV trials

Phases of Clinical Trials

Clinical trials of experimental drug, treatment, device or behavioural intervention may proceed through four phases (Fig. 11.2):

Phase I clinical trials test a new biomedical intervention in a small group of people (e.g. 20–80) for the first time to evaluate safety (e.g. to determine a safe dosage range, toxic levels and to identify side effects).

Phase II clinical trials study the biomedical or behavioural intervention in a larger group of people (several hundred) to determine efficacy and to further evaluate its safety.

Phase III studies are large multi-institutional studies that investigate the efficacy of the biomedical or behavioural intervention in large groups of human subjects (from several hundred to several thousand) by comparing the intervention to other standard or experimental interventions as well as to monitor adverse effects, and to collect information that will allow the intervention to be used safely.

Phase IV studies are conducted after the intervention has been marketed. These studies are designed to monitor effectiveness of the approved intervention in the general population and to collect information about any adverse effects associated with widespread use.

A much more inclusive and general approach that subsumes the four phases of clinical trials is put forth by Piantadosi (1997), who defines the four phases as (1) early-development studies (testing the treatment mechanism), (2) middle-development studies (treatment tolerability), (3) comparative (pivotal, confirmatory) studies, and (4) late-development studies (extended safety or post-marketing studies).[4]

RANDOMIZED CONTROLLED TRIAL (RCT)

This is an experimental design in which we randomly allocate individuals to intervention group (study group) and non-intervention group (control group) without the ability to predict who is in which group, and then compare their outcomes (Fig. 11.3). Randomization is the process by which allocation of subjects to treatment groups is done by chance. Random allocation aims to achieve similar balanced/equivalent groups. RCTs serve as the ***gold standard***, and serves as a benchmark against which other trial designs can be measured. A randomized controlled trial gives the strongest form of evidence when compared against any epidemiological study and helps in establishing a cause–effect relationship. When whole communities or groups of people are randomized, we term that design as a 'cluster randomized controlled trial' or cluster RCT. Randomized controlled trials, when appropriately designed, conducted, and reported, represent the gold standard in evaluating healthcare interventions. The randomized trial design has major applicability.

RCTs are mostly used to study a new therapeutic or preventive regimen. The specific criteria for the condition under investigation must be met by the trial participants, so that the group is fairly homogenous. If randomly allocated groups are sufficiently large, they will be equivalent and hence directly comparable. Valid methods of randomization include flipping a coin, rolling a die, using a table of random numbers, or running a computerized random allocation generator (e.g. http://www. random.org). Parallel and crossover designs are the two standard designs for RCTs.[5] Randomization is a powerful tool to ensure validity in parallel-designed studies, special precautions have to be considered in crossover studies to avoid or at least account for possible carryover effects.

Randomization has three major advantages[6] (Table 11.2). Firstly, if implemented

	FDA approved to test the drug(s) in human drugs			At the end of phase III application submitted for FDA approval	FDA approved drug(s)
	Preclinical trial (usually done on animals to determine the drug is safe enough for human testing)	**Phase I** (determine pharmacological actions and tolerability*)	**Phase II** (evaluate safety and efficacy)	**Phase III** (evaluate effectiveness** and risk–benefit ratio)	**Phase IV** (monitor long-term effects and effectiveness)
Duration	3–6 years since the drug discovery	Months	Months–Years	Years	Ongoing following FDA approval
Sample size	Not specific	Small	Large	Larger	Impacting larger beyond
Population	*In vitro* and *in vivo* animals	Healthy population/may be with targeted disease, e.g. cancer, TB, etc.	Population with target disease	Diverse population with target disease	Diverse population with target disease and new age groups, gender
Types of studies	Not specific	Unblinded and uncontrolled	May be placebo (inactive substance) and active, controlled	Randomized and controlled	Expended safety comparison
Factors to be identified	Mechanism of action, efficacy (ability of drug to act against pathogen /disease), safety (concerns the medical risk to the patient)	Pharmacodynamics (side effect/desire effect, mechanism of action of drug), pharmacokinetics (absorption, distribution, metabolism and elimination of drug), tolerated dose	Drug–drug and Drug–disease interaction, efficacy at various doses, patient safety	Dosage intervals, risk–benefit information, efficacy and safety for subgroups	Epidemiological data, efficacy and safety within large diverse populations, pharmacoeconomics (comparison of value of one pharmacentical drug or drug therapy to another)

*Tolerability: Represents the degree to which overt advese effects can be tolerated by the patient.
**Effectiveness: The extent to which a drug achieves its intended effects

Fig. 11.2: Phases of clinical trials

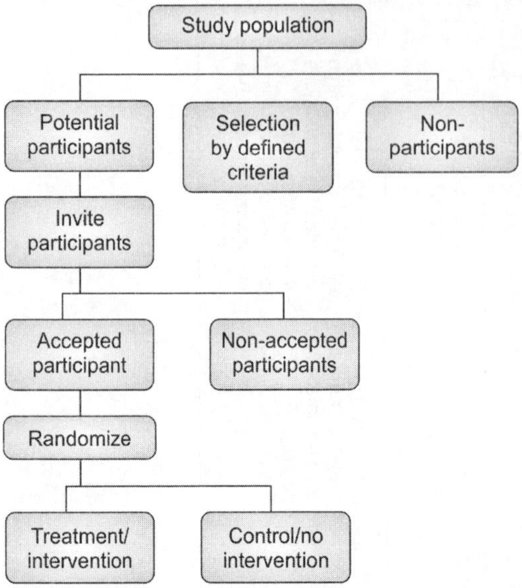

Fig. 11.3: Design of a randomized controlled trial[7]

well, it eliminates selection bias, in the assignment of treatments, without which selection of participants to receive a particular treatment may be prejudiced. Secondly, random assignment permits the use of probability theory to express the likelihood that any difference in outcome between intervention groups merely reflects chance and thirdly, random allocation, facilitates blinding thus reducing bias, which is very important.[7]

If random assignment is used, we call the design a randomized experiment or true experiment. If random assignment is not used, then we have to ask a second question: Does the design use either multiple groups or multiple waves of measurement? If the answer is yes, we would label it a quasi-experimental design. If no, we would call it a non-experimental design.

The sample size should be large enough for the study to have sufficient statistical power to detect important differences. Sample size calculations can be done depending on:

- required level of statistical significance of the ability to detect a difference
- acceptable error, or chance of missing a real effect
- magnitude of the effect under investigation
- amount of disease in the population
- Relative sizes of the groups being compared.

Control Groups

- No treatment concurrent controls
- Concurrent placebo controls
- Wait list comparison controls
- Controls with dose comparison
- Active treatment concurrent control (superiority/inferiority/equivalence trial)
- Historical control

Table 11.2: Advantages and disadvantages of RCT[14]

Advantages	*Disadvantages*
• Allows rigorous evaluation of a single variable • Prospective design (data is collected on events that happen after you decide to do a study) • Uses hypothetic–deductive reasoning (seeks to falsify rather than confirm, its own hypothesis) • Potentially eradicates bias by comparing two otherwise identical groups. • Allows for meta-analysis (combining the numerical results of several similar trials at a later date.	• Expensive and time consuming hence: – many RCT are never done – are performed on too few patients or – are undertaken for too short a time period • Most are funded by large research bodies (university or government sponsored) or drug companies, who ultimately dictate the research agenda • Surrogate end-points are often used in preference to clinical outcome measures and may introduce 'hidden bias' through improper randomization • Failure to blind assessors to randomization status of patients

Bradford-Hill Criteria for Casual Inference[8]

- Strength of the association
- Temporal relationship
- Biologic plausibility
- Dose–response relationship
- Replication of the findings
- Effect of removing the exposure
- Alternate explanations considered
- Specificity of the association
- Consistency with other knowledge

Once the design has been determined, there are four elements of true experimental research that must be considered:

1. ***Manipulation:*** Here the treatment or condition that is to be applied to the experimental groups (independent variable) is manipulated purposefully. It is important to establish clear procedural guidelines for application of the treatment to promote consistency and ensure that the manipulation itself does affect the dependent variable.
2. ***Control:*** Control is used to prevent the influence of outside factors (extraneous variables) from influencing the outcome of the study. This ensures that outcome is caused by the manipulation of the independent variable. Therefore, a critical piece of experimental design is keeping all other potential variables constant. For example, if testing the effects of fertilizer on plant height, all other factors such as sunlight, soil type and water would have to be constant (controlled).
3. ***Random assignment*:** A key feature of true experimental design is the random assignment of subjects into groups. Participants should have an equal chance of being assigned into any group in the experiment. This further ensures that the outcome of the study is due to the manipulation of the independent variable and is not influenced by the composition of the test groups. Subjects can be randomly assigned in many ways, some of which are relatively easy, including flipping a coin, drawing names, using a random table, or utilizing a computer assisted random sequencing.
4. ***Random selection*:** In addition to randomly assigning the test subjects in groups, it is also important to randomly select the test subjects from a larger target audience. The respondents of the trial are selected in such a way that all eligible population has an equal chance of being selected for the study. This ensures that the sample population provides an accurate cross-sectional representation of the larger population including different socio-economic backgrounds, races, intelligence levels, and so forth.

Randomization

Randomization refers to how subjects are assigned to study groups (Fig. 11.4). Designs in which randomization is used provide each subject with a known probability of being assigned to each of the study groups, (e.g. experimental or control). In most studies the probability of assignment to the two groups is equal.[9]

- ***Simple randomization:*** Pure randomization based on a single allocation ratio is known as simple randomization. Simple randomization with 1:1 an allocation ratio is analogous to a coin toss, although we do not advocate coin tossing for randomization in an RCT. Other methods include using a shuffled deck of cards (e.g. even-control, odd-treatment) or throwing a dice (e.g. below and equal to 3-control,

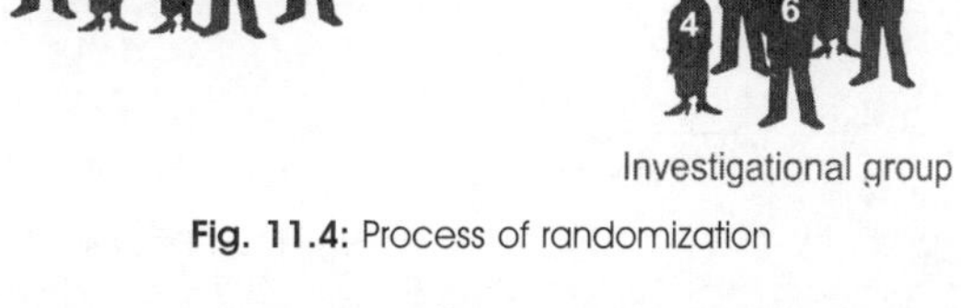

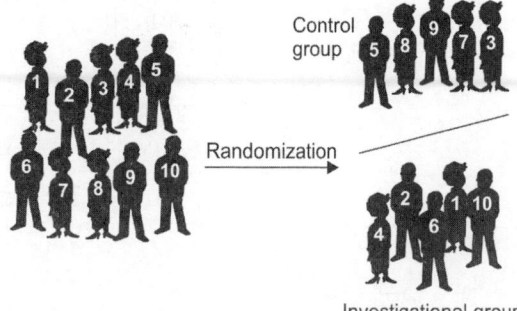

Fig. 11.4: Process of randomization

over 3-treatment). A random number table found in a statistics book or computer-generated random numbers can also be used for simple randomization of subjects. 'Simple' is somewhat of a misnomer. While other randomization schemes sound complex and more sophisticated, in reality, simple randomization is elegantly sophisticated in that it is more unpredictable and surpasses the bias prevention levels of all other alternatives.

- ***Restricted randomization:*** Blocked randomization is the most common form. Other means of restricted randomization include replacement, biased coin, and urn randomization, although these are used much less frequently.
- ***Blocked randomization:*** Blocking is used to ensure that comparison groups are generated according to a predetermined ratio, usually 1:1 or groups of approximately the same size. Instead of randomizing each patient individually, this scheme randomizes several patients at a time in such a way as to ensure that equal numbers are allocated to each group. For example, if the block size is four, we randomize four patients at a time ensuring that two patients are allocated to the treatment group and two patients to control. There are six different possible ways we could randomize four patients equally to two treatments. Blocking can be used to ensure close balance of the numbers in each group at any time during the trial. Improved balance comes at the cost of reducing the unpredictability of the sequence. If he or she knew the block size, a person running the trial could deduce the next treatment allocations. Blinding or using larger block sizes, and randomly varying the block size can ameliorate the bias due to this.[10]

Allocation				
	Patient 1	Patient 2	Patient 3	Patient 4
1	Treatment	Treatment	Control	Control
2	Treatment	Control	Treatment	Control
3	Treatment	Control	Control	Treatment
4	Control	Control	Treatment	Treatment
5	Control	Treatment	Control	Treatment
6	Control	Treatment	Treatment	Control

- ***Stratified randomization:*** Stratified randomization (Fig. 11.5) is achieved by first stratifying the study population by each important variable, and then performing a randomization procedure within each of two or more subsets of participants (for example, those defining each study centre, age, or disease severity). Stratification by centre is common in multicentre trials. Stratification helps to ensure good balance of participant characteristics in each group so that the groups are similar for an

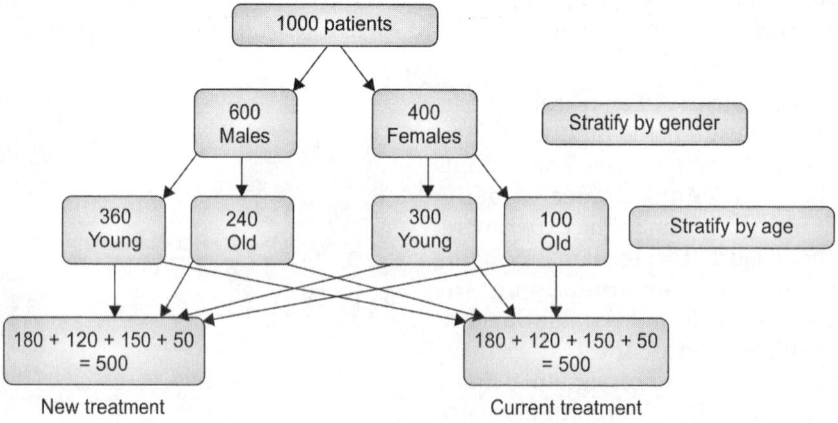

Fig. 11.5: Process of stratified randomization[11]

important prognostic feature. The credibility of small trials may be weakened as study groups may not be well matched for baseline characteristics, such as age and stage of disease. Stratification ensures that the numbers of participants receiving each intervention are closely balanced within each stratum. Stratification requires some form of restriction (such as blocking within strata). Stratification without blocking is ineffective.

- ***Minimization***: Minimization ensures balance between intervention groups for several selected patient factors (such as age). The first patient is truly randomly allocated; for each subsequent participant, the treatment allocation that minimizes the imbalance on the selected factors between groups at that time is identified. The use of a random component is generally preferable. Minimization has the advantage of making small groups closely similar in terms of participant characteristics at all stages of the trial. Minimization offers the only acceptable alternative to randomization, and some have argued that it is superior. On the other hand, minimization lacks the theoretical basis for eliminating bias on all known and unknown factors. Nevertheless, in general, trials that use minimization are considered methodologically equivalent to randomized trials, even when a random element is not incorporated.
- ***Adaptive randomization***: Another strategy to minimize imbalances in prognostic factors is to use an adaptive randomization scheme when randomization is influenced by analysis of either the baseline characteristics or outcomes of previous patients. When treatment assignment is based on patient characteristics, the adaptive randomization procedure known as minimization assigns the next treatment to minimize any imbalance in prognostic factors among previously enrolled patients.[12]

The two fundamental characteristics of randomization are:[10]

Researchers must be unable to predict the group to which a patient will be randomized until the patient is unambiguously registered on study

- Researchers must be unable to change a patient's allocation after they are randomized.
- A trial meeting these criteria is said to have adequate 'allocation concealment'.

Results of RCTs

Hazard ratio: Hazard ratios have also been used to describe the outcome of therapeutic trials where the question is to what extent treatment can shorten the duration of the illness. Clinical trials commonly record the length of time from study entry to a disease end-point for a treatment and a control group. These data are commonly depicted with a Kaplan-Meier curve from which the median (time at which 50% of cases are resolved) and the mean (average resolution time) can be derived. The groups are compared by a time-to-event analysis (survival analysis).[13]

Absolute risk reduction (ARR): Cumulative incidence (CI) in control group minus cumulative incidence in the experimental group.

Relative risk reduction: ARR divided by cumulative incidence in the control group.

Number needed to treat (NNT) is expressed as a reciprocal of the difference in test and control treatments. NNT = 1/ARR, or 1/(CI control—CI treatment). The NNT indicates the number of patients whom the new treatment has to be given in place of standard treatment to get one additional patient to benefit. The NNT can also be obtained for survival analysis.

Compliance is the willingness of the participants to carry out the procedures according to the established protocols (adherence).

Drop-outs are the participants who do not adhere to the experimental regimen during follow-up.

SUPERIORITY, INFERIORITY AND EQUIVALENCE TRIALS

A superiority trial aims to demonstrate the superiority of a new therapy compared to an established therapy or placebo.

Equivalence Trials

The purpose of an equivalence trial is to establish identical effects of the therapies being compared. An equivalence trial would be relevant if the new therapy is simpler, associated with fewer side-effects or less expensive, even if it is not expected to have a larger therapeutic effect than the control therapy. The two treatments could be called equivalent if the observed difference and its 95% CI are completely inside the interval of clinical equivalence. In terms of null and alternative hypotheses, proving equivalence boils down to rejecting the non-inferiority trial, which is related to the equivalence trial, aims not at showing equivalence but only at showing that the new therapy is no worse than the reference therapy.

EXPERTISE-BASED TRIALS

An expertise-based trial differs from a conventional RCT because surgeons perform only the procedure at which they believe they are most skilled. Proponents argue that expertise-based trials minimize bias resulting from differences in technical competency and surgeon preference, decrease crossover from one intervention to the other, and can be more ethical than conventional RCTs.[15]

FIELD TRIAL

Field trials are conducted on people who are presumed to be at risk but disease-free unlike clinical trials and they are much larger than clinical trials as they study therapeutic interventions. This method can be used to evaluate interventions meant for reducing exposure. They are usually carried out in the field among non-institutionalized people. The largest field trial was the use of Salk vaccine for prevention of poliomyelitis conducted on one million children. As the risk of people to have a particular disease is usually low, a very large sample of individuals is necessary to test the efficacy of a vaccine.

COMMUNITY TRIAL

An extension of field trials that involves allocation of treatment to communities rather than individuals. Community trials are conducted for diseases that have a social origin and can be influenced by intervention for group or individuals.[7] For example, water fluoridation was tested by exposing some communities to it and comparing to other communities without this exposure.

SOLOMON FOUR GROUP DESIGN

Subjects are randomly assigned into one of four groups. There are two experimental groups and two control groups. Only two groups are pre-tested. One pre-tested group and one untested group receive the treatment. All four groups will receive the post-test. The effects of the dependent variable originally observed are then compared to the effects of the independent variable on the dependent variable as seen in the post-test results. This design assesses the plausibility of pre-test sensitization effects, that is, taking a pre-test influences scores on subsequent administration of the test by priming the respondent with answers and they fare better than if they did not do the pre-test. This method is really a combination of the previous two methods and is used to eliminate potential sources of error.

FACTORIAL DESIGN

To test for treatment effects of combined interventions, factorial study designs have been proposed where individuals are randomly assigned to receive two or more interventions.[16] The factorial study design increases the study efficiency because it allows for assessment of multiple interventions within the same trial. The researcher manipulates two or more independent variables (factors) simultaneously to observe their effects on the dependent variable. This design allows for the testing of two or more hypotheses in a single project. One example would be a researcher who wanted to test two different protocols for burn wounds with the frequency of the care being administered in 2-, 4-, and 6-hour increments.

RANDOMIZED BLOCK DESIGN

This design is used when there are inherent differences between subjects and possible differences in experimental conditions. If there are a large number of experimental groups, the randomized block design may be used to bring some homogeneity to each group. For example, if a researcher wanted to examine the effects of three different kinds of cough medications on children ages 2–16, the research may want to create age groups (blocks) for the children, realizing that the effects of the medication may depend on age. This is a simple method for reducing the variability among treatment groups.

CROSSOVER DESIGN (also known as repeat measures design)

Subjects in this design are exposed to more than one treatment and the subjects are randomly assigned to different orders of the treatment. The groups compared have an equal distribution of characteristics and there is a high level of similarity among subjects that are exposed to different conditions (Fig. 11.6).

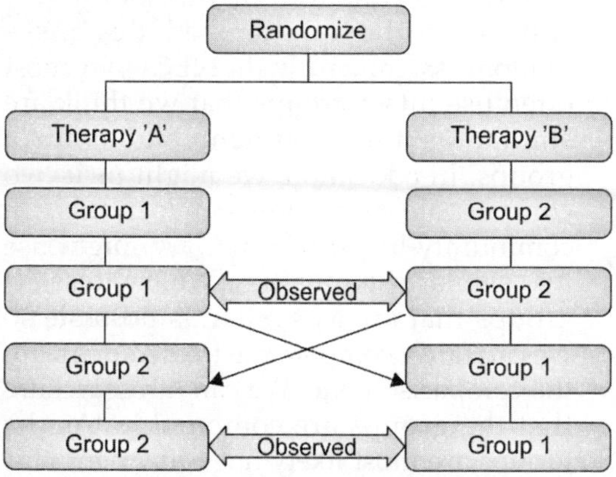

Fig. 11.6: Planned crossover[11]

The crossover design has the advantage that each subject becomes its own control, thereby directly controlling formost extraneous variables. Crossover designs are excellent research tools, however, there is some concern that the response to the second treatment or condition will be influenced by their experience with the first treatment. In this type of design, the subjects serve as their own control groups. Carryover effects are defined as effects that 'carry over' from one condition, e.g. exposure or treatment, to another. Besides randomization of the treatment sequence, wash-in and wash-out periods of appropriate length are commonly used in crossover studies to avoid carryover effects.

Unplanned Crossover

In unplanned crossover, participants in the surgical group may not want to have surgery and switch over to the medical group, and others in the medical group may worsen and go over to the surgical group. The problem is compounded if there is a large crossover (Fig. 11.7).

QUASI-EXPERIMENTAL DESIGNS

Quasi-experimental designs (QED) try to duplicate experimental designs, but there is no random allocation of subjects to intervention/control groups. There are many different QEDs—some involve comparison or control groups, some only involve single groups, some involve baseline (pre-test) and post-intervention (post-test) measures, while others only have post-test outcome measures.

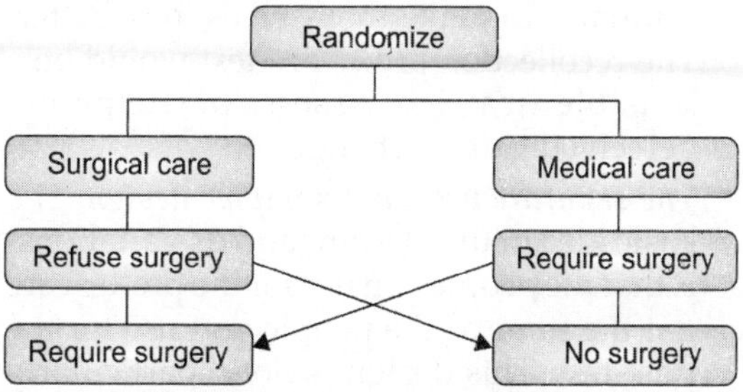

Fig. 11.7: Unplanned crossover

Comparison Group Post-test Design

This type of design has two randomly assigned groups—an experimental group and a control group. Neither group is pre-tested before the implementation of the treatment. This design can be used to demonstrate a difference in the outcome between the two groups, to assess the effect of the manipulation but any observed difference can not be interpreted as 'actual' program effects. This design reduces the likelihood of instrumentation and testing threats (as no pre-test data) but can be affected by attrition and selection threats (comparison group differs systematically from the intervention group) can affect this design. This type of design is common when it is not possible to pre-test the subjects.

Pre-test–post-test Only Design

The subjects are randomly assigned to either the experimental or the control group. Both groups are pre-tested for the independent variable. The experimental group receives the treatment and both groups are post-tested to examine the effects of manipulating the independent variable on the dependent variable.

Other Quasi-experimental Designs

- *The proxy pre-test design*: 'Recollection' proxy pre-test design and 'Archived' proxy pre-test design. The pre-test in this design is collected after the program is given estimating how you would have answered the questions 6 months ago. This type of proxy pre-test is not very good for estimating actual pre-post changes because people may forget where they were at some prior time or they may distort the pre-test estimates to make themselves look better. The recollection proxy pre-test would be a sensible way to assess participants' perceived gain or change.
- *The separate pre–post samples design:* The basic idea in this design (and its variations) is that the people you use for the pre-test are not the same as the people you use for the post-test. This design is not a particularly strong one. Because you cannot match individual participant responses from pre to post, you can only look at the change in average customer satisfaction. Here, you always run the risk that you have non-equivalence not only between the agencies but that within agency the pre- and post-groups are non-equivalent.
- *The double pre-test design*: The double pre-test is a very strong quasi-experimental design with respect to internal validity.
- *The switching replications design*: The switching replications quasi-experimental design is also very strong with respect to internal validity. And, because it allows for two independent implementations of the program, it may enhance external validity or generalizability. The design has two groups and three waves of measurement. In the first phase of the design, both groups are pre-tests, one is given the program and both are post-tested. In the second phase of the design, the original comparison group is given the program while the original program group serves as the 'control'.
- *The non-equivalent dependent variables (NEDV) design*:[16] One of the most commonly used quasi-experimental designs because it is the most internally valid design that can be implemented in applied settings where random assignment is not possible. A control group is used but there is no randomization. It is the most frequently used design in social research. It is structured like a pre-test–post-test randomized experiment, but it lacks the key feature of the randomized designs—random assignment. In the NEGD, we most often use intact groups that we think are similar as the treatment and control groups. In education, we might pick two comparable classrooms or schools. In community-based research, we might use two similar communities. We try to select groups that are as similar as possible so we can fairly compare the treated one with the comparison one. We can never be sure that the groups are comparable. As the groups are most likely not equivalent, this design was named the non-equivalent groups design.

- ***The regression point displacement (RPD) design***: The regression point displacement (RPD) design is a simple quasi-experimental strategy that has important implications, especially for community-based research. The problem with community-level interventions is that it is difficult to do causal assessment, to determine if your program made a difference as opposed to other potential factors.

Programme trials are experiments or quasi experiments that test hypothesis concerning the effects of health programs. The main focus of programme trials is usually the outcome of care, and its variation in different population groups or different circumstances. These are done for economic efficiency, performance appraisal, satisfaction, compliance, and usually have the specific purpose of explaining effectiveness or its lack, feasibility or acceptability.

CATEGORIZATION OF STUDY DESIGNS ACCORDING TO THE QUALITY OF EVIDENCE

Trials

a. Randomized, double-blind, placebo-controlled with sufficient power appropriately analyzed.
b. Randomized, but blindness not achieved.
c. Non-randomized trials with good control of confounding that are well conducted in other respects.
d. Randomized, but with deficiencies in execution or analysis (insufficient power, major losses to follow-up, suspect randomization, analysis with exclusions).
e. Non-randomized trials with deficiencies in execution or analysis.

Among other issues that must be considered in reviewing the evidence are the precision of definition of the outcome being measured, the degree to which the study methodology has been described, adequacy of the sample size, and the degree to which characteristics of the population studied and of the intervention being evaluated have been described.

A study can be well designed and carried out in an exemplary fashion (internal validity), but if the population studied is an unusual or highly selected one, the results may not be generalizable (external validity).

Validity

Validity is the extent to which an instrument actually measures what it purports to measure. Internal validity is essentially concerned with detecting change and being able to attribute it to the intervention. External validity is concerned with whether the results are generalizable to other populations and is influenced by your sample selection. An example would be how well a questionnaire measures exposure or outcome in a prospective cohort study, or the accuracy of a diagnostic test.

Assessing Validity

Assessing validity requires that an error free reference test or gold standard is available to which the measure can be compared.

Reliability (Repeatability)

Reliability refers to the consistency of the performance of an instrument over time and among different observers.

Assessing Reliability

1. Intra-measurement reliability: Repeated measurements by the same observer on the same subject.
2. Inter-observer measurement carried out on the same subject by two or more observers and the results compared.

   Efficacy = Reduction in risk

   Efficacy = (Rate in placebo – Rate in treated)/rate in placebo

   = 1 – Rate in treated/rate in placebo

Even though subjects are assigned to treatment at random, there may be some concern that any difference in the post-test measurements might be due a failure in the randomization. Perhaps the groups differed in their pre-test measurements.

One way around the problem is to compare the groups on differences between post-test and pretest, sometimes called **change scores** or **gain scores**. The test can be carried out in a number of equivalent ways:

- t-test of the differences;
- 2-group ANOVA of the differences,
- repeated measures analysis of variance.

Another approach that could be used—analysis of covariance, in which

- The post-test measurement is the response,
- Treatment is the design factor, and the pretest is a covariate.

Number needed to treat (NNT):[17] Number needed to treat is a way to communicate the effectiveness of a treatment. It is used to assess beneficial and harmful effects of medical interventions. It is often reported in RCTs and systematic reviews on therapy. It signifies how many patients would need to be treated to get one additional patient better who would not have gotten better without this particular treatment.

Patient information necessary for informed consent:[17]

- Diagnosis
- Available treatments and treatment on trial
- Potential risks and benefits of treatment
- Concept of a clinical trial (including randomization, use of placebos, double-blind procedures
- Discomforts or inconveniences associated with assessments
- Number of follow-up visits or extra travel for trial.

THE CONSORT STATEMENT

Critical appraisal of the quality of clinical trials is possible only if the design, conduct, and analysis of RCTs are thoroughly and accurately described in the report. Randomized trials can yield biased results if they lack methodological rigor.[18] The CONSORT Statement[19] is an evidence-based checklist (Table 11.3) of essential items for reporting randomized trials that should be included in reports of RCTs and a diagram for documenting the flow of participants through a trial. It is aimed at primary reports of RCTs with two-group parallel designs, but also used to report other trial designs, such as non-inferiority, equivalence, factorial, cluster, and crossover trials. The CONSORT statement comprises a 25-item checklist and a flow diagram. The flowchart proposed by the CONSORT 2010 guideline. This flowchart shows the recommended design and structure of a clinical trial.

CONSORT 2010 focuses predominantly on the two-group parallel randomized controlled trial, which accounts for over half of trials in the literature.[18] It offers a standard way for authors to prepare reports of trial findings, facilitating their complete and transparent reporting, and aiding their critical appraisal and interpretation. The CONSORT Statement comprises a 25-item checklist and a flow diagram (Table 11.3 and Fig. 11.8).[19]

Flowchart shows the recommended design and structure of a clinical trial.

Good clinical practice (GCP)[20] is an international ethical and scientific quality standard for designing, conducting, recording and reporting trials that involve the participation of human participants. The ICH GCP E6 Guideline (ICH GCP) was published in 1996. The International Conference on Harmonisation of Technical Requirements for Registration of Pharmaceuticals for Human Use brought together the European Union, Japan and the United States.

1. The principles of ICH GCP clinical trials should be conducted in accordance with the ethical principles that have their origin in the declaration of Helsinki, and that are consistent with GCP and the applicable regulatory requirement(s).
2. Before a trial is initiated, foreseeable risks and inconveniences should be weighed against the anticipated benefit for the individual trial subject and society. A trial should be initiated and continued only if the anticipated benefits justify the risks.

Table 11.3: CONSORT checklist

Section/topic	*Item no.*	*Checklist item*
Title and abstract	1a	Identification as a randomized trial in the title
	1b	Structured summary of trial design, methods, results, and conclusions (for specific guidance see CONSORT for abstracts)
Introduction		
Background	2a	Scientific background and explanation of rationale
Objectives	2b	Specific objectives or hypotheses
Methods		
Trial design	3a	Description of trial design (such as parallel, factorial) including allocation ratio
	3b	Important changes to methods after trial commencement (such as eligibility criteria) with reasons
Participants	4a	Eligibility criteria for participants
	4b	Settings and locations where the data were collected
Interventions	5	The interventions for each group with sufficient details to allow replication, including how and when they were actually administered
Outcomes	6a	Completely defined pre-specified primary and secondary outcome measures, including how and when they were assessed
	6b	Any changes to trial outcomes after the trial commenced, with reasons
Sample size	7a	How sample size was determined?
	7b	When applicable, explanation of any interim analyses and stopping guidelines
Randomization		
Sequence generation	8a	Method used to generate the random allocation sequence
	8b	Type of randomization; details of any restriction (such as blocking and block size)
Allocation	9	Mechanism used to implement the random allocation
Concealment		Sequence (such as sequentially numbered containers), mechanism describing any steps taken to conceal the sequence until interventions were assigned
Implementation	10	Who generated the random allocation sequence, who enrolled participants, and who assigned participants to interventions
Blinding	11a	If done, who was blinded after assignment to interventions (for example, participants, care providers, those assessing outcomes) and how
	11b	If relevant, description of the similarity of interventions

Contd...

Table 11.3: CONSORT checklist (*Contd...*)

Section/topic	*Item no.*	*Checklist item*
Statistical methods	12a	Statistical methods used to compare groups for primary and secondary outcomes
	12b	Methods for additional analyses, such as subgroup analyses and adjusted analyses
	13a	For each group, the numbers of participants who were randomly assigned, received intended treatment and were analysed for the primary outcome
Results participant flow (a diagram is strongly recommended)	13b	For each group, losses and exclusions after randomization, together with reasons
Recruitment	14a	Dates defining the periods of recruitment and follow-up
	14b	Why the trial ended or was stopped
Baseline data	15	A table showing baseline demographic and clinical characteristics for each group
Numbers analyzed	16	For each group, number of participants (denominator) included in each analysis and whether the analysis was by original assigned groups
Outcomes	17a	For each primary and secondary outcome, results for estimation each group, and the estimated effect size and its precision (such as 95% confidence interval)
	17b	For binary outcomes, presentation of both absolute and relative effect sizes is recommended
Ancillary analyses	18	Results of any other analyses performed, including subgroup analyses and adjusted analyses, distinguishing pre-specified from exploratory
Harms	19	All important harms or unintended effects in each group (for specific guidance see CONSORT for harms)
Discussion		
Limitations	20	Trial limitations, addressing sources of potential bias, imprecision, and, if relevant, multiplicity of analyses
Generalisability	21	Generalisability (external validity, applicability) of the trial findings
Interpretation	22	Interpretation consistent with results, balancing benefits and harms, and considering other relevant evidence
Other information		
Registration	23	Registration number and name of trial registry
Protocol	24	Where the full trial protocol can be accessed, if available
Funding	25	Sources of funding and other support (such as supply of drugs), role of funders

Note: All experimental studies must follow the good clinical practice, so as to get authentic observations and implementation thereof.

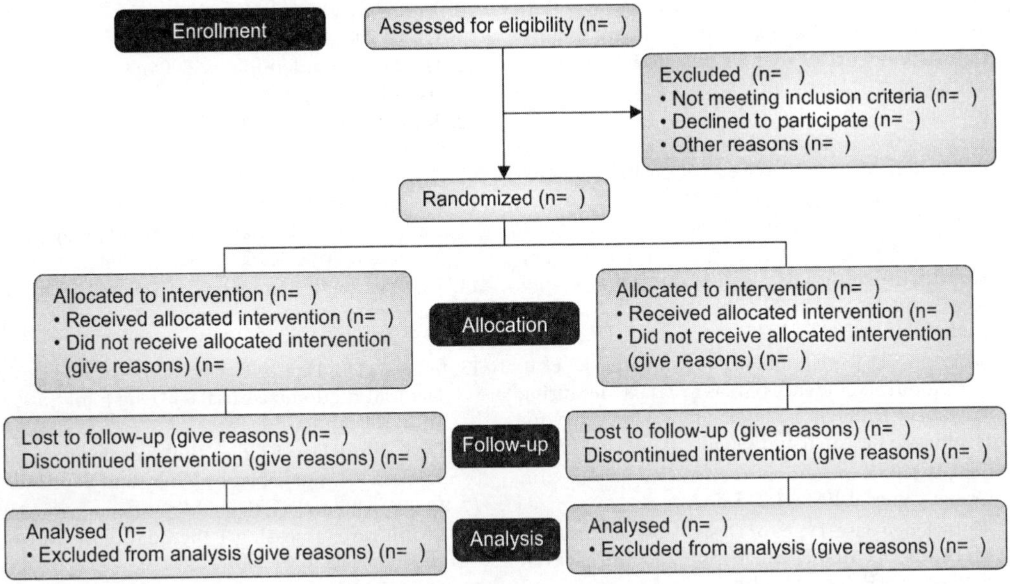

Fig. 11.8: Flow diagram CONSORT 2010

3. The rights, safety, and well-being of the trial subjects are the most important considerations and should prevail over interests of science and society.
4. The available non-clinical and clinical information on an investigational product should be adequate to support the proposed clinical trial.
5. Clinical trials should be scientifically sound, and described in a clear, detailed protocol.
6. A trial should be conducted in compliance with the protocol that has received prior institutional review board (IRB)/independent ethics committee (IEC) approval/favourable opinion.
7. The medical care given to, and medical decisions made on behalf of, subjects should always be the responsibility of a qualified physician or, when appropriate, of a qualified dentist.
8. Each individual involved in conducting a trial should be qualified by education, training, and experience to perform his or her respective task(s).
9. Freely given informed consent should be obtained from every subject prior to clinical trial participation.
10. All clinical trial information should be recorded, handled, and stored in a way that allows its accurate reporting, interpretation and verification.
11. The confidentiality of records that could identify subjects should be protected, respecting the privacy and confidentiality rules in accordance with the applicable regulatory requirement(s).
12. Investigational products should be manufactured, handled, and stored in accordance with applicable good manufacturing practice (GMP). They should be used in accordance with the approved protocol.
13. Systems with procedures that assure the quality of every aspect of the trial should be implemented."

References

1. Bull JP. The historical development of clinical therapeutic trials. J Chronic Dis 1959;10:218.

2. Lind J, James Lind. A Treatise of the Scurvy in Three Parts. Containing an inquiry into the Nature, Causes and Cure of that Disease, together with a Critical and Chronological View of what has been published on the subject. A. Millar, London, 1753.
3. Thompson CB, Edward A. Basics of Research Part 3, RN, PhD, and Panacek, MD, MPH. Research Study Designs: Experimental and Quasi-Experimental. Air Medical Journal 25:6.
4. Charles H Evans (Jr), Suzanne T Ildstad (Eds). Small Clinical Trials: Issues and Challenges. Available from: https://books.google. co.in/books?isbn = 0309073332. Accessed on: 7.7.18.
5. Berkman ND, Santaguida PL, Viswanathan M, et al. The Empirical Evidence of Bias in Trials Measuring Treatment Differences. Rockville, MD: Agency for Healthcare Research and Quality (US); 2014.
6. Schulz KF. Randomized controlled trials. Clin Obstet Gynecol 1998;41:245–56.
7. Knowledge Base-Types of Designs-Social Research Methods. Available at: https://socialresearch methods.net › destypes.php.
8. Austin Bradford Hill. "The Environment and Disease: Association or Causation?" Proceedings of the Royal Society of Medicine, 1965;58:295–300.
9. Suresh KP. An overview of randomization techniques: An unbiased assessment of outcome in clinical research. J Hum Reprod Sci 2011; 4(1):8–11.
10. Andrew J Vickers. How to randomize. J Soc Integr Oncol 2006;4(4):194–98.
11. Gordis L. Epidemiology 2004. 3rd edn. Elsevier Saunders.
12. Kao LS, Tyson JE, Blakely ML, Lally KP. Clinical Research Methodology I: Introduction to Randomized Trials. J Am Coll Surg 2008;206(2):361–69.
13. Spruance SL, Reid JE, Grace M, Samore M. Hazard Ratio in Clinical Trials. Antimicrobial agents and chemotherapy 2004;2787–92.
14. Devereaux PJ, Bhandari M, Clarke M, et al. Need for expertise based randomized controlled trials. BMJ 2005; 330:88. [PubMed: 15637373]
15. Whelan DB, Dainty K, Chahal J. Efficient designs: factorial randomized trials. J Bone Joint Surg Am. 2012;94(Suppl 1):34–38.
16. D Machin, S Day, S Green (Ed). Textbook of Clinical Trials. 2004, Published by Wiley and Sons Ltd.
17. Jüni P, Altman DG, Egger M. Systematic reviews in health care: assessing 1 the quality of controlled clinical trials. BMJ 2001;323:42–6.
18. Chan AW, Altman DG. Epidemiology and reporting of randomized trials published in PubMed journals. Lancet 2005;365:1159–62.
19. CONSORT Transparent Reporting of Trials. Available from: http://www.consort-statement.org/
20. ICH e6: GCP consolidated guidelines 1996. www.ich.org. assessed on July 2017.

Chapter

12

Confounding Including Errors in Epidemiological Studies

Paramita Sengupta

CONFOUNDING

Randomized controlled trial or randomized clinical trial is the gold standard of all epidemiological studies, yet even these may be fraught with errors. While studying the association between exposure to a cause (or risk factor) and the occurrence of disease, confounding can occur when another exposure exists in the study population and is associated both with the disease and the exposure being studied. A problem arises if this extraneous factor itself a determinant or risk factor for the health outcome is unequally distributed between the exposure subgroups is also associated with the outcome and thus can change the direction of the study. Confounding occurs when the effects of two exposures (risk factors) have not been separated, thus provides misleading estimates of effect due to one variable rather than the other.[1]

Common confounders are age and sex, followed by which is a common cause of both exposure and outcome, many disease outcomes vary by age, as do the exposures or potential risk factors, and a failure to adjust for age in an analysis is likely to distort the results. For example, if we look at age an example of confounding is: When we try to find the association of alcoholism on esophageal cancer, smoking can behave as a confounder, as we know that those who drink alcohol, often smoke cigarettes as well and smoking is an independent risk factor for esophageal cancer.

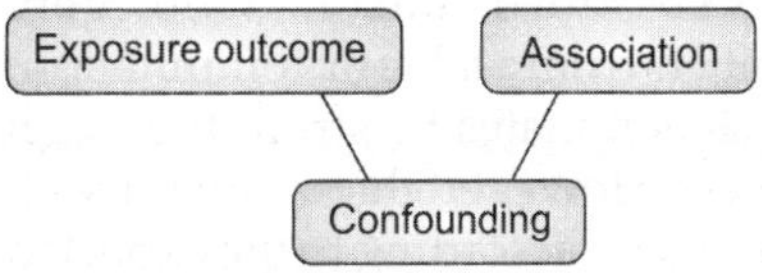

Effects of Confounding

Role of chance, bias and confounding in epidemiological studies (role of chance, bias and confounding in epidemiological studies.[2] Confounding factors can cause bias in the estimate of the exposure if not controlled for. The effects of confounding may be:

- An observed association when no real association exists.
- No observed association when a true association does exist.
- Underestimating the association (negative confounding)
- Overestimating the association (positive confounding).

Controlling for Confounding

Confounding can be addressed either at the study design stage, or adjusted for at the analysis stage providing sufficient relevant data have been collected. A number of methods can be applied to control for potential confounding factors and the aim of all of them is to make the groups as similar as possible with respect to the confounder(s).

Controlling for Confounding at the Design Stage

Potential confounding factors may be identified at the design stage based on previous studies or because a link between the factor and outcome may be considered as biologically plausible. Methods to limit confounding at the design stage include randomization, restriction and matching.

- **Randomization:** This is the best way of controlling for confounding by random allocation (e.g. using a table of random numbers) so that all potential confounding variables are distributed equally between the intervention and control groups. The best method of randomization is by a blinded third party, who generates numbers from a table or computer program, which eliminates biasfrom the assignment process. However, the sample sizes have to be adjusted according to the expected effect of the intervention, with smaller the expected effect, larger is the sample size needed to be able to conclude, with enough power that the differences are unlikely to be due to chance.[3]
- **Restriction:** Restriction limits participation in the study to individuals, who are similar in relation to the confounder. For example, if participation in a study is restricted to non-smokers only, any potential confounding effect of smoking will be eliminated. However, a disadvantage of restriction is that it may be difficult to generalize the results of the study to the wider population if the study group is homogenous.
- **Matching:** Matching involves selecting controls so that the distribution of potential confounders (e.g. age or smoking status) is as similar as possible to that amongst the cases. In practice this is only utilized in case-control studies, but it can be done in two ways:
  Pair matching—selecting for each case one or more controls with similar characteristics (e.g. same age and smoking habits).
  Frequency matching—ensuring that as a group the cases have similar characteristics to the controls.

Detecting and Controlling for Confounding at the Analysis Stage

The presence or magnitude of confounding in epidemiological studies is evaluated by observing the degree of discrepancy between the crude estimate (without controlling for confounding) and the adjusted estimate after accounting for the potential confounder(s). If the estimate has changed and there is little variation between the stratum specific ratios (*see* below), then there is evidence of confounding.

It is inappropriate to use statistical tests to assess the presence of confounding, but the following methods may be used to minimize its effect.

- **Stratification:** Stratification allows the association between exposure and outcome to be examined within different strata of the confounding variable, for example by age or sex. The strength of the association is initially measured separately within each stratum of the confounding variable. Assuming the stratum specific rates are relatively uniform, they may then be pooled to give a summary estimate as adjusted or controlled for the potential confounder. An example is the Mantel-Haenszel method. One drawback of this method is that the more the original sample is stratified, the smaller each stratum will become, and the power to detect associations is reduced.
- **Multivariate analysis:** Statistical modelling (e.g. multivariate regression analysis) is used to control for more than one confounder at the same time, and allows for the interpretation of the effect of each confounder individually. It is the most

commonly used method for dealing with confounding at the analysis stage.

- **Standardization:** Standardization accounts for confounders (generally age and sex) by using a standard reference population to negate the effect of differences in the distribution of confounding factors between study populations.
- **Residual confounding:** It is only possible to control for confounders at the analysis stage if data on confounders were accurately collected. Residual confounding occurs when all confounders have not been adequately adjusted for, either because they have been inaccurately measured, or because they have not been measured (for example, unknown confounders). An example would be socio-economic status, because it influences multiple health outcomes but is difficult to measure accurately. Small sample size in a randomized clinical trial can also lead to residual confounding. In a stratified or regression analysis there could be residual confounding if data on confounding variable was not precise enough, e.g. age was simply classified as 'young' or 'old'.
- **Interaction (effect modification):** Interaction occurs when the incidence rate of a disease in the presence of two or more risk factors differs from the incidence rate expected to result from their individual effects. For example, aspirin can be used to manage the symptoms of viral illnesses, such as influenza. However, while it may be effective in adults, aspirin use in children with viral illnesses is associated with liver dysfunction and brain damage (Reye's syndrome).[4] In this case, the effect of aspirin on managing viral illnesses is modified by age.

Where interaction exists, calculating an overall estimate of an association may be misleading. Unlike confounding, interaction is a biological phenomenon and should not be statistically adjusted for. A common method of dealing with interaction is to analyse and present the associations for each level of the third variable. In the example above, the odds of developing Reye's syndrome following aspirin use in viral illnesses would be far greater in children compared to adults, and this would highlight the role of age as an effect modifier. Interaction can be confirmed statistically, for example using a chi-square test to assess for heterogeneity in the stratum-specific estimates. However, such tests are known to have a low power for detecting interaction and a visual inspection of stratum-specific estimates is also recommended.

Risk of Bias in Randomized Controlled Trials

Bias in a RCT can be introduced even before the trial is started, in the type of problem to research on, or in the study design chosen, during the allocation of participants into study groups, the delivery of intervention, in the measurement of outcomes or during analysis. These biases can have a profound influence in the interpretation of an RCT and so treated with caution. The Cochrane Collaboration has prepared the Cochrane Risk of Bias Tool[5] to assess bias in a RCT. It comprises of six bias domains—selection bias, reporting bias, performance bias, attrition bias, detection bias and other bias, and assesses seven potential sources of bias as low risk, high risk or unclear risk of bias. The seven potential sources of bias are:

1. Random sequence generation
2. Allocation concealment
3. Blinding of participants and personnel
4. Blinding of outcome assessment
5. Incomplete outcome data
6. Selective reporting
7. Other sources of bias

Confounding by indication can occur in observational studies on the effects and side effects of drugs. This confounding arises from the fact that individuals who are prescribed a medication or who take a given medication are inherently different from those who do not take the drug because they are taking the drug for a reason. In medical terminology, such individuals have an 'indication' for use of the drug.

ERRORS IN EPIDEMIOLOGICAL STUDIES

All measurements are prone to error. Understanding common errors and the means to reduce them improves the precision of estimates.

Types of error are:

Random error: Type I error and Type II error

Type I error: Incorrect rejection of the null hypothesis and concluding that a relationship exists between two variables when actually it does not.[6]

Type II error: Incorrect acceptance of the null hypothesis even though a relationship exists between the two variables leads to type II error.

Systematic error: Bias, confounding

Random error mostly occurs due to chance and portrays the divergence of an observation from its true value leading to lack of precision in a measurement. Random errors can be estimated by statistical analysis.

Systematic errors may be of four kinds:

1. Instrumental.
2. Observational.
3. Environmental.
4. Theoretical.

Bias has been defined as "any systematic error in the design, conduct or analysis of a study that results in a mistaken estimate of an exposure's effect on the risk of disease.[7] Bias is lack of internal validity or incorrect measurement of an association between an exposure and its effect in the target population."[8]

Common Types of Bias in Epidemiological Studies

Selection Bias

Selection bias occurs when the study population does not represent the target population and there is systematic difference between selecting one or more of the study groups that will be compared. Proper randomization removes selection bias in a manner in which each study participant gets an opportunity to be allocated to either the intervention or control arm. Non-response of potential study subjects may lead to selection bias. More diseased people who were exposed to the risk factor may turn up than diseased people who were not exposed to the factor thus an apparent association could be observed even if in reality there is no association. The non-responders often differ from responders in socio-demographic, cultural, lifestyle, behavioural, socio-economic and medical characteristics. As non-response may introduce bias, it is important to keep non-response to a minimum. Selection bias can lead to invalid inferences regarding associations of exposure and disease. There is a clear cut difference between errors in selecting a study population and selection bias. Volunteers for studies mostly cause selection bias. Selection bias is an error in selecting a study group or groups within the study itself and affects internal validity whereas when we select a study population from a larger reference population, a systematic error in selecting subjects in one or more of the study groups, such as exposed or non-exposed, and may lead to loss of external validity or generalizability.

Incidence–Prevalence Bias

Incidence–prevalence bias is a type of selection bias particularly common in cross-sectional studies. This bias is also known as the Neyman bias or survival bias.

Exclusion Bias

It results when investigators apply different eligibility criteria to the cases and to the controls in regard to which clinical conditions in the past would permit eligibility in the study and which would serve as the basis for exclusion.

Random error (chance): Chance is a random error appearing to cause an association between an exposure and an outcome. A principal assumption in epidemiology is that we can draw an inference about the experience of the entire population based on the evaluation of a sample of the population. However, a problem with drawing such an inference is that the play of chance may affect the results of an epidemiological study because of the effects of random variation from sample to sample. The effect of random error may produce an estimate that is different from the true underlying value. The effect of random error may result in either an under-estimation or over-estimation of the true value.

Information Bias

Information bias arises due to errors in measuring exposure or disease. Information bias occurs in data collection stage. Misclassification bias, ecological fallacy and regression to the mean are three important types of information bias.

Misclassification refers to the classification of an individual, a value or an attribute into a category other than that to which it should be assigned.[9]

Observer Bias

Observer bias occurs when there are systematic differences in the way information is collected for the groups being studied. Observer bias may occur as a result of the investigator's prior knowledge of the hypothesis under investigation or knowledge of an individual's exposure or disease status. Such information may result in differences in the way information is collected, measured or interpretation by the investigator for each of the study groups.

Recall Bias

In a case-control study data on exposure is collected retrospectively. The quality of the data is therefore determined to a large extent on the patient's ability to accurately recall past exposures. Recall bias may occur when the information provided on exposure differs between the cases and controls. For example, an individual with the outcome under investigation (case) may report their exposure experience differently than an individual without the outcome (control) under investigation. Recall bias may result in either an under-estimate or over-estimate of the association between exposure and outcome.

Sampling bias is when the sample in question is not representative of the general population.

Measurement Errors

Measurement bias occurs when the individual measurements or classifications of disease or exposure are inaccurate—that is, they do not measure correctly what they are supposed to measure. "This may be random error due to biological/natural variation, sampling error, or non-random systematic measurement error which leads to bias may be random error due to biological/natural variation, sampling error, or non-random systematic measurement error which leads to bias.

Response Bias

Response bias (also known as 'self-selection bias') occurs when only certain types of people respond to a survey or study. When this occurs, the resulting data is biased towards those with the motivation to answer and submit the survey or participate in the study. Randomization can help in removing selection bias. RCTs are the best study designs in which selection bias does not occur.

Reducing Sampling Error

Sampling error cannot be eliminated but with an appropriate study design can be reduced to an acceptable level. The size of the expected effect of the intervention is one of the major determinants of the sample size necessary to conduct a successful trial.[10] In general, sampling error decreases as the sample size increases. The smaller the expected effect of the intervention, the larger the sample size needed to be able to conclude, with enough power, that the differences are unlikely to be due to chance. Therefore, use of an appropriate sample size will reduce the degree to which chance variability may account for the results observed in a study.

The role of chance can be assessed by performing appropriate statistical tests and by calculation of confidence intervals. The p value will depend on both the magnitude of the association and on the study size. Confidence intervals are more informative than p values because they provide a range of values, which is likely to include the true population effect. They also indicate whether a non-significant result is or is not compatible with a true effect that was not detected because the sample size was too small.

Blinding

Blinding is the purposeful concealment of the group allocation from one or more individuals involved in a clinical research study, most commonly a randomized controlled trial. Blinding helps in removing placebo effect, which has a significant impact on the measured outcomes. Blinding patients to the treatment they have received in a controlled trial is particularly important when the response criteria are subjective, such as alleviation of pain, but less important for objective criteria, such as death. If two active compounds are to be used, blinding is possible using the 'double dummy' method. Two active medicines can be compared by giving two different coloured tablets to both the groups, one given as active compound, the other as placebo and vice versa.[11]

In a single blind trial, either the investigator or participant is unaware of which treatment the participant is taking. In a double blind trial neither patient nor the caregivers are aware of the treatment assignment. Blinding means more than just keeping the name of the treatment hidden. Triple blind study is where the treatment is unknown to the research participant, the investigators and also the assessors of the outcome (Table 12.1).

Hawthorne Effect

The Hawthorne effect is a change in the trial respondents' behaviour or outcomes that is not directly attributable to the therapeutic treatment regimen received, but simply to the awareness of being in a research study. The Hawthorne effect derived its name from a study of the psychological aspects plus physical and environmental influences in the workplace at the Hawthorne Plant of the Western Electric Company in Cicero, Illinois, during the 1920s.

Workers increased their productivity when they were studied, but it declined when the study finished.[12] This may be random error due to biological/natural variation, sampling error, or non-random systematic measurement error which leads to bias.

Heuristics and Cognitive Biases

When interpreting data, a researcher must avoid cognitive bias and be aware of the use of heuristics to avoid drawing incorrect conclusions. Heuristics are defined as mental shortcuts developed by a clinician over time and include recognizing patterns of disease, case experience, intuitive judgment, and 'rule-of-thumb' applications.[13] This is useful in assimilating large amounts of information and summarizing these into salient points. Study publication bias and outcome reporting bias—studies that report positive or significant results are more likely to be published and outcomes that are statistically significant have higher odds of being fully reported (Table 12.2).

Table 12.1: Types of blinding and their description

Type	*Description*
Unblinded or open label	All are aware of the treatment the participant receives
Single blind or single-masked	Only the participant is unaware of the treatment they receive
Double blind or double-masked	The participant and the clinicians/data collectors are unaware of the treatment the participant receives
Triple blind	Participant, clinicians/data collectors and outcome adjudicators/data analysts are all unaware of the treatment the participant receives.

Table 12.2: Cognitive biases and descriptions[16]

Cognitive bias	*Description*
Anchoring	Placing emphasis on salient features too early in the diagnostic process with a failure to adjust the initial impression in light of new information.
Ascertainment bias	Occur when a physician's thinking is shaped by prior expectation (gender or stereotyping are examples).
Availability	A disposition to considering diagnoses which more readily come to mind (sometimes dictated by recent experience). If a disease has not been seen for a long time (less available), it may be missed.
Confirmation bias	The tendency to look for evidence 'confirming' a diagnosis rather than disconfirming evidence to refute it.
Diagnostic momentum	Once diagnostic labels are attached to the patient, they can gather momentum and make it harder to change course
Hindsight bias	An inability to realistically appraise past events once the outcome becomes known. This compromises learning in the context of diagnostic error.
Omission bias	A tendency toward inaction grounded in the principle of 'Do No Harm.' Progression of disease is then attributed to its natural history rather than physician inaction.
Overconfidence bias	A common tendency to believe "we know more than we do." This can be augmented by anchoring and availability biases.
Premature closure	Cognitive error in diagnosis (CDR) accounts for a high proportion of missed diagnoses. "When the diagnosis is made, the thinking stops."
Representativeness restraint	Restraining decision-making along pattern recognition only may miss atypical disease.
Triage cueing	Either through patient self-triaging or within the healthcare system, this sends the patient in a particular direction and may start the process of diagnostic momentum.
Visceral bias	A 'first impression' on meeting the patient may generate positive or negative feelings which may affect decision-making.
Zebra retreat	The hesitation with which one may consider a rare diagnosis even though it may be the most likely.

The Pygmalion effect,[14] or Rosenthal effect, is the phenomenon whereby higher expectations lead to an increase in performance. Participants receiving **positive feedback perform well.** The **Pygmalion effect** (also called the ***Galatea effect***) originates with researchers Robert Rosenthal and Lenore Jacobsen in 1968. The **Rosenthal effect,** also called the ***experimenter expectancy effect,***[15] is a special case of the Pygmalion effect that pertains to experiments and experimenter bias. If a researcher believes that their experiment is likely to results in a particular outcome, that bias will have an effect how the researcher conducts their work. The results will very likely sway towards the direction the researcher wanted, invalidating any study results.

- Design the experiment properly.
- Have clear rules and procedures in place.
- Make sure behaviours are clearly defined.
- Set a time frame for—data collection, for the duration of the experiment, and for experimental parts.

Placebo effect: It is a beneficial effect produced by a placebo drug or treatment, which cannot be attributed to the properties of the placebo itself, and must therefore, be due to the patient's belief in that treatment.

Placebo is a substance with no known medical effects, such as sterile water, saline solution, or a sugar pill. When this response to a fake treatment occurs, many patients have no idea that they are responding to what is essentially a 'sugar pill.' Placebos are often utilized in medical research to help doctors and scientists discover and better understand the physiological and psychological effects of new medications.

Internal validity is concerned with the rigor (and thus the degree of control) of the study design. Threats to internal validity compromise our confidence in saying that a relationship exists between the independent and dependent variables. Eight threats to internal validity have been defined: History, maturation, testing, instrumentation, regression, selection, experimental mortality, and an interaction of threats. Threats to external validity compromise our confidence in stating whether the study's results are applicable to other groups.

Threats to External Validity

External validity is related to generalizing. An externally valid study is one in which the data and conclusions gathered from the results of an experiment can be applied to the general population outside of the experiment itself. A study's external validity can be threatened by such factors as small sample sizes, high variability, and sampling bias. A threat to external validity is an explanation of how you might be wrong in making a generalization. There are three major threats to external validity because there are three ways you could be wrong—people, places or times. Critiques may argue that the results of your study are due to the unusual type of people who were in the study, or the unusual place where the study was conducted, or a peculiar time.

Improving External Validity

Random selection, rather than a non-random procedure is important for drawing a sample from a population. Keeping the dropout rates low, or using the theory of proximal similarity more effectively, by describing the ways the contexts differ, providing lots of data about the degree of similarity between various groups of people, places, and even times. The external validity (ability to generalize) will be stronger if we are able to replicate our study.

The Single Group Threats

Single group threats occur if there is a certain level of post-test achievement or a change or gain from pre-test to post-test. Here are some of the ways, some of the threats to interval validity that your critics might raise, some of the plausible alternative explanations for your observed effect:

- **History threat:** If any unanticipated event has occurred during the progress of the experiment and these events affected the dependent variable, a history threat occurs. History is a threat for the one group design but not for the two-group design. If the history threat occurs for both groups, the difference between the two groups will not be due to the history event. In a one group pre-post test design, the treatment effect is the difference in the pre-test and post-test scores which may be due to the treatment or history.
- **Maturation threat:** Here the changes in the dependent variables are due to normal developmental processes operating within the subject as a function of time. For example, if we are looking at the effect of food supplementation on malnutrition, the effect may be due to normal development of the child rather than to food supplementation. In general, if we're talking about a specific event or chain of events that could cause the outcome, we call it a history threat. If we're talking about all of the events that typically transpire in one's life over a period of time, we call it a maturation threat.
- **Testing threat:** This threat only occurs in the pre-post design. Sometimes appearing for a pre-test in a training program for health workers makes some of them more aware of the contents of the training and it

'primed' them for the program so that when the said training is conducted, they are ready for it in a way that they wouldn't have been without the pre-test. This is what is meant by a testing threat—taking the pre-test (not getting your program) affects how participants do on the post-test.

- **Instrumentation threat:** Like the testing threat, this threat only operates in the pre-test–post-test situation, if any change occurred during the study in the way the dependent variable was measured or a change in the test that was used. It can also happen if there was contamination and the comparison group found out about the experimental group or wanted to make the research succeed or fail. Pre-post gain is attributable to the change in instrument, not to the program or intervention. Instrument threat mostly occurs if the 'instrument' is a human observer, either because they don't use the exact same test but 'alternate forms' of the same tests, or if two examiners administered the post-test with different instructions and procedures, or there is different difficulty level in the tests or if the observers get tired or bored with the repeated observations, or even the older observers may be better at making the observations as they have more practice.
- **Selection threat:** This appears if the groups are not equivalent at the beginning of the study. If one group is better off than the other group in some manner like in their level of skills, then there will be selection threat. If subjects were selected by random sampling and random assignment, all would have equal chance of being in treatment or comparison groups, and the groups would have been equivalent.
- **Mortality threat:** Mortality threat is due to people dropping out of the study. There should be same number of participants during the entire study period in both experimental and comparison groups. For example, if a study involves pre-test and post-test scores, the score in pre-test would be lower and may dropout. The potential low scorers who had dropped out after pre-test, will not be appearing for the posttest, or, one would be artificially inflating the post-test average over what it would have been if no students had dropped out. This problem would not be solved by comparing pre–post averages for only those kids who stayed in the study. This subsample would certainly not be representative even of the original entire sample. Furthermore, we know that because of regression threats (see below) these students may appear to actually do worse on the post-test, simply as an artifact of the non-random dropout or mortality in your study. When mortality is a threat, the researcher can often gauge the degree of the threat by comparing the dropout group against the non-dropout group on pre-test measures. If there are no major differences, it may be more reasonable to assume that mortality was happening across the entire sample and is not biasing results greatly. But if the pre-test differences are large, one must be concerned about the potential biasing effects of mortality.
- **Regression threat:** Statistical regression—in an experiment involving reading instruction, subjects grouped because of poor pre-test reading scores show considerably greater gain than do the groups who scored average and high on the pre-test. A regression threat, also known as a 'regression artifact' or 'regression to the mean' is a statistical phenomenon that occurs whenever you have a non-random sample from a population and two measures that are imperfectly correlated. The regression threat means that the pre-test average for the group in your study will appear to increase or improve (relatively to the overall population) even if you don't do anything to them—even if you never give them a treatment. Regression is a confusing threat to understand at first. It is 'you can only go up from here' phenomenon. If you include in your program only the kids who constituted the lowest 10% of the class on the pre-test, what are the chances that they

would constitute exactly the lowest 10% on the post-test? Not likely. Most of them would score low on the post-test, but they aren't likely to be the lowest 10% twice. For instance, maybe there were a few kids on the pre-test who got lucky on a few guesses and scored at the eleventh percentile who would not get so lucky next time. No, if you choose the lowest 10% on the pre-test, they can not get any lower than being the lowest—they can only go up from there, relative to the larger population from which they were selected. This purely statistical phenomenon is what we mean by a regression threat.

Removal of single group threats to internal validity is by incorporating a good research design, which can be done by introducing a control group. Out of the two groups one will receive the intervention and the other one doesn't. In this way, the control group will experience the same history and maturation threats, would have the same testing and instrumentation issues, and would have similar rates of mortality and regression to the mean. Hence, the most effective way of ruling out single-group threats to internal validity is a good control group.

Multiple Group Threats to Internal Validity

A multiple-group design typically involves at least two groups and before-after measurement. Most often, one group receives the program or treatment while the other does not and constitutes the 'control' or comparison group. But sometimes one group gets the program and the other gets either the standard program or another program you would like to compare. In this case, you would be comparing two programs for their relative outcomes. Typically you would construct a multiple group design so that you could compare the groups directly. In such designs, the key internal validity issue is the degree to which the groups are comparable before the study. If they are comparable, and the only difference between them is the program, post-test differences can be attributed to the program. But that is a big if the groups are not comparable to begin with, you would not know how much of the outcome to attribute to your program or to the initial differences between groups.

There really is only one multiple group threat to internal validity: That the groups were not comparable before the study. We call this threat a **selection bias** or **selection threat**. A selection threat is any factor other than the program that leads to post-test differences between groups.

Whenever we suspect that outcomes differ between groups not because of our program but because of prior group differences we are suspecting a selection bias. Although the term 'selection bias' is used as the general category for all prior differences, when we know specifically what the group difference is, we usually hyphenate it with the 'selection' term. The multiple-group selection threats directly parallel the single group threats. For instance, while we have 'history' as a single group threat, we have 'selection-history' as its multiple-group analogue.

As with the single group threats to internal validity, we'll assume a simple example involving a new compensatory mathematics tutoring program for first graders. The design will be a pre-test–post-test design, and we will divide the first graders into two groups, one getting the new tutoring program and the other not getting it.

The multiple-group threats to internal validity are:

- **Selection-history threat:** A selection-history threat is any event occurring differently in the pre-test and post-test groups that the groups experience differently. A selection threat, indicates that the groups differ in some way. And a 'history' threat indicates that the groups differ is with respect to their reactions to history events. If we are measuring hemoglobin status of children, but the eating habits of the two groups of children are different, leading one group to have more iron rich foods, thus affecting their hemoglobin status.

- **Selection-maturation threat:** A selection-maturation threat results from differential rates of normal growth between pre-test and post-test for the groups. In this case, the two groups are different in their different rates of maturation with respect to math concepts. It is important to distinguish between history and maturation threats. In general, history refers to a discrete event or series of events whereas maturation implies the normal, ongoing developmental process that would take place. In any case, if the groups are maturing at different rates with respect to the outcome, we cannot assume that pos-test differences are due to our program—they may be selection-maturation effects.
- **Selection-testing threat:** A selection-testing threat occurs when there is a differential effect between groups on the post-test of taking the pre-test. Perhaps the test 'primed' the children in each group differently or they may have learned differentially from the pre-test. In these cases, an observed post-test difference cannot be attributed to the program, they could be the result of selection-testing.
- **Selection-instrumentation threat:** Selection-instrumentation refers to any differential change in the test used for each group from pre-test and post-test. In other words, the test changes differently for the two groups. Perhaps the test consists of observers who rate the class performance of the children. What if the program group observers, for example, get better at doing the observations while, over time, the comparison group observers get fatigued and bored. Differences on the post-test could easily be due to this differential instrumentation—selection-instrumentation—and not to the program.
- **Selection-mortality threat:** Selection-mortality arises when there is *differential* non-random one group is more extreme on the pre-test than the other. If we take malnourished and normally nourished children, mostly the malnourished ones will appear to improve because of regression to the mean and they will appear to gain more than their normal counterparts. This is not a real program gain, it is just a selection-regression threat. To remove this threat, the groups have to be comparable. If we randomly assign persons in our sample into the two groups, and thus conduct a randomized or 'true' experiment, then we can say that they are comparable. In some cases we can't randomly assign because of financial constraints or ethical issues. Studies in which random assignment has not been used may not be equivalent such designs are called quasi-experimental designs.

Social Threats to Internal Validity

Though multiple group designs assure that the groups are comparable, it cannot be assumed that there is strong internal validity as there are a number of social threats to internal validity. Here the treatment itself does not directly cause the post-test differences. Social threats to internal validity occur when the different program and comparison groups carrying out the research are aware of each other's roles in the research. Isolating the two groups from each other can be minimize this type of threats.

- **Diffusion or imitation of treatment:** This occurs when a comparison group learns about the program either directly or indirectly from program group participants. In a school context, children from different groups within the same school might share experiences during lunch hour. Students of comparison group might set-up their own experience to try to imitate that of the program group. In either case, if the diffusion of imitation affects the post-test performance of the comparison group, it can have jeopardize your ability to assess whether your program is causing the outcome. Notice that this threat to validity tends to equalize the outcomes between groups, minimizing the chance of seeing a program effect even if there is one.

- **Compensatory rivalry:** Here, the comparison group knows what the program group is getting and develops a competitive attitude with them. The students in the comparison group might see the special math tutoring program, the program group is getting and feel jealous. This could lead them to deciding to compete with the program group 'just to show them' how well they can do. Sometimes, in contexts like these, the participants are even encouraged by well-meaning teachers or administrators to compete with each other (while this might make educational sense as a motivation for the students in both groups to work harder, it works against our ability to see the effects of the program). If the rivalry between groups affects post-test performance, it could make it more difficult to detect the effects of the program. As with diffusion and imitation, this threat generally works in the direction of equalizing the post-test performance across groups, increasing the chance.
- **Resentful demoralization:** This is almost the opposite of compensatory rivalry. Here, students in the comparison group know what the program group is getting. But here, instead of developing a rivalry, they get discouraged or angry and they give up (sometimes referred to as the 'screw you' effect!). Unlike the previous two threats, this one is likely to exaggerate post-test differences between groups, making your program look even more effective than it actually is.
- **Compensatory equalization of treatment:** This is the only threat of the four that primarily involves the people who help manage the research context rather than the participants themselves. When program and comparison group participants are aware of each other's conditions they may wish they were in the other group (depending on the perceived desirability of the program it could work either way). Often they or their parents or teachers will put pressure on the administrators to have them reassigned to the other group. The administrators may begin to feel that the allocation of goods to the groups is not 'fair' and may be pressured to or independently undertake to compensate one group for the perceived advantage of the other. If the special math tutoring program was being done with state-of-the-art computers, you can bet that the parents of the children assigned to the traditional non-computerized comparison group will pressure the principal to 'equalize' the situation. Perhaps the principal will give the comparison group some other good, or let them have access to the computers for other subjects. If these 'compensating' programs equalize the groups on post-test performance, it will tend to work against your detecting an effective program even when it does work. For instance, a compensatory program might improve the self-esteem of the comparison group and eliminate your chance to discover whether the math program would cause changes inself-esteem relative to traditional math training. The threats described here can often be minimized by constructing multiple groups that are not aware of each other (e.g. program group from one school, comparison group from another) or by training administrators in the importance of preserving group membership and not instituting equalizing programs. But we will never be able to entirely eliminate the possibility that human interactions are making it more difficult for us to assess cause–effect relationships.

References

1. Bonita R, Beaglehole R, Kjellström T. Basic epidemiology, WHO 2006. 2nd edn.
2. Epidemiology for Practitioners. Available from: https://www.healthknowledge.org.uk/e-learning/.../chance-bias-confounding. Accessed on: 25/8/18
3. Freedman KB, Back S, Bernstein J. Sample size and statistical power of randomized, controlled trials in orthopaedics. J Bone Joint Surg Br 2001;83(3): 397–402.

4. MacMohan B. Concepts of multiple factors. In: Lee DH, Kotin P (Eds). Multiple factors in the causation of environmentally induced disease. New York, Academic Press, 1972.
5. Dwan K, Altman DG, Arnaiz JA, et al. Systematic review of the empirical evidence of study publication bias and outcome reporting bias. PLoS One 2008;3(8):e3081.
6. Bhandari M, Sanchet IPK. Clinical research made easy-A guide to publishing in medical literature. 2nd edn. Jaypee, New Delhi, India.
7. Leon Gordis. Epidemiology. 5th edn.
8. Miguel Delgado-Rodriguez, Javier Llorca. Bias. J Epidemiol Community Health 2004;58:635–41.

9a. Hennekens CH, Buring JE. Epidemiology in Medicine, Lippincott Williams and Wilkins, 1987.

9b. Carneiro I, Howard N. Introduction to Epidemiology. Open University Press, 2011. http://www.edmundjessop.org.uk/fulltext.doc-Accessed 20/02/16.

10. Kirkwood B. Essentials of Medical Statistics. Blackwell Science, 2003.
11. Day SJ, Altman DG. Statistics Notes. Blinding in clinical trials and other studies. BMJ 2000;321: 19–26.
12. Sedgwick Philip. The Hawthorne effect. BMJ 2011; 344:d8262 doi: 10.1136/bmj.d8262.
13. Harvey N. Use of heuristics: Insights from forecasting research, Think Reason 2007;13(1):5–24.
14. Cohen JM, Burgin S. Cognitive biases in clinical decision making: A primer for the practicing dermatologist. JAMA Dermatol 2016;152(3):253–254.
15. Pygmalion Effect/Rosenthal Effect: Definition, Examples. Available at: www.statisticshowto.com/pygmalion-effect-rosenthal/. Accessed on: 12.7.18.
16. Rosenthal R, Fode KL. The effect of experimenter bias on the performance of the albino rat. Behavioral science 1963;8:183–89.

Chapter

13

Epidemiological Statistics

Ram Chandra Goyal

BACKGROUND

Basic forms of statistics have been used since the beginning of civilization. Early empires often collated censuses of the population or recorded the trade in various commodities. The general principles of the science of health statistics, as of most others, were foreshadowed by the ancient Greeks, who carefully observed, recorded and analyzed natural phenomena, and applied the inductive method of reasoning in a search for natural rather than supernatural causes, treating the unproven with skepticism.

The use of statistical methods dates back to least to the 5th century BCE. The historian Thucydides in his History of the Peloponnesian War describes how the Athenians calculated the height of the wall of Platea by counting the number of bricks in an unplastered section of the wall several times. The most frequent value (in modern terminology—the **mode**) was taken as final count. Multiplying this value by the height of the bricks used in the wall allowed the Athenians to determine the height of the ladders necessary to scale the walls.[1]

In the Mahabharata, the Story of Nala-King Rtuparna estimated the number of fruit and leaves (2095 fruit and 50,000,000—five crore leaves) on two great branches of a Vibhitaka tree by counting them on a single twig. This number was then multiplied by the number of twigs on the branches. This estimate was later checked and found to be very close to the actual number. With knowledge of this method Nala was subsequently able to regain his kingdom.

Collection, classification, presentation, analysis and interpretation of the data and correlation concepts in statistics will be taken into consideration and they will be related with the concepts, instances mentioned in Ayurvedic authoritative textbooks like Charaka Samhita, Sushruta Samhita, and Ashtanga Hrudaya, hence proving the essence of statistics in Ayurveda.[2]

The earliest writing on statistics was found in a 9th-century book entitled: "Manuscript on Deciphering Cryptographic Messages", written by Al-Kindi (801–873 CE). In his book, Al-Kindi gave a detailed description of how to use statistics and analysis to decipher encrypted messages. This text arguably gave rise to the birth of both statistics and cryptanalysis.

The **arithmetic mean**, although a concept known to the Greeks, was not generalised to more than two values until the 16th century. The invention of the decimal system by Simon Stevin in 1585 seems likely to have facilitated these calculations. This method was first adopted in astronomy by Tycho Brahe who was attempting to reduce the errors in his estimates of the locations of various celestial bodies.

The idea of the **median** originated in Edward Wright's book on navigation (Certain Errors in Navigation) in 1599 in a section concerning the determination of location with a compass. Wright felt that this value was the most likely to be the correct value in a series of observations.

The *science* of epidemiology, which took shape in the wake of the great epidemics of the 1800s, developed analytical tools and statistical methods in order to trace the health and disease profile in small or large population groups. From a modest beginning in the 19th century, epidemiology developed in four phases, but phases that have overlapped one other:

1. The Era of Sanitary Epidemiology from the 1850s.
2. The Era of Infectious Disease Epidemiology from the 1880s.
3. The Era of Chronic Disease Epidemiology from the 1950s.
4. The Era of Risk Factor Epidemiology from the 1980s.[3]

So far in the 21st century, epidemiology – which currently deals to a great extent with *Risk Factor Epidemiology*—is extremely specialized and requires insight into complicated mathematical methods and statistical analyses. As such, it is as a rule inaccessible to the ordinary citizen, and furthermore, many of us demand broader analyses of epidemiological data related to qualitative assessments.[3]

John Graunt, a British merchant, categorized the cause of death of the London populace using statistical sampling, noting that "considering that it is esteemed an evenly, whether any man lived 10 years longer, supposed it was the same, that one of any 10 might die within 1 year." He also noted the reason for doing this—to "set down how many died of each (notorious disease)... those persons may better understand the hazard they are in. Graunt's statistics can be compared to recent data from the United States in 1993. As a result of this work, the government of the United Kingdom set-up the first government-sponsored statistical sampling service.[4]

The seventeenth and eighteenth century witnessed the growth of sanitary engineering and public health. This improvement had the greatest impact on human health through improved water supplies, waste removal, and living and working conditions.

John Snow performed the first recorded modern epidemiological study in 1854 during a cholera epidemic in London. He found that a particular water pump was the source of the epidemic and was being contaminated by sewage dumped into the River Thames. This type of data gathering in medicine was rare up to that time.

The nineteenth century saw the development of modern physiology (Bernard) anesthesia (Morton), antisepsis (Lister and Semmelweis), X-rays (Roentgen), the germ theory (Pasteur and Koch), and psychiatric theory (Freud).

The twentieth century saw an explosion of medical technology. Specifics include the discovery of modern medicines (Erlich), antibiotics (sulfanilamide by Domagk and penicillin by Fleming), and modern hemotherapeutic agents to treat ancient scourges like diabetes (insulin by Banting, Best, and McLeod), cancer, and hypertension. The modern era of surgery has led to open-heart surgery, joint replacement, and organ transplantation. Advances in medicine continue a tan ever-increasing rate. Why weren't physicians using statistics in medicine?[4]

Before the middle of the twentieth century, advances in medicine and conclusions about human illness occurred mainly through the study of anatomy and physiology. The **case study** or **case series** was a common way to 'prove' that a treatment was beneficial or that a certain aetiology was the cause of an illness. The use of statistical sampling techniques took a while to develop. There were intense battles between those physicians who wanted to use statistical sampling and those who believed in the power of inductive reasoning from physiological experiments.

Pierre Simon Laplace put forward the idea (1814), that essentially all knowledge was uncertain and therefore, probabilistic in nature. The work of Pierre Charles Alexandre Louis (1838) on typhoid and diphtheria showed that bleeding (the most important medical therapeutic tool of the time) was not beneficial in the treatment of these diseases. On the other side was Francois Double (1835) who felt that treatment of the individual was more important that knowing what happens to groups of patients. The art of medicine was defined as deductions from experience and induction from physiologic mechanisms. These were felt to be more important than the 'calculus of probability.' This debate continued for over 100 years in France, Germany, Britain, and the United States.

To summarize, the tradition of epidemiological study through observation and the use of vital statistics dates back to the 18th century in Britain. At the close of the 19th century, however, a new and more sophisticated statistical approach emerged, from a base in the discipline of mathematics, which was eventually to transform the practice of epidemiology.[4]

WHAT AND WHY EPIDEMIOLOGICAL STATISTICS?[5]

Epidemiological statistics is a subset of statistics with its applications to epidemiological studies wherein systematic collection, analyses, interpretation and drawing conclusions from information.

The information so generated may be used for the following.

Design: Planning and carrying out research studies.

Description: Summarizing and exploring data.

Inference: Making predictions and generalizing about phenomena represented by the data.

Epidemiological statistics is being used to study the efficiency, effectiveness, impact of various health programs, demography issues and not only limited to epidemics/clinical trials.

Categories of Statistics

The data collected in the study need to be systematically analyzed so that trend and patterns of relationship can be detected. Statistical procedures enable the investigator to summarize, organize, interpret and communicate numeric information. The statistics are classified in the following categories.

Descriptive statistics: Descriptive statistics consist of methods for organizing and summarizing information (Weiss, 1999).

Inferential statistics: Inferential statistics consist of methods for drawing and measuring the reliability of conclusions about population based on information obtained from a sample of the population. (Weiss, 1999).

In epidemiology, variables are considered in terms of description or presentation, and relationships. The allocation of specific variables into the specific classes is relative. It depends upon the level of knowledge, study questions and methodology (Table 13.1 and Fig. 13.1).

Variable

Variable is a characteristic of a person, object or phenomenon which can take on different values. These may be in the form of numbers (e.g. age, height, weight) or non-numerical characteristics (e.g. sex, race, colour of eyes, marital status, etc.).[5–7]

Independent Variables and Dependent Variables

The independent variable is called 'independent', because it is independent of the outcome being measured. More specifically, the independent variable is what causes or influences the outcome. The dependent variable is called 'dependent' because it is influenced by the independent variable.

In other terms: **Dependent variable** (syn—effect, criterion, criterion measure, outcome, output variable) is a response that the researcher wanted to predict.

Independent variable (syn—treatment, experimental. predictor, input, exposure.

Table 13.1: Types of variables and their sub-types

Types of variable	*Sub-types*	*Examples*
Quantitative (numerical)	Discrete	No. of children, no. of vehicles, no. of trees, etc.
	Continuous	Height, weight, temperature, etc.
Qualitative (non-numerical)	Categorical	
	i. Nominal	Ordinal: Stages of cancer, low or high education
	ii. Ordinal	Nominal: Opinion of people

explanatory variable) is a stimulus or activity that is identified or manipulated to predict the dependent variable.

The assumptions regarding the association that the independent precedes the dependent variable and there is a cause and effect relationship between the two (Fig. 13.1).

Controlled extraneous variables are recognized before the study is initiated and are controlled in the design and selection criteria.

Uncontrolled extraneous variables (confounding) are recognized before the study is initiated or, sometimes, even if recognized cannot be controlled in the design and selection phase.

Details of the variables are beyond the scope of this chapter, readers are advised to read from the references given at the end of the chapter.

ORGANIZATION OF THE DATA

Keen observation is the key determinant in epidemiology so in statistics. Observation of any values of the variables results in data and collection of all observations for particular variables is called a data set or data matrix.

Data set are the values of variables recorded for a set of sampling units. Values of the qualitative variable are often coded by assigning numbers to the different categories and thus converting the categorical data to numerical data.

For example, educational status might be coded as 1, 2, 3, and 4 depicts primary, secondary, graduate, and postgraduate still continues to be nominal data.

In data matrix, all the values of variables are organized in column and observations form a row.

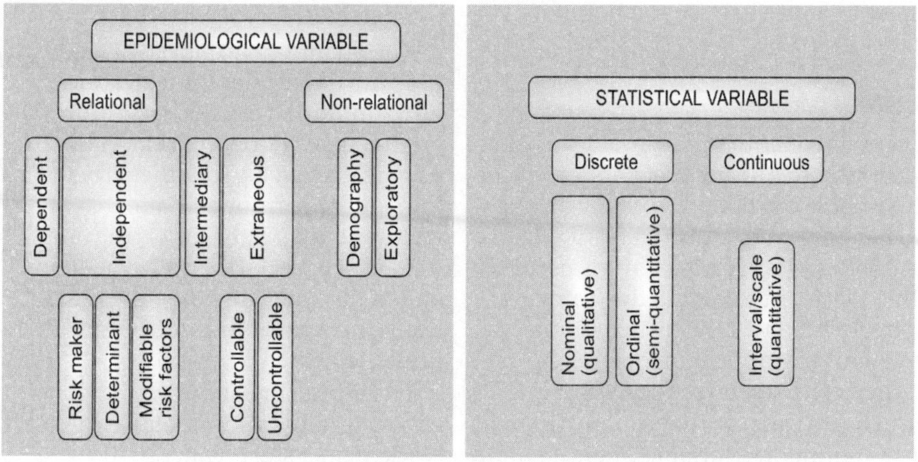

Fig. 13.1: Dependent and independent variables and their subtypes[7]

DESCRIBING THE DATA[5,6]

Descriptive Statistics

These are used to describe and synthesize data. It includes frequency counts, tables, graphs, averages, minimum, maximum, range, SD, and percentages are some examples of the descriptive statistics.

Qualitative Variable

The number of observations that fall into particular class (or category) of the qualitative variable is called the **frequency (or count)** of that class. A table listing all classes and their frequencies is called a frequency distribution.

The **percentage** can be calculated by dividing the frequency of the class by the total number of observations and multiplying the result by 100. The percentage of the class, expressed as a decimal, is usually referred to as the **relative frequency** of the class.

A table listing all classes and their relative frequencies is called a relative frequency distribution, which is sum to 1 (100%).

A **cumulative frequency** (cumulative relative frequency) is obtained by summing the frequencies (relative frequencies) of all classes up to the specific class. In a case of qualitative variables, cumulative frequencies generally used for ordinal variables, not for nominal variables.

The qualitative data are presented graphically either as a pie chart or as a horizontal or vertical bar graph.

Quantitative Variable

The data of the quantitative variable can also presented by a frequency distribution. If the discrete variable can obtain only few different values, then it can be summarized in a same way as qualitative variables in a frequency table. In a place of the qualitative categories, list in a frequency table the distinct numerical measurements that appear in the discrete data set and then count their frequencies.

If the discrete variables have more different values or continuous variable, then the data must be grouped into classes (categories) before the table of frequencies can be formed.

The main steps in a process of grouping quantitative variable into classes are:

Step 1: Find the minimum and the maximum values variable have in the data set

Step 2: Choose intervals of equal length that cover the range between the minimum and the maximum without overlapping. These are called **class intervals**, and their end points are called **class limits**.

Step 3: Count the number of observations in the data that belongs to each class interval. The count in each class is the class frequency.

Step 4: Calculate the relative frequencies of each class by dividing the class frequency by the total number of observations in the data.

The number in the middle of the class is called **class mark of the class**. The number in the middle of the upper class limit of one class and the lower class limit of the other class is called the real class limit. As a rule of thumb, it is generally satisfactory to group observed values of numerical variable in a data into 5 to 15 class intervals.

A smaller number of intervals is used if number of observations is relatively small; if the number of observations is large, the number on intervals may be greater than 15.

The quantitative data are usually presented graphically either as a **histogram or as a horizontal or vertical bar graph**. The histogram is like a horizontal bar graph except that its bars do touch each other. The histogram is formed from grouped data, displaying either frequencies or relative frequencies (percentages) of each class interval. If quantitative data is discrete with only few possible values, then the variable should graphically be presented by a bar graph.

Example: Frequency distribution table showing educational status of the factory workers in a steel plant.

Educational status	*Frequency*	*Percentage*
Illiterate	650	24.07
Primary	750	27.78
Secondary	550	20.37
Higher secondary	400	14.82
Graduate	235	08.70
Postgraduate	115	04.26
Total	**2700**	**100.00**

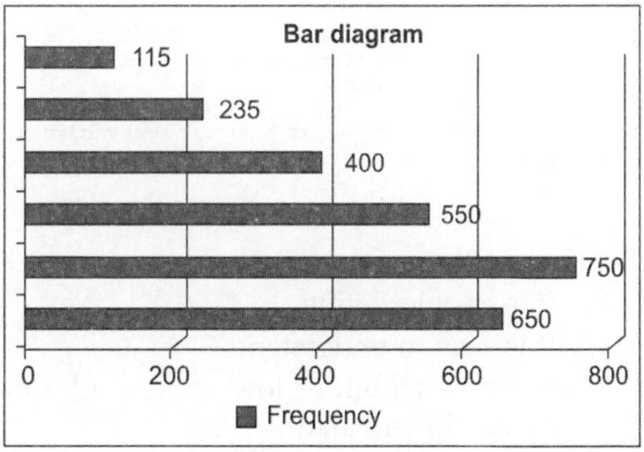

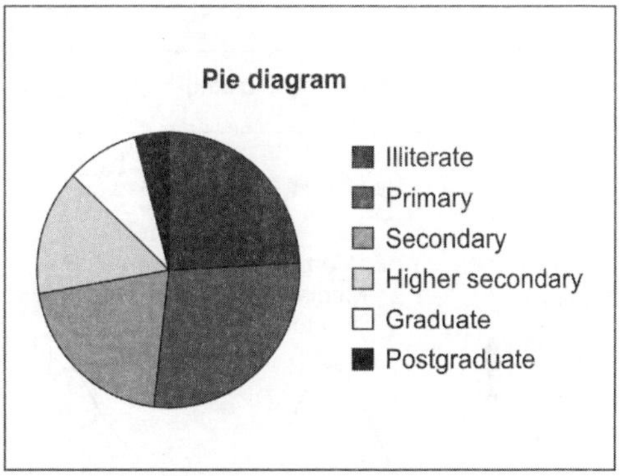

Example: Age-wise distribution of patients admitted in a tertiary care hospital

Age groups (in years)	*Frequency*	*Percentages*	*Cumulative %*
0–10	75	06.00	06.00
11–20	180	14.40	20.40
21–30	275	22.00	42.40
31–40	325	26.00	68.40
41–50	190	15.20	83.60
51–60	85	06.80	90.40
61–70	55	04.40	94.80
71–80	40	03.20	98.00
80–90	25	02.00	100.00
Total	**1250**	**100.00**	

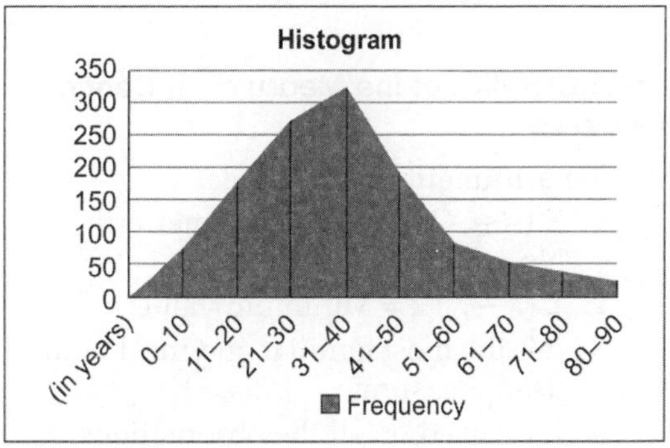

Sample and Population Distributions

Population distribution: Frequency distributions for a variable apply to a population.

Sample distribution: Frequency distributions for a variable apply to samples. As the sample size increases, we are closer to the true population. There are symmetrical distribution (bell shaped—normal distribution curve and U-shaped—distribution curve) (Fig. 13.2) and asymmetrical distribution (positive and negative distribution curve) (Fig. 13.3).[5,6]

MEASURES OF CENTRAL TENDENCY[6,8–11]

Average is a general term which describes the centre of a series. There are three common types of average or measures of central position or central tendency. The median and the mean apply only to quantitative data, whereas the mode can be used with either quantitative or qualitative data.

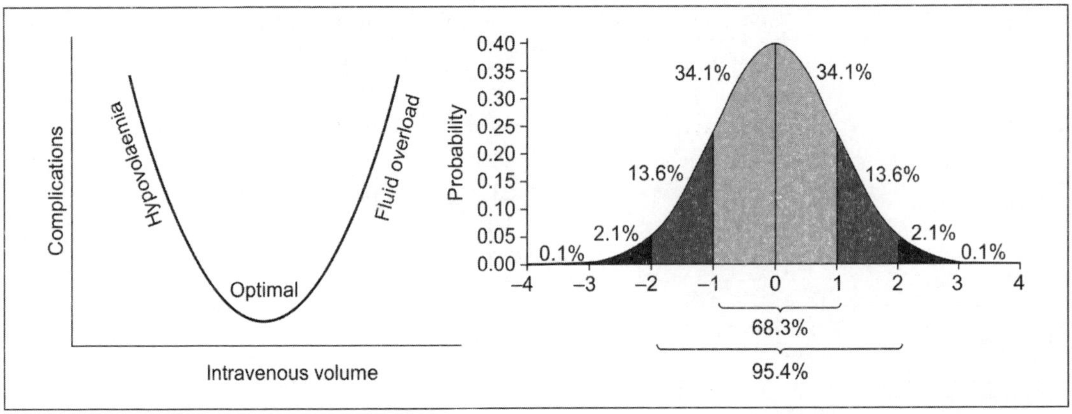

Fig. 13.2: Symmetrical distribution

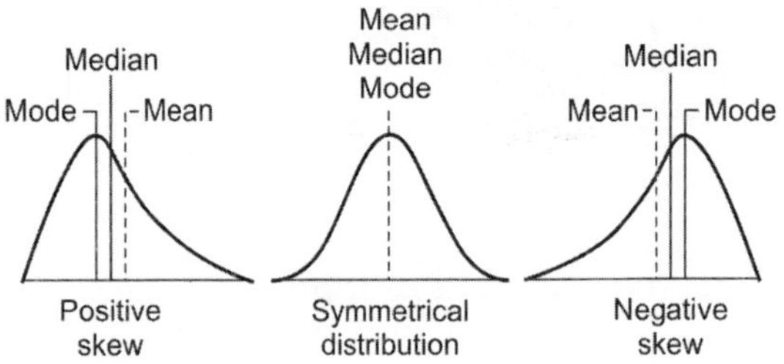

Fig. 13.3: Asymmetrical distribution

Characteristics of the Measures of Central Tendency

A. The arithmetic mean

1. Σ (X – X) = 0; {Σ = summation}, {X = No. of observation}
2. Σ (X – X) 2 = Minimum value;
3. It is the most familiar and most widely used measure;
4. It is based on all the observations;
5. It is rigidly defamed;
6. It is easily calculated and understood;
7. It is least affected by the fluctuations of sampling;
8. It is most suitable for further algebraic treatment;
9. It may be greatly affected by extreme values.
10. When the distribution has open-ended classes, its computation would be based on assumption and therefore, may not be valid.

B. The median

1. It is easy to define.
2. It is easy to understand.
3. Extremely high or low values will not distort the median.
4. Median is a better choice than the mean when a distribution is badly skewed.
5. It may be computed in an open-ended distribution.
6. It is generally less reliable than the mean for statistical inference purposes.

C. The mode

1. It may not exist in some sets of data. Or there may be more than one mode in other set of grouped data.
2. It can be located in an open-ended distribution.
3. It is not affected by extreme values in a distribution.
4. It is less popular measure than the mean or median.
5. In a small number of items the mode may not exist.
6. It is not capable of mathematical treatment.

Mean

The commonly used measures of central tendency for quantitative variable is the (arithmetic) sample mean. Arithmetic mean (AM) or arithmetic averages is obtained by summing up all the observations and dividing the total by number of observations.

The AM of a population is denoted by the symbol μ and AM of a sample is denoted by the symbol $\bar{x}$.

Mean for Ungrouped Data

Let $x_1, x_2, x_3, ..., x_n$ be the sample observation, i.e. x_1 is the 1st observation, x_2 be the 2nd observation, x_n be the *n*th observation and so on. Then

Mean = Sum of all observation ÷ Total no. of observation or $x_1 + x_2 + ... + x_{n/n}$

Example: 10 students in maths obtained following marks out of 30. Calculate the mean.

28, 22, 26, 29, 21, 23, 24, 20, 15, 30 = 238/10 = 23.8

Mean for Grouped Data

When a particular value (x) occurs more than once, the AM is then obtained by multiplying each value of x by frequency of its occurrence adding together these products and then dividing by the total number of observation.

Symbolically $x_1, x_2, ..., x_k$ be the no. of observations with frequencies $f_1, f_2, ..., f_k$ then arithmetic mean is given by

$$\text{Mean} = x_1 f_1, + x_2 f_2 + ... + x_k f_k \div f_1 + f_2 + ... + f_k$$

Examples

Calculate the average income per person/day from the following data.

Income (₹):	100	150	200	225	250	300	350
No. of persons:	50	60	60	40	35	20	20

Calculation has been done as per the formula given under heading mean.

x_i	f_i	$x_i f_i$
100	50	5000
150	60	9000
200	60	12000
225	40	9000
250	35	8750
300	20	6000
350	20	7000
Total	**275**	**56750**
Mean	₹ 206.37 person/day	

Median

The sample median of a quantitative variable is that value of the variable in a data set that divides the set of observed values in half, so that the observed values in one half are less than or equal to the median value and the observed values in the other half are greater or equal to the median value. Median is a position average whereas the arithmetic mean is the calculated average. It is generally denoted by **'M'**.

Median for Ungrouped Data

Arrange the *n* values in the ascending (or descending) order of magnitude.

Case 1: When *n* is odd, in this case: Md = (*n* + 1 ÷ 2)th term, value is median

Case 2: When *n* is even, then median is the average value of *n* ÷ 2th and (*n* ÷ 2 + 1)th term

Md = (*n* ÷ 2)th + (*n* ÷ 2 + 1)th ÷ 2 term, value is median

Median for Discrete Data

For such data, we follow the following steps.

1. Arrange the data in an ascending order.
2. Find the cumulative frequencies.
3. Calculate the median by applying the formula. Md = (*n* + 1 ÷ 2)th value of term where, *n* = total frequencies.
   $= \Sigma f$

Median for Continuous Data

Step 1. Compute the cumulative frequencies.

Step 2. Determine value one half of number of item.

Step 3. Find the interval in which the middle values falls, and exact limits of this interval.

Step 4. Calculate median by using the formula.

$$\text{Median} = L + \frac{\frac{n}{2} - F}{f_M} \times h$$

where, L = Lower limit of the interval containing median.

f_M = Frequency of the interval containing median.

F = Sum of all the frequencies above the interval containing median.

n = Total no. of frequencies is Σf.

Example: Pulse rate of 10 students in years is as follows:

Pulse rate: 70 80 76 78 82 86 90 82 88 94

Calculate median.

Solution:

Arrange in ascending order.

70 76 78 80 82 82 86 88 90 94

Here n (number of observation) = 10 (even number)

The average of ($n \div 2$)th term (i.e. 5th term = 82) and ($n \div 2 + 1$)th term (i.e. 6th term = 82) = median = 82

Mode

Mode is defined as that value in a series which occurs most frequently. In a frequency distribution mode, the variate which has the maximum frequency.

To obtain the mode(s) of a variable, we first construct a frequency distribution for the data using classes based on single value. The mode(s) can then be determined easily from the frequency distribution.

a. **Mode for simple series:** In the case of simple series the value which is repeated maximum no. of times is the mode of the series. Sometimes in simple series more than one mode exists.

b. **Mode for discrete frequency distribution series:** In the case of discrete frequency distribution mode is the value of the variable corresponding to the maximum frequency.

c. **Mode for continuous frequency distribution:** We calculate the mode by following formula

$$\text{Mode} = L + \frac{f_M - f_1}{2f_M - f_1 - f_2} \times h$$

where

L → Lower limit of the modal class.

h → Class-width of modal class.

f_1 → The frequency of the class preceding modal class.

f_M → The frequency of the modal class.

f_2 → The frequency of the class succeeding modal class.

Modal class is the class in which the maximum frequency occurs.

Examples for calculation of mode are given in the following box.

Example: The following is the frequency distribution of the duration (in days) from the 1st day of the last menstruation period and the childbirth from 2000 records. Obtain the value of mode.

Duration:	240–250	250–260	260–270	**270–280**	280–290	290–300
Frequency:	150	200	450	**600**	500	100

Solution:

Maximum frequency = 600; Modal class = 270–280 (600 corresponding to 270–280)

Given: $L = 270$; $f_1 = 450$; $f_2 = 500$; $h = 10$; $f_M = 600$

∴ ***Mode* = 276**

Example: Pulse rate of 10 students in years is as follows:

Pulse rate: 70 80 76 78 82 86 90 82 88 94

Calculate mode.

Solution:

Arranging in ascending order:

70 76 78 80 82 82 86 88 90 94

Mode for above data is ***82*** because 82 is repeated maximum number of times.

MEASURE OF DISPERSION/VARIATION

In the measure of central tendency (Fig. 13.4), averages represent the central position of data, but it does not tell us about how the measurements are arranged from the centre. It is also unable to describe scatterings of the observation. To study the scatterings of the observation in the data are studied through measure of dispersions. Measures of variation are used mostly only for quantitative variables.

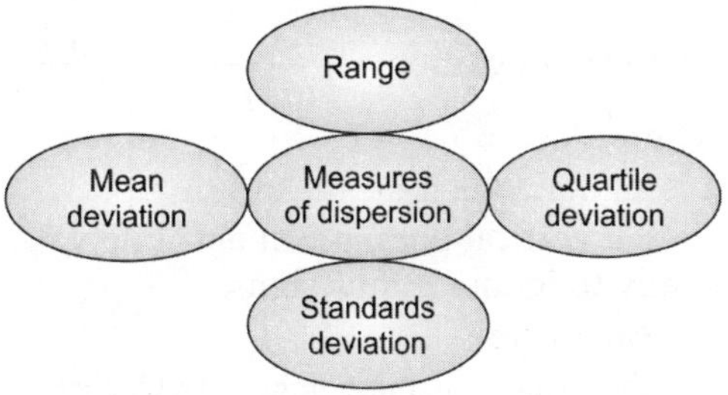

Fig. 13.4: Measures of dispersion/variation

Range

It is the simplest measure of dispersion. The range is defined as the difference between the highest and the lowest values.

Example: Range (R) for the these 5 observations (10, 20, 25, 45, 95) = Highest value–Lowest value, i.e. 95–10 = 85, shows greater variability. Range may vary from sample to sample. Range is not independent of sample size.

It is easy to understand, compute and units are the same as the units of the variables being noted. The drawbacks are that it considers only the highest and lowest observation in the data and does not depend upon the number of observation noted for analysis point of view.

QUARTILE DEVIATION/INTERQUARTILE RANGE (IQR)[5,6]

For better understanding of the interquartile range, we must define the percentiles, the deciles and the quartiles of the variable in a data set. The median of the variable divides the observed values into two equal parts—the bottom 50% and the top 50%.

The percentiles of the variable divide observed values into hundredths, or 100 equal parts, the first percentile, P_1, is the number that divides the bottom 1% of the observed values from the top 99%; second percentile, P_2, is the number that divides the bottom 2% of the observed values from the top 98%; and so forth. The median is the 50th percentile.

The deciles of the variable divide the observed values into tenths, or 10 equal parts. The variable has nine deciles, denoted by D_1, D_2,..., D_9. The first decile D_1 is 10th percentile, the second decile D_2 is the 20th percentile, and so forth.

The most commonly used percentiles are quartiles. The quartiles of the variable divide the observed values into quarters, or 4 equal parts.

The first quartile, Q_1, is the number that divides the bottom 25% of the observed values from the top 75%; second quartile, Q_2, is the median, which is the number that divides the bottom 50% of the observed values from the top 50%; and the third quartile, Q_3, is the number that divides the bottom.

75% of the observed values from the top 25%.

IQR = $Q_3 - Q_1$. The IQR gives the range of the middle 50% of the observed values.

where

Q_1 = 1st quartile and Q_3 = 3rd quartile

Thus, it gives more idea about the distribution of the individual observation by showing that the distributions are actually different.

Method for Determining the Interquartile Range (IQR)

Step 1: Arrange the observations in increasing order.

Step 2: Find the position of the 1st and 3rd quartiles with the following formulas. Divide the sum by the number of observations.

Position of 1st quartile (Q_1) = 25th percentile = $(n + 1)/4$

Position of 3rd quartile (Q_3) = 75th percentile = $3(n + 1)/4 = 3 \times Q_1$

Step 3: Identify the value of the 1st and 3rd quartiles.

a. If a quartile lies on an observation (i.e. if its position is a whole number), the value of the quartile is the value of that observation. For example, if the position of a quartile is 20, its value is the value of the 20th observation.

b. If a quartile lies between observations, the value of the quartile is the value of the lower observation plus the specified fraction of the difference between the observations. For example, if the position of a quartile is 20¼, it lies between the 20th and 21st observations, and its value is the value of the 20th observation, plus ¼ the difference between the value of the 20th and 21st observations.

Step 4: Calculate the interquartile range as Q_3 minus Q_1.

Example. Calculate various quartile deviations for the following fasting blood glucose values (in mg%) in 10 diabetics.

110 120 100 90 95 80 105 115 125 100

Solution: Ascending order of data: 80, 90, 95, 100, 100, 105, 110, 115, 120, 125

$Q_1 = (N + 1)/4 = (10 + 1)/4 = 2.75$,

Position of Q_1 = 2¾, the value of Q_1 is equal to the value of the 2nd observation plus ¾ of the 2nd and 3rd observation = 90 + ¾ (95–90) = 90 + ¾ (5) = 90 + 3.75 = 93.75

$Q_3 = 3(N + 1)/4$ = 3¾ = 8.25, position of Q_3 = 8¼, value of Q_3 is equal to the value of the 8th observation plus ¼ of the 8th and 9th observation = 115 + ¼ (125–115) = 115 + ¼ (10) = 115 + 2.5 = 117.5

IQR = 117.5 – 93.75 = 24.25

Quartile deviation =

$$\frac{\text{Third quarttile} - \text{first quartile}}{2}$$

$$\text{Quartile deviation } (Q, D) = \frac{Q_2 - Q_2}{2}$$

Quartile deviation = $Q_3 - Q_1 \div 2$

= 117.5 – 93.25

= 24.25/2 = 12.125

Mean Deviation or Average Deviation

Mean deviation is also called average deviation. It is defined as the arithmetic mean of the absolute deviation from its mean

$$\text{i.e. Mean deviation} = \frac{\Sigma|x_i - \bar{x}|}{n} = \frac{\Sigma|d|}{n}$$

where,

Σ is sigma, which means to sum up.

|| (the vertical bars) mean absolute value, basically to ignore minus signs.

x is each value.

μ is the mean, n is the number of values.

|d| is the deviation without considering the algebraic sign (plus or minus).

Similarly, mean deviation about median and mode. It defined as

$$\text{MD about median} = \frac{1}{n}\,\Sigma\,(x_i - \text{median})$$

$$\text{MD about mode} = \frac{1}{n}\,\Sigma\,(x_i - \text{mode})$$

In case of frequency distribution means deviation defined as

$$\text{MD about A} = \frac{1}{N}\,\Sigma\,(x_i - \text{A})$$

where A is the absolute value.

$$\text{MD about mean} = \frac{1}{N}\,\Sigma f_i|x_i - \bar{x}|$$

$$\text{MD about median} = \frac{1}{N}\,\Sigma f_i|x_i - median|$$

$$\text{MD about mode} = \frac{1}{N}\,\Sigma f_i|x_i - mode|$$

Steps to calculate mean deviation

1. Find the mean of all values

2. Find the distance of each value from that mean (subtract the mean from each value, ignore minus signs)
3. Then find the mean of those distances

Example: Calculate mean deviation of the following data.

Data series: 3, 6, 6, 7, 8, 11, 15, 16

Solution:

Step 1: Mean of all values = Mean = 72 ÷ 8 = 9

Step 2: Distance of each value from that mean

Value	3	6	6	7	8	11	15	16
Difference from mean	6	3	3	2	1	2	6	7

Step 3: Sum of all difference ignoring plus/ minus sign = 30 ÷ 8 = 3.75

So, the mean = 9 and mean deviation = 3.75

Example: Calculate the mean deviation for following data.

Age group	*No. of mean*
20–30	61
30–40	132
40–50	153
50–60	57
60–70	36
70–80	140
80–90	03

Solution:

CI	f_i	x_i = mid-point	x_if_i	$\sqrt{X_i - \bar{X}}$	$f_i(x_i - x)$
20–30	61	25	1525	25.27	1541.47
30–40	132	35	4620	15.27	2015.64
40–50	153	45	6885	5.27	806.31
50–60	57	55	3135	4.73	269.61
60–70	36	65	2340	14.73	530.28
70–80	140	75	10500	24.73	3462.2
80–90	3	85	255	34.73	104.19
Total	582		29260	124.73	8729.7
Mean = 50.27	Mean deviation = 8729.7/582 = 14.99				

Standard Deviation

Whereas range is unstable, quartile deviation excludes half the data arbitrarily and mean deviation neglects algebraic signs of the deviation, a measure of dispersion that does not suffer from any of these defects and is at the same time useful in statistical work is standard deviation. It is represented by **(σ)**. Standard deviation is least affected from sample to sample as compared with other three measures of dispersion.

The square of the standard deviation is called variance (σ^2). It is a square root of the arithmetic mean of the standard deviation of individual items from their arithmetic mean.

Method for Calculating the Standard Deviation

Step 1. Calculate the arithmetic mean.

Step 2. Subtract the mean from each observation. Square the difference.

Step 3. Sum the squared differences.

Step 4. Divide the sum of the squared differences by $N - 1$ (for sample data)

Step 5. Take the square root of the value obtained, is the standard deviation.

Note: When you have **'*N*'** data values that are:

The population: Divide by ***N*** when calculating variance

A sample: Divide by ***N* – 1** when calculating variance

Example: Respiratory rate (RR) of eight patients were as under (see on next page):

Standard Deviation and Normal Distribution (Gaussian distribution)

A bell-shaped symmetric distribution (**the normal distribution**), empirical rule relates the standard deviation to the proportion of the observed values of the variable in a data set that lie in a interval around the mean (Fig. 13.5).

Example: Respiratory rate (RR) of eight patients were as under.

Values	RR	16	20	18	14	18	20	22	16
Step 1	Mean	16 + 20 + 18 + 14 + 18 + 20 + 22 + 16 = 144 ÷ 8 = 18							
Step 2	Difference from mean	+ 2	− 2	0	+ 4	0	−2	− 4	+ 2
Step 3	Square of difference	4	4	0	16	0	4	16	4
Step 4	Sum of difference	4 + 4 + 0 + 16 + 0 + 4 + 16 + 4 = 48							
		Variance = 48 ÷ 7 (N − 1 = 8 − 1) = 6.86							
Step 5	Square root of the variance	√6.86 = 2.62 RR							

Formula for Variance and Standard Deviation

The 'population variance' $\sigma^2 = \frac{\Sigma(x_i - \bar{x})^2}{N}$

σ^2 = Variance

x_i = The value of the ith element

$\bar{X}$ = The mean of X

N = The number of elements

The '**population** standard deviation' $\sigma = \sqrt{\frac{1}{N}\sum_{i=1}^{N}(x_i - \mu)^2}$

The '**sample** standard deviation' $\sigma = \sqrt{\frac{1}{N-1}\sum_{i=1}^{N}(x_i - \bar{x})^2}$

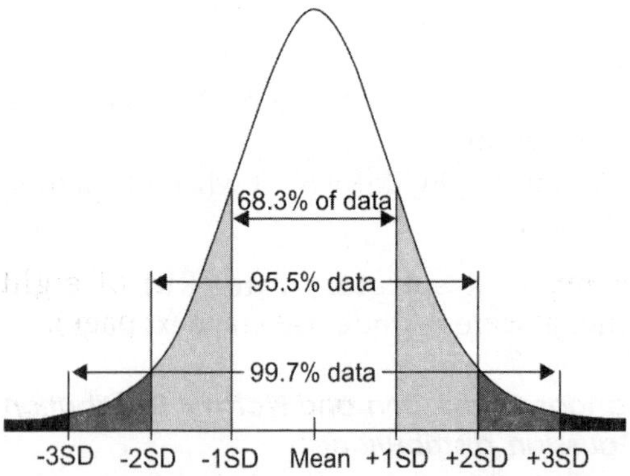

Areas included in normal distribution:

+ 1 SD includes 68.3%

+ 1.96 SD includes 95.0%

+ 2 SD includes 95.5%

+ 3 SD includes 99.7%

Fig. 13.5: Bell-shaped symmetric distribution

Coefficient of Variation

By computing the variance of a variable, we may have an idea about the extent of variability. Now often occasions arise when two or more sets are to be compared as regards their variability. When the units of the variable under comparison are different by computing the means or variances of the variables, comparison is not possible. Even for two or more sets of values of a variable, simple means or variances may not give adequate information about variability of the different sets.

The **coefficient of variation (CV)** is the ratio of the standard deviation to the mean. The higher the coefficient of variation, the greater the level of dispersion around the mean. It is generally expressed as a percentage. Without units, it allows for comparison between distributions of values whose scales of measurement are not comparable.

When we are presented with estimated values, the CV relates the standard deviation of the estimate to the value of this estimate. The lower the value of the coefficient of variation, the more precise the estimate.

CV = [Standard deviation (σ) ÷ Mean (μ)] × 100.

CV is important in the field of probability and statistics to measure the relative variability of the data sets on a ratio scale. In probability theory and statistics, it is also known as unitized risk or the variance coefficient.

Steps to Calculate CV of the Sample Data

1. Calculate the mean of the data set.
2. Calculate the sample SD for the data set.
3. Finding the ratio of sample standard deviation to mean brings the CV of the data set.

Example: Following are the number of people had diarrhoea in a village in last 10 months in 2017.

Village	120	115	105	70	75	120	125	60	80	100

Solution:

Mean = (120 + 115 + 105 + 70 + 75 + 120 + 125 + 60 + 80 + 100)/10 = 970/10 = 97

Standard deviation = σ = √ 567.78 = 23.83

Variance = σ_2 = 23.83 × 23.83 = 567.78

CV = 23.83 ÷ 97 × 100 = 24.57%

Standard Error of the Mean

The standard deviation describes variability in a set of data, whereas the standard error of the mean refers to variability we might expect in the arithmetic means of repeated samples drawn from the same population.

The standard error assumes that the data is actually a sample from a larger population. According to the assumption, sample drawn is just one of an infinite number of possible samples that could be taken from the source population. Thus, the mean for sample drawn is just one of an infinite number of other sample means. The standard error quantifies the variation in those sample means.

The primary practical use of the standard error of the mean is in calculating confidence intervals around the arithmetic mean.

Steps to Calculate the Standard Error of the Mean

Step 1: Calculate the standard deviation.

Step 2: Divide the standard deviation by the square root of the number of observations (n).

Example (hypothetical): Serum cholesterol levels of 500 persons above the age of 40 years were measured, the mean cholesterol level was 213, with a standard deviation of 42.

Solution: Calculate the standard error of the mean: SE of mean = σ | $\sqrt{n}$ = 42 | $\sqrt{500}$ = 1.88

Confidence Interval/Confidence Limits

Study results on sample population will always have qualifiers into reports, warn about all sorts of assumptions, and never admit to anything more extreme than probable.

There's a famous saying: ***"Statistics means never having to say you're certain."***

Any kind of statements must be qualified, of course, because we are always dealing with imperfect information. In particular, it is often necessary to make statements about a population using information from a sample. No matter how carefully this sample is selected to be a fair and unbiased representation of the population, relying on information from a sample will always lead to some level of uncertainty. Studies not only to measure characteristics in the subjects studied, but also to make generalizations about the larger population from which subjects/sample is selected. This process is called inference.

Usually, the inference includes some consideration about the precision of the measurement.

In epidemiology, a common way to indicate a measurement's precision is by providing a confidence interval. A narrow confidence interval indicates high precision; a wide confidence interval indicates low precision.

So, a confidence interval is an interval within which we can estimate, with some confidence that the true population parameter lies.

Statistical definition of a confidence interval is that 95% of the confidence intervals from an infinite number of similarly conducted samples would include the true population values.

Confidence interval = Mean ± Standard error/margin of error

Method for calculating a 95% confidence interval for a mean

Step 1. Calculate the mean and its standard error.

Step 2. Multiply the standard error by 1.96.

Step 3. Lower limit of the 95% confidence interval = mean minus 1.96 × standard error.

Upper limit of the 95% confidence interval = mean plus 1.96 × standard error.

Example (hypothetical): Serum cholesterol levels of 500 persons above the age of 40 years were measured, the mean cholesterol level was 213, with a standard deviation of 42. Calculate 95% confidence interval for a mean.

Solution:

Mean = 213, standard deviation = 42 and **SE of mean =** $\sigma \div \sqrt{n}$ **= 42 | √500 = 1.88**

CI = 213 + 1.96 × 1.88 = 216.68 (upper limit) and CI = 213–1.96 × 1.88 = 209.31 (lower limit)

So, 95% confidence value lies between 209.31–216.68, means we are 95% confident to have our values represents the true population.

Box 13.1: Point to remember

Confidence intervals are commonly calculated for mean, proportions, rates, risk ratios, odds ratios, and other epidemiologic measures when the purpose is to draw inferences from a sample survey or study to the larger population. All are calculated using different formulas. Confidence intervals serve guide rather than as a strict range of values.

INFERENTIAL STATISTICS[5,6,12–14]

It includes methods like point estimation, interval estimation and hypothesis testing, which are all based on probability theory.

Probability (randomness or 'chance'): The probability of a particular outcome is the proportion of times that outcome would occur in a long run of repeated observations.

Random variable: A random variable is a variable whose value is a numerical outcome of a random phenomenon.

A. The probabilities $P(x_i)$ must satisfy two requirements for discrete random variable:
   1. Every probability $P(x_i)$ is a number between 0 and 1.
   2. $P(x_1) + P(x_2) + \ldots + P(x_k) = 1$.
B. The probabilities $P(x_1 \leq X \leq x_2)$ must satisfy two requirements:
   1. For every interval $[x_1, x_2]$, the probability $P(x_1 \leq X \leq x_2)$ is a number between 0 and 1.
   2. $P(a \leq X \leq b) = 1$.

Standard normal distribution and probabiltiy (Fig. 13.6): A continuous random variable Z is said to have a standard normal distribution if Z is normally distributed with mean ì = 0 and standard deviation σ = 1, the standardized value Z tells how many standard deviations below or above the mean the original value is, and is calculated as: Z score = x – μ/σ (0, 1).

Estimation

Statistical inference uses sample data to form two types of estimators of parameters. **A point**

estimate consists of a single number, calculated from the data, for the unknown parameter. An **interval estimate** consists of a range of numbers around the point estimate, within which the parameter is suppose to be included.

A. **Point estimation:** A point estimator of a unknown population parameter is defined as the statistic that estimates the value of that parameter. A point estimate of a parameter is the value of a statistic that is used to estimate the parameter. (Agresti and Finlay, 1997 and Weiss, 1999)

B. **Interval estimation:** A confidence interval for a parameter is defined the range of numbers within which the parameter is believed to fall. The probability that the confidence interval contains the parameter is called the confidence coefficient. This is a chosen number close to 1, such as 0.95 or 0.99 (Agresti and Finlay, 1997). The details described earlier in this chapter.

C. **Hypotheses testing:** A hypothesis is a statement about some characteristic of a variable or a collection of variables. (Agresti and Finlay, 1997)

A tests of significance analyzes the strength of sample evidence against the null hypothesis. Most of the major inferential statistics come from a general family of statistical model known as the general linear model. This includes the *t*-test, analysis of variance (ANOVA), analysis of covariance (ANCOVA), regression analysis and many of the multivariate methods like factor analysis, multi-dimensional scaling, cluster analysis, discriminate function analysis, population parameters from observing the sample values (Table 13.2).

TESTS OF SIGNIFICANCE

A significance test is a way of statistically testing a hypothesis by comparing the data to values predicted by the hypothesis. Data that fall far from the predicted values provide evidence against the hypothesis. All significance tests have ***five elements—assumptions, hypotheses, test statistic, P-value, and conclusion.***

All significance tests require certain assumptions for the tests to be valid. These assumptions refer to the type of data, the form of the population distribution, method of sampling, and sample size.

Hypothesis

It is prediction about the parameter before the test applies and assertion or statement about the parameter.

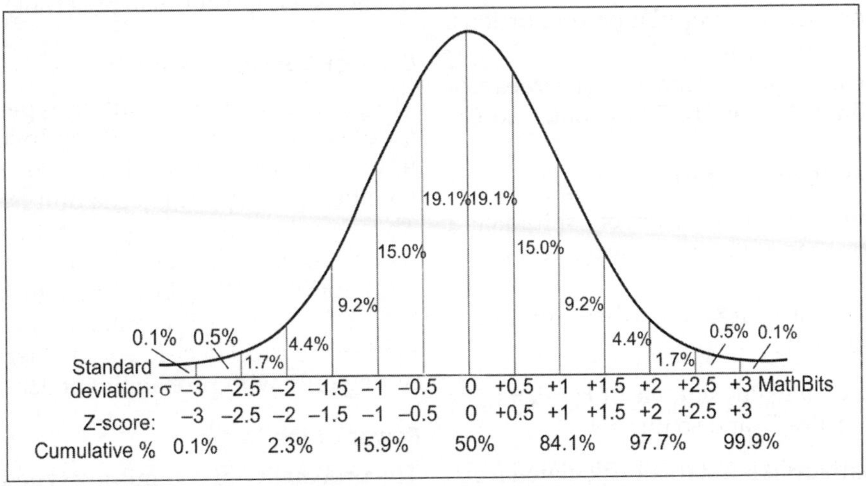

Fig. 13.6: Standard normal deviation—bell curve

Table 13.2: Hypotheses testing

Population	*Null hypothesis (based on sample)*	
	Rejected	*Accepted*
Null hypothesis—true	Type I error (α)	Correct decision
Null hypothesis—false	Correct decision	Type II error (β)

OR

Results	*Truth*	
	H_0 correct	H_0 wrong
Accept H_0	Right	Type II or β-error
Reject H_0	Type I or α error	Right

Hypothesis is a tentative or working proposition suggested as a solution to a problem, and the theory as the final hypothesis which is defensibly supported by all the evidence (Koul 2009).

A research hypothesis is a formal affirmative statement predicting a single research outcome, a tentative explanation of the relationship between two or more variables (Best and Kahn, 2009).

There are two types of hypotheses—the null hypothesis (non-directional) and the alternative hypothesis (directional).

Null Hypothesis (H_0)

It is hypothesis which assumes that there is no difference between two values such as population means or population proportions. It is denoted by H_0: $\mu_1 = \mu_2$

H_0: Mean of population A (P_1) = Mean of population B (P_2), i.e. H_0: $P_1 = P_2$ and so on.

Alternative Hypothesis (H_1)

A hypothesis that differs from or contradicts a null hypothesis is called an alternative hypothesis.

In other words, it is true when null hypothesis is false. It is denoted by H_1.

H_1: $\mu_1 \neq \mu_2$ or $\mu_1 < \mu_2$ or $\mu_1 > \mu_2$ or H_1: $P_1 \neq P_2$ or $P_1 < P_2$ or $P_1 > P_2$ and so on.

Test statistic: It is a statistic calculated from the sample data to test the null hypothesis. This statistic typically involves a point estimate of the parameter for which the hypotheses is established.

It is a rule which tells us whether to accept or reject null hypothesis (H_0) on the basis of a sample data.

The *p*-value: It is the probability, when H_0 is true, of a test statistic value is false to H_0 as the value actually observed, the smaller the *p*-value, the more strongly the data to reject H_0.

Conclusion: Most studies require very small *p*-value, such as $p \leq 0.05$, before concluding that the data disagrees with H_0. In such cases, results are said to be significant at the 0.05 level. This means that if the null hypothesis were true, the chance of getting such extreme results as in the sample data would be no greater than 5% (Table 13.2).

Level of Significance (α)

The probability of committing **type I error** is called level of significance (LoS). Investigators have used probability levels for deciding whether to accept or reject a null hypothesis. These probability levels are called level of significance. It is usually denoted by $\alpha = 0.05$ (5%) and 0.01 (1%). Level of significance of 0.05 (5%) means, 95% confident, i.e. we have made the correct decision or in other word we wrong only with probability of 0.05.

Power of the Test

The probability of committing **type II error** is denoted by β and $1-\beta$ is called the power of the test. It depends on the alternative hypothesis. Power is probability of rejecting H_0 when H_0 is false. Thus, it is probability of taking correct decision.

Tests Used for Testing Hypothesis

There are two types of statistical tests **(parametric and non-parametric)** for testing hypothesis

Parametric Tests

Following conditions are to be fulfilled for testing the hypotheses[12]

- Randomly selected sample
- The variances of the various groups are equal or near equal
- The data should be of interval scale or ratio scale
- The observations are independent
- The sample size is more than 30
- The data follow a normal distribution

This includes the *t*-test, analysis of variance (ANOVA), analysis of covariance (ANCOVA), regression analysis and multivariate analysis meyhods.

Non-parametric Tests

The tests which allows to compare samples and make inferences or tests of significance without having to assume normality in the populations are known as non-parametric.

Tests: Some of the non-parametric techniques are the chi-square test, the rank difference correlation coefficient, the sign test, the median test and the sum-of-ranks test.

Procedure for Testing of Hypothesis

The steps for testing of hypothesis are given below.

Step 1: Set-up null hypothesis H_0.

Step 2: Set-up the alternative hypothesis H_1. This gives the idea whether we have used one tailed or two tailed test.

Step 3: Choose the appropriate level of significance ( ).

Step 4: Compute the value of test statistic 'Z' = Observed difference ÷ Standard error

Step 5: Obtain the table value at given level of significance (LoS)

Step 6: Compare the value of Z calculated with that of table value.

Step 7: Draw the conclusion.

Large and Small Sample Test

Tests based on large sample (n >30) are called large sample tests then Z-statistics used for testing significance and tests based on small samples ($n \leq 30$), are called small sample tests, *t*-test (statistics) is appropriate test for testing significance.

LARGE SAMPLE TESTS (Z-STATISTICS)

Sample of variables/tests for quantitative data:

H_0: X = μ, i.e. Z = Sample mean – Population mean ÷ SE of mean

$$Z = \frac{\bar{X} - \mu}{\frac{\sigma}{\sqrt{n}}}$$

Test for single proportion: $H_0 = p = P$ *vs.* H_1: $p \neq P$

$$Z = \frac{p - P}{SE(p)} = \frac{p - P}{\sqrt{\frac{PQ}{n}}}$$

where,

p—sample proportion or percentage of positive characteristic

q—sample proportion or percentage of negative characteristics, i.e. $q = 1 - p$

P—population proportion of positive characteristics

Q—population proportion of negative characteristics

n—sample size.

Test for two sample proportion H_0: $p_1 = p_2$ *vs.* H_1: $p_1 \neq p_2$

The test statistics $Z = \dfrac{p_1 - p_2}{SE(p_1 - p_2)}$

where, SE (p_1, p_2) $\sqrt{PQ\left[\dfrac{1}{n_1} + \dfrac{1}{n_2}\right]}$

where, $$P = \frac{n_1 p_1 + n_2 p_2}{n_1 + n_2}$$

Confidence interval: The 95% confidence interval for population mean is sample mean ±1.96 × SE of mean. Symbolically the population means μ will be lie between—

$$\bar{X} - 1.96 \times \frac{\sigma}{\sqrt{n}} \text{ and } \bar{X} - 1.96 \times \frac{\sigma}{\sqrt{n}}$$

Similarly, 99% confidence interval is given by

$$\bar{X} - 2.58 \times \frac{\sigma}{\sqrt{n}} \text{ and } \bar{X} + 2.58 \times \frac{\sigma}{\sqrt{n}}$$

Test about two population's means:

$$z = \frac{\bar{x}_1 - \bar{x}_2}{\sqrt{\frac{\sigma_1^2}{n_1} + \frac{\sigma_2^2}{n_2}}}$$

Exercise

1. In a medical college out of 120 admissions of 1st year MBBS, 35 are girl students. Check whether the proportion of girl students is 40% in the college.

   Let p be the sample proportion of girl students.

   $p = 35/120 = 0.29$

   P (which is given) = 40% = 0.40

   H_0—the proportion of girl students is 40%

   The statistic $Z = (p - P)/\text{sqrt}(PQ/n) = (0.29 - 0.40)/\text{sqrt}(0.40 * 0.60/120) = 2.46$

   Reject the null hypothesis at 5% level of significance since absolute value of Z = 2.46 is greater than 1.96 (tabulated value)

   Conclusion: The proportion of girl students is not 40%.

2. In a large city A, 20% of a random sample of 900 school boys had defective eyesight in another large city B, 15.5% of a random sample of 1600 school boys had the same defect. Is the difference between the two proportions significant?

   n_1 = size sample of 1st sample = 900, n_2 = size sample of 2nd sample = 1600

   p_1 = sample proportion of 1st sample = 20/100 = 0.20

   p_2 = sample proportion of 2nd sample = 15.5/100 = 0.155

   $Z = (p_1 - p_2)/\text{SE}(p_1 - p_2) = (p_1 - p_2)/\text{Sqrt}\{P \times Q [(1/n_1) + (1/n_2)]\}$

   $P = (n_1 p_1 + n_2 p_2)/(n_1 + n_2) = 0.17, Q = 1 - P = 0.63$

   By using defined formula for test of two proportions, Z = 2.81

   Z cal = 2.81 > 1.96 at 5% level of significance, Reject H_0.

SMALL SAMPLE TEST (*T*-STATISTICS)

It was first derived by WS Gosset in 1908, who published statistical papers under the pen name of 'student'. Thus the test is known as student's *t*-test.

Assumption for t-test

The assumption used for *t*-test is as below.

- The sample must be random.
- Unknown population standard deviation.
- The distribution of population from which the sample is drawn is normal.

Uses of t-test

The *t*-test is used for testing the significance of:

- The mean of sample
- The difference between means or to compare two samples.
- Correlation coefficient.

Types of t-test

There are three main types of *t*-test:

1. An independent sample *t*-test compares the means for two groups (unpaired *t*-test).
2. A paired sample *t*-test compares means from the same group at different times (say, one year apart).
3. A one sample *t*-test the mean of a single group against a known mean.

Test Regarding Single Mean

(One sample *t*-test)

For testing the significance of difference between sample mean and population mean or whether sample has been drawn from the population with mean in case of small sample (n <30), the test statistics is

$$t = \frac{\bar{X} - \mu}{\frac{S}{\sqrt{n}}}$$

where,

$$S^2 = \frac{\Sigma(X - \bar{X})^2}{n - 1}$$

Steps in Calculating One Sample t-test

Step 1: Find out the sample mean ($\bar{x}$), the population mean (μ), the sample standard deviation (s) and number of observations (n)

Step 2: Insert the items from above into the t-test formula.

Step 3: Find the t (table value). You need two values to find this:

The alpha level—given as 5% in the question and degrees of freedom, which is the number of items in the sample ($n-1$).

Step 4: Compare the calculated and table value and conclude.

The test statistics 't' has $n - 1$ degrees of freedom. Calculated value of 't' with table value at certain level of significance (Generally 5% and 1% LoS). If absolute value of 't' obtained is greater than table value then reject the null hypothesis and if it is less than table value then H_0 may be accepted.

Tests Regarding two Means

i. Unpaired t-test

ii. Paired t-test

Unpaired t-test

Two data samples are independent from different population and the samples does not affect each other. Here, we assume that the data populations follow the normal distribution. Using the unpaired t-test, we can obtain an interval estimate of the difference between two population means.

$$t = \frac{X_1 - X_2}{S\sqrt{\frac{1}{n_1} + \frac{1}{n_2}}}$$

where,

$$S^2 = \frac{\Sigma(X_1 - \bar{X}_2)^2 + \Sigma(X_2 - \bar{X}_2)^2}{n_1 + n_2 - 2}$$

Degrees of freedom (df):

df = $(n_1 - 1) + (n_2 - 1) = n_1 + n_2 - 2$

Steps in calculating unpaired t-test:

Step 1: Sum the two groups, i.e. sum of X and sum of Y

Step 2: Square the sums from Step 1:

Step 3: Calculate the means for the two groups X and Y

Step 4: Square the individual scores and then add them up

Step 5: Insert numbers into the formula and solve

Step 6: Find the degrees of freedom ($nX - 1 + nY - 1$)

Step 7: Look up your degrees of freedom (Step 6) in the t-table. Use 5% (0.05) with degrees of freedom at an alpha level of 0.05

Step 8: Compare your calculated value (Step 5) to your table value (Step 7)

Examples: Apgar scores in two groups of newborn, one born to high risk mothers and other to normal mothers are given below. Comments whether there is significant difference in the apgar scores of these two groups.

Newborn of high risk mothers (X)	5	3	2	4	7	6	3
Newborn of normal mothers (Y)	1	1	2	1	1	3	5

Solution:

Mean for x = 4.28, SD = 1.79 and mean for y = 1.87, SD = 1.45

Calculated 't' value = 2.825, table 't' value at df 13 = 2.16, significant difference was found.

Paired 't'-Test

Steps in calculating paired t-test:

Step 1: Subtract each Y score from each X score

Step 2: Add up all of the values from Step 1. Set this number aside for a moment.

Step 3: Square the differences from Step 1.

Step 4: Add up all of the squared differences from Step 3.

Step 5: Use the following formula to calculate the *t*-score.

Step 6: Subtract 1 from the sample size to get the degrees of freedom. We have 11 items, so 11 – 1 = 10.

Step 7: Find the *p*-value in the *t*-table, using the degrees of freedom in Step 6. If you don't have a specified alpha level, use 0.05 (5%). For this sample problem, with df = 10, the *t*-value is 2.228.

Step 8: Compare your *t*-table value from Step 7 (2.228) to your calculated *t*-value (–2.74). The calculated *t*-value is greater than the table value at an alpha level of 0.05. The *p*-value is less than the alpha level: $p < 0.05$. We can reject the null hypothesis that there is no difference between means.

$$t = \frac{(\Sigma D)/N}{\Sigma D^2 - \left(\frac{(\Sigma D)^2}{N}\right)/(N-1)(N)}$$

ΣD: Sum of the differences (sum of $X - Y$), ΣD^2: Sum of the squared differences $(\Sigma D)^2$: Sum of the differences, squared.

$$t = \frac{(\Sigma D)/N}{\Sigma D^2 - \left(\frac{(\Sigma D)^2}{N}\right)/(N-1)(N)}$$

$$t = \frac{-73/11}{\sqrt{\dfrac{1131 - \left(\dfrac{(-73)^2}{11}\right)}{(11-1)(11)}}}$$

$$t = \frac{-73/11}{\sqrt{\dfrac{1131 - \left(\dfrac{(5329)}{11}\right)}{(110)}}}$$

$$t = -2.74$$

Example

Patient number	*Pre-test result (X)*	*Post-test result (Y)*	*X – Y*	*X – Y²*
1	3	20	– 17	289
2	3	13	– 10	100
3	3	13	– 10	100
4	12	20	– 8	64
5	15	29	– 14	196
6	16	32	– 16	256
7	17	23	– 6	36
8	19	20	– 1	1
9	23	25	– 2	4
10	24	15	+ 9	81
11	32	30	– 2	4
			– 73	1131

Note: You can ignore the minus sign when comparing the two *t*-values, as ± indicates the direction; the *p*-value remains the same for both directions.

Chi-square Test[13,14]

Chi-square test is one of the important non-parametric tests that is used to compare more than two variables for a randomly selected data. The chi-square test is based on the difference between the observed and the expected values for each category. The expected frequencies are calculated based on the conditions of null hypothesis. The rejection of null hypothesis is based on the differences of actual value and expected value. The data can be examined by using the two types of Chi-square test.

1. Chi-square goodness of fit test: It is used to observe that the closeness of a sample matches a population. The Chi-square test statistic is,

$$\chi^2 = \Sigma \frac{(O_i - E_i)^2}{E_i}$$

with $k - 1$ degrees of freedom.

where O_i is the observed value, k is categories, and E_i is the expected value.

2. Chi-square test for independence of two variables: It is used to check whether the variables are independent of each other or not. The Chi-square test statistic is,

$$\chi^2 = \Sigma \frac{(O_i - E_i)^2}{E_i}$$

with $(r - 1)(c - 1)$ degrees of freedom

where O_i is the observed value, r is number of rows, c is the number of columns, and E_i is the expected value.

The test for independence of X and Y begins by assuming that there is no relationship between the two variables. The alternative hypothesis states that there is some relationship between the two variables. If the two variables in the cross classification are X and Y, the hypotheses are

- H_0: No relationship between X and Y
- H_1: Some relationship between X and Y

In terms of independence and dependence these hypotheses could be stated

- H_0: X and Y are independent
- H_1: X and Y are dependent

For both the goodness of fit test and the test for independence, the chi-square statistic is the same. For both of these tests, all the categories into which the data have been divided are used. The data obtained from the sample are referred to as the **observed** numbers of cases. The goodness of fit test examines only one variable, while the test of independence is concerned with the relationship between two variables.

Steps for chi-square test:

- Write down the null hypothesis.
- Obtain the expected frequencies
- Compute the values of chi-square test statistics

$$\chi^2 = \frac{\Sigma(\text{Observed} - \text{Expected})^2}{\text{Expected}}$$

- Find out the degrees of freedom.
- Obtain the table value from chi-square table
- Compare chi-square calculated with table value. If calculated value of χ^2 is greater than table value of χ^2 reject the null hypothesis otherwise accept it.
- Write down the conclusion.

Contingency table: The chi-square test for independence of two variables is a test which uses a cross classification table to examine the nature of the relationship between these variables. These tables are sometimes referred to as contingency tables.

Expected frequencies: Expected frequencies are the frequencies which are obtained from model.

$$E = \frac{RT \times CT}{GT}$$

where RT is row total, CT is column total and GT is grand total.

Degrees of freedom: When contingency table has 'c' column and 'r' row, the degrees of freedom is $(r - 1) \times (c - 1)$.

2×2 Contingency table:

Factor A	*Factor B*		*Total*
	Present	*Absent*	
Present	a	b	$a + b$
Absent	c	d	$c + d$
Total	$a + c$	$B + d$	$a + b + c + d = N$

The chi-square value for testing the independence of characters A and B simplifies to

$$X^2 = \frac{(ad - bc)^2 N}{(a + b)(c + d)(a + c)(b + d)}$$

where $N = a + b + c + d$

Expected cell frequency = (Row total × Column total)/N

(Assumptions about E: No expected case, E should be less than 1. No more than 20% of the cells should have less than 5 expected cases).

Using the same procedure to compute all the expected cell frequencies—each of the squared differences is then divided by the expected cell frequency for each cell.

The chi-square test of significance is useful as a tool to determine whether or not it is worth the researcher's effort to interpret a contingency table. A significant result of this test means that the cells of a contingency table should be interpreted. A non-significant test means that no effects were discovered and chance could explain the observed differences in the cells. In this case, an interpretation of the cell frequencies is not useful.

Example: Chi-square goodness of fit test

Age-wise distribution of male population (15–54 yrs) in a village	*Sample population (observed)*	*Population as per census (in percentage)*	*Expected population (Sample total × Census% ÷ 100)*	*O – E*	*(O – E)²*	*(O – E)² ÷ E*
15–24	650	25	575	75	5625	9.78
25–34	500	22	506	6	36	0.07
35–44	600	28	644	44	1936	3.01
45–54	550	25	575	25	625	1.08
	2300	100	2300			13.94

H_0: The age distribution of respondents in the sample is the same as the age distribution in the census.

H_1: The age distribution of respondents in the sample differs from the age distribution in the census.

Calculate X_2 value = 13.94, df = 3, table value = 7.81, a chi-square value larger than this leads to rejection of the null hypothesis, and a chi-square value from the data which is smaller than 7.81 means that the null hypothesis cannot be rejected.

Since 13.94 > 7.81, the null hypothesis can be rejected, and the research hypothesis accepted at the 0.05 level of significance.

Example: Chi-square test for independence of two variables

Treatment of diabetes with drug *'A'* was in 200 cases and drug *'B'* was 300 cases, find out the most effective drug on diabetes.

	Blood glucose level controlled		*Total*
	Yes	*No*	
Drug *'A'*	$O_1 = 125$ ($E_1 = 120$)	$O_3 = 75$ ($E_3 = 80$)	200
Drug *'B'*	$O_2 = 175$ ($E_2 = 180$)	$O_4 = 125$ ($E_4 = 120$)	300
Total	**300**	**200**	**500**

Solution:

H_0 = there is no difference between drug *'A'* and drug *'B'*

H_1 = there is a difference between drug *'A'* and drug *'B'*

Expected values for each cell = Row total × Column total ÷ Grand total

$E_1 = 200 \times 300 \div 500 = 120$, $E_2 = 300 \times 300 \div 500 = 180$, $E_3 = 200 \times 200 \div 500 = 80$, $E_4 = 300 \times 200 \div 500 = 120$

$O_1 - E_1 = 125–120 = \mathbf{5}$, $O_2 - E_2 = 175–180 = \mathbf{5}$, $O_3 - E_3 = 15–80 = \mathbf{5}$, $O_4 - E_4 = 125–120 = \mathbf{5}$

$(O - E)^2$ of each cell = $(O_1 - E_1)^2 = 25$, $(O_2 - E_2)^2 = 25$, $(O_3 - E_3)^2 = 25$, $(O_4 - E_4)^2 = 25$

$(O - E)^2 \div E$ of each cell = 0.21, 0.14, 0.31, 0.21, sum of these values is (calculated X_2 value) = 0.87

Df = $(r - 1)(c - 1) = (2 - 1)(2 - 1) = 1$, Table X_2 value = 3.84

The calculated chi-square value is smaller (0.87) than table value 3.84, hence that the null hypothesis cannot be rejected null hypotheses is accepted). Means there is no difference between two drugs.

CORRELATIONS AND REGRESSION [6,7,15]

Concept of Correlation for Bi-variate Data

When more than one variable are related or correlated with each other, then their relationship is only studied through the help of correlation analysis. The study of the relationship between the two variables, then the correlation analysis is called bivariate analysis. In correlation change in the value of one variable affects the change in the value of another variable, then such variables are called correlated variables.

The scatter-plot provides a visual impression of the nature of relation between the x and y values in a bivariate data set. Our visual impression of the closeness of the scatter to a linear relation can be quantified by calculating a numerical measure, called the **sample correlation coefficient.** The sample correlation coefficient, denoted by 'r', is a measure of the strength of the linear relation between the x and y variables.

The sample correlation coefficient is also called Pearson correlation coefficient. As it is clear now that Pearson correlation coefficient can be calculated only when both variables are quantitative, i.e. defined at least on interval scale. When variables are qualitative ordinal scale variables, then **Spearman correlation coefficient** can be used as a measure of association between two ordinal scale variables. Spearman correlation coefficient is based on ranking of subjects, but the more accurate description of the properties of Spearman correlation coefficient is not within the scope of this course.

Types of Correlation

i. Positive correlation
ii. Negative correlation

Positive Correlation

If the increase (decrease) in the value of one variable affects the increase (decrease) in the value of another variable, then the correlation is said to be positive correlation. In other words changes in both the variables are in the same direction then it is positive correlation, e.g. height and weight, income and expenditure (Fig. 13.7).

Negative Correlation

If increase (or decrease) in the value of one variable affects the decrease (or increase) in the value of another variable then the correlation is said to be negative correlation. In other words changes of variables are in opposite direction then it is negative correlation, e.g. price and demand (Fig. 13.7).

Karl-Pearsonís Coefficient of Correlation

The coefficient of correlation calculated by using the formula

Karl-Pearson's coefficient, $r =$

$$\frac{\text{cov}(x,y)}{\sigma x \cdot \sigma y} = \frac{\Sigma(x_i - \bar{x})(y_i - \bar{y})}{\sqrt{\Sigma(x_i - \bar{x})^2 (y_i - \bar{y})^2}}$$

where, $\bar{x}$ = means of X variable and $\bar{y}$ = means of Y variable.

Alternative formula,

$$r = \frac{\frac{1}{N}\Sigma x_i y_i - \bar{x} \cdot \bar{y}}{\sqrt{\frac{1}{n}\Sigma x_i^2 - \bar{x}^2}\sqrt{\frac{1}{n}\Sigma y_i^2 - \bar{y}^2}}$$

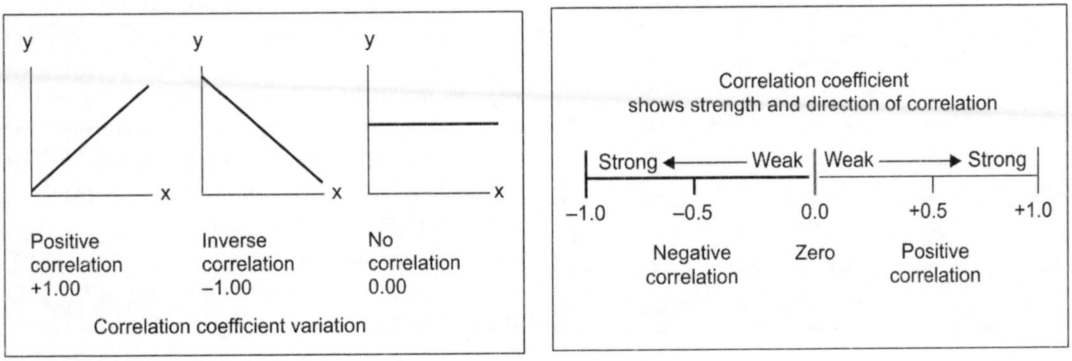

Fig. 13.7: Types of correlation

Properties of Coefficient of Correlation

Correlation coefficient always lies between –1 and + 1, i.e.

1. The correlation is perfect and positive if $r = 1$ and it is perfect and negative if $r = -1$.
2. If $r = 0$, then there is no correlation between the two variables and thus the variables are said to be independent.

Interpretation of the Correlation Coefficient

Correlation analysis is a measure of relationship between two variables. The higher value of 'r' establishes high degree of relationship only and it should not be taken as a measure of cause and effect relationship. In some cases a casual relation may exist between two variables whereas in other a relationship may exists between two variables because both are related to a third variable. Sometimes the relationship may be purely due to chance, if another set of data is collected and a Pearson 'r' is calculated the resulting 'r' may be meaningless. For example, one may measure height of student and correlate it with their marks obtained. Even if $r = 0.77$, still it is meaningless, such high positive relationships are purely result of chance.

Testify correlation coefficient:

$T = r\sqrt{(n-2)} \quad \sqrt{(1-r^2)}$

If $t_{cal} \leq t_{tab}$ at α (alpha) level of significance for $(n - 2)$ df then H_0 is accepted, otherwise rejected, i.e. correlation is not significant.

Example

Subjects	*Age 'x'*	*Glucose level 'y'*	xy	x^2	y^2
1	43	99	4257	1849	9801
2	21	65	1365	441	4225
3	25	79	1975	625	6241
4	42	75	3150	1764	5625
5	57	87	4959	3249	7569
6	59	81	4779	3481	6561
Σ	**247**	**486**	**20485**	**11409**	**40022**

Kerl-Pearson's coefficient, $r =$

$$\frac{\text{cov}(x,y)}{\sigma x \cdot \sigma y} = \frac{\Sigma(x_i - \bar{x})(y_i - \bar{y})}{\sqrt{\Sigma(x_i - \bar{x})^2 (y_i - \bar{y})^2}}$$

r **= 0.5298:** The range of the correlation coefficient is from – 1 to 1. Our result is 0.5298 or 52.98%, which means the variables have a moderate positive correlation.

REGRESSION ANALYSIS

Regression analysis is a form of predictive modelling technique which investigates the relationship between a **dependent** (target) and **independent variable(s)** (predictor). This technique is used for forecasting, time series modelling and finding the causal effect relationship between the variables.

It is used to indicate the significant relationships between dependent variable and independent variable and the strength of impact of multiple independent variables on a dependent variable.

The regression techniques are mostly driven by three metrics (number of independent variables, type of dependent variables and shape of regression line). Some of the techniques are: Linear regression, logistic regression, polynomial regression, stepwise regression, ridge regression, lasso regression, ElasticNet regression, etc.

Most commonly used regression analysis is linear regression for continuous variable and for binary—use logistic regression!

Linear Regression[15]

In this technique, the dependent variable is continuous, independent variable(s) can be continuous or discrete, and nature of regression line is linear. Linear regression establishes a relationship between **dependent variable (*Y*)** and one or more **independent variables (*X*)** using a **best fit straight line** (also known as regression line).

It is represented by an equation $Y = a + b*X + e$, where a is intercept, b is slope of the line and e is error term. This equation can be used to predict the value of target variable based on given predictor variable(s).

Logistic Regression

Logistic regression is used to find the probability of event = success and event = failure. We should use logistic regression when the dependent variable is binary (0/1, True/False, Yes/No) in nature. Here the value of Y ranges from 0 to 1 and it can represented by following equation.

Odds = $p/(1-p)$ = Probability of event occurrence/probability of not event occurrence

$\ln(\text{odds}) = \ln[p/(1-p)]$

$\text{logit}(p) = \ln[p/(1-p)] = b_0 + b_1X_1 + b_2X_2 + b_3X_3 + \ldots + b_kX_k$

- It is widely used for classification problems.
- Logistic regression doesn't require linear relationship between dependent and independent variables. It can handle various types of relationships because it applies a non-linear log transformation to the predicted odds ratio.
- To avoid over-fitting and under-fitting, we should include all significant variables. A good approach to ensure this practice is to use a step-wise method to estimate the logistic regression.
- It requires large sample sizes because maximum likelihood estimates are less powerful at low sample sizes than ordinary least square.
- The independent variables should not be correlated with each other, i.e. no multi co-linearity. However, we have the options to include interaction effects of categorical variables in the analysis and in the model.
- If the values of dependent variable is ordinal, then it is called ordinal logistic regression.

REGRESSION COEFFICIENT

Regression coefficient is a statistical measure of the average functional relationship between two or more variables. In regression analysis, one variable is considered as dependent and other(s) as independent. Thus, it measures the degree of dependence of one variable on the other(s). It is customary to denote the independent variable by ***X*** and dependent variable by ***Y*** and expressed in terms of original unit of data.

Regression coefficients are classified as:

1. Simple, partial and multiple
2. Positive and negative and
3. Linear and non-linear.

The formula for obtaining the regression coefficient is as follows:

$Y = Y + b(X - X)$, where, Y = Mean of $Y_1, Y_2, \ldots, Y_n$ and X = Mean of $X_1, X_2, \ldots, X_n$

$b = (X_i - X) \times (Y_i - Y) \div \sqrt{(X_i - X)^2}$

b is called regression coefficient of ***Y*** upon **X**.

Similarly, we obtain the regression of X upon Y.

$X = X + b^1(Y - Y)$, $b^1 = (X_i - X) \times (Y_i - Y) \div \sqrt{(Y_i - Y)^2}$

where b^1 is called regression coefficient of ***X*** upon ***Y***.

Properties of Regression Coefficient

The correlation coefficient is the geometric mean of the regression coefficient.

If one of the regression coefficient is less than unity then other must be greater than unity.

Arithmetic mean of regression coefficient is greater than the correlation coefficient provided $r > 0$.

Regression coefficients are independent of the change of origin but not the scale.

Example

No.	*Age (X)*	*Sys BP (Y)*
1	45	150
2	48	153
3	46	148
4	45	150
5	46	147
6	48	153
7	46	149
8	55	159
9	51	157
10	56	160
11	53	158
12	60	165
13	53	157
14	54	158
15	49	154

BP = Response (dependent) variable; Age = Predicator (independent) variable

REGRESSION MODEL

We can perform a 'regression of BP on age', to derive a straight line that gives an estimated value of BP for any given age.

The general equation of a linear regression line is: $Y = a + bX + e$, where, a = intercept, b = regression coefficient, e = statistical error

Precautions

Adequate sample size should be ensured. Prediction should be made within the range of the observed values. No extrapolation should be attempted. The equation, $Y = a + bX$ should not be used to predict X for a given Y and model adequacy should be verified.

Results of Regression Analysis

Ind. variable	Reg. coeff.	SE	*t*	*P*-value
Age	1.08	0.08	14.16	< 0.0001
Constant	100.34			

$R_2 = 93.99\% \approx 94\%$, systolic $BP = 100.34 + 1.08$ Age

95% CI for $b = b \pm 1.96$ SE(b) $= 1.08 \pm 1.96 \times 0.08 = (0.92, 1.24)$

Interpretations

1. Change in age by one year results in a change of 1.08 mm Hg in Sys BP
2. When age = 0, $BP = 100.34$, which is absurd *BP* of a 50-year-old individual is: $100.24 + 1.08 \times 50 = 154.34 \approx 154$ mm Hg
4. 94% of the variation in BP is explained by age alone

References

1. Stephen M Stigler. History of statistics: The Measurement of Uncertainty before 1900. http://www.hup.harvard.edu/catalog.php?isbn=9780674403413&content=bios.
2. Kamath Nagaraj, Shetty Suhas Kumar, Chiplunkar Shivprasad. Critique on biostatistical concepts in ayurveda. UJAHM 2013, 01 (03): Page 44–47; HYPERLINK "http://www.ujconline.net" www.ujconline.net.
3. Aina Schiøtz. Medical statistics and epidemiology–the early history. Norsk Epidemiologi 2015;25(1–2): 3–9).
4. Dan Mayer. Essential Evidence-based Medicine: Ch 1: A brief history of medicine and statistics, Cambridge University Press. Jun-2004.
5. Jarkko Isotalo (auth). Basics of Statistics, ch 2 and 3. https://www.mv.helsinki.fi/home/jmisotal/BoS.pdf
6. Goyal RC. Research Methodology for Health Professionals Including Proposal, Thesis and Article Writing. 1st edition, published by Jaypee Brothers, New Delhi, 2013.
7. Avan BI, White. Perspective on Variables in Medical Research. JPMA 51: 94, 2001 http://www.jpma.org.pk/full_article_text. php?article_id=2516
8. Principles of Epidemiology in Public Health Practice. 3rd edn., An Introduction to Applied Epidemiology and Biostatistics. October 2006. Updated May 2012. U.S. Centers for Disease Control and Prevention (CDC). Office of Workforce and Career Development. Atlanta, GA30333: https://www.cdc.gov/ophss/csels/dsepd/ss1978/ss1978.pdf. Assessed on 10th June 2018
9. Bonita R, Beaglehole R, Kjellström T. Basic epidemiology, 2nd edn, WHO Press, World Health

Organization, 20 Avenue Appia, 1211 Geneva 27, Switzerland.

10. Wolfgang Ahrens, Iris Pigeot (Ed.). Handbook of Epidemiology, Published by Springer-Verlag Berlin Heidelberg, 2005.
11. McNeil, Don. Chapter on Epidemiological Statistics–II. 10.1002/0471667196.ess019. Macquarie University, Sydney, New South Wales, Australia, 2004. https:www.researchgate.net/publication/228018339-Epidemiological_Statistics-11/citation/download
12. Inferential Analysis of Data, Chapter 8, http://shodhganga.inflibnet.ac.in/bitstream/10603/31029/15/15_chapter%208.pdf, Assessed on 9th July 2018
13. Gabrenya WJ (Jr). Inferential Statistics: Basic Concepts. 2003, version 1.0 http://my.fit.edu/~gabrenya/IntroMethods/eBook/inferentials.pdf. Assessed on 10th July 2018.
14. Chi-square test. http://uregina.ca/~gingrich/ch10.pdf, HYPERLINK "http://websupport1.citytech.cuny.edu/Faculty/mbessonov/MAT1272/Worksheet%20November%2021%252" http://websupport1.citytech.cuny.edu/Faculty/mbessonov/MAT1272/Worksheet%20November%2021%2, http://www.statisticshowto.com/probability-and-statistics/chi-square/
15. Logistic regression. Ch 12. http://www.stat.cmu.edu/~cshalizi/uADA/12/lectures/ch12.pdf. Assessed on 10th July 2018.

Chapter
14

Principles of Screening of Diseases

Ram Chandra Goyal

INTRODUCTION

Ideally, the control of a disease should be achievable, either by preventing the disease from occurring (primary prevention) or, if it does occur, by curing those who develop it by appropriate early disease detection and treatment (secondary prevention) and rehabilitation after treatment or disability and palliative care (tertiary prevention). "Early disease detection" generically includes both screening and periodic physical examination. Generally, epidemiological surveys are conducted to establish the prevalence and incidence of conditions, as well as to study longitudinally the natural history of developing disease, and case-finding is a natural by-product of surveys.

At present, neither the prevention nor the treatment is completely successful for most diseases; they will continue to complement each other for a number of conditions, while screening can be regarded as complementary to one or both of the other approaches.

In reality, screening may not be feasible for all diseases due to very nature of the diseases itself and limited resources, especially in developing low income countries where much of the resources are still spent curative services and whatever left is on environmental modifications as preventive measures. There are no time and resources to spend on looking for disease in its incipient stages (mostly applied to detect the hidden part of an 'iceberg' of diseases). On the other hand developed countries where infectious diseases have less mortality than chronic diseases and also with adequate resources can plan and practice screening programmes for disease.

Most of the screening programmes may be cost effective if widely applied and requires little physician time for interpretation as paramedical staff may be trained to conduct these programmes. Screening will help to improve the life expectancy and quality of life by avoiding late detection and early therapeutic interventions.

DEFINITIONS

Screening

The Commission on Chronic Illness (CCI) on Preventive Aspects of Chronic Disease (1957), defined screening as "the presumptive identification of unrecognized disease or defect by the application of tests, examinations, or other procedures which can be applied rapidly".[1–3]

The group's working definition of the term **screening** is based on that used in the WHO 'principles of screening' document (September 2001 draft): "screening is the process of identifying those individuals who are at sufficiently high risk of a specific disorder to warrant further investigation or direct action".

The definition goes on to say: "it [screening] is systematically offered to a population of people who have not sought medical attention on account of symptoms of the disease for which screening is being offered and is normally initiated by medical authorities and not by a patient's request for help on account of a specific complaint. The purpose of screening is to benefit the individuals being screened".[4]

Screening tests is applied to apparently healthy persons (who do not suspect that they may have a disease). A screening test is not intended to be diagnostic. A diagnostic test is applied to apparently sick persons. Persons with symptoms or suspicious findings must be referred for diagnosis and necessary treatment. Although it is usual to make the assumption that participants in screening programmes are asymptomatic/pre-symptomatic, this is not a necessary nor an absolute prerequisite for participation in public health based screening programmes.

Screening Program

It is a comprehensive disease control activity based on the identification and treatment of persons with either unrecognized disease or unrecognized risk factors for disease.

Surveillance

Surveillance is French word which means—**sur** (over) and **veiller** (to watch): So it is the "close and continuous observation of one or more persons for the purpose of direction, supervision, or control".[5]

In 1968, at the 21st World Health Assembly, surveillance was defined as "the systematic collection and use of epidemiologic information for the planning, implementation, and assessment of disease control".[6]

In the 1980s and 1990s, Thacker expanded the term to encompass not just disease, but any outcome, hazard, or exposure. In fact, the term **surveillance** is often applied to almost any effort to monitor, observe, or determine health status or event, diseases, or risk factors within a population.[7]

Surveillance should include—(1) identification, defining, and measuring the health problem of interest; (2) collection and compilation of data about the problem; (3) analyzing and interpreting these data; (4) providing these data and their interpretation to those responsible for controlling the health problem; and (5) monitoring and periodically evaluating the usefulness and quality of surveillance to improve it for future use. Surveillance of a problem does *not* include actions to control the problem.

Case-finding

It is one of the forms of screening of which the main object is to detect disease and bring patients to treatment, in contrast to epidemiological surveys.[1]

Epidemiological Surveys

It is a method of finding out the prevalence, incidence and natural history of the variable or variables under study, however these survey may findout cases, e.g. malnutrition during anthropometric survey, hypertension during blood pressure measurement, dental caries in children during school health check-up, etc. Examples of epidemiological surveys are Framingham study of ischemic heart disease, US Nurses' Health Study, etc.

Early Disease Detection

It refers to "all forms of early detection whether by screening, physical examination or other means (Tables 14.1 and 14.2)".[1]

Purpose of screening

1. Detection of those diseases in early stages for which early treatment is available and shown to be effective. This is also known as 'prescriptive screening.' It is defined as the presumptive identification of unrecognized disease, which does not arise from a patient's request. For example, people are examined primarily for their own benefit, e.g. examination of antenatal mothers

Table 14.1: Difference between screening and diagnostic test

Screening test	*Diagnostic test*
1. Done on apparently healthy	1. Done on those with indication or sick
2. Applied on groups	2. Applied on single patient when all diseases are under consideration
3. Test results are arbitrary and final	3. Diagnosis is not final but modified in light of new evidence, diagnosis is sum of all evidence
4. Based on one criteria or cut-off point	4. Based on evaluation of a number of symptoms, signs and lab findings
5. Less accurate	5. More accurate
6. Less expensive	6. More expensive
7. Not the basis for treatment	7. Used as a basis for treatment
8. The initiative comes from investigator	8. The initiative comes from patient

Table 14.2: Some examples

Disease	*Screening tests*	*Diagnostic tests*
Diabetes	Urine sugar and blood sugar	Oral glucose tolerance test
Hypertension	Measurement of blood pressure	Measurement of blood pressure
Cervical cancer	PAP smear	Biopsy
Tuberculosis	Mass miniature radiography (MMR)	Sputum examination
HIV	ELISA test	Western blot test
Breast cancer	Self breast examination, mammography	Biopsy, mammography

for anemia, blood pressure, syphilis, diabetes, etc.

2. To lower morbidity and mortality of the disease in a population (control, rather than elimination of disease).
3. It provides access to the medical care system which is not an actual goal of screening, but is a benefit.
4. People are examined primarily for the benefit of others (prevention of disease transmission), e.g. examination of immigrants for communicable diseases such as TB, hepatitis 'B' and 'C' to protect unaffected population. This is also known as 'proscriptive screening'.
5. Screening (epidemiological survey) is also done to study the incidence, prevalence and natural history of the disease to acquire more knowledge for prevention and control of diseases.

Types of Screening

Primarily the type of screening depends on the disease and its outcome, i.e. morbidity and mortality and its impact on the quality of life. Other than these factors, sociological factors like the level of education and awareness, availability of medical care, standard of living, etc. have also been important in the development of screening. In developing countries, most efforts are directed at relatively simple screening tests for infection and signs of poor growth and development in babies and young children, or for chronic conditions such as tuberculosis and HIV/AIDS. Developed countries test for these conditions too, but a lot of screening is directed at middle-aged or older people where cancers, heart disease and high blood pressure are most common. Whatever the cost and complexity of the test, the rationale for all screening methods is either to prevent disease from occurring in the first place. Basically, there are three broad categories of screening as discussed below.

Mass screening: It is offered to whole or subgroup of population irrespective of special risk. In this context, 'population' rarely means every citizen of a country. Population screening usually identifies a particular target population group—for example, everyone over the age of 50 years, or all newborn babies or all women of reproductive age—and attempts are made to screen everyone in that category, sometimes at regular intervals. Now a day's scope of mass screening is limited to those disease having high endemicity usually to control the spread of communicable disease, however indiscriminate mass screening is not a useful preventive measure unless it is backed-up by suitable treatment and follow-up facilities for positive screeners. It has been recognized that this approach gives rise to operational and financial problems and of late it has declined in popularity as a means of early disease detection.

Selective screening: The aim is to find out high risk population so as to reduce morbidity and mortality in a select group. It is done by combining a number of tests and applying them all at the one examination, providing each has been shown to be medically worthwhile. For example at antenatal, post-natal and infant welfare clinics, where conditions such as pre-eclampsia, anemia, diabetes, hepatitis/HIV infection and congenital conditions are sought by the application of simple tests. This kind of screening may be applied to school children, elderly, living in disease prone geographical areas, etc.

High-risk screening: High-risk screening is a type of selective screening offered to those thought to be at special risk, e.g. screening of close relatives of known diabetics, hypertension, breast cancer, hereditary/familial diseases. This way a greater number of cases can be identified at less cost.

Targeted screening: For occupational exposures—this is also in a way kind of selective screening. When targeted screening is done in groups with occupational exposures, the criteria for screening are not necessarily as strict as those for general population screening. Screening may be a high priority if the health effects reduce the patient's ability to work. Targeted screening can be legally required, e.g. in miners, people working with lead or chromium, etc. 'Targeted' screening for diabetes, dyslipidemia, other cancers like prostate, colon and transient ischaemic attacks to be carried out.[8]

Multiphase screening: It is the most efficient and economical method of screening. It uses several screening tests at the same time to screen variety of diseases at one time rather than to carryout separate screening tests for a single disease.

In 1957, the commission on chronic illness (CCI) accepted the value of multiple screenings as 'contributing to good medical practice' and considered that it "constitutes a practical means for early detection of a number of important chronic diseases and impairments". The CCI considered at that time that screening might profitably be carried out for the pulmonary tuberculosis, visual defects (including chronic glaucoma), hearing defects, syphilis, diabetes, cancers of skin, mouth, breast, cervix and rectum, hypertensive diseases, ischaemic heart disease.[1]

In 1960, the American Public Health Association strongly endorsed multiple screening in a publication entitled chronic disease and rehabilitation—a program guide for state and local health agencies. In India, evaluation of conventional risk factors like hypertension, diabetes mellitus, obesity, dyslipidaemia, and smoking must be done in men from the age of 30 years onwards and in women of post-menopausal age.[9]

Opportunistic Screening or Case-finding

It is aimed at patients who consult a health practitioner for some other purpose, e.g. patient seeking physician's advice for diabetes may also be screened for hypertension, obesity, cardiovascular diseases, etc. In India, 'opportunistic' screening for tobacco consumption, high blood pressure, overweight, central obesity, COPD, cervical cancer and oral cancer to be done.

Principles of introduction of screening program: It is based on the disease to be screened and test to be applied for screening the disease under study.

Disease to be Screened

Disease must be an important public health problem—the prevalence of the disease should be high and the cause of substantial mortality and/or morbidity. The level of morbidity and mortality considered to be important will depend on a combination of factors such as the age distribution of the population affected, or the severity of the illness. Sometimes, the screening may not reduce death rates, but may alter the natural history of the diseases by identifying the diseases in early stage and instituting the treatment at an early stage so as to get cure or may reduce the suffering. The importance of the problem needs to be considered for screening should be looked into the perspectives of both the individual and the community. Those conditions with serious consequences (inborn metabolic defects) to the individual and their family in general may necessitate relatively costly screening measures; while some diseases (tuberculosis) having serious consequences for the community if not discovered early and treated, will justify screening on these grounds.

Disease should have latent pre-symptomatic stage—there must clearly be a reasonable period in the natural history of the condition during which symptoms are either not present or not reported. The disease should have a reasonably long lead time; that is, the interval between the time when the disease can be first diagnosed by screening and when it is usually diagnosed in patients presenting with symptoms. If the disease is detected well in early stage then only screening is meaningful (Figs 14.1 to 14.3).

Facilities for diagnosis and treatment—it is a pre-requisite for screening that persons found in need of treatment should be able to obtain the same and the disease should be treatable. There should be evidence of the effectiveness of treatment in reducing disease incidence and/or mortality and the subjective improvement. For example, availability of the definitive diagnostic and treatment facilities for those found to be positive on cytological examination is necessary before introducing the nationwide cytological screening program for all women with a risk of developing cervical cancer.

Availability of suitable test and acceptability to the population—the screening should be safe, easy and quick to perform. It may have higher margin of error and may be less valid than a diagnostic test.

A test or series of tests must be acceptable to the population to which it is offered.

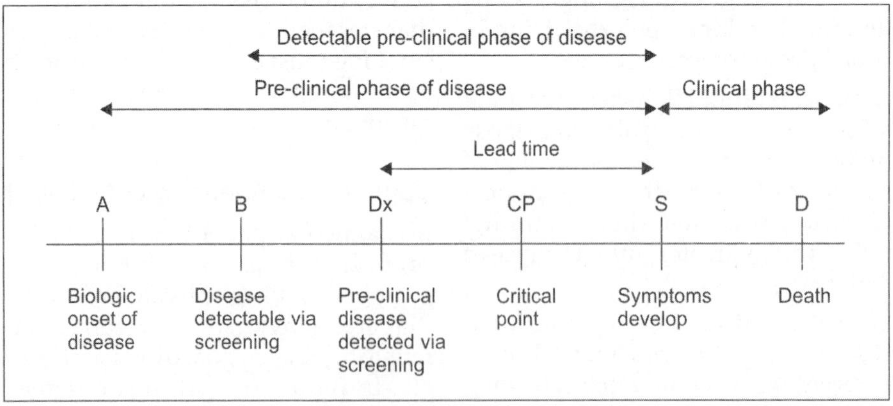

Fig. 14.1: Concept of lead time

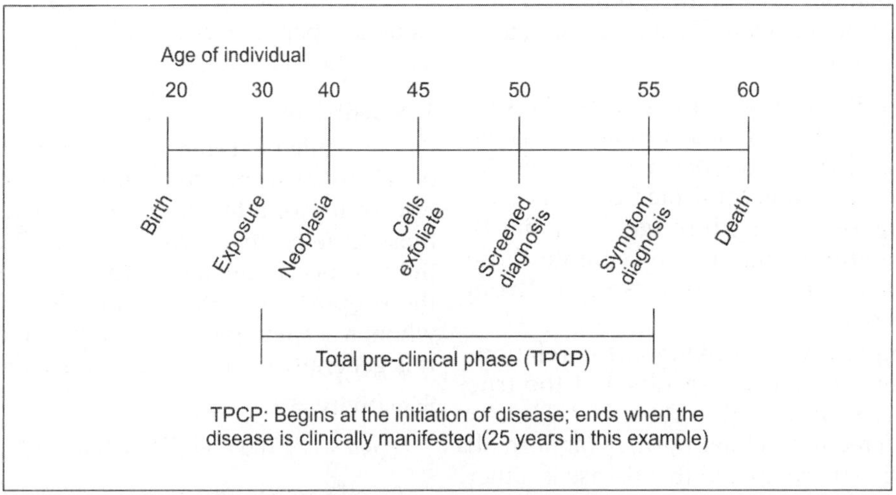

Fig. 14.2: Natural history of disease

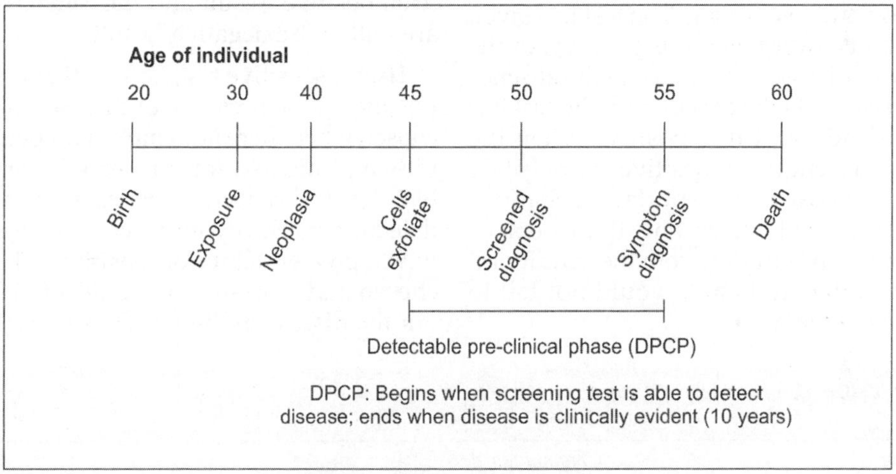

Fig. 14.3: Natural history of disease

Acceptability is related to the nature of the risk and psychological preparation. For example, the risk prenatal is well accepted by all the sections of the society but prophylactic vaginal and cytological examination is not well accepted in many low socio-economic women.

Cost of screening programs—the costs of a screening programme must be cost effective, i.e. balanced against the number of cases detected and the consequences of not screening. The CCI, states that: "Multiple screening, by combining several disease-detection tests, is a streamlined process assuring speed, efficiency and economy. Multiple screening contributes to good medical practice".

The primary aim is to improve the health of a population by the early detection and treatment of illness; while the immediate socio-economic aim is to spare the time of highly trained people by using technicians, and automated methods, as a first line in disease detection, hence reducing the cost.

Test Used for Screening

Apart from the screening test criteria like cost effectiveness, easy to apply and acceptable to the population—the validity, reliability and yield must be considered while choosing for a screening test.

The validity of a screening test—the CCI defines the validity of a screening test as the measure of the frequency with which the result of that test is confirmed by an acceptable diagnostic procedure (gold standard), i.e. the ability of the test to separate those who have the condition sought from those who do not.

A simple way of looking at the relationships between a test's results and the true diagnosis is mentioned in Table 14.3. The test is considered to be either positive (abnormal) or negative (normal) and the disease is either present or absent. There are then four possible interpretations of the test results, two of which are correct and two wrong. The test has given the correct answer when it is positive, in the presence of disease or negative in the absence of the disease. On the other hand, the test has been misleading, if it is positive when the disease is absent (false positive) or negative when the disease is present (false negative). An ideal test would detect only those persons in a population suffering from the condition/ diseases under study and would not fail to detect any of them.

From the Tables 14.3 and 14.4, following statistical parameters of validity of screening test can be calculated.

1. Sensitivity

It is also called 'PiD rate (positivity in disease)' or 'TP rate (true positive rate)'. It is defined as 'the ability of a test to identify correctly all those (true positive) who have the disease' in the screened population. This is expressed as the proportion of those with the disease in whom a screening test gives a positive result. It is generally expressed as percentages.

Sensitivity =

$$a/a + c \times 100 = 40/50 \times 100 = 80\%$$

An 80% sensitivity mean that 80% of people with disease screened by the test will give 'true positive' result and the remaining 20% are with 'false negative' result.

Use: A sensitive test, i.e. one that is usually positive in the presence of disease, should be chosen when there is an important penalty for missing a disease. If the disease is very lethal (e.g. cervical cancer, breast cancer) and early detection markedly improves prognosis, test with a greater degree of sensitivity should be chosen and work-up can be relied on to rule out the disease in the false positives. That is,

Table. 14.3: The relationship between sensitivity, specificity, and positive and negative predictive value (the gold standard)

Screening test results	*Gold standard (True disease classification of apparently well population)*			
	Disease			
	Present	*Absent*	*Total*	
Positive	a **True positive** (with disease and positive test)	b **False positive** (without disease but with positive test)	$a + b$ (total persons with positive test)	Positive predictive value (PPV) = $a/b + b$
Negative	c **False negative** (with disease but with negative test)	d **True negative** (without disease and with negative test)	$c + d$ (total persons with negative test)	Negative predictive value (NPV) = $d/c + d$
Total	$a + c$ (total unknown cases of disease)	$b + d$ (total persons without disease)	$a + b + c + d$ (total persons)	
	Sensitivity = $a/a + c$	Specificity = $d/b + d$		

Table 14.4: Distribution of pap smear results for screening of cervical cancer among 200 women aged between 50 and 55 years (a hypothetical example)

Screening test results	*Gold standard (true disease classification of apparently well population)*		
	Disease		
	Present	*Absent*	*Total*
Positive	$a = 40$ **True positive**	$b = 5$ **False positive**	$a + b = 45$ Total positive tests
Negative	$c = 10$ **False negative**	$d = 145$ **True negative**	$c + d = 155$ Total negative test
Total	$a + c = 50$	$b + d = 150$	$a + b + c + d = 200$

proportion of false positives are tolerable but not false negatives. However, there are several other criteria, which need to be taken into consideration while choosing optimal sensitivity of a test.

Specificity

It is also known as 'NiH rate (negativity in health)' or 'TN rate (true negative rate)'. It is defined as 'the ability of a test to identify correctly those who do not have the disease or free of diseases, that is, 'true negatives' in the screened population. This is expressed as the proportion of people free of the disease in which the screening test gives a negative result and expressed as percentages.

Specificity =

$$d/b + d \times 100 = 145/150 \times 100 = 96.7\%$$

A total of 96.7% specificity means that 96.7% of the persons without diseases screened by the test will give 'true negative' result, and the remaining 3.3% 'false positive' result. In other words, 3.3% of persons without diseases screened by the test will be wrongly classified as 'having disease' when actually they do not have disease.

Use: Specific tests are useful to confirm (or 'rule in') a diagnosis that has been suggested by other data. This is because a highly specific test is rarely positive in the absence of disease, i.e. it gives few false positive results. Highly specific tests are recommended in following situations.

For diseases like diabetes for which treatment does not markedly alter outcome, specificity must be high and early cases may be missed, but false positives should be limited; otherwise the health system will be overburdened with diagnostic demands on the positives, both true and false.

Highly specific tests are particularly needed when false positive result can harm the patient physically, or financially. Thus, before patients are subjected to cancer chemotherapy, with all its attendant risks, emotional trauma, and financial costs, true diagnosis is generally required instead of relying upon less specific tests. That is, high specificity is necessary when false positive errors must be avoided.

False negatives and false positives: Quest for ideal screening test should take in consideration both pre-test probabilities (sensitivity and specificity of a test) and post-test probabilities (false negative and false positives results). To estimate the post-test probability, predictive values are horizontally calculated operating characteristics, which incorporate both false-positive and false-negative results into disease probability. The positive predictive value (PPV) is the probability of a patient actually having the disease if the test result is positive. The probability of the patient being free of the disease after a negative test result is given by the negative predictive value (NPV).

False-negative rate: The term 'false negative' means that patients who actually have the disease are told that they do not have the disease (test result negative). A screening test, which is very sensitive, has few 'false negatives'. The lower the sensitivity, the larger will be the number of 'false negatives'.

False-negative rate =
$c/a + c \times 100 = 10/50 \times 100 = 20\%$

Of all the people with diseased screened by the test, 20% showed false negative results. The sensitivity of a test is 80% and false negative rate is 20%.

Implications: False-negative result means giving 'false reassurance'. The persons with a 'false negative' test result might ignore the development of signs and symptoms and may delay the treatment. This could be detrimental if the disease in question is a serious one and the test is unlikely to be repeated within a short period of time.

False-positive rate: The term 'false positive' means that persons who do not have the disease (gold standard) are told that they have disease (test result positive). A screening test with high specificity will have few false positives.

False-positive rate =
$b/b + d \times 100 = 5/150 \times 100 = 3.3\%$

Out of all the persons without disease screened by the test, 3.3% showed false-positive results. The specificity of a test is 9.7% and false-positive rate is 3.3%.

Implications: In this case, normal healthy people may be subjected to further diagnostic tests, at some inconvenience, discomfort, anxiety and expense—until their freedom from disease is established. Thus, false positives not only burden the diagnostic facilities, but they also bring discredit to screening programme.

Positive predictive value

Synonyms:
- Predictive value of a positive test.
- Post-test likelihood of the target disorder following a positive test
- Posterior probability of the target disorder following a positive test
- Post-test probability of the target disorder following a positive test

The 'predictive value of positive test' indicates the probability that a patient with a positive test result has, in fact, the disease in question or this is the proportion of patients with positive test results who have the target disorder.

Positive predictive value = $a/a + b \times 100 = 40/45 \times 100 = 88.9\%$; means nearly 89% of patients with positive test results had really the disease.

Features:
- It reflects the screening power of a test.
- The more specific the test is, the better will be the positive predictive value of the test.
- It depends on sensitivity, specificity and disease prevalence.
- The positive predictive value is directly proportional to the disease prevalence in population.

Effect of disease prevalence: The predictive value of a test is not a property of the test alone; it is determined by the sensitivity and the prevalence of disease in the population being tested, where prevalence has its customary meaning—the proportion of persons in a defined population at a given point in time with the condition in question. Prevalence is also called prior (pre-test) probability of disease before the test result is known. The mathematical formula relating sensitivity, specificity, and prevalence to positive predictive value is derived from the Bayes' theorem of conditional probabilities:

Positive predictive =
(Sensitivity × Prevalence/value)/
[(Sensitivity × Prevalence) +
(1 – Specificity) × (1 – Prelevance)]

The more sensitive a test is, the better will be its negative predictive value (the more confident the investigator can be that a negative test result rules out the disease being sought) conversely the more specific the test is, the better will be its positive predictive value (the more confident the investigator can be that a positive test confirms or rules in the diagnosis being sought). Because predictive value is also influenced by prevalence, it is not independent of the setting in which the test is used. As the prevalence of disease in a population approaches zero, the positive predictive value of a test also approaches zero. Conversely, if everyone in a population tested has the disease, all negative results will be false negative even for a sensitive test. As prevalence approaches 100%, negative predictive value approaches zero.

Negative predictive value: This is also called predictive value of a negative test or post-test likelihood of not having the target disorder following a negative test or posterior probability of not having the target disorder following a negative test or post-test probability of not having the target disorder following a negative test.

The 'predictive value of negative test' indicates the probability that a patient with a negative test result does not in fact, have the disease in question or this is the proportion of patients with negative test results who do not have the target disorder.

Negative predictive value

= $d/c + d \times 100$

= $145/155 \times 100$

= 93.5% (means 93.5% of persons with negative test results did not have the disease)

Features:

- It reflects the screening power of a test.
- The more sensitive a test is, the better will be the negative predictive value of the test (the more confident the investigator can be that a patient with a negative test result does not have the disease being sought).
- It depends on sensitivity, specificity and disease prevalence.
- It is inversely proportional to the disease prevalence in population.

Sensitivity and specificity variation: Sensitivity and specificity can be varied reciprocally according to the 'setting' of the test. This may be due to variation of the method and the variation of the observer. The example of intra-observer bias while screening for tuberculosis by X-ray chest examination among contacts of active tuberculosis patients is as under.

Radiologists are frequently subject to this kind of bias when they read X-ray. Because X-ray interpretation is somewhat subjective, it is easy to be influenced by the clinical information provided. All clinicians experience the situation of having X-rays over read because of a clinical impression, or conversely, of going back over old-X-ray in which a finding was missed because a clinical event was not known at that time and therefore attention were not directed to the particular area in the X-ray. Because of these biases, some radiologists prefer to read X-rays twice, first without and then with the clinical information. All of these biases tend to increase the agreement between the test and the standard of validity (Table 14.5).

A number of studies in different populations have reported on the performance of a **fasting plasma glucose** of 6.1 mmol/L. They report sensitivities ranging from 58–87% (median—81%) and specificities ranging from 75–98% (median—92%).

Random blood glucose (RBG) as a screening test have mostly used random capillary blood glucose (RCBG) measured with a blood glucose meter. Rolka *et al*. reported that RCBG

Table 14.5: An example variation of the method

Total population	*Diabetics*	*Screening method for type-2 diabetes*							
400	40	*Venous fasting plasma glucose*				*Random capillary blood glucose (RCBG)*			
		Positive		*Negative*		*Positive*		*Negative*	
		True	*False*	*True*	*False*	*True*	*False*	*True*	*False*
		32	35	325	08	22	15	345	18
Sensitivity		$32/40 \times 100 = 80\%$				$22/40 \times 100 = 55\%$			
Specificity		$325/360 \times 100 = 90.2\%$				$345/360 \times 100 = 95.8\%$			

of 6.7 mmol/L had sensitivity of 56% and specificity of 96%, respectively.[10]

Likelihood ratio: As the prevalence of disease in a population approaches zero, the positive predictive value of a test also approaches zero and if the prevalence of disease in a population approaches 100%, the positive predictive value of a test also approaches 100%. However, as prevalence approaches 100%, negative predictive value approaches zero and if prevalence approaches zero, negative predictive value approaches 100%. Thus, predictive values are quite susceptible to prevalence. But, sensitivity and specificity are usually not affected by varying prevalence rates, even if they are affected, much less than the predictive values. In most situations sensitivity and specificity are stable.

Likelihood ratios more stable than sensitivity and specificity and are therefore likely to become more popular as test evaluation statistics.

Likelihood ratio of a positive test result—this is the ratio of the proportion with a positive test result in those with disease to the proportion with a positive test result in those without disease.

Likelihood ratio of a positive test result = $[a/a + c]/[b/b + d]$

Or Sensitivity/1 – Specificity
Or True positives/False positives

Calculation and interpretation—(Table 14.4)—0.80/0.33 = 2.42

The likelihood ratio for a positive test result is 2.42, means that screening test of this nature is 2.42 times as likely to come from patients with diseases as from patients without disease.

Likelihood ratio of negative test result—this is the ratio of proportion with a negative test result in those with disease to the proportion with a negative test result in those without disease, i.e. the odds that a negative test result would be expected in a patient with disease as opposed to one without it.

Estimation—likelihood ratio of a negative test result = $[c/a + c]/[d/b + d]$

Or 1 – Sensitivity/Specificity
Or False negatives/True negatives

Calculation and interpretation—(Table 14.4)—0.200/0.967 = 0.21

The likelihood ratio for a negative test result is 0.21, means that screening test of this kind is 0.21 times as likely to come from patients with disease as opposed to patients without diseases.

One can define likelihood ratios for any number of test results, over the entire range of possible values. In this way, information represented by the degree of abnormality, rather than the crude presence or absence of it, is not discarded. In computing likelihood ratios across a range of test result, sensitivity refers to the ability of that particular test result to identify people with the disease, not individuals with that result or worse. The same is true for the calculation of specificity. Thus, likelihood ratios can accommodate the common and reasonable clinical practice of putting more weight on extremely high (or low) test result than on borderline ones when estimating the probability (or odds) that a particular disease is present.

Receiver Operating Characteristic (ROC) Curve

When the test result is expressed as a continuous variable (mg% or international units), there are obviously varying sensitivity and specificity rates for differing values of the test. The choice of cut-off points usually depends on the relative merits of sensitivity and specificity of the screening test of the disease in question. What is plotted is the sensitivity in the vertical axis and 1 – specificity (the false positive rate) in the horizontal axis. The point on the curve that is chosen as optimal is often that furthest from the 45° diagonal, labelled 'chance' as this represents a test with no better sensitivity or specificity than could be expected by chance (Fig. 14.4).

The ideal cut-off values are those with the greatest net benefits of screening, making a diagnosis and instituting therapy. However,

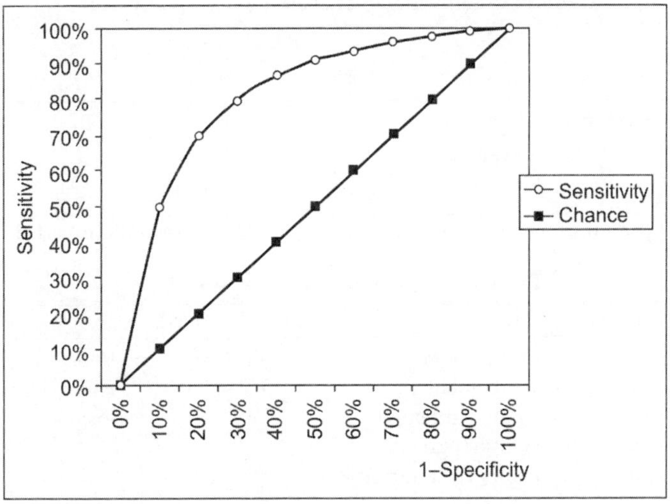

Fig. 14.4: ROC curve

generally there is a trade-off between the sensitivity and specificity of a screening test. It is obviously desirable to have a test, which is both highly sensitive and highly specific. Unfortunately, this is frequently not possible. In order to evaluate the performance of a test over a range of possible cut-off values and also to compare different screening tests, the receiver operating characteristic (ROC) curve is a very useful mode of analysis.

Properties of ROC Curve

a. Best cut-off—the upper left-hand corner of ROC denotes a perfect screening test—a TP rate of 100% and FP rate of 0%. It follows that the points on ROC curve that is closest to this upper left-hand corner is the 'best' cut-off in terms of making the fewest mistakes when prevalence is around 50% (i.e. its use minimizes the sum of false-positives and false-negatives). It is where (sensitivity + specificity)/2 attain its highest value. The screening test whose ROC curve encloses the largest area is the most accurate one.
b. Area under ROC curve—area under ROC curve can be calculated by either Wilcoxon statistics or trapezoidal rule. It indicates the overall predictive accuracy of a test.
c. Comparison of different screening tests for the same disease.
d. Such curves cannot be applied to a test with a dichotomous outcome if the boundaries defining positive and negative are invariant. Further they imply a similar weight to sensitivity and specificity, which may not be ideal.

Agreement

When a screening test is being compared with a gold standard, establishment of agreement between two is important (Table 14.6). How much is the agreement between positive and negative results of two tests, has to be answered. It is also essential to evaluate the reproducibility of test interpretation by different observers. If there is a wide disagreement between observers in interpreting the same set of test results, it renders the test useless for widespread application. If the results are dichotomous, a chance-corrected index of agreement like Cohen's Kappa should be calculated (Tables 14.6 and 14.7).

$P_0 = a + d$ and $P_e = P_1 \times P_2 + Q_1 \times Q_2$, so kappa = $(P_0 - P_e)/(1 - P_e)$

Sources of Bias

Lead-time: The interval between the time of detection by screening and the time diabetes would have been diagnosed in the absence of screening. Thus, lead-time bias prolongs the apparent duration of survival and/or

Table 14.6: Agreement between two tests/observers

		Gold standard/second test		
	Test results	*Positive*	*Negative*	
First test	Positive	*a*	*b*	P_1
	Negative	*c*	*d*	Q_1
·	Total	$P_2(a+c)$	$Q_2(b+d)$	$N = 1$

$P_o = a + d$, proportion observed and $P_e = P_1 P_2 + Q_1 Q_2$, proportion expected

Table 14.7: Quantitative terms to kappa's

Landis and Koch		*Fleiss*	
0–0.2	Slight agreement	<0.4	Poor
0.2–0.4	Fair agreement	0.4–0.75	Fair to good
0.4–0.6	Moderate agreement	>0.75	Excellent
0.6–0.8	Substantial agreement		
0.8–1.0	Almost perfect agreement		

complication-free period simply by advancing the diagnosis.

Selection bias: People who enter screening programmes are volunteers who are almost always more health conscious than the rest of the population. Thus they are more likely to have a better disease outcome even without screening.

Length-time bias: This relates to the fact that individuals with rapid deterioration will tend to develop symptoms that prompt them to contact health services. Thus, only people with slowly progressing and milder disease remain to be identified by screening. These people are likely to have a better clinical outcome than rapidlyprogressing cases, regardless of the treatment.

Over-diagnosis bias occurs when enthusiastic screening results in diagnosing the diseases in people that do not have it. Since healthy individuals have a more favourable life course than persons with disease, this difference in the outcome may be erroneously attributed to screening.

Unregulated Screening Tests (Are they Useful?)[11]

Whole-body Computerized Tomography (CT) Screening

This is being promoted, particularly in the USA, as a 'useful' screening test for apparently healthy. In April 2002, the American Food and Drug Administration (FDA) stated that—(1) no manufacturer has submitted data to the FDA supporting the safety and efficacy of screening claims for whole-body CT; (2) The radiation exposure of a CT exam can be several hundred times that of a chest X-ray; and (3) A CT scan is not helpful for ruling out disease.

Whole-body Magnetic Resonance Imaging (MRI) Screening

As public awareness of the high radiation dose from whole-body CT screening has grown, commercial providers are moving into the field of whole-body MRI screening for healthy people. Although there is no radiation dose, the usefulness of this as a screening procedure is completely unproven. Full-body MRI is likely to produce many false alarms as it shows up minor 'lumps and bumps' within the body. For example, in people over 50 years of age, half will have one or more cysts found in the kidneys. To then establish that these cysts are not harmful may require expensive and hazardous further tests. A study published in 2005 concluded that costs and benefits are uncertain.

Exercise Electrocardiogram (ECG) Screening (exercise stress test)

Some commercial companies in developed countries like in the UK offer exercise ECG as part of well-person screening. Yet in people without symptoms or signs of heart disease this is far more likely to do harm than good. Authoritative recommendations from heart specialists' professional organizations, even in the USA, say that this test is valuable for some people with heart disease but **not** for people without.

Prostate Cancer Screening Using Prostate Specific Antigen (PSA) Testing

If there was certain evidence that prostate screening could successfully cut deaths from prostate cancer without causing too much harm, then the government would introduce screening without delay. Unfortunately, this is not the case. There is no evidence to say that you will succeed in cutting the deaths.

Breast Screening with Mammography (breast X-ray) Under Age 50 Years

Private screening providers often advise mammography under 50, although the NHS breast screening programme only starts screening from 50. The NHS policy is based on the balance of benefit and harm. For example, if 1,000 women in their 40s are screened for 10 years, it may prevent one death from breast cancer and 250 of the 1,000 women will suffer false alarms, with most needing biopsy investigations and many having mastectomy 'just in case'.

Table 14.8: Screening test validity criteria, formula and definitions

Validity criteria	*Formula*	*Definition*
Sensitivity = True - positive rate (TPR)	TP/(TP + FN)	The probability that a patient with the disease will have a positive test result
1 – Sensitivity = False - negative rate (FPR)	FN/(TP + FN)	The probability that a patient with the disease will have a negative test result
Specificity = True - negative rate (TNR)	TN/(TN + FP)	The probability that a patient without the disease will have a negative test result
1 – Specificity = False - positive rate (FPR)	FP/(TN + FP)	The probability that a patient without the disease will have a positive test result
Positive predictive value (PPV)	TP/(TP + FP)	The probability that a patient with a positive test result will have the disease
Negative predictive value (NPV)	TN/(TN + FN)	The probability that a patient with a negative test result will not have the disease
Accuracy	(TP + TN)/(TP + TN + FP + FN)	The probability that the results of a test will accurately predict presence or absence of disease
Bayes' theorem	Post-test odds = Pre-test odds × Likelihood ratio	The odds of having or not having the disease after testing
Likelihood ratio of a positive test result (LR+)	Sensitivity/(1 – Specificity)	The increase in the odds of having the disease after a positive test result
Likelihood ratio of a negative test result (LR–)	(1 – Sensitivity)/Specificity	The decrease in the odds of having the disease after a negative test result
Cohen's kappa test (refer Tables 14.6 and 14.7)	$P_0 = a + d$ and $P_e = P_1 \times P_2 + Q_1 \times Q_2$, kappa = $(P_0 - P_e)/(1 - P_e)$	It is a measure of agreement for a screening test which gives a categorical result

Summary

- Screening for disease involves a test to identify individuals at sufficient risk of a specific disorder to warrant further investigation, preventive action or treatment; the aim is to detect and treat the condition more successfully at an earlier stage.
- Screening tests must be simple, safe, accurate and acceptable to the public and health professionals; the benefits of screening must outweigh the potential harms or risks.

Screening test validity criteria, formula and definitions are mentioned in Table 14.8.

List of screening recommendations for older adults, USA is mentioned in Table 14.9 and chronic diseases in India are mentioned in Table 14.10.

Table14.9: List of screening recommendations for older adults, USA[12]

	CANCER
Breast	USPSTF: Women aged 50–74 years—biennial mammography; before age 50, the decision to start regular, biennial screening mammography should be an individual one and take patient context into account, including the patient's values regarding specific benefits and harms; no upper age limit suggested although limited evidence >75
	ACS: CBE every 3 years for women in 20s and 30s; mammography yearly for women ≥40 with annual CBE; no upper age limit suggested. Some women, because of their family history, a genetic tendency, or other factors, should be screened with MRI in addition to mammograms; discuss with healthcare provider.
Cervical	Yearly regular Pap test beginning latest age 21. At age 30, change to every 2–3 years if had 3 normal Pap tests in a row stopping at:
	USPSTF: Age 65
	ACS: Age 70 if had 3 or more normal Pap tests in a row and no abnormal Pap tests in last 10 years
Colon	USPSTF: FOBT yearly or flexible sigmoidoscopy every 5 years or colonoscopy every 10 years starting at age 50 and continuing until age 75 (unless a primary relative was diagnosed with colorectal cancer <60, then screen earlier)
	ACS: Beginning at age 50, both men and women at average risk. FOBT yearly, fecal immunochemical test, or stool DNA (time interval not defined), or flexible sigmoidoscopy every 5 years (if positive, do colonoscopy) or colonoscopy every 10 years starting at age 50 or double contrast barium enema every 5 years (if positive, do colonoscopy) or CT colonography every 5 years (if positive, do colonoscopy) (unless a primary relative was diagnosed with colorectal cancer <60 or >2 or more primary relatives of any age, then screen earlier).
	ACS does not impose an upper age limit to stop screening.
Prostate	Yearly digital rectal exam (DRE) as part of yearly physical examination.
	USPSTF: Older men, African–American men, and men with a family history of prostate cancer are at increased risk of prostate cancer. Evidence insufficient for screening men <75; recommend against screening men >75.
	ACS: Evidence insufficient for screening. Beginning at age 50, discuss screening with healthcare provider. Begin discussion at age 45 if at higher risk (African–American or have first degree relatives with prostate cancer before age 65).

Contd...

	CARDIOVASCULAR DISEASE AND DIABETES
CHD	ACC/AHA: Exercise stress testing in selected men >45 and women >55 with multiple cardiac risk factors or diabetes and discuss aspirin chemoprevention in high-risk patients; no upper age limit suggested
Hypertension	JNC-7: BP reading every 2 years in all adults if <120/80, otherwise yearly
Dyslipidemia	USPSTF: Routine screen (TC and HDL-C) in women >45 if at increased risk of CHD and all men >35 NCEP: Age ≥20 (TC, LDL, and HDL) No upper age limit suggested; approximately every 5 years, depending on levels
Obesity	USPSTF: All adults screened for obesity (BMI >30 kg/m^2) and offer counselling and behavioural interventions; no upper age limit suggested
Tobacco	USPSTF: Screen all adults and provide cessation interventions for those who use tobacco; no upper age limit suggested
Diabetes	ADA: Adults ≥45 and repeated every 3 years with fasting blood sugar; more frequently if high risk; no upper age limit suggested USPSTF: Screen in presence of hypertension or dyslipidemia to reduce cardiovascular disease risk

ACC = American College of Cardiology; ACS = American Cancer Society; ADA = American Diabetes Association; AHA = American Heart Association; CBE = Clinical breast exam; CHD = Coronary heart disease; DRE = Digital rectal exam; FOBT = Fecal occult blood testing; HDL-C = High-density lipoprotein cholesterol; JNC-7 = Seventh Report of the Joint National Committee on Prevention, Detection, Evaluation, and Treatment of High Blood Pressure; LDL-C = Low-density lipoprotein cholesterol; MRI = Magnetic resonance imaging; NCEP = National Cholesterol Education Panel; PSA = Prostatic specific antigen; TC = Total cholesterol; USPSTF = US Preventive Services Task Force

Table 14.10: List of screening tests for chronic diseases in India[9,13–15]

	CANCER
Breast	• Regular breast self examination by women themselves. • Mammographic screening (if feasible).
Oral	• Visual examination of oral cavity by trained health professionals.
Cervical	• Visual inspection of the cervix after swabbing it with acetic acid (VIA) beginning age of 35 years. • Yearly regular cervical cytology (Pap test) beginning age of 35 years (if feasible).
Prostate	• Yearly digital rectal exam (DRE) beginning at age 50 years. • Serum prostate specific antigen (PSA) measurement, if facilities available
Colon	• Fecal occult blood test (FOBT) starting at age 50 yearly or flexible sigmoidoscopy or colonoscopy (if facilities available)
	CHRONIC DISEASES OTHER THAN CANCER
Hypertension	JNC-7: BP reading (at first opportunity) every 2 years in all adults if <120/80, otherwise yearly
Overweight/obesity	Height and weight measurement of all adults for obesity (BMI >30 kg/m^2) at first opportunity and then at regular interval (may be biannually)
Diabetes	Random blood sugar by glucometer or oral glucose tolerance test (OGTT) yearly after the age of 40 years (targeted group)
CHD	ECG, exercise stress testing in selected men >45 and women >55 (targeted group)
Dyslipidemia	HDL-C, LDL-C, total cholesterol and triglycerides (if facilities available) beginning at age 35 years every 5 years (targeted group)

References

1. Commission on Chronic Illness. Chronic illness in the United States: Volume I. Prevention of chronic illness, Cambridge, Mass, Harvard University Press, 1957, p. 45.
2. Wilson JMG , Jungner G. Principles and practice of screening for Disease.Public health papers No. 34. World Health Organization, Geneva, 1968.
3. Anthony B Miller. Screening (Ch III 10) in Ahrens W, Pigeot I (Eds). Handbook of Epidemiology. Springer-Verlag Berlin Heidelberg 2005, pp 1267–1304.
4. World Health Organization. Principles of Screening (draft). Geneva: World Health Organization, 2001.
5. Merriam-Webster. Merriam-Webster's Dictionary of English Usage. Springfield (MA): Merriam-Webster, Inc. 1976.
6. World Health Organization. Report of the technical discussions at the twenty-first World Health Assembly on 'national and global surveillance of communicable diseases.' Geneva: World Health Organization; 18 May 1968, p. A21.
7. Thacker SB, Berkelman RL. Public health surveillance in the United States. Epidemiol Rev 1988;10:164–190.
8. Srinath K Reddy. Prevention and control of non-communicable diseases: Status and strategies. Working paper no. 104. Indian Council for Research on International Economic Relations, New Delhi, 2003 pp-14.
9. Rissam HS, Kishore S, Trehan N. Coronary Artery Disease in Young Indians—The Missing Link. Journal, Indian Academy of Clinical Medicine 2001;2(3):128–132.
10. World Health Organization. Definition, Diagnosis and Classification of Diabetes Mellitus and its Complications. Report of a WHO Consultation. Geneva: World Health Organization, 1999.
11. Angela E Raffle. Types of screening that can do more harm than good. NHS Evidence—screening. National Screening Committee, UK. April 2006
12. Kimberly TH, Deborah AC. General Screening Recommendations for Chronic Disease and Risk Factors in Older Adults. Try this—general assessment series. The Hartford Institute for Geriatric Nursing, New York University 2010;27.
13. Partha Basu, Debjani Chowdhury. Cervical cancer screening and HPV vaccination: A comprehensive approach to cervical cancer control. Indian J Med Res 130, September 2009, pp 241–246.
14. Cherian Varghese. CANCER PREVENTION AND CONTROL IN INDIA. 50 Years of Cancer Control in India. Mohfw, pp 48–59.
15. Lizzy Sunny. Prostate cancer: An epidemiological study in India (Academic Dessertation). University of Tampere, Finland, 2005 pp 23, downloaded from http://acta.uta.fi/pdf/951-44-6377-3.pdf

Chapter

15

Causation and Association

Vinay Rao

A major focus of epidemiology is to make informing efforts to prevent and control disease and promote health. To do this, we need to know the causes of disease or injury and the ways in which these causes can be modified. In this chapter, we discuss the *epidemiological approach* to causation.

The Concept of Cause

An understanding of the causes of disease or injury is important not only for prevention, but also for correct diagnosis and treatment. The concept of cause is the source of much controversy in epidemiology. The process by which we make causal inferences—judgements linking postulated causes and their outcomes—is a major theme of the general philosophy of science, and the concept of cause has different meanings in different contexts.

Sufficient or Necessary

A cause of a disease or injury is an event, condition, characteristic or a combination of these factors which plays an important role in producing the health outcome. Logically, a cause must precede an outcome. *A cause is termed* ***sufficient when it inevitably produces or initiates an outcome*** *and is termed* ***necessary if an outcome cannot develop in its absence.*** Some diseases are caused completely by genetic factors in the individual, and other causes of a disease interact with genetic factors in making certain individuals more vulnerable than others. The term environmental causes is often used to distinguish these other causes from the genetic causes. It has been pointed out that there are nearly always some genetic and some environmental component causes in every causal mechanism.

Multiple Factors

A sufficient cause is not usually a single factor, but often comprises several components (multi-factorial causation). In general, it is not necessary to identify all the components of a sufficient cause before effective prevention can take place, since the removal of one component may interfere with the action of the others and thus prevent the disease or injury. For example, cigarette smoking is one component of the sufficient cause of lung cancer. Smoking is not sufficient in itself to produce the disease: Some people smoke for 50 years without developing lung cancer. Other factors, mostly unknown, are involved and genetic factors may play a role. However, the cessation of smoking reduces the number of cases of lung cancer greatly in a population even if the other component causes are not altered.

Attributable Fraction

The attributable fraction can be used to quantify the likely preventive impact of eliminating a specific causal factor. For instance, what would be expected if smoking asbestos workers had either never smoked or never been exposed to asbestos: Never smoking would have decreased the lung cancer death rate substantially from 602 per 100,000 to 58 per 100,000 (a 90% reduction) and never exposed to asbestos, but still smoking, would have reduced the rate to a lesser extent from 602 to 123 per 100,000 (an 80% reduction).[1]

Sufficient and Necessary

Each sufficient cause has a necessary cause as a component. For example, in a study of an outbreak of food borne infection, it may be found that chicken salad and creamy dessert were both sufficient causes of *Salmonella* diarrhoea. However, the ingestion of *Salmonella* bacteria is a necessary cause of this disease. Similarly, there are different components in the causation of tuberculosis, but the infection with *Mycobacterium tuberculosis* is a necessary cause but not sufficient. However, a causal factor on its own is often neither necessary nor sufficient, such as tobacco use as a factor for cerebro-vascular disease.

The usual approach in epidemiology is to begin with a disease and search for its causes, although it is also possible to start with a potential cause (such as air pollution) and search for its effects. Epidemiology encompasses a whole set of relationships. For example, social class is associated with a range of health problems. Low social class, as measured by income, education, housing and occupation, leads to a general susceptibility to poor health, rather than to a specific effect. A gamut of specific causes of disease could explain why poor people have poor health, among them excessive exposure to infectious agents due to over-crowding, lack of clean water and sanitation, insufficient and unsafe food, and dangerous working conditions. In addition, being at the bottom of the social ladder is in itself associated with poorer health even after taking all the other factors into account.

A causal pathway: Epidemiologists have been criticized, particularly by laboratory scientists, for not using the concept of cause in the sense of being the sole requirement for the production of disease. Such a restrictive view of causation, does not take into account the fact that diseases commonly have *multiple* causes. Prevention strategies often need to be directed simultaneously at more than one factor. In addition, causes can be linked to a causal pathway where one factor leads to another until eventually the specific pathogenic agent becomes present in the organ that gets damaged; this can also be called a hierarchy of causes. Laboratory scientists might, for example, suggest that the basic cause of coronary heart disease relates to cellular mechanisms involved in the proliferation of tissue in the arterial wall (Fig. 15.1).

Research directed at determining pathogenic relationships is obviously important, but concepts of causation need to be understood in a wider epidemiological context.

It is often possible to make major progress in prevention by dealing only with the more remote or 'upstream' causes. It was possible

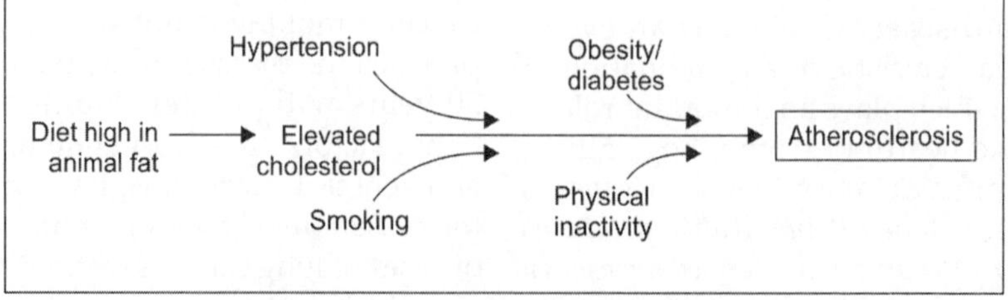

Fig. 15.1: Causal process in atherosclerosis

to prevent cholera cases decades before the responsible organism—let alone its mechanism of action—had been identified. **However, it is of interest that even in 1854, John Snow thought that a living organism was responsible for the disease.**

Single and Multiple Causes

Pasteur's work on microorganisms led to the formulation, first by Henle and then by Koch, of the following rules for determining whether a specific living organism causes a particular disease:

- The organism must be present in every case of the disease;
- The organism must be able to be isolated and grown in pure culture;
- The organism must, when inoculated into a susceptible animal, cause the specific disease;
- The organism must then be recovered from the animal and identified.

Anthrax was the first disease demonstrated to meet these rules, which have since proved useful with many other infectious diseases and with chemical poisoning.

However, for many diseases, both communicable and non-communicable, Koch's rules for determining causation are inadequate. Many causes act together, and a single factor such as tobacco use, may be a cause of many diseases. In addition, the causative organism may disappear when a disease has developed, making it impossible to demonstrate the organism in the sick person. Koch's postulates are of most value when the specific cause is a highly pathogenic infectious agent, chemical poison or other specific factor, and there are no healthy carriers of the pathogen—a relatively uncommon occurrence.

Factors in Causation

Four types of factors play a part in the causation of disease, all may be necessary but they are rarely sufficient to cause a particular disease or state:

- **Predisposing factors**, such as age, sex, or specific genetic traits that may result in a poorly functioning immune system or slow metabolism of a toxic chemical. Previous illness may also create a state of susceptibility to a disease agent.
- **Enabling (or disabling) factors** such as low income, poor nutrition, bad housing and inadequate medical care may favour the development of disease. Conversely, circumstances that assist in recovery from illness or in the maintenance of good health could also be called enabling factors. The social and economic determinants of health are just as important as the precipitating factors in designing prevention approaches.
- **Precipitating factors** such as exposure to a specific disease agent may be associated with the onset of a disease.
- **Reinforcing factors** such as repeated exposure, environmental conditions and unduly hard work may aggravate an established disease or injury.

The term *'**risk factor**'* is commonly used to describe factors that are positively associated with the risk of development of a disease, but that are not sufficient to cause the disease. This concept has proved useful in several practical prevention programs. Some risk factors (such as tobacco smoking) are associated with several diseases, and some diseases (such as coronary heart disease) are associated with several risk factors.

Epidemiological studies can measure the relative contribution of each factor to disease occurrence, and the corresponding potential reduction in disease from the elimination of each risk factor. However, multi-causality means that the sum of the attributable fractions for each risk factor may be greater than 100%.

Interaction

The effect of two or more causes acting together is often greater than would be expected on the basis of summing the individual effects. This phenomenon, called interaction, is illustrated by the particularly high risk of lung cancer in people who both smoke and are exposed to asbestos dust. The risk of lung cancer in this group is much higher than would be indicated by a simple addition of the risks from smoking (ten times) and exposure to asbestos dust (five times); the risk is multiplied, i.e. fifty times (Figs 15.2 and 15.3).

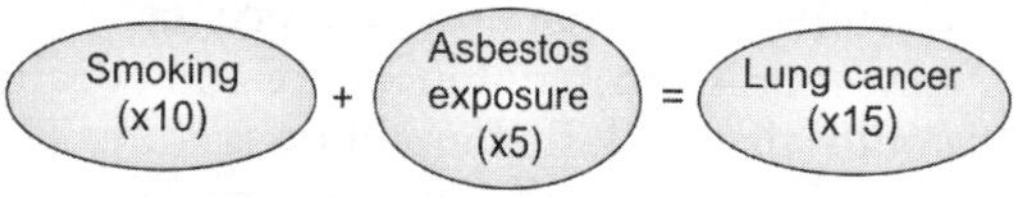

Fig. 15.2: Additive effect

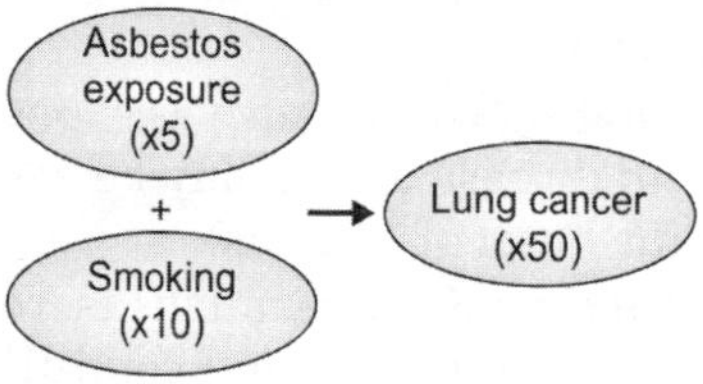

Fig. 15.3: Multiplicative effect

A Hierarchy of Causes

Multiple causes and risk factors can often be displayed in the form of a hierarchy of causes, where some are the proximal or most immediate causes (precipitating factors) and others are distal or indirect causes (enabling factors). Inhaled tobacco smoke is a proximal cause of lung cancer, while low socio-economic status is a distal cause that is associated with smoking habits and indirectly with lung cancer.

The WHO Global Burden of Disease project, the multiple exposures, multiple effects framework emphasizes the complex relationships between environmental exposures and child health outcomes. This model takes into account that individual exposures can lead to many different health outcomes, and specific health outcomes can be attributed to many different exposures.[2]

In epidemiological studies linking one or more causes to a health outcome, it is important to consider to what extent different causes are at the same or different levels in the hierarchy. If a 'cause of a cause' is included in the analysis together with the cause itself, the statistical method of analysis has to take this into account. The identification of the hierarchy of causes and the quantitative relationships between them will provide one way of describing the mechanism of causation. For example, low socio-economic status is associated in many industrialized nations with more tobacco smoking, which is associated with higher blood pressure, which in turn increases the risk of stroke.

Establishing the Cause of a Disease

Association and Causation

Association is the occurrence of two variables or factors more often than would be expected by chance. The measure of association in terms of statistics is called 'correlation'. It is the degree of association between two characteristics. The value of correlation coefficient ranges from negative (–1.0) to positive (+1.0). The coefficient value of 1 indicates perfect linear relationship.

Types of association (Fig. 15.4)

1. Spurious (artificial).
2. Indirect (confounding).
3. Direct (causal or aetiological)
   a. One-to-one causal association
   b. Multi-factorial association

1. ***Spurious (artificial) association:*** Sometimes an observed association between a suspected factor and disease may turn out to be false due to biased methods of selecting cases and controls, e.g. in 1929, Poarl identified 816 individuals with a malignant tumour, and 816 control patients who did not have a malignant tumour. Both groups were observed for age, sex, colour

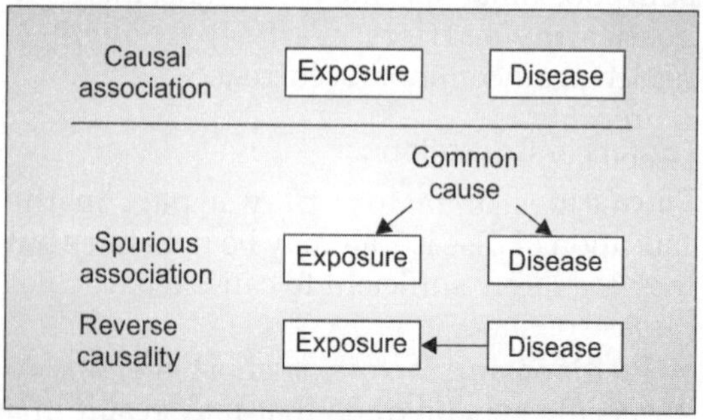

Fig. 15.4: Types of association

and date of death and autopsies performed. At autopsy, 16.3% of control group showed active tuberculosis lesions as against 6.6% in the study group. The difference was statistically significant. The hypothesis drawn was that TB was inversely related to malignancy (the association was false). On further study, it was found that the control group included a considerable number of individuals who died of TB (selection bias).

2. ***Indirect association:*** This type of association is a statistical association between a characteristic (variable) of interest and a disease due to the presence of another factor which is common to both the characteristic and disease. This factor is known as confounding variable.
3. ***Direct (causal) association***
   a. ***One-to-one causal relationship***: The two factors are casually related (**AB**), means a change in factor **A** will always cause change in **B.** If disease **B** is present then there must be factor **A** responsible for it, e.g. *Mycobacterium tuberculosis* bacilli. **(A)** ——→ Tuberculosis **(B).**
   b. ***Multi-factorial causation association***: Non-communicable or chronic diseases have several factors in causation of these diseases. Sometimes, these factors act independently while at other these factors show combined effect.

Causal inference is the term used for the process of determining whether observed associations are likely to be causal; the use of guidelines and the making of judgements are involved. The process of judging causation can be difficult and contentious. Causal inference should not be restricted to the measurement of an effect, rather a criterion-guided process for deciding whether an effect is present or not should be used. Before an association is assessed for the possibility that it is causal, other explanations, such as chance, bias and confounding, have to be excluded (Fig. 15.5).

Role of Chance

One of the major problems in evaluating an entire population based on the findings in a sample of the population is that chance always plays a role because of the random variation from sample to sample.

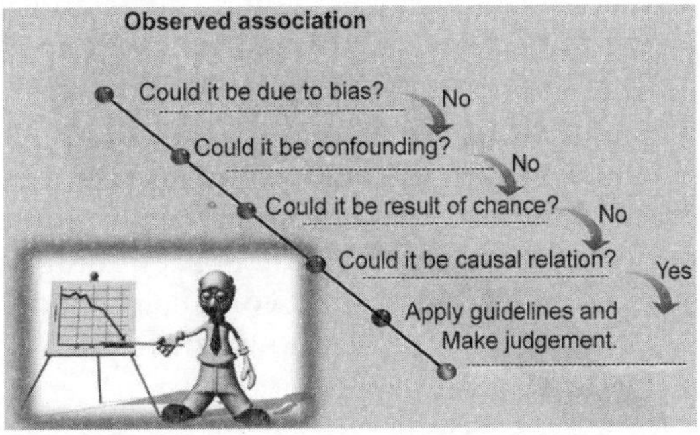

Fig. 15.5: Factors influencing causal inference of an association

Role of Bias

It is possible that some aspect of the study design or conduct of the study has introduced a systematic error or bias into the result.

Types of biases frequently encountered—*selection bias*; this type of bias is encountered when non-comparable criteria are used to enroll participants in the study. *Observation biases*—these arise either the investigator eliciting or interpreting the information differently *(interviewer bias*) or the study subjects themselves reporting events in a non-comparable manner (*recall bias*).

Role of Confounding

Confounding occurs due to the mixing of effect of a third factor (***confounding factor***) with the exposure and the disease. A confounding factor is one that is independently *associated with the cause as well as the disease*, and such a factor is *unequally distributed among the exposed and the non-exposed*. In studying the causation of myocardial infarction, due to smoking, coffee drinking may be a confounding factor as coffee drinkers are known to smoke and coffee drinking, by itself is, known to be a risk factor for myocardial infarction.

Additional Criteria for Judging Causality

A systematic approach to determining the nature of an association was used by the

United States Surgeon General to establish that cigarette smoking caused lung cancer.

This approach was further elaborated by Hill **(Hill's criteria of association).**[3]

On the basis of these concepts, a set of 'considerations for causation,' *listed in the sequence* of testing that the epidemiologist should follow to reach a conclusion about a cause of disease, is shown in following Table 15.1.

A. Temporal Relationship

The temporal relationship is crucial—the cause must precede the effect. This is usually self-evident, although difficulties may arise in case-control and cross-sectional studies when measurements of the possible cause and effect are made at the same time. In cases where the cause is an exposure that can be at different levels, it is essential that a high enough level be reached before the disease occurs for the correct temporal relationship to exist. Repeated measurement of the exposure at more than one point in time and in different locations may strengthen the evidence.

In a time series of measurements of exposure and effect, high daily temperatures (above 30°C) in Paris during a 2-week period in August 2003 and the increase of daily mortality during this period. This relationship between heat waves and increased urban mortality has been documented previously in several other cities and is expected to occur with increased frequency as a result of global climate change.[4]

A statistically significant association was demonstrated by a case-control study between the use of a drug for asthma and young people's risk of dying from asthma. However, we do need to know if there was a temporal relation between the use of the drug and deaths in those children before, we can recommend the withdrawal of the drug.

B. Biological Plausibility

An association is plausible, and thus more likely to be causal, if consistent with other knowledge. For instance, laboratory experiments may have shown how exposure to the particular factor could lead to changes associated with the effect measured. However, biological plausibility is a relative concept, and seemingly implausible associations may eventually be shown to be causal. For example, the predominant view on the cause of cholera in the 1830s involved 'miasma' rather than contagion. Contagion was not supported by evidence until Snow's work was published; much later, Pasteur and his colleagues identified the causative agent. Lack of plausibility may simply reflect lack of scientific knowledge. Doubts about the therapeutic effects of acupuncture and homeopathy may be partly attributable to the absence of information about a plausible biological mechanism. A recent example of plausibility being the main reason for a conclusion about causality is variant Creutzfeldt-Jakob disease.

Table15.1: Evidence that an association is cause and effect

Criteria	*Comments*
Temporal relation	Does the cause precede effect? (necessary)
Biological plausibility	According to biological knowledge of the time
Consistency	Similar results obtained by different studies
Strength of association	Association with a large relative risk
Dose–response relationship	Larger exposure related to higher rates
Specificity	One cause leads to one effect
Reversibility	Reduction in exposure leads to decreased rates
Analogy	Cause–effect relationship known for other similar illness

Example 1: BSE and vCJD

Variant Creutzfeldt-Jakob disease (vCJD) is the human form of 'mad cow disease' or bovine spongiform encephalopathy (BSE). There was an epidemic of BSE in the United Kingdom in 1987. Both diseases are invariably fatal and there are similar pathological changes in the brains of humans with vCJD and cows with BSE. These diseases are examples of transmissible spongiformencephalopathies, which are caused by an infectious agent called a prion. The epidemic in cattle had been caused by feed contaminated with infected carcasses of other cattle, and was finally controlled by banning the use of ruminant proteins as cattle feed. In 1995, there were three cases of vCJD in young people, and by 2002 a total of 139 human cases had been reported. *Despite a lack of evidence for an oral route of transmission in humans*, many experts concluded that the human epidemic was related to the bovine epidemic and caused by the same infective agent. Concerns about human transmission led to changes in blood donation policies and greater use of disposable surgical instruments.[5]

Example 2: Lead exposure in children

The study of the health consequences of low-level lead exposure is another example of the initial difficulties in getting conclusive epidemiological evidence, even when animal experiments indicate an effect of lead on the central nervous system. Similar effects in an epidemiological study of children are therefore plausible but, because of potential confounding factors and measurement difficulties, epidemiological studies originally showed conflicting results.

However, assessment of all the available epidemiological data leads to the conclusion that children are affected at a low level of exposure to lead.

In the United States of America, regular monitoring of lead exposure in hundreds of thousands of children's blood samples has shown that, while average levels are decreasing since lead was banned from motor-fuels, many children still have elevated levels. For children, there are sources of lead exposure other than motor-fuels and the blood lead level at which a risk for damage to the child's brain is considered to occur could be as low as 100 mcg/L. It is plausible that with more precise measurement tools, it may be found that some children are affected at still lower levels. More research on this lingering environmental health problem has to be carried out in low- and middle-income countries.[6]

C. Consistency

Consistency is demonstrated by several studies giving the same result. This is particularly important when a variety of designs are used in different settings, since the likehood that all studies are making the same 'mistake' is thereby minimized. However, a lack of consistency does not exclude a causal association, because different exposure levels and other conditions may reduce the impact of the causal factor in certain studies. *Systematic review* uses standardized methods to select and review all relevant studies on a particular topic with a view to eliminating bias in critical appraisal and synthesis. Systematic review as part of the Cochrane Collaboration is sometimes, but not always, coupled with meta-analysis. Furthermore, when the results of several studies are being interpreted, the best-designed ones should be given the greatest weight. Techniques are available for pooling the results of several studies that have examined the same issue, particularly randomized controlled trials. This technique is called ***meta-analysis*** and is used to combine the results of several trials, each of which may deal with a relatively small sample, to obtain a better overall estimate of effect.

In a systematic review, the results of 113 case-control studies and two cohort studies on the relationship between oral clefts in babies and tobacco use among women who smoked during pregnancy were studied. One important reason for the apparent inconsistency of the results is that several of the early studies were based on small samples. For the aggregated data from all the trials, covering a large number of events, the 95% confidence interval was very narrow. Overall, maternal smoking was associated with a 22% increase in cleft palates and the 95% confidence interval showed that the increase could be at least 10% and as much as 35%.[7]

Meta-analysis can also be used to pool results from other types of epidemiological studies such as time-series studies of daily air pollution (particulate matter) and total mortality.

D. Strength of Association

A strong association between possible cause and effect, as measured by the size of the risk ratio (*relative risk*), is more likely to be causal than is a weak association, which could be influenced by confounding or bias. ***Relative risks greater than 2 can be considered strong.*** For example, cigarette smokers have a two-fold increase in the risk of acute myocardial infarction compared with non-smokers. The risk of lung cancer in smokers, compared with non-smokers, has been shown in various studies to be increased between fourfold and twentyfold. However, associations of such magnitude are rare in epidemiology.

The fact that an association is weak does not preclude it from being causal; the strength of an association depends on the relative prevalence of other possible causes.

For example, weak associations have been found between diet and risk of coronary heart disease in observational studies; and although experimental studies on selected populations have been done, no conclusive results have been published. Despite this lack of evidence, diet is generally thought to be a major causative factor in the high rate of coronary heart disease in many industrialized countries. The probable *reason* for the difficulty in identifying diet as a risk factor for coronary heart disease is that *diets in populations are rather homogeneous* and variation overtime for one individual is greater than that between people. If everyone has more or less the same diet, it is not possible to identify diet as a risk factor. Consequently, ecological evidence gains importance. This situation has been characterized as one *of sick individuals and sick population*, meaning that in many high-income countries, whole populations are at risk from an adverse factor.[8]

Air pollution and total mortality: The results of a large number of time-series studies in different cities in the USA were combined; although some of the studies had conflicting results, a statistically significant association between the exposure and effect was observed. This strengthens the impression that particulate matter air pollution is causing increased mortality, even though the exact mechanism is unclear. However, such meta-analysis are limited by 'publication bias', meaning that studies which did not achieve statistical significance, or the desired effect, are not published

E. Dose–response Relationship

A dose–response relationship occurs when changes in the level of a possible cause are associated with changes in the prevalence or incidence of the effect. Table 15.2 below illustrates the dose–response relationship between noise and hearing loss—the prevalence of hearing loss increases with noise level and exposure time. The demonstration of such a clear dose—response relationship in unbiased studies provides strong evidence for a causal relationship between exposure and disease.

Table 15.2: Dose–response relationship: Percentage of people with hearing loss due to workplace noise exposure

Average noise level during 8 hours (decibels)	*Exposure time (years)* 5	10	40
<80	0	0	0
85	1	3	10
90	4	10	21
95	7	17	29
100	12	29	41
105	18	42	54
110	26	55	62
115	36	71	64

Lung cancer deaths show an increase as the number of cigarettes smoked per day by an individual. This number increases incrementally as the number of cigarettes smoked increases (Fig. 15.6).

F. Specificity

The criterion of specificity requires that a cause leads to a single effect, not multiple effects. We must also keep in mind that diseases may have more than one cause. One-to-one relationships are not frequent. Indeed, multi-causation is generally more likely than single causation though possibly if we knew all the answer we might get back to a single factor. In short, if specificity exists we may be able to draw conclusions without hesitation; if it is not apparent, we are not thereby necessarily left sitting irresolutely on the fence.

G. Reversibility

When the removal of a possible cause results in a reduced disease risk, there is a greater likelihood that the association is causal. For example, the cessation of cigarette smoking is associated with a reduction in the risk of lung cancer relative to that in people who continue to smoke. This finding strengthens the likelihood that cigarette smoking causes lung cancer. If the cause leads to rapid irreversible changes that subsequently produce disease whether or not there is continued exposure, then reversibility cannot be a condition for causality.

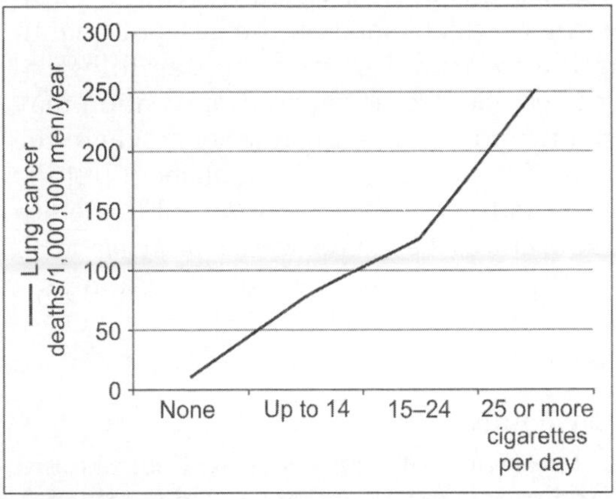

Fig. 15.6: Number of lung cancer deaths per 1,000,000 men/year according to the number of cigarettes smoked per day

H. Analogy

Refers to cause–effect relationship known for other similar illness. In the endosulphan tragedy that is seen in southern India, there has been an increase in the incidence of congenital deformities in areas where endosulphan spraying is being conducted over the cashew plantations. Consumption of groundwater in these areas by the pregnant women living in the area has been linked to the particular tragedy. Although the same water may be consumed by all others without any serious illness, the foetus is more vulnerable to the even small doses of the pesticide. This association was strengthened by the thalidomide tragedy which established the ill effects on the foetus by consumption of the drug by the mother.

I. Study Design

The ability of a study design to prove causation is an important consideration. Figure 15.7 outlines the different types of study and relative strengths in establishing causality. These study designs were discussed in previous chapters; their use in providing evidence for causal relationships is discussed in (Fig. 15.7).

Ecological studies: Ecological studies provide the weakest evidence for causality because of the danger of incorrect extrapolation to individuals from regional or national data. However, for certain exposures that cannot normally be measured individually (such as

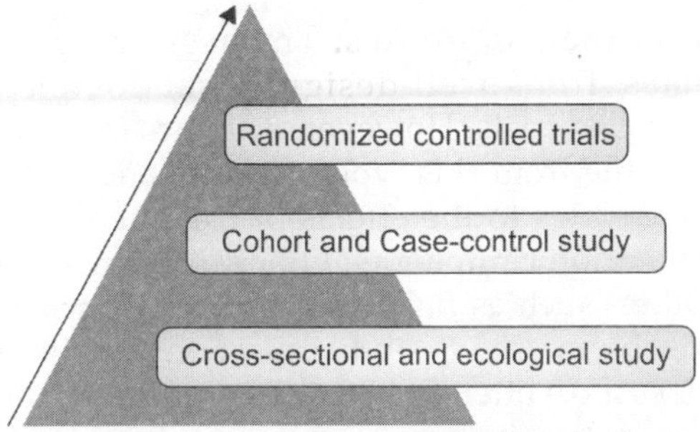

Fig.15.7: Hierarchy of different study designs used to prove causation

air pollution, pesticide residues in food, fluoride in drinking water), evidence from ecological studies is very important. When causal relationships have already been established, well-designed ecological studies, particularly *time-series studies*, can be very useful to quantify effects observational studies; almost all the evidence on the health consequences of smoking comes from observational studies.

Cross-sectional studies: Cross-sectional studies are less able to prove causation as they provide no direct evidence on the time sequence of events. However, the time sequence can often be inferred from the way exposure and effect data is collected. For instance, if it is clear that the health effect is recent and the exposure to the potential causes is recorded in a questionnaire, questions about the past may clearly identify exposures before the effect occurred.

Cohort and case-control studies: However, there are occasions when ecological studies provide good evidence for establishing causation. One such example relates to epidemics of asthma deaths. In 1968, the sale of inhaled bronchodilators without prescription in England and Wales was stopped because the increase in asthma deaths in the period 1959–66 had been shown to coincide with a rise in bronchodilator sales.[9] After the availability of inhaled bronchodilators was restricted, the death rate fell. A similar pattern was observed, following restrictions on the availability of the inhaled bronchodilator fenoterol in New Zealand in 1989.

Experimental studies: The best evidence comes from well-designed randomized controlled trials. However, evidence is rarely available from this type of study, and often only relates to the effects of treatment and prevention campaigns. Other experimental studies, such as field and community trials, are seldom used to study causation. Evidence comes most often from Cohort studies are the next best design because, when well conducted, bias is minimized. Again, they are not always available. Although case-control studies are subject to several forms of bias, the results from large, well-designed investigations of this kind provide good evidence for the causal nature of an association; judgements often have to be made in the absence of data from other sources.

Judging the Evidence

Regrettably, there are no completely reliable criteria for determining whether an association is causal or not. Causal inference is usually tentative and judgements must be made on the basis of the available evidence: uncertainty always remains. Evidence is often conflicting and due weight must be given to the different types when decisions are made. *In judging the different aspects of causation referred to above,* ***the correct temporal relationship is essential****; once that has been established, the greatest weight may be given to plausibility, consistency and the dose–response relationship.* The likelihood of a causal association is heightened when many different types of evidence lead to the same conclusion.

Evidence from well-designed studies is particularly important, especially if they are conducted in a variety of locations. The most important use of information about causation of diseases and injuries may be in the area of prevention, which we will discuss in the following chapters. When the causal pathways are established on the basis of quantitative information from epidemiological studies, the decisions about prevention may be uncontroversial. In situations, where the causation is not so well established, but the impacts have great potential public health importance, the *'precautionary principle'* may be applied to take preventive action as a safety measure; this is called *'precautionary prevention'*.

Key points

1. The study of causation of diseases and injuries is fundamental to epidemiology.
2. There is seldom one single cause of a specific health outcome.

3. Causal factors can be arranged into a hierarchy from the most proximal to the distal socio-economic factors.
4. Criteria for judging the evidence of causality include—*temporal relationship, plausibility, consistency, strength, dose–response relationship, specificity, reversibility, analogy and study design.*

References

1. Hammond EC, Selikoff IJ, Seidman H. Asbestos exposure, cigarette smoking and death rates. Ann N Y Acad Sci 1979;330:473–90.
2. Briggs D. Making a difference: Indicators to improve children's environmental health. Geneva, World Health Organization, 2003.
3. Hill AB. The environment and disease: association or causation? Proc R Soc Med 1965;58:295–300.
4. McMichael AJ, Campbell-Lendrum DH, Corvalan CF, Ebi KL, Githeko AK, Scheraga JD, et al. Climate change and human health, risks and responses. Geneva, World Health Organization, 2003.
5. Smith PG. The epidemics of bovine spongiform encephalopathy and variant Creutzfeldt-Jakob disease: current status and future prospects. Bull World Health Organ 2003;81:123–30.
6. Tong S, Baghurst P, McMichael A, Sawyer M, Mudge J. Low-level exposure to lead and children's intelligence at ages eleven to thirteen years: the Port Piriecohort study. BMJ 1996;312:569–75.
7. Little J, Cardy A, Munger RG. Tobacco smoking and oral clefts: a meta-analysis. Bull World Health Organ 2004;82:213–8.
8. Rose G. Sick individuals and sick populations. Int J Epidemiol 1985;14:32–8.
9. Pearce N, Hensley MJ. Beta agonists and asthma deaths. Epidemiol Rev 1998;20:173–86.

Chapter

16

Basics of Infectious Disease Modelling

Ram Chandra Goyal

"Mathematical model is a lie that helps us to discover the truth."
"I simply wish that, in a matter which so closely concerns the well-being of the human race, no decision shall be made without all the knowledge which a little analysis and calculation can provide."

—Daniel Bernoulli

INTRODUCTION

Infectious diseases have ever been a great concern of human kind since the very beginning of our history. Millions of people die annually from measles, malaria, tuberculosis, AIDS, Ebola, SARS, Nipah ... and billions of others are infected.

There was a belief in early nineties that infectious diseases would be soon eliminated with the improvement in sanitation, discovery of antibiotics and vaccines, improved medical care services. However, they are still the major causes of deaths in low- and middle-income group countries.[1]

We also know that infectious disease agents are mutating, adapting and evolving with environment milieu, as a result new infectious diseases emerging re-emerging. It was the need of the hour to understand the spread and control of infectious diseases and their nature of transmission.

(Natural history of diseases, dynamics of disease transmission, etc. are covered in earlier chapters on basics of communicable disease epidemiology and the transmissibility of infections.)

A model is a simplified representation of a complex system, designed to focus in on a specific question. In general, modelling techniques used in health are adaptations from other fields such as telecommunications and traffic engineering.

In health service planning, modelling techniques derived from queuing theory can be used to forecast the effects of changes on access to services and to calculate the required capacity of services given assumptions about patterns of demand and levels of utilization; techniques derived from the physics of gravitation may be used to estimate catchment areas of new facilities; models utilizing network analysis may be used to study patients' travel requirements to services; models based on Markov chains can be used to assess patients' progress though through treatment and also in economic assessments.[2]

Epidemiological models should facilitate to understand biomedical phenomenon of a diseases process into simple and understandable way of its complexities so that the relationships among the components of the phenomenon can be studied mathematically.

The evolution of causal models in epidemiology has led to the concept of 'systems'—a set of assembly of factors connected with each other in some coherent relationship. A useful modelling technique for use in epidemiological studies is systems analysis. Although the mathematical aspect of this technique are quite complex, the underlying requirement for its use require a thorough understanding of the epidemiology of the disease(s).

Once the components of the system are identified, appropriate mathematical equations are established to represent the system and reasonable estimates for the parameters in use are obtained. Then the model could be programmed and put on a computer. This would then facilitate the manipulation of the model using a computer so that various alternatives for disease control or prevention could be evaluated and detailed research on various hypothesis pertaining to the infections process could be examined.

In many cases, since manipulating the disease and the environment in the field is not an easy task, with the aid of an epidemiologic model such a task is simplified. However, it is important to emphasize that without a proper knowledge of the epidemiology of the disease of interest and without a detailed understanding of the complexities of the mathematics involved in the model, major errors and fallacies could result. With this caution, epidemiologic and other biomedical models and the use of computers to study such phenomenon is unlimited.

At this stage, then, it should become apparent that what is required for maximal utilization of epidemiologic techniques (especially to evaluate disease control alternatives) are—a detailed analytic understanding of the epidemiology of disease(s) under study; and expertise in utilizing mathematical and computer methods to design, collect, analyze and interpret results. This is an important domain of analytic epidemiology.[1,2]

Other modelling techniques are used in epidemiology and in health impact assessment, and in clinical audit. They can also help to identify where there may be problems or pressures, identify priorities and focus efforts, where the mathematics results in equations that are too complex to solve directly modellers have recourse to simulation.

Modelling is important in a range of areas such as:[3]

- Understanding the biomedical mechanism that underlie infections processes, epidemic processes, etc.
- Preparing for outbreak-modelling the impact of an epidemic, Nipah, SARS, H1N1 ('swine flu') etc.
- Models for infectious diseases are helpful for prevention and control of emerging infectious diseases.
- Useful for studying the development and spread of drug resistant strains, e.g. malaria, tuberculosis, MRSA, ..., etc.
- Predicting health needs in the future such as the long-term health service resource requirements.
- Depicting what could happen with important public health issues if no interventions are undertaken. For example, projecting year on year increase in non-communicable diseases prevalence has helped to identify this issue as a national priority and allocate resources to tackle it.
- Understanding the impact of service redesign on different areas such as general practice waiting times, hospital bed occupancy.
- Estimating prevalence when detailed data are not available.
- Predicting demand on services from subgroups of the population, such as those at risk of emergency admissions or re-admissions.

Models of Infectious Disease Transmission[4]

Models of infectious disease transmission, in which the human population is located within a broader system with which it interacts; models that integrate the emission and dispersion of pollutants with their impacts on health; and the relationship of social factors to specific risk factors and to selection effects.

A number of investigators have analyzed systems and/or used causal diagrams. For developing models. The most important of these are:

- Path diagram analysis, which was devised by the geneticist Sewall Wright but which has mainly been employed in quantitative social science analysis, and
- The similar but more general method of structural equation modelling, which also systematically analyses measurement error including the use of latent
- Variables that represent theoretical constructs, estimated from several measured variables;
- Diagrams of metabolic pathways in biochemistry;
- Infectious disease epidemiology modelling based on demographic and ecological models;
- Various systems modelling, including cybernetics, dynamical systems modelling, and system dynamics and open systems theory.

How Epidemiological Modelling Started?[1]

The first major epidemic which we can find in the records of historians and scholars is the Plague of Athens (430–428 BC). Hippocrate's (459–337 BC) work, 'On the Epidemics', described the factors which were affecting the disease spreading and ways of the spreading at that time.

In 14th century, 25 million people die due to bubonic plague (Black Death, 1347–1350) and in 16th century—smallpox killed 35 million in Aztecs population. Many such epidemics occurred and took millions of life for the want of clear understating of the mechanism by which epidemics spread.

Modern mathematical biology begins with Hamer in 1906, first applied the 'simple mass action principle' for a deterministic epidemic model in discrete time. Ross's Simple Epidemic Model was published in 1911 and Generalized Epidemic Model produced by Kermack and McKendrick in 1927. These models have deterministic character and are still widely used although new models were created taking into consideration various factors like migration, vaccination and its gradual loss, chemotherapy, quarantine, passive immunity, genetic heterogeneity, non-uniformly distribution of population, etc.

Mathematical epidemiology contributed to the understanding of the behaviour of infectious diseases, its impacts and possible future predictions about its spreading. Mathematical models are used in comparing, planning, implementing, evaluating and optimizing various detection, prevention, therapy and control programs.

Types of Mathematical Modelling

1. **Deterministic *vs.* stochastic models:** Deterministic models have no components that are inherently uncertain, i.e. no parameters in the model are characterized by probability distributions, as opposed to stochastic models. For fixed starting values, a deterministic model will always produce the same result. A stochastic model will produce many different results depending on the actual values that the random variables take in each realization.
2. **Static *vs.* dynamic models:** Static models are at an equilibrium or steady state, as opposed to dynamic models which change with respect to time.
3. **Continuous *vs.* discrete models:** Differential *vs.* difference equations
4. **Individual *vs.* structured models:** Structured models based on age, size, stage, etc.
5. **Mechanistic *vs.* statistical models:** Statistical or empirical models are usually regression based. They provide a quantitative summary of the observed relationships among a set of measured variables. A mechanistic or scientific model begins with a description of how nature might work, and proceeds from this description to a set

of predictions relating the independent and dependent variables.

6. **Qualitative *vs.* quantitative models:** Qualitative models lead to a detailed, numerical prediction about responses, whereas qualitative models lead to general descriptions about the responses.

Although many types of the mathematical modelling in epidemiology are described, however this section will be dealing only with the basics of the deterministic and stochastic models.

STOCHASTIC VERSUS DETERMINISTIC MODELS[6]

Two types of model are useful in the study of infectious diseases at the population scale—these are stochastic and deterministic models.

A stochastic model represents a situation where uncertainty is present. In other words, it is a model for a process that has some kind of randomness. The word stochastic comes from the Greek word *stokhazesthai* meaning to aim or guess. In the real word, uncertainty is a part of everyday life, so a stochastic model could literally represent *anything*. The opposite is a **deterministic model, which predicts outcomes with 100% certainty**. Deterministic models always have a set of equations that describe the system inputs and outputs exactly. On the other hand, stochastic models will likely produce different results every time the model is run.

Stochastic models: 'Stochastic' means *random*, so a 'stochastic process' could more simple be called a *random process*. It relies on among individual chance variation in risks of exposure, disease, and other factors. They are used when chance fluctuations or known heterogeneities are important as in small or isolated populations. Stochastic models have advantages like allow follow-up of each individual in the population on a chance basis. Stochastic models, however, difficult to set-up and need many simulations to yield useful predictions. Notwithstanding, incorporating chance variation into transmission processes provides a range of possible outcome-based probabilities.

Deterministic models (compartmental models): The word 'deterministic' signifies that the predictions of these models are determined entirely by their initial conditions, the set of underlying equations, and the input parameter values (Fig. 16.1).

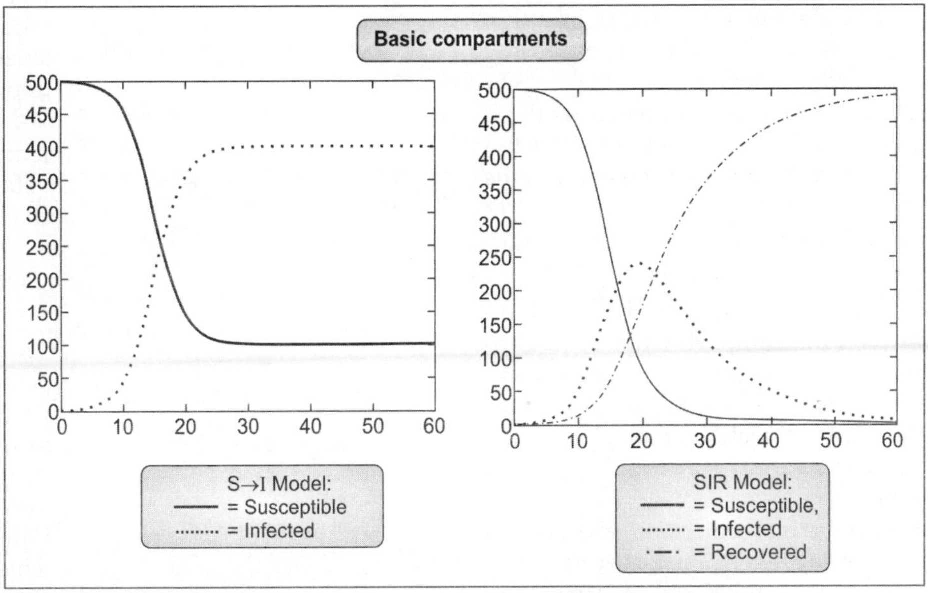

Fig. 16.1: Basic compartment in deterministic model[1,4–6]

Basic Ideas and Assumptions[5]

- Populations under study are divided into compartments.
- Rates of transfer between compartments are expressed mathematically as derivatives with respect to time of the sizes of the compartments—systems of ordinary differential equations.
- The community size is constant over the duration of the epidemic.
- The infection is transmitted primarily by person-to-person contacts.
- Individuals are homogeneous and mix uniformly.
- It ignores demography, i.e. births and deaths.

It attempts to describe and explain what happens on the average at the population scale. These models categorize individuals into different subgroups (compartments). In SEIR model basically individuals are classified in the following groups.[7,8]

- **Susceptible**—initially, individual/host is susceptible to infection: No pathogen is present; just a low-level non-specific immunity within the host.
- **Exposed**—in early stages, the host may or may not exhibit obvious signs of infection and abundance of pathogen may be too low to allow further transmission.
- **Infectious**—host encounters infectious individual and becomes infected with a infective agent; abundance of the infectious agent grows with time.
- **Recovered**—the host is either no longer infectious or 'removed' (dead).

Further, the models specify the transition rates between the compartments as susceptibles may become exposed, exposed infectious, and so on. The best known transition rate is the force of infection or attack rate that measures the rate at which susceptibles become infected.

Most models of infectious disease processes used until now are deterministic because they require less data, are relatively easy to set-up, and because the computer software are widely available and user-friendly. The dynamics of the SEIR model are now well understood so that deterministic models are commonly used to explore whether a particular control strategy will be effective.

Various epidemiology models based on the transition between these compartments are: SI, SIS, SIR, SIRS, SEIR, SEIRS MSEIR, and MSEIRS[2,6] (Figs 16.2–16.4).

If a newborn baby is delivered by an infected women, the newborn will have antibodies which provide temporary passive immunity to that infection. The class **'M'** represents these infants with the passive immunity and when the infant looses passive immunity, then enters in the class of susceptible **'S'**. If these babies exposed to an infective individual for an adequate time then only move from '**S →E**'.

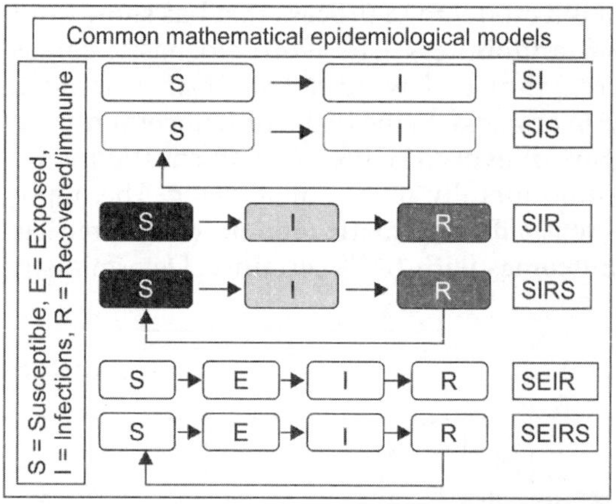

Fig. 16.2: Common mathematical epidemiological modelling

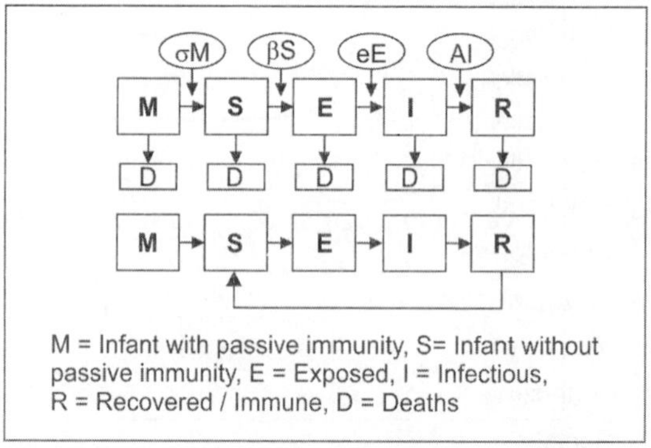

Fig. 16.3: Compartment with stages of infections

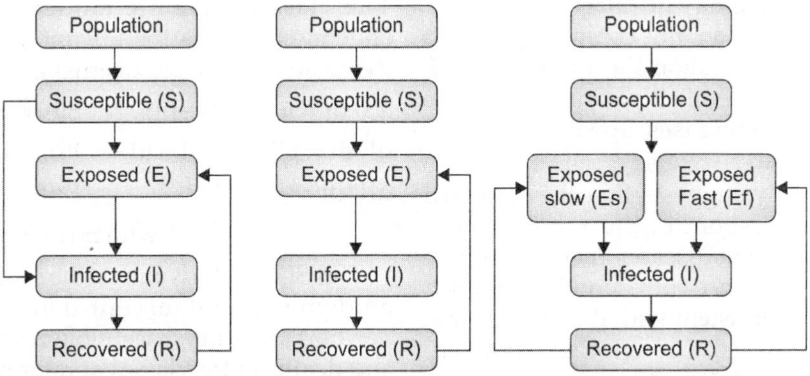

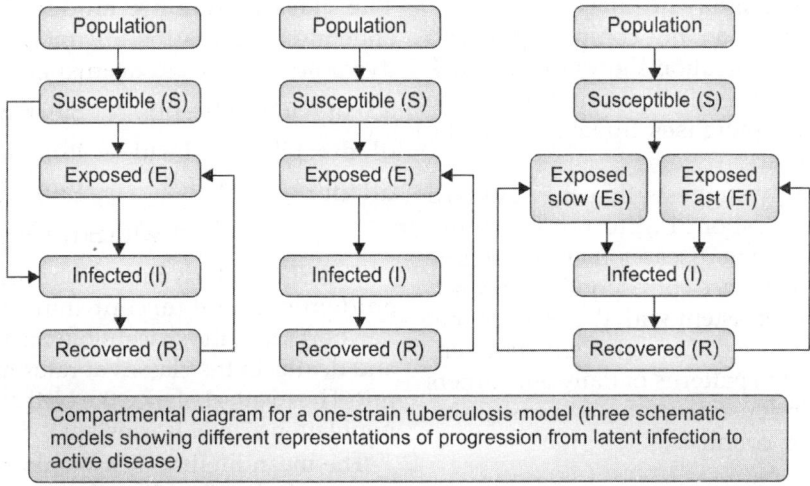

Compartmental diagram for a one-strain tuberculosis model (three schematic models showing different representations of progression from latent infection to active disease)

Fig. 16.4: SEIR model with progression from exposed/latent to active disease

These are the babies in latent period who are infected but not yet infectious. When they become infectious, then they enter class **'I'**—infectious. And finally, they enter the class **'R'**—recovered and have permanent immunity (Box 16.1).[1,2]

The basic reproduction number **(R_0)**—this is a measure of the force of infection/transmissibility, i.e. the rate at which susceptible become infected. R_0 implies that susceptible get in contact with infectious individuals and that the contact can lead (with a probability *b*) to effective transmission of the infectious agent (this takes account of the type of contact and the duration of the period of infectivity). A mass action principle (everyone can contact anyone in the population) is involved in determining the frequency of infections that denies heterogeneity in the contact rate.

Box 16.1: Symbols and their meaning

M (m) = Passive immune infants (fraction of M)

S (s) = Susceptible (fraction of S)

E (e)/I (i) = Exposed (fraction of E/I)

R (r) = Recovered with acquired immunity (fraction of R)

β = Contact rate

1/§ = Average period of passive immunity

1/e = Average latent period

$1/\lambda$ = Average infectious period

R_0 = Basic reproduction number

σ = Contact number

R = Replacement number

Interpretation of Various Deterministic Models

SI Model ($S \rightarrow I$)

The horizontal incidence is the infection rate of susceptible individuals through their contacts with infective. If S(t) is the number of susceptible at time t, I(t) is the number of infective, and N is the total population size, then s(t) = S(t)/N and i(t) = I(t)/N are the susceptible and infectious fractions, respectively.

If β is the average number of adequate contacts (i.e. contacts sufficient for transmission) of a person per unit time, then $\beta I/N = \beta i$ is the average number of contacts with infectives per unit time of one susceptible, and (bI/N) S = βN is the number of new cases per unit time due to the S = Ns susceptibles. This form of the **horizontal incidence is called the standard incidence**, because it is formulated from the basic principles.

The simple mass action law $\eta IS = \eta(Ni)(Ns)$, with η as a mass action coefficient, has sometimes been used for the horizontal incidence.

The parameter η has no direct epidemiological interpretation, but comparing it with the standard formulation shows that $\beta = \eta N$, so that this form implicitly assumes that the contact rate β increases linearly with the population size.

This strongly suggests that the standard incidence corresponding to $v = 0$ is more realistic for human diseases than the simple mass action incidence corresponding to $v = 1$. This result is consistent with the concept that people are infected through their daily encounters and the patterns of daily encounters are largely independent of community size within a given country.

SIR Model

The SIR model is sometimes known as the compartmental model, generalised model or Kermack-McKendrick's Model after two mathematicians who formulated it first in 1927.

There are two classic SIR models are formulated and analyzed. Epidemic models are used to describe rapid outbreaks that occur in less than one year, while endemic models are used for studying diseases over longer periods of time, during which there is a renewal of susceptibles by births or recovery from temporary immunity. The two classic SIR models provide an intuitive basis for understanding more complex epidemiology modelling results and are still widely used in practice.[2]

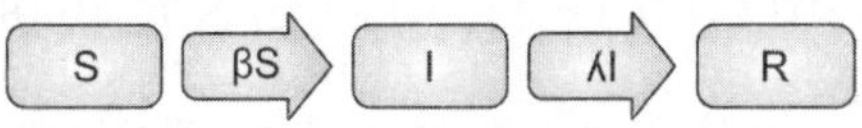

The classic epidemic model: The classic epidemic model is the SIR model given by the initial value as

$$dS/dt = \beta IS/N, \qquad S(0) = S_0 \geq 0,$$
$$dI/dt = \beta IS/N - \gamma I \qquad I(0) = I_0 \geq 0,$$
$$dR/dt = \gamma I, \qquad R(0) = R_0 \geq 0,$$

where $S(t)$, $I(t)$, and $R(t)$ are the numbers in these classes, so that $S(t) + I(t) + R(t) = N$.

This SIR model is a special case of the MSEIR model, in which the passively immune class **M** and the exposed class **E** are omitted.

The classic endemic model: The classic endemic model is the SIR model with vital dynamics (births and deaths) given by

$$dS/dt = \mu N - \mu S - \beta IS/N \qquad S(0) = S_0 \geq 0,$$
$$dI/dt = \beta IS/N - \gamma I - \mu I \qquad I(0) = I_0 \geq 0,$$
$$dR/dt = \gamma I - \mu R \qquad R(0) = R_0 \geq 0,$$
$$\text{with } S(t) + I(t) + R(t) = N$$

This SIR model is almost the same as the SIR epidemic model, except that it is adding newborns into the susceptible class at rate mN and deaths in the classes at rates mS, mI, and mR. The deaths balance the births, so that the population size N is constant.

The mean lifetime $1/\mu$ would be about 65 years in India. Dividing the equations in by the constant total population size N yields

$$ds/dt = \beta IS + \mu - \mu s \qquad s(0) = s_0 \geq 0,$$
$$di/dt = \beta IS - (\gamma + \mu)i, \quad i(0) = I_0 \geq 0$$
$$\text{with } r(t) = 1 - s(t) - i(t)$$

The Threshold Phenomenon and R_0[5]

The threshold for many epidemiology models is the basic reproduction number $\mathbf{R_0}$, which is defined as the average number of secondary infections produced when one infected individual is introduced into a host population where everyone is susceptible. For many deterministic epidemiology models, an infection can get started in a fully susceptible population if and only if $\mathbf{R_0 > 1}$. Thus, the basic reproduction number $\mathbf{R_0}$ is often considered as the threshold quantity that determines when an infection can invade and persist in a new host population.

Realistic infectious disease models include both time (t) and age (a) as independent variables, because age groups mix heterogeneously, the recovered fraction usually increases with age, risks from an infection may be related to age, vaccination programs often focus on specific ages, and epidemiologic data is often age specific.

Consider initial stages after I(0) infectives introduced into a population of S(0) susceptibles.

The question is whether an epidemic will occur or invasion fade?

Rewrite equation: $dI/dt = I(\beta S - r)$. If $S(0) < r/\beta$ then $dI/dt < 0$ and infection dies out. this is known as 'threshold phenomenon' (Kermack and McKendrick, 1927) since susceptibles must exceed a critical threshold for an infection to invade.

Another important interpretation—need β/r, the relative removal rate, to be small enough.

Basic reproductive ratio, $R_0 = \beta/r$ = average number of secondary cases arising from an average primary case in a completely susceptible population.

If everyone in the population is initially susceptible [$S(0) = 1$], a pathogen can invade only if $R_0 > 1$. R_0 = rate at which new cases are produced by an infectious individual (when population is completely susceptible), multiplied by the average infectious period.[7]

HERD IMMUNITY MODEL[9]

Herd immunity occurs for a disease if enough people have disease-acquired or vaccination-acquired immunity, so that the introduction of one infective into the population does not cause an invasion of the disease.

Naturally, if the contact number is σ, so that the typical infective has adequate contacts with σ people during the infectious period, then the replacement number σs must be less than 1, so that the disease does not spread. This means that 's' must be less than $1/\sigma$, so the immune fraction 'r' must satisfy $r > 1 - 1/\sigma = 1 - 1/R_0$.

For example, if $R_0 = \sigma = 20$, then the immune fraction must satisfy $r > 1 - 1/8 = 0.88$, so that the replacement number (R) is less than 1 and the disease does not invade the population.[9]

Conclusions

Modelling clarifies what the underlying assumptions are, model analysis and simulation predictions suggest crucial data that should be gathered model analysis and simulation suggest control strategies that could be implemented. Modelling is not prefect and usually is a simplification of reality.

Limitations of Models

Modelling is essentially a transaction between the generality, realism and precision, hence the interpretation should be made in judicious manner.

The usefulness of any particular model depends on its aims and objectives.

To describe general ecological principles, it is usually necessary to sacrifice realism and precision.

To describe a particular population, it is usually necessary to sacrifice generality.

Further discussion on models and their variants are beyond the scope of this chapter, readers are suggested to go through the reference cited below for details.

Reference

1. Lenka Bubniakov, The Mathematics of Infectious Diseases, Master's Thesis, Comenius University, Bratislava, 2007.
2. Herbert W Hethcote. The Mathematics of Infectious Diseases, SIAM REVIEW, 2000;42(4):599–653.
3. Congdon P. The development of gravity models for hospital patient flows under system change: a Bayesian modelling approach, Health Care Management Science 2001;4:289–304.
4. Joffe, et al. Causal diagrams in systems epidemiology, emerging themes in epidemiology 2012;9:1, http://www.ete-online.com/content/9/1/1
5. Bokil VA. Mathematical modeling and analysis of infectious disease dynamics, MTH 323: Mathematical Modeling, Oregon State University, Corvallis, OR; May 22, 2017, http://math.oregonstate.edu/~gibsonn/Teaching/MTH323-010S18/Supplements/Infectious.pdf
6. Trottier H, Philippe P. Deterministic modeling of infectious diseases: Theory and methods. The Internet Journal of Infectious Diseases 2000;1(2):2000.
7. Murali Haran. An introduction to models for disease Dynamics. Spatial Epidemiology, SAMSI, Dec. 2009, https://www.unc.edu/~rls/s940/samsidisdyntut.pdf
8. Anderson RM, May RM. Infectious Diseases of Humans–Dynamics and Control. Oxford, New York: Oxford University Press, 1991.
9. Levins, R. The strategy of model building in population biology. Am Sci 1966;54:421–31.

Chapter

17

Integrated Diseases Surveillance Program

Ram Chandra Goyal

"There is no value to surveillance system unless the information is used for action that prevent or control diseases".

Surveillance for diseases is essential for health system for early detection of outbreaks, measuring disease burden, and change in morbidity and mortality patterns; and for timely implementation of control and preventive measures. Today most surveillance activities are supported and managed by a variety of vertical disease-control programs. Many developing countries are only having disease-specific programs were not cost effective in long run.

Surveillance is the backbone of public health program and provides information so that effective action can be taken in controlling and preventing diseases of public health importance. In some cases action must be immediate—within hours—in order to prevent large scale epidemics and deaths, e.g. cholera, food poisoning, etc. The frequency of the occurrence of epidemics is an indication of the inadequacy of the surveillance system and preparedness to identify and control outbreaks in a timely manner.[1]

Effective disease control relies on effective response systems and effective response systems rely on effective disease surveillance. A functional surveillance system is essential in providing information for action on country's priority diseases; it is a crucial tool for public health decision-making in all countries. Surveillance data provide information, which can be used, for priority setting, policy decisions, planning, implementation, resource mobilization and allocation, and prediction and early detection of epidemics.[2,3]

A surveillance system can also be used for monitoring, evaluation and improvement of disease prevention and control programs. Disease surveillance is thus a critical component of the health system since it provides essential information for optimal healthcare delivery and a cost-effective health strategy.[3]

Integrated disease surveillance is 'a combination of active and passive systems that use a single infrastructure to gather information about multiple diseases or behaviours of interest using similar structures, personnel and processes.[4]

Definition of Surveillance

Surveillance is defined as "the ongoing systematic collection, collation, analysis, and interpretation of data and dissemination of information to those who need to know in order that action is taken".

A more complete definition of surveillance is "the ongoing systematic collection, analysis and interpretation of health data essential to planning, implementation, and evaluation of public health practice closely integrated with timely dissemination of these date to those who need to know." The final link in the surveillance chain is the application of these data to prevention and control. A surveillance system includes a functional capacity for data collection, analysis and dissemination linked to public health programs (CDC 1988) (Fig. 17.1).[1]

Need for Integration of Various Surveillance Systems

There are various activities for measuring the high burden, detect outbreaks of epidemic-prone disease and monitor progress at national and international level, however, these activities have not shown the desires outcome for prevention, control or eradication of the targeted diseases. Moreover, financially, operationally and administratively, it was difficult to have a dedicated program for each and every important disease and newly emerging diseases. Following are some of the reasons to undertake integrated diseases surveillance.

- Uneven surveillance activities and multiple surveillance systems
- Only vertical disease-control programs included
- Lost momentum for previously designed programs over the period of time.
- Programs were poorly maintained or collapsed
- Continuation of outdated surveillance systems
- Multiple channels for collection of data without integration
- Non-involvement of private sector and non-governmental organizations
- Inadequate training of health personnel leads to ineffective and inefficient outcome.
- Duplication of data and availability of huge data without expected analysis.
- Feedback were scanty and very less attention for usage of data for decision-making.

INTEGRATED DISEASES SURVEILLANCE PROGRAM IN INDIA

Historical Perspective

Although the health infrastructure in India has grown immensely over the years, disease surveillance system has not been developed with that pace. The outbreaks of plague (1994,

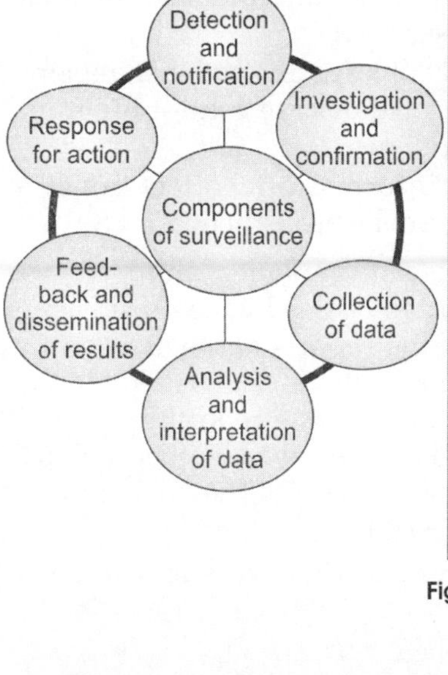

Components of surveillance system	
Surveillance system structure • Legislation (laws and regulations); including IHR (2005) • Surveillance strategy • Improve preparedeness for surveillance and response • Surveillance implementation and stakeholders • Networking and partnerships	**Core functions of surveillance** • Case detection, registration and confirmation • Reporting • Data analysis and interpretation • Epidemic preparedness • Response and control • Feedback and evaluate
Surveillance quality • Completeness and timeliness • Usefulness and simplicity • Acceptability and flexibility • Sensitivity and specificity • Positive predictive value • Representativeness	**Surveillance support functions** • Standards and guidelines • Trainings • Supervisions • Communication facilities • Resources (including logistics) all type • Monitoring and evaluation (M and E) and coordination

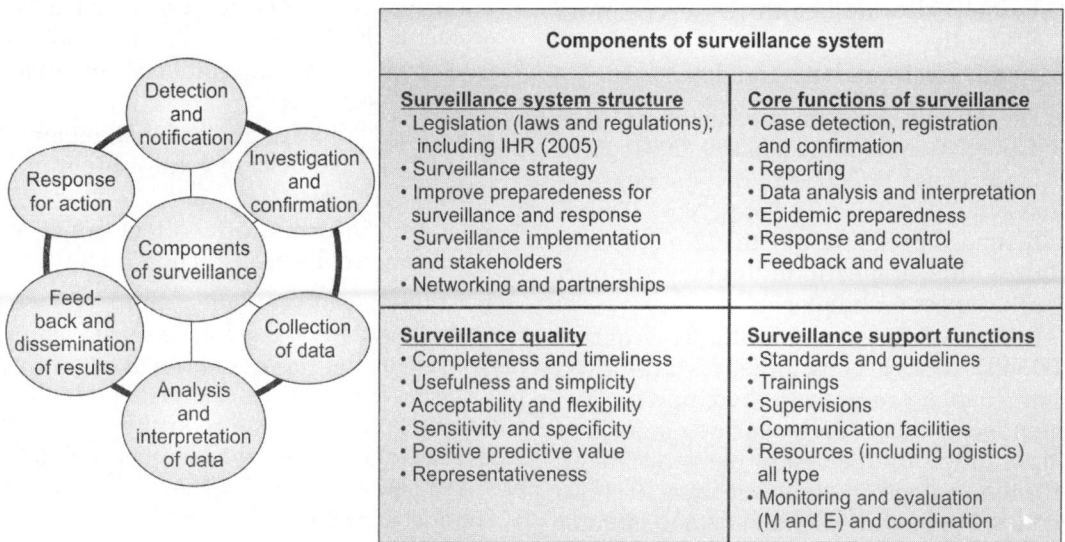

Fig. 17.1: Components of surveillance

2002), malaria (1995), dengue hemorrhagic fever (1996) and recent chikungunya fever (2006) in different parts of the country further highlighted the weaknesses in the surveillance system.

Government of India constituted a number of high-powered committees from time to time and they recommended strengthening of disease surveillance activities across the country.

On recommendations of National Apical Advisory Committee (NAAC), Government of India launched National Surveillance Program for Communicable Diseases (NSPCD) as a pilot project in 1997–98 with the overall goal of improving the health status of the people and was in operation in 101 districts.

With the encouraging results of the program, Government of India expanded the program as an integrated disease surveillance project (IDSP) on 8th November 2004. Integrated disease surveillance project is a decentralized, state-based surveillance program with **broad objectives:**

- To detect early warning signals of impending outbreaks
- To provide essential data to monitor progress of on-going disease control program
- To help allocate health resources more efficiently
- To take decisions based on data.[5]

The IDSP was implemented in three phases by Government of India: Phase I (2004–05) in 9 states, Phase II (2005–06) in 14 states, and Phase III (2006–07) in 12 states. Now IDSP is fully funded program since the 12th Five Year Plan with a domestic budgetary support worth Rupees 6.4 billion.

Integrated disease surveillance program (IDSP)[1] is a decentralized, state-based surveillance program in the country. It is intended to detect early warning signals of impending outbreaks and help initiate an effective response in a timely manner. It is also expected to provide essential data to monitor progress of on-going disease control program and help allocate health resources more efficiently (Tables 17.1 and 17.2).

In the integrated disease surveillance system:

- The district level is the focus for integrating surveillance functions.
- All surveillance activities are coordinated and streamlined. Rather than using scarce resources to maintain vertical activities, resources are combined to collect information from a single focal point at each level.
- Several activities are combined for similar surveillance to optimally usage of skills, resources and target populations.
- The IDSP integrates public, private sector and academia with community participation.
- The IDSP is for both communicable and non-communicable diseases.
- Integration of both rural and urban health systems.

Criteria for Selection of Diseases for Surveillance[1]

It is impossible to include all diseases prevalent in the country for the surveillance, therefore, following questions to be answered before the inclusion under IDSP:

1. Does the disease condition have high health impact (morbidity, mortality, disability)—malaria, NCD risk factors, road traffic accidents (RTA)?
2. Does it have significant epidemic potential? (cholera, measles)?
3. Is it a target of a specific national, regional or international disease control program? (HIV, TB, polio)?
4. Will the information collect lead to significant public health action?

For effective surveillance standard case definitions are to be used. One must ensure regularity of the reports and action on the reports. Several methods can be used for data collection. While routine reporting (passive surveillance) is universalized, other methods are need and area specific. These include:

1. Sentinel surveillance
2. Active surveillance (active search for cases)

3. Vector surveillance
4. Laboratory surveillance
5. Sample surveys
6. Outbreak investigations
7. Special studies

Who should be involved in surveillance activities (Fig. 17.2)?

1. Sub-center and village level—health worker/ANM/AWW/ASHA reports all patients fulfilling the clinical syndrome from PHC, private clinic, hospital, etc.
2. PHC/CHC medical officers report all probable cases of interest where this cannot be confirmed by laboratory tests at the peripheral reporting units and as confirmed when the laboratory information is available as in case of blood smear positive malaria and sputum AFB positive tuberculosis.
3. Sentinel private practitioners, district hospitals, municipal hospitals, medical colleges, sentinel hospitals, NGOs' medical officers report as probable cases of interest.

Table 17.1: Types of surveillance in IDSP

Type	*Characteristics*	*Diseases*
Syndromic	Diagnosis made on the basis of clinical pattern by paramedical personnel and members of the community.	1. Fever 2. Cough more than 3 weeks duration 3. Acute flaccid paralysis 4. Diarrhoea 5. Jaundice 6. Unusual events causing death or hospitalization
Presumptive	Diagnosis made on typical history and clinical examination by medical officers (MOs)	MOs of PHC, CHC, medical colleges and sentinel surveillance to conduct presumptive surveillance routinely. This will be supplemented by confirmation of diseases by laboratory reporting.
Confirmed	Clinical diagnosis confirmed by an appropriate laboratory test	

Table 17.2: Core conditions under surveillance in IDSP[1]

Type of surveillance	*Core conditions*
Vector-borne disease	Malaria
Water-borne disease	Acute diarrheal disease (cholera), typhoid
Respiratory diseases	Tuberculosis
Vaccine preventable diseases	Measles
Diseases under eradication	Polio
Other conditions	Road traffic accidents
Other international commitments	Plague, yellow fever
Unusual clinical syndromes	Meningo-encephalitis/respiratory distress (causing death/hospitalization), hemorrhagic fevers, other undiagnosed conditions
Sexually transmitted diseases/blood	HIV/HBV, HCV
Other conditions related to	Water quality, outdoor air quality
NCD risk factors	Anthropometry, physical activity, blood pressure, tobacco, nutrition
State specific diseases	Dengue, Japanese encephalitis, leptospirosis

4. Other sentinel sites like ANC sites under NACO—HIV/HBV/HCV surveillance, water board, pollution control board and district police office for road traffic accidents.
5. Participating labs will report confirmed cases when they get positive diagnostic tests especially in PHC, CHC, medical colleges, district hospitals, private hospitals, etc.
6. Community bases organizations like SHG leaders, health club/youth members club/farmer's club leaders, etc.

NON-COMMUNICABLE DISEASE RISK FACTOR SURVEILLANCE UNDER IDSP

- Of the 56 million deaths occurring globally in 2012, NCDs were responsible for 38 million (68%). By 2030, these figures are expected to rise to 52 million deaths.
- Age-standardized NCD death rates are highest in low-income, and lowest in high-income countries.
- Approximately 42% of all NCD deaths are premature, occurring before the age of 70 years. The majority of premature deaths (82%) are in low- and middle-income countries. Especially in developing countries, the burden of NCDs is increasing rapidly and will have significant social, economic, and health consequences.[6]

The key to the control of epidemics of NCDs is primary prevention. The basis of prevention of NCDs is therefore identification of the major risk factors and their prevention

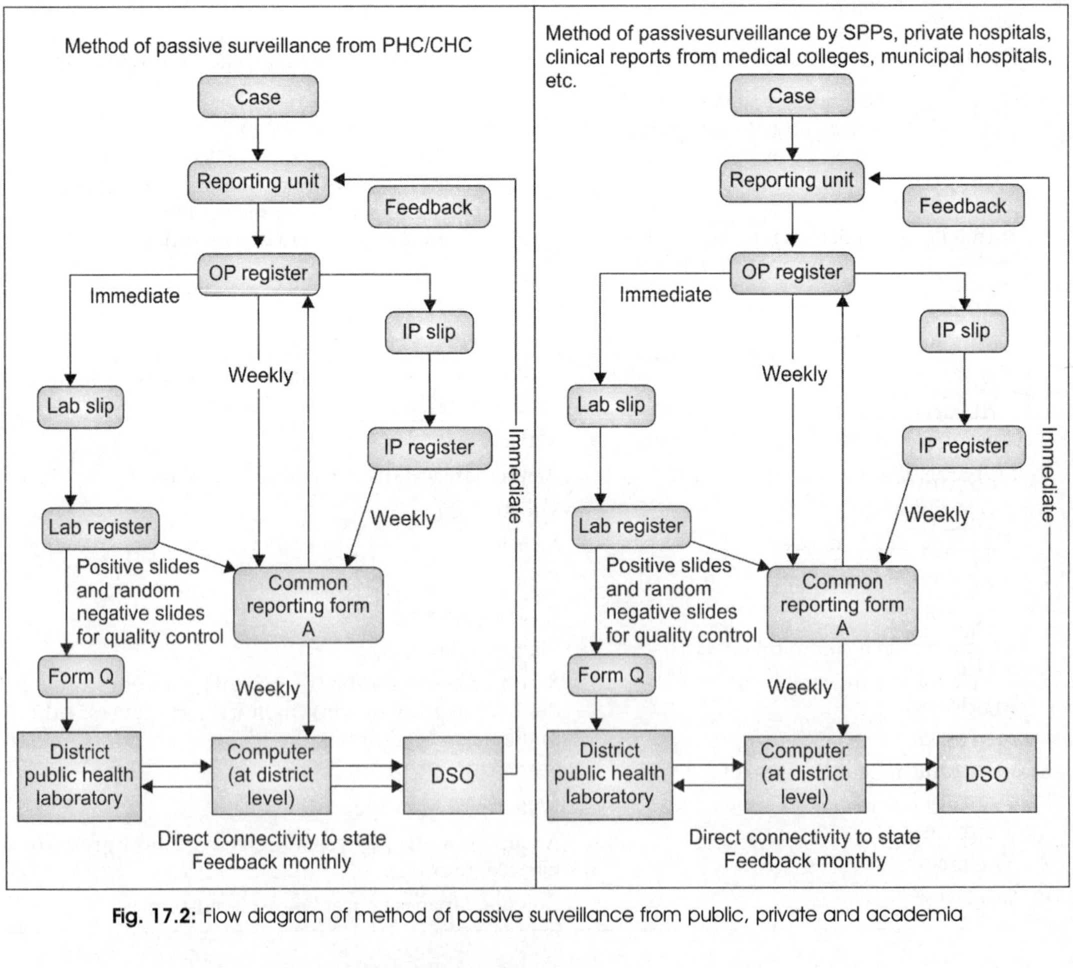

Fig. 17.2: Flow diagram of method of passive surveillance from public, private and academia

and control. Population measurements of these risk factors are used to describe the distribution of disease in a population, rather than predicting the health of a specific individual.

Around the world **WHO STEPwise approach to surveillance (STEPS)** is being followed with modification suited to local area (Fig. 17.3).

The **objectives of surveillance** of the most common NCD risk factors and NCDs are therefore to:

- Collect consistent data across and within countries;
- Develop standardized tools to enable comparisons over time and across countries;
- Prevent NCD epidemics before they occur;
- Help health services plan and determine public health priorities;
- Predict future caseloads of NCDs;
- Monitor and evaluate population—wide interventions.

The following major risk factors are measured under IDSP by conducting periodic surveys in the population in a state every 5 years:[6,7]

i. Tobacco use
ii. Alcohol consumption
iii. Raised blood pressure (systolic and diastolic)
iv. Obesity (height, weight, BMI, waist circumference)
v. Diet (low fruit, high fat, added salt to served food)
vi. Physical inactivity
vii. Diabetes mellitus (fasting plasma glucose)
viii. High serum cholesterol

In addition, demographic (age, sex, urban/rural residence), socio-economic variables (educational level, occupation, income), past and family history of cardiovascular diseases, diabetes, and hypertension are also measured.

The target population for the survey is from 15 years to 64 years. As a standard, 10-year age groups (15–24, 25–34, 35–44, 45–54, 55–64) are included as participants.

The NFHS sampling technique is used for selection of sample. Proportionate to population cluster survey technique is used to draw the sample. While estimating sample the following recommendations of the WHO STEPS approach to NCD surveillance should be considered.

"It is recommended that a minimum sample of 2500 persons each from urban and rural area across the recommended core age range of 15–64 years (equivalent to 250 participants in each 10-years age- and sex group) is undertaken for additional variable of interest such as ethnicity, area or urban–rural differences, the sample will need to be increased where an additional variable is of interest, which is based dealt with by stratification of the total population, the same number of cases in each age and sex groups needs to be added for each level of the additional variable". It is important to detect urban–rural differences and hence 2500 individuals from urban area and further 2500 from rural area will be required.

WHO (STEPS) tool is modified for the Indian scenario and already in use for sentinel surveillance for cardiovascular risk factors in 10 selected industrial populations all over India. The questionnaire basically includes socio-demographic data of the participant, assesses the tobacco habits and alcohol consumption pattern and records the measured data (height, weight and blood pressure) and biochemical results (fasting blood glucose and serum cholesterol).

STEPS core, expanded and optional levels of detail gathered for each step are briefly described in Table 17.3.

WHO STEPS includes specific software and supporting materials to undertake data collection electronically **(eSTEPS)**, such as with android devices. The benefits of electronic data collection include:

- Immediate error checking during data collection (e.g. inadvertently);
- Skipped questions or out of range responses);

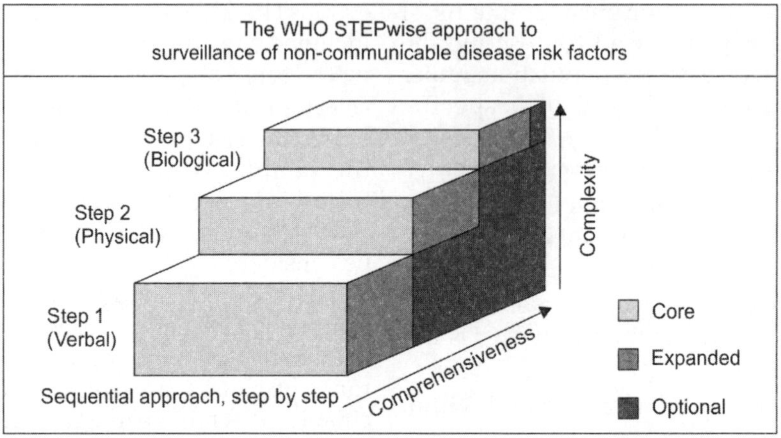

Fig. 17.3: WHO STEPwise approach to NCD surveillance

Table 17.3: STEPS core, expanded and optional items[6]

	Core items	*Expanded items*	*Optional items*
STEP 1 Behavioural	Basic demographic information including age, sex, and years at school	Expanded demographic information including highest level of education, ethnicity, marital status, employment status, household income	Cervical cancer Mental health/ suicide Oral health
	Tobacco use, duration and quantity of smoking, quit attempts, past smoking, smokeless tobacco use	Cessation, exposure to environmental tobacco smoke	Sexual health Tobacco policy
	Alcohol consumption, cessation, binge drinking, past 7 days drink ing, consumption of un-taxed Alcohol	Alcohol use disorders	Violence and injury
	Fruit and vegetable consumption, consumption of salt and processed food high in salt	Awareness of too much salt as a health problem, control of salt intake	
	Physical activity at work/in the household, for transport and during leisure time	Sedentary behaviour	
	History of raised blood pressure, diabetes, raised total cholesterol and cardiovascular diseases		
	Lifestyle advice Cervical cancer screening		
STEP 2 Physical measurements	Blood pressure Height and weight Waist circumference	Hip circumference Heart rate	Objective measurement of physical activity
STEP 3 Biochemical measurements	Fasting blood sugar Total cholesterol Urinary sodium and creatinine	HDL-cholesterol Fasting triglycerides	

- Marked reduction of materials to be carried by data collectors;
- Remote data submission;
- No additional data entry from paper-based questionnaires is needed, and therefore, it will reduce cost, errors for data entry and final dataset can be created quickly.

It is computer friendly and it can easily feed into the software program to generate the necessary analysis of trends and patterns of NCD risk factors in the community surveyed.

District level is the focus for integrated disease surveillance system. At sub-centre levels multi-purpose health workers (MPHW), accredited social health activist (ASHA) and auxiliary nurse midwifery (ANM) are involved in data collection through **Form-S (based on syndromic approach)** on weekly basis. **Form-P (presumptive cases)** is used by the clinicians for provisional diagnosis and **Form-L (laboratory cases)** for the lab-confirmed cases. This approach is based on detection of early warning signals of impending outbreaks and helps initiating an effective response in a timely manner.

Through the provision of **L-, S- and P-form** detection of early warning signals of impending outbreaks and initiation of an effective response in a timely manner is ensured. Computerization of data collection, compilation and reporting were established down to primary healthcare level with web-enabled databases and connectivity with the district surveillance units. The IDSP integrates both public and private sector by capturing data from private practitioners as well.

The data thus collected is analyzed and shared with stakeholders for further planning and action thereof.[1,7]

Details of the data collection, questionnaire, measurement and risk factors are beyond the scope of this chapter.

Monitoring of the Progress of IDSP[1,7]

All surveillance activities should be constantly monitored using standard performance indicators. If the performance of surveillance does not meet the necessary standards, prompt action should be taken to improve it. Thus, constant monitoring ensures that the surveillance system is effective. Indicators should be developed for each level. Indicators may also be classified according to the periodicity of review, e.g. weekly, monthly and yearly (Table 17.4).

Good supervision helps health staff to perform their best. During supervision one must just observe and reinforce stipulated practices in surveillance. The crux of supervisory visits should be on education, coordination, motivation, facilitation and guidance with the overall objective of implementing corrective action. Monitoring is also

Table 17.4: Indicators and frequency of monitoring

Event	*Frequency of monitoring*
Timeliness of reporting	Weekly/monthly/quarterly/annually
Completeness of reporting units (separately for public and private sector)	Weekly/monthly/quarterly/annually
Percentage of outbreaks detected by the reporting units	Quarterly/annually
Percentage of MPWs with annual supervisory reports, Case definitions and using them	Annually
Percentage of MPWs annual supervisory reports whose reports are in concurrence with their registers	Annually
Percentage of private sector enrolled as reporting units	Annually
Number of outbreaks prevented, annual comparison of previous year's reports	Annually

a vital component of any surveillance program and would determine the efficacy and effectiveness of the surveillance mechanisms in place. The various indicators should be continuously and vigorously monitored at different levels.

FEEDBACK UNDER IDSP

It is essential that feedback loops be in-built in the system. Invariably data that originates from the peripheral health facility is compiled and forwarded to the next higher level without any feedback being given to the originator. This results in de-motivation of the reporting unit and unreliability, sluggishness/falsification of data (non-reporting of suspect cases), as they would not know if the information they provided was utilized or not. Feedback helps to inform the peripheral staff the value of the work that they have performed.

Uses of feedback

- Feedback opens up channels of communication between the various levels and is helpful in strengthening the working relationships between the levels.
- Feedback allows the staff at various levels to understand the progress of the performance and provide opportunity to compare with other colleagues and do SWOT analysis.
- Motivates staff for better performance while learning from the process and other staff.

Administrative Structure Under IDSP[1]

In all multi-sectoral programs coordination between them is the hallmarks of the program. All diseases occurrence is basically the domain of other development departments, e.g. diseses transmitted through faeco–oral route, the state and local government departments and public at large is responsible for poor water quality and supply and sanitation.

It was proposed to set-up steering committees at central, state and district levels to perform coordination functions between various stakeholders, review the surveillance activities at regular intervals (monthly), identify trouble shooters and suggest mechanisms to rectify them, initiate internal and external evaluations of the IDSP activities at different levels. These committees will advise the surveillance officers (i.e. the nodal officer) at all the three levels to operationalize the suggestions of the steering committees and also manage the program on a day-to-day basis (Fig. 17.4).

PROGRESS OF IDSP IN INDIA

Integrated disease surveillance project/ program (IDSP) was launched with World Bank assistance in November 2004 to detect and respond to disease outbreaks quickly. The project was extended for 2 years in March 2010. From April 2010 to March 2012, World Bank funds were available for Central Surveillance Unit (CSU) at NCDC and 9 identified states (Uttarakhand, Rajasthan, Punjab, Maharashtra, Gujarat, Tamil Nadu, Karnataka, Andhra Pradesh and West Bengal) and the rest 26 states/UTs were funded from domestic budget.

The program continues during 12th plan under NRHM with outlay of Rs. 640 Crore from domestic budget only. Surveillance units have been established in all states/districts (SSU/DSU).

Central surveillance unit (CSU) established and integrated in the National Centre for Disease Control, Delhi. Training of state/ district surveillance teams and rapid response teams (RRT) have been completed for all 35 states/UTs. IT network connecting 776 sites in states/district HQ and premier institutes has been established with the help of National Informatics Centre (NIC) and Indian Space Research Organization (ISRO) for data entry, training, video conferencing and outbreak discussion.

Under the project weekly disease surveillance data on epidemic prone disease are being collected from reporting units such as subcentres, primary health centres, community health centres, hospitals including government and private sector hospitals and medical colleges. States/districts have been asked to notify the outbreaks immediately to the system.

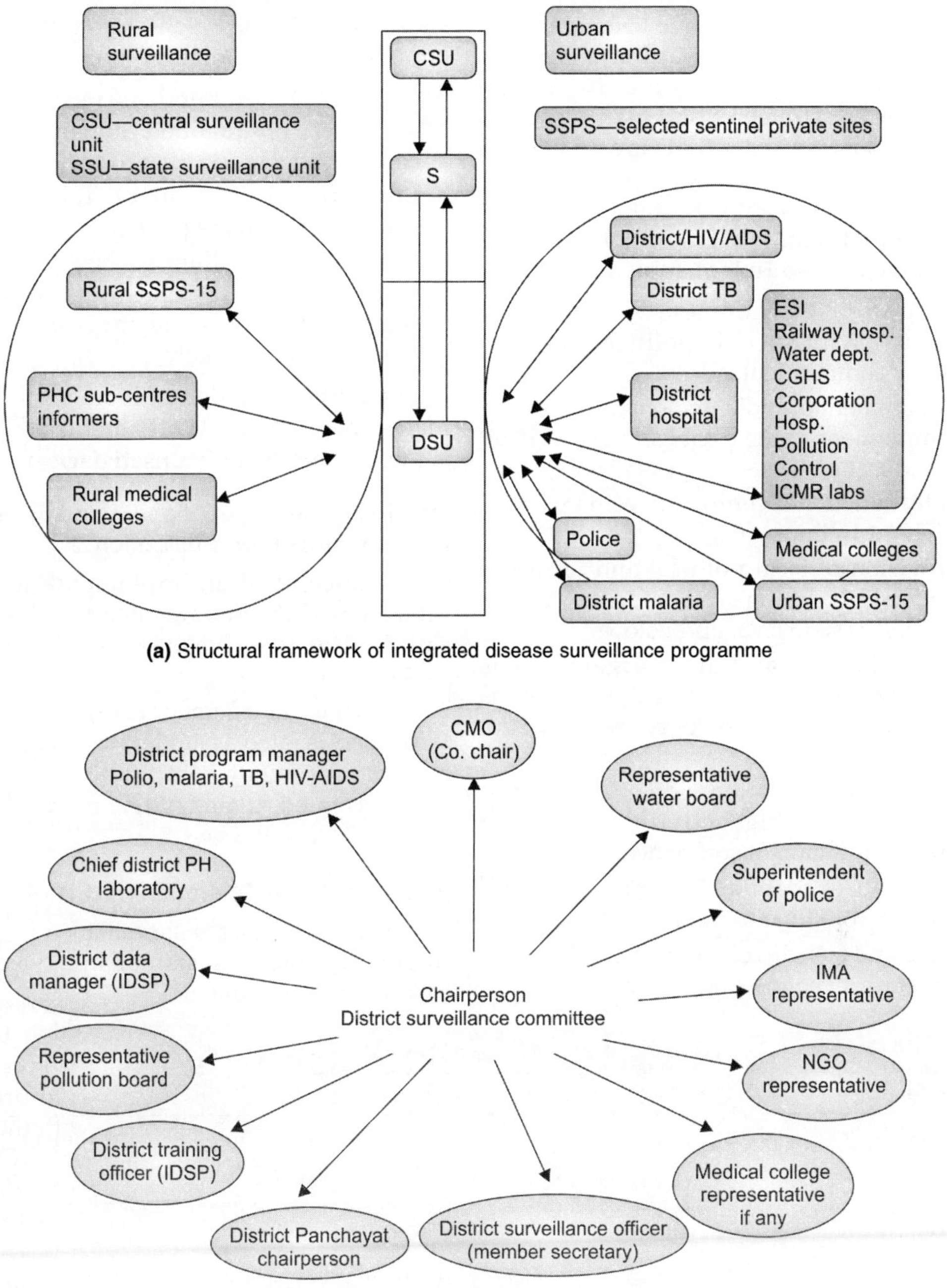

(a) Structural framework of integrated disease surveillance programme

(b) Organogram for district

Fig. 17.4: Administrative organization framework

On an average, 30–40 outbreaks are reported every week by the states. 553 outbreaks were reported and responded to by states in 2008, 799 outbreaks in 2009, 990 in 2010, 1675 outbreaks in 2011, 1584 outbreaks in 2012 and in 2013, 1898 outbreaks have been reported till 8th December 2013.[7]

Various stakeholders have been assessing the progress of the IDSP in India since its inception from time-to-time to understand current strategies and plan for better strategies. Some of the reports are mentioned in Table 17.5.[8]

Factors and Events that Favourably Contributed to the Project Implementation

- Supportive environment at global and country with specific political and economic commitment.
- Government of India demonstrated strong commitment to the establishment of IDSP in India at all levels.
- Fully-functional central surveillance unit (CSU) at Delhi.
- Provision of local political and technical leadership was imperative for the success of IDSP at state level and below
- WHO, SEARO and other organizations provided the technical assistance in terms of guidelines, manpower recruitment and training.
- Conduction of nationwide adequate and effective training activities including human and animal component.
- Flexibility in adapting to changing circumstances from time to time.
- Tremendous development of IT infrastructure, even in remote areas.

Factors and Events which Negatively Impacted Project Achievements

- **Chronic HR-related issues:** Lack of adequate and qualified human resources constantly plagued the project.
- **Low capacity of project financial and procurement management**
- **Safeguard compliance:** There was significant delay in implementing the agreed safeguard actions and the actions were implemented partially.

The implementation of biomedical waste management plan (BWMP) and tribal TDAP is rated as **moderately unsatisfactory**.

Monitoring and Evaluation (M and E) Design, Implementation and Utilization[8]

On balance, design, implementation and utilization of M and E are rated as **moderately satisfactory** given steady progress over the project period.

Financial management compliance under the project is rated as **moderately satisfactory** and procurement compliance under the project is rated as **moderately unsatisfactory** (Table 17.6).

Post-completion Operation/Next Phase

The integrated disease surveillance system is **highly likely to be sustained** in India due to following development.

Table 17.5: Highlights from World Bank report 2012[8]

Original components	*Revised components*
Year 2004	Additional component 2007—Avian Influenza and Restructuring of Components 2010
Establishing and operating a central-level disease surveillance unit (US$ 2.02 million)	Central surveillance monitoring and oversight (US$ 6.01 million)
Integrating and strengthening disease surveillance at the state and district levels (US$ 40.54 million)	Improving state/district surveillance and response capacity (US$ 22.66 million).
Improving laboratory support (US$ 22.67 million)	Flu surveillance and response (US$ 30.53 million). Human health and animal health
Training for disease surveillance and action (US$ 2.77 million).	Modified implementation arrangements and schedule
	Partial cancellation of the credit

Table 17.6: Rating of selected risks to development outcome

Criteria	*Explanation*	*Rating*
Technical	• Innovation—integrated system, web-based reporting, event-based surveillance; lack of GIS functionality; automatic warning/alert; powerful analytical functions; coverage in remote or difficult to access areas/populations.	M
Financial	• Government has committed to IDSP • Financial management capacity was improved	M
Economic	• Cost for maintaining the functioning IDS is low • Economic growth is expected	L
Social	• Challenges for IDS in tribal groups and remote areas remain • Inclusion of local stakeholders in the surveillance and response	S
Political	• Disease surveillance is a public good, and politically neutral; therefore, there is limited political risk • Improving social services wins support from constituencies	L
Environmental	• Improved disease surveillance increases sample transportation, medical waste, exposure of health workers which increases environmental risk; although guidelines for infection control and bio-security measures were developed, they are still not adequately practiced	M
Government ownership	• Government ownership is high as documented in certain sections in the report	L
Stakeholder ownership	• Stakeholder ownership is high as documented in certain sections in the report	L
Institutional support: project entities and legal/legislative framework	• Legal framework exists—mandatory disease reporting, issuance of public health bill, but enforcement of legal framework is challenging for urban centers, private service providers, etc.	M
Governance	• The system is transparent—community-based disease reporting, call centers, media rumor scanning, willingness to report by districts and states • Information from IDSP has been used for designing disease prevention and control programs and for results verification	M
Natural disaster exposure	• Back-up plans need to be worked out in case of IT system breakdown during natural disasters, etc.	M

Note: L—negligible or low; M—moderate; S—significant.
World Bank report, 2012

- **IDSPs were operated in all states in India.**
- **The NCDC and the states have developed basic technical expertise in a functioning integrated disease surveillance and response system.**
- **Integration with the existing health programs**—Government of India has integrated the national disease surveillance project under the NRHM.
- **Secured funding**—for the human health components, after the project restructuring in 2010, MOHFW assumed all the funding responsibility for the integrated disease surveillance in 26 states and union territories that were not included in the restructured project. Funding beyond 2012 for the project has been planned by GoI under the budgetary provision in the 12th Five Year Plan (2012–2017).

- Overall, efficiency is rated as **satisfactory.**
- The overall risk to development outcome is rated as **moderate.**

GOVERNMENT OF INDIA REPORT ON IDSP (2015–2016)[9]

The Government of India conducted an assessment of achievements of IDSP and progress made in 12th Five Year Plan period. Findings depicted as SWOT analysis are mentioned in Tables 17.7 to 17.9.

Various studies conducted on evaluation of IDSP have indicated the following.

- Lack of integration of private sector in surveillance activity,
- Poor laboratory capacity,
- Lack surveillance infrastructure in the tribal, remote rural and urban regions,
- Slow and inefficient sharing of surveillance information at the district level,
- Limited capacity to undertake analysis and response at the district level,

Table 17.7: SWOT analysis of the indicator-based surveillance—IDSP review, 2015–16

Strengths	*Weaknesses*
1. Strong ownership and steering by CSU.	1. Inadequate efforts in using the IBS for timely and appropriate response.
2. The sustainability of the IDSP is the improved political and bureaucratic response from MoHFW.	2. Lack of integration of private sector in surveillance activity.
3. Management of capacity building for HR	3. Lower number of outbreaks detected through IBS
4. Oversight of field investigations.	4. Insufficient data analysis by some states and many districts.
5. Good data analysis by CSU and some states.	5. Limited capacity to undertake analysis and response at the district level.
6. Timely reporting has progressively increased.	6. Poor urban infrastructure for surveillance.
	7. Lack of data on mortality.
	8. No SOPs for feedback at the district level.
	9. Varied quality of reporting system
	10. Poor supportive supervision and communication at district and state levels.
	11. Absence of strong monitoring and evaluation system.
	12. Frequent transfers of key officials.
	13. Duplication and multiplicity of data collection and reporting from the level of SCs, districts and states.
Opportunities	*Threats*
1. Mobile phone-based applications, such as Apps, can be used to develop and sustain universal reporting (including from private health facilities).	1. The entire system works with contractual staff. The system can collapse at any time if the funding dwindles or the political will continues to fade off.
2. Greater potential for generation of in-built warning signals within the system.	2. Funding is barely enough to manage salaries of contractual staff (vacancies), and needs to be made available.
3. Form S can be used for greater efficiency including use in urban areas. Apps can use form S for generating effective data.	3. Disease burden at local levels to be monitored.
4. Linking response to IBS data analysis is needed.	4. Importance of data-driven or evidence-based policy making is not realized.
5. A dashboard comprising several surveillance platforms is needed.	
6. Strengthening the SSUs and DSUs to be done.	

Table 17.8: SWOT analysis of event-based surveillance—IDSP review, 2015–16

Strengths	*Weaknesses*
1. Surveillance functions started in 1998 in the country	1. Media scanning and verification function concentrated at CSU
2. Functional surveillance units are present in each district of the country	2. Quality of events/outbreak identification, reporting, response and data analysis at the state and district levels
3. Regular and continuous media scanning and monitoring at the CSU since 2009	3. Competence of epidemiologists and data managers in event/outbreak information management
4. Strategic health operations centre (SHOC) in place since 2013—emergency operations plan and SOPs being developed by the SHOC	4. EWS/outbreak reports information management is HR intensive
5. Entomologists and veterinary consultants posts for state surveillance units	5. Discontinuity in 24 × 7 toll free number for EBS reporting
Opportunities	*Threats*
1. Strengthen media scanning and verification at state and district level	1. India is one of the global hot spots for emerging and re-emerging zoonotic diseases
2. Strengthening of information collection from all possible sources, including the community	2. High frequency of travel of population to ongoing foci of transmission of ebola. Middle eastern respiratory syndrome coronavirus (MERS-CoV) and other emerging pathogens
3. Strengthening of portal entry of events/EWS/outbreak data and web analytical features	3. Long porous borders with neighbouring countries where formal points of entry (PoE) surveillance and screening are not possible
4. Integration of veterinary and entomological information with human health information	4. Diversity of health systems capacity across the country and within states and districts
5. To expand the training for EBS with other partner agencies, e.g. Food Safety and Standards Authority India (FSSAI) National Disaster Management Authority (NDMA), etc.	
6. To include EBS indicators in key surveillance quality indicators	
7. Operationalization of the 24 × 7 toll free number	

- Inadequate human capacity building
- Inadequate supervision and monitoring, etc.

Evaluation of thirty-three IDSP assessment studies by Revati *et al.* showed that IDSR strategy has been best adopted and implemented in the WHO–AFRO region. Although significant progress is made in overcoming the challenges identified with vertical disease surveillance strategies, gaps still exist. Mixed challenges with core and support IDSR functions were observed across countries. Main issues identified include non-sustainable financial resources, lack of co-ordination, inadequate training and turnover of peripheral staff, erratic feedback, inadequate supervision from the next level, weak laboratory capacities coupled with unavailability of job aids (case definitions/reporting formats), and poor availability of communication and transport systems particularly at the periphery. Best outcomes in core functions and system attributes were reported when support surveillance functions performed optimally.

Apart from technical and technological issues, human resources and the healthcare system structures were also issues for proper implementation of IDSP.[10]

Table 17.9: SWOT analysis of special surveillance—IDSP review, 2015–16

Strengths	*Weaknesses*
1. Sample collection and transport system in place. 2. Integration of influenza surveillance in national reporting system. 3. Good intersectoral coordination with department of animal husbandry for containment of avian influenza. 4. Demonstration of Manipal hospital in Karnataka as a successful public-private partnership in influenza surveillance. 5. Initiation of sentinel surveillance through IDSP laboratory network.	1. Epidemiological data analysis needs to be strengthened. 2. Quality of testing needs to be maintained at all laboratories. 3. Influenza subtyping algorithm must be standardized. 4. Delay in supply of consumables. 5. Quality of training to be improved. 6. Quality of data collected needs improvement. 7. Limited capacity of the system to detect emergence of new subtypes of influenza virus A in human populations unless the transmission is sustained.
Opportunities	*Threats*
1. Aligning with the global health security agenda and expediting IHR-2005 core capacity requirements for laboratory surveillance. 2. Collaboration with CDC, transfer of technology and sharing of sequences for seasonal flu viruses. 3. The influenza network can be utilized to monitor other emerging/re-emerging infections and viruses such as MERS and Zika. 4. Strengthening training components and support from WHO and partners in capacity building.	1. India is a global hot spot for emergence and re-emergence of zoonotic diseases. 2. States and districts have weak health systems and poor laboratory network.

A study undertaken by Eva Pilot, *et al.* on syndromic surveillance under IDSP by the Triple S project: "A real-time (or near-real time) collection, analysis, interpretation, and dissemination of health-related data to enable the early identification of the impact (or absence of impact) of potential human or veterinary public health threats that require effective public health action.[11]

The study highlighted the need and potential of early warning capacity via enlisting the currently untapped (for surveillance) standardized data sources. The implementation of a sustainable, cost-effective intervention has the potential to improve infectious disease surveillance in the immediate future and help the government to appropriately prioritize timely interventions. The use of routinely-collected health data for syndromic surveillance is sowing the seeds for responsible and sustainable public health decision-making.

DK Srivastava, *et al.* found that reporting was incomplete (syndromic surveillance 13.7% and of presumptive surveillance was 87.5%) and not on time. Laboratory surveillance from rural reporting units had not been started yet.[12]

GLOBAL DISEASE DETECTION (GDD) PROGRAM: INDIA—AN ASSESSMENT BY CDC[13]

In 2009, the India Global Disease Detection (GDD) Regional Center was established to build capacity with local and regional public health entities to detect and respond to disease outbreaks. The center works to strengthen surveillance networks and public health laboratory systems, provide technical assistance to improve outbreak response, and detect emerging zoonotic disease threats.

The GDD center in India helps contain outbreaks close to the source by building up local resources, drawing on combined expertise in:

- Emerging infectious disease detection and response
- Field epidemiology and laboratory training
- Pandemic influenza preparedness and response
- Zoonotic disease research and control

In collaboration with India's National Centre for Disease Control, CDC India established and is expanding the India **Epidemic Intelligence Service** (EIS) which has increased local and regional capacity to better detect, identify, and contain threats to public health. Through the India EIS Program, GDD India participates in non-communicable disease projects like studying road traffic accidents, measuring the air quality index, and assessing acute cardiac and respiratory illness.

From 2009–2016, the GDD Center in India supported:

- Effective response to 91 outbreaks, including hepatitis A, dengue, measles, avian flu, anthrax, cholera, and malaria
- Training of over 4,017 public health officials in short-term public health exercises
- Graduation of 24 future global health leaders as part of the 2-year India Epidemic Intelligence Service (EIS) Program, with plans to train 100 future officers per year.
- Conducted a 3-month frontline epidemiology training for all 50 districts of the state of Rajasthan, with plans to expand to 100 districts throughout India per year.

INDIA'S IDSP PROGRESS REPORT IN 2017[14]

Outbreaks Reported in 2017

India's Central Surveillance Unit, IDSP receives disease outbreak reports from the states/UTs on weekly basis. On an average 30–35 outbreaks are reported to CSU weekly.

A total of 1562 outbreaks were reported in 2014, 1935 outbreaks in 2015, 2679 outbreaks reported in 2016 and 1714 outbreaks reported from 2nd January 2017 till 31st December 2017. Majority of outbreaks reported in 2017 were of acute diarrheal disease (21%), food poisoning (15%), followed by chickenpox and measles (13% each).

Labs Strengthening

So far, 138 district laboratories in 29 states are functional and supported by trained manpower, funds for essential equipment and reagents and consumables.

A state-based referral laboratory network has been established through existing functional labs in the medical colleges and other major centers in the states and linking them with adjoining districts for providing diagnostic services for epidemic prone diseases during outbreaks. Presently this network is functional in 23 states/UTs involving 108 labs.

Media Scanning and Verification Cell

Media scanning is an important component of surveillance to detect the early warning signals. Media scanning and verification cell (MSVC) daily receives an average of 2–3 media alerts of unusual health events which are detected and verified. A total of 4157 health alerts have been detected since July 2008. Majority of them were acute diarrheal disease, measles and dengue. A total of 650 media alerts were scanned in 2017. Three most common conditions scanned in MSVC were dengue, food poisoning and fever. The process of establishing media scanning and verification cells in all 29 states and 7 UTs is being undertaken right now.

Surveillance Report of Selected Diseases

Seasonal influenza (H1N1): IDSP compiles year-wise cases and deaths from seasonal influenza (H1N1) on behalf of MoHFW. This has become increasingly important in view of increase in number of cases which is seen from time to time. It was observed that in 2017, Seasonal influenza (H1N1) previously called Swine flu had a spurt from mid-June and started declining from Sept. 2017.

Measles: Measles is an important vaccine preventable disease (VPD) reported under IDSP. In 2015, 279 outbreaks of measles were reported from all over the country which increased to 294 in 2016. However, in 2017, there was a decline in the number of outbreaks with total of 231 outbreaks in IDSP system. Using standardized case definitions, measles is reported in P ('Probable') form by PHC/CHC medical officers and doctors in tertiary care institutes.

Dengue: With rapid urbanization, dengue has emerged as an important disease in recent years, causing outbreaks in many parts of the country. Under IDSP system, dengue is reported in both P ('probable') and L ('lab confirmed') forms. In 2015, 152 outbreaks of dengue were reported; while in 2016, there were 177 outbreaks. In 2017, 164 total outbreaks have been reported (including 10 mixed dengue and chikungunya outbreaks, and 2 dengue and leptospirosis outbreaks).

Leptospirosis: Leptospirosis has emerged as an important emerging disease. Transmitted by urine of infected rats, humans become infected through contact with water or soil which has been seeded with infected urine. In India, leptospirosis is predominantly seen in southern states like Tamil Nadu, Kerala and Karnataka. In addition, large number of cases are also increasingly reported from Maharashtra, Gujarat and Uttar Pradesh. In IDSP system, leptospirosis is reported in P ('probable') form by PHC/CHC medical officers and doctors in tertiary care institutes and 'L' (lab confirmed) forms.

Other diseases under surveillance

- Acute febrile illness (AFI),
- Acute encephalitis syndrome/Japanese encephalitis (AES/JE),
- Viral hemorrhagic fever (VHF) and respiratory virus (RV) surveillance,
- Acute diarrheal diseases (ADD) and food poisoning,
- Healthcare associated infections (HAIs) and antimicrobial resistance (AMR)

OUTBREAKS INVESTIGATED BY CENTRAL TEAM OF IDSP AND NCDC IN 2017 IN INDIA

- Central team assisted Kerala state in outbreak investigation of H1N1, leptospirosis, and dengue.
- Chickenpox outbreak in Maharajganj district, Uttar Pradesh.
- Measles outbreak in Longding district Arunachal Pradesh.
- Central team visit to review rising trends of cases and deaths related to H1N1 in the State of Maharashtra.
- Central team visit to review rising trend of H1N1 cases and deaths in Gujarat state.
- NCDC team visit to Noida, Uttar Pradesh to investigate hand, foot and mouth disease.
- Central team investigated dengue upsurge in Karnataka.
- Central team investigated outbreak of febrile illness in Varadaiahpalem, Chittoor, Andhra Pradesh.
- Outbreak investigation of glanders in horses in Delhi, Uttar Pradesh, Haryana, Rajasthan and Punjab.

A BRIEF NOTE ON IDSP STRATEGY FOR TRIBAL POPULATIONS[15]

The integrated disease surveillance project (IDSP) covering all states in India and implemented by the states, districts and communities. The tribal development plan was proposed as an integral part of IDSP. **World Bank's Operational Directive 4.20** related to indigenous people triggered in IDSP.

There are over 700 scheduled tribes notified under Article 342 of the Constitution of India and account for 8.6% of the country's population. Population of scheduled tribes (STs) in the country is 10.45 crore as per Census 2011.[7] Indian states account for more than 75% of the tribal population. The main concentration of tribal people is the central tribal belt in the middle part of the India and in the north-eastern states.

Integrated Tribal Development Project

Integrated tribal development project (ITDP) is an area of size of one or more development blocks in which ST population is 50% or more of total population of such blocks. Complete development block/*Panchayat Samiti* is the minimum constituent unit of an ITDP. There can be more than one ITDP in a district.[16]

Tribals in IDSP

Widespread poverty, illiteracy and malnutrition, lack of personal hygiene, absence of drinking water, sanitary living conditions and health education, poor maternal and child health services, and ineffective coverage by national health and nutritional services, have been identified as conditions responsible for poor health status of the poor. Tribal settlements tend to be small and isolated and difficult to reach with facilities and services.

The project involves all stakeholders including tribals in disease surveillance for rapid identification of disease conditions and outbreaks to prevent large scale impacts and a quick response from the health system.

One need to:

i. Strengthen link between the tribal communities and the health system for enhancing credibility of the health system,
ii. Reaching to unreached areas
iii. Increased disease identification and reporting by tribal communities overcoming their socio-cultural and economic barriers;
iv. Improved health awareness and
v. improved surveillance in tribal areas.

Project Benefits

The integration of the various disease surveillance programs would provide more complete and coherent health information, better monitoring of disease burden and improved health system response in the tribal areas too. In the tribal areas also, community-based information is a key input to the district surveillance unit (DSU) which will coordinate all the analysis, response and feedback of information. These should have a positive impact on the tribals and their health status.

Major findings: During the FGDs with women in the tribal areas, the rural and urban areas are given below.

1. **Socio-cultural and economic barriers**
2. **Decision making process about health issues:** Elders in the families influenced decisions regarding the place, type and timing of seeking healthcare especially in tribal areas.
3. **Seeking healthcare:** Due to poverty, poor accessibility to health facilities and various socio-cultural beliefs, home remedies are first resort.
4. **Socio-cultural factors in the care of sick:** Illnesses are often viewed as a curse for which Gods have to be placated by making offerings at the local temple. The offerings ranged from fruit and flowers to goat, chicken and liquor.
5. **Gender barriers:** Discussions with women in tribal areas consistently brought out the gender disparity to seek healthcare.
6. **Credibility of health system:** Tribal women perceived that doctors in public sector health facilities did not provide good care to them because they were poor.
7. **Information sharing:** While there was no voluntary sharing of information on symptoms and diseases, on enquiry there was sharing of information.
8. **Participation in surveillance:** Greater involvement of Panchayats, overall improvement in government health services in their area, greater awareness generation on disease surveillance through campaigns, were identified as important steps in enthusing communities for getting involved in reporting of various health conditions of public health significance.

Focal social mobilization, training and involvement of local tribal, sensitization of health system staff, design and use of culturally-compatible IEC material and monitoring and evaluation will be for the IDSP among tribal groups.

Study of Community-based Disease Surveillance Systems

In order to better understand the basic principles that would govern the setting-up of community-based surveillance systems under this project. A study, pointed out the following basic tenets as critical for involving communities including tribals' in disease surveillance under the IDSP. Some of the key findings related to:

- People's collectives like self help groups could be effective partners and their involvement could help sustain the process;
- Local volunteers could be trained to assist in disease surveillance;
- Training of health staff for collection of high quality data, proper supervision;
- Integration of communicable and non-communicable diseases in the program;
- Selection of conditions that have significant association with public health action;
- Translation of information into public health action initiation;
- Integration of private practitioners and medical colleges in disease control efforts;
- Higher level of technology—computerization with networking across at all levels;
- Appropriate automated and predetermined responses built into the system;
- Establishing systems for efficient sharing of information across vertical disease control-programs and stakeholders belonging to departments other than health;
- Good laboratory support.

Institutional Mechanism

The national and state-level project implementation plans identify tribal populations as a target group with unique problems of physical and social access requiring culturally sensitive strategies.

The project emphasizes two institutional initiatives which would address the needs of the tribal people:

1. Decentralization of planning and implementation to the state and district levels.
2. Better relationship between the health system and the tribals through volunteers.

Implementation and Local Participation

The project seeks to address this by:

- Social mobilization strategies
- Preparation of simple case definitions for diseases
- Sensitization and training programs
- IEC

Monitoring and evaluation: Capturing unrecorded information (due to socio-cultural barriers and gender discrimination faced by communities, especially vulnerable groups) from tribal population may reveal the extent of participation in and benefited from the project.

THE FUTURE STRATEGIES TO IMPROVE IDSP IN INDIA[1,8,9]

Much progress has been made in IDSP in India, however, some of the areas mentioned below to be focused for optimum benefit from this project:

Surveillance

- Electronic medical records (EMRs), hospital management information systems and geographical information system (GIS) are possible solutions for the problem of ineligible or missing information in the outdoor registers of clinicians in hospitals.
- Conducting high-impact public health surveillance of disease syndromes such as acute febrile illness and acute encephalitis syndrome. Strengthening viral hemorrhagic fever and respiratory disease surveillance.
- Enhancing surveillance platforms to detect vaccine-preventable bacterial disease in young children.
- Supporting surveillance of healthcare associated infections and antimicrobial resistance.

Lab Strengthening

- Enhancing the quality and capacity of public health laboratories by supporting the national laboratory strengthening initiative of the national centre for disease control.

- This initiative strengthens the capacity of all district and state laboratories beginning in the states of Gujarat, Tamil Nadu, Jharkhand and Madhya Pradesh.
- Government of India to build bio-risk management (BRM) capacities in the public health laboratories of India.
- Implementing a district model of integrated lab services in the states of Rajasthan, Maharashtra, Telangana, Andhra Pradesh, West Bengal, and Assam through labs for life.
- Expanding laboratory-enhanced disease surveillance for improved outbreak response.
- Developing rapid diagnostic capabilities and whole genome sequencing methodology to be used for drug-resistant TB, and to diagnose known and unknown pathogens.

Workforce Development

- Strengthening national epidemiologic capacity through the 2-year India Epidemic Intelligence Service (EIS) EIS program, 3-month frontline epidemiology trainings, and rapid response team trainings, including for veterinarians.
- Rapid response team (RRT) training enhances health security by increasing emergency response capacity as well as the efficiency and effectiveness of the responses.
- Evaluating laboratories on techniques including for antimicrobial resistance, and hospital staff on infection control practices and healthcare-associated infection surveillance.

Emergency Preparedness

- Providing training for disaster response and mass casualty events.
- Supporting the national Indian Emergency Operations Centers (EOC)/Strategic Health Operations Centers (SHOC) with emergency response training and facilitating development of these centers at the state level.
- Training laboratory staff in safe handling and rapid transportation of clinical specimens and of potentially infectious waste during public health emergencies.

Technical Advisory Group

In order to review the progress of the program, periodic independent external evaluation of the program and strengthening the integrated disease surveillance in India, it is also suggested there should be constituted a technical advisory group constituting of all important stakeholders in public health surveillance.

References

1. GoI-MoHFW. Integrated disease surveillance project operations manual for district surveillance unit. Government of India, Directorate General of Health Services, Ministry of Health and Family Welfare, Nirman Bhavan, New Delhi 2005.
2. WHO. An Integrated Approach to Communicable Disease Surveillance, Epidemiological Bulletin/ PAHO, Vol. 21, No. 1, (2000).
3. Raut DK, Bhola AK. Integrated disease Surveillance in India: Way forward. Global Journal of Medicine and Public Health, Vol. 3, No. 4 2014. www.gjmedph.org
4. Nsubuga P, White M, Evans E, Jha P, Mills A, Musgrove P, (Eds). 2006 Ch-53: Public health surveillance: A tool for targeting and monitoring interventions. Available at http://files.dcp2.org/ pdf/DCP/DCP53.pdf)
5. Thakur JS. Integrated disease surveillance—A key step to improve public health in India; Editorial, Indian J of Community Medicine 2006;31(4):215.
6. WHO STEPS surveillance manual: http://www. who.int/ncds/surveillance/steps/en/Last Updated: 26 January 2017.
7. MoSP. Manual on Health Statistics In India, Central Statistical Office Ministry of Statistics and Programme Implementation, Government of India, New Delhi May, 2015. http://www.mospi.gov. in/ sites/default/files/publication_reports/Manual-Health-Statistics_5june15.pdf.
8. World Bank. 2012 India - Integrated Disease Surveillance Project (IDSP) (English). Washington DC: The World bank.http://documents. world bank.org/curated/en/395451468051013436/ India-Integrated-Disease-Surveillance-Project-IDSP
9. http://www.searo.who.int/india/publications/ jmm_idsp_2015_part_2a.pdf?ua = 1

10. Revati K Phalkey, Shelby Yamamoto, Pradip Awate, Michael Marx. Challenges with the implementation of an integrated disease surveillance and response (IDSR) system: systematic review of the lessons learned. Health Policy and Planning 2015; 30:131–143. doi:10.1093/heapol/czt097
11. Eva Pilot, et al. Towards Sustainable Public Health Surveillance in India: Using Routinely Collected Electronic Emergency Medical Service Data for Early Warning of Infectious Diseases. Sustainability 2017, 9, 604; doi:10.3390/su9040604 www.mdpi.com/journal/sustainability
12. Srivastava DK, et al. Completeness and timeliness of reporting under IDSP in Rural Surveillance Unit of Nanital District. Indian J Prev Soc Med 2009;40 (3,4).
13. CDC, Division of Global Health Protection, Global Disease Detection Program: India. https://www.cdc.gov/globalhealth/healthprotection/gdd/india.html
14. IDSP Annual Report, 1st edn, Vol. 1, 2017. https://www.dhskashmir.org/pdf/IDSP%20Annual%20Report%202017.pdf
15. MOHFW. Integrated Disease Surveillance project. Draft Tribal Development Plan (RTI ACT, 2005). https://mohfw.gov.in/.../8945026795Draft Tribal Development Plan.
16. GoI-MoTA. Annual Report 2016-17. Ministry of Tribal Affairs, Govt. of India, Shastri Bhawan, New Delhi. www.tribal.gov.in

Chapter

18

International Health Regulations

Purushottam Giri

The international health regulations (IHR) are legally binding set of regulations adopted by World Health Organization (WHO) which helps countries to save lives caused by diseases spread internationally and other health risks.[1]

HISTORY OF THE IHR

The IHR's origins can be traced to a series of sanitary conferences beginning in 1851 to forge an international agreement to curb the spread of infectious diseases (originally cholera, followed by plague and yellow fever) entering Europe from Asia, particularly India and the Levant. The cholera epidemics that over-ran Europe between 1830 and 1847 were catalysts for intensive infectious disease-diplomacy and multilateral cooperation in public health. This led to the first International Sanitary Conference in Paris in 1851. In 1948, the WHO Constitution entered into force and in 1951 WHO member states adopted the International Sanitary Regulations, which were replaced by and renamed the International Health Regulations in 1969. The 1969 Regulations were subject to minor modifications in 1973 and 1981.[1,2]

The 1969 IHR were primarily intended to monitor and control six serious infectious diseases—cholera, plague, yellow fever, smallpox, relapsing fever and typhus. Under the IHR (1969), only cholera, plague and yellow fever remain notifiable, meaning that states are required to notify WHO if and when these diseases occur on their territory.[3]

In the early 1990s, the resurgence of some well known epidemic diseases, such as cholera in parts of South America, plague in India and the emergence of new infectious agents such as Ebola haemorrhagic fever, resulted in a resolution at the 48th World Health Assembly in 1995 calling for there vision of the Regulations.

In May 2001, the World Health Assembly adopted resolution WHA 54.14, global health security—epidemic alert and response, in which WHO was called upon to support its member states in strengthening their capacity to detect and respond rapidly to communicable disease threats and emergencies.

In May 2003, resolution WHA56.28 on revision of the international health regulations, established an intergovernmental working group (IGWG) open to all member states to review and recommend a draft revision of the international health regulations for consideration by the World Health Assembly. The IGWG held two sessions in November 2004 and February/May 2005 with a view to endorsing a final text for consideration by the World Health Assembly at its 58th meeting. The World Health Assembly adopted the IHR (2005) on 23 May 2005 by way of resolution WHA58.3. The IHR (2005) entered into force on 15 June 2007.

International Health Regulations (2005) or 'IHR 2005' are an international law which helps countries work together to save lives and livelihoods caused by the international spread of diseases and other health risks. They entered into force on 15 June 2007 and are binding on 194 countries across the globe, including all WHO member states.[1]

The IHR (2005) establish a set of rules to support the global outbreak alert and response system and to require countries to improve international surveillance and reporting mechanisms for public health events and to strengthen their national surveillance and response capacities.[1]

Major changes since 1969 are:

- IHR 1969 consisted of 9 parts with 94 articles, 4 appendices and 6 annex.
- IHR 2005 consists of 10 parts with 66 articles, no. 10 appendix and 9 annex.
- Basic changes from IHR 1969 to IHR 2005 are following.
  1. From control at border to (also) containment at source,
  2. From limited list of diseases to all infectious and non-infectious public health hazards and
  3. From preset measures to response according to condition.[3]

PURPOSE AND SCOPE OF IHR

To prevent, protect against, control and provide a public health response to the inter national spread of disease in ways that are commensurate with and restricted to public health risks, and which avoid unnecessary interference with international traffic and trade.[2]

FUNCTIONS OF IHR

Notification

The IHR (2005) require states to notify WHO of all events that may constitute a public health emergency of international concern and to respond to requests for verification of information regarding such events. This enables WHO to ensure appropriate technical collaboration for effective prevention of such emergencies or containment of outbreaks and, under certain defined circumstances, inform other states of the public health risks where action is necessary on their part.

National IHR Focal Points and WHO IHR Contact Points

Under the IHR (2005), countries are required to notify and report events and other information through their national IHR focal points to a regional WHO IHR contact points. Focal points and contact points must be available on a 24 hour-a-day basis, 7 days a week.[3] There are currently 193 national IHR focal points and six corresponding WHO IHR contact points.

Requirements for National Core Capacities

Under the IHR (2005), each state party is required to develop, strengthen and maintain core public health capacities for surveillance and response by using existing national resources, such as the national plans for influenza pandemic preparedness. Key sanitary and health services and facilities are also to be developed at international airports, ports and ground crossings designated for this purpose by states parties.

External Advice Regarding the IHR

The IHR (2005) include procedures for obtaining independent technical advice concerning IHR implementation. One context is the process for the establishment of an emergency committee to advise the Director General of WHO in determining whether a particular event is, in fact, a public health emergency of international concern and to provide advice on any appropriate temporary recommendations. An IHR review committee is tasked with advising the Director General on technical matters relating to standing recommendations, the functioning of the regulations and amendments thereto.

Public Health Emergency of International Concern (PHEIC)[2]

According to the IHR (2005) a public health emergency of international concern refers to an extraordinary public health event which is determined under specific procedures—(a) to constitute a public health risk to other states through the international spread of disease; and (b) to potentially require a coordinated international response.

To ensure adequate and early communications with WHO about potential international public health emergencies, the IHR (2005) include a decision instrument ***(Annex 2 of the Regulations)*** (Fig. 18.1) which sets the parameters for notification to WHO of all

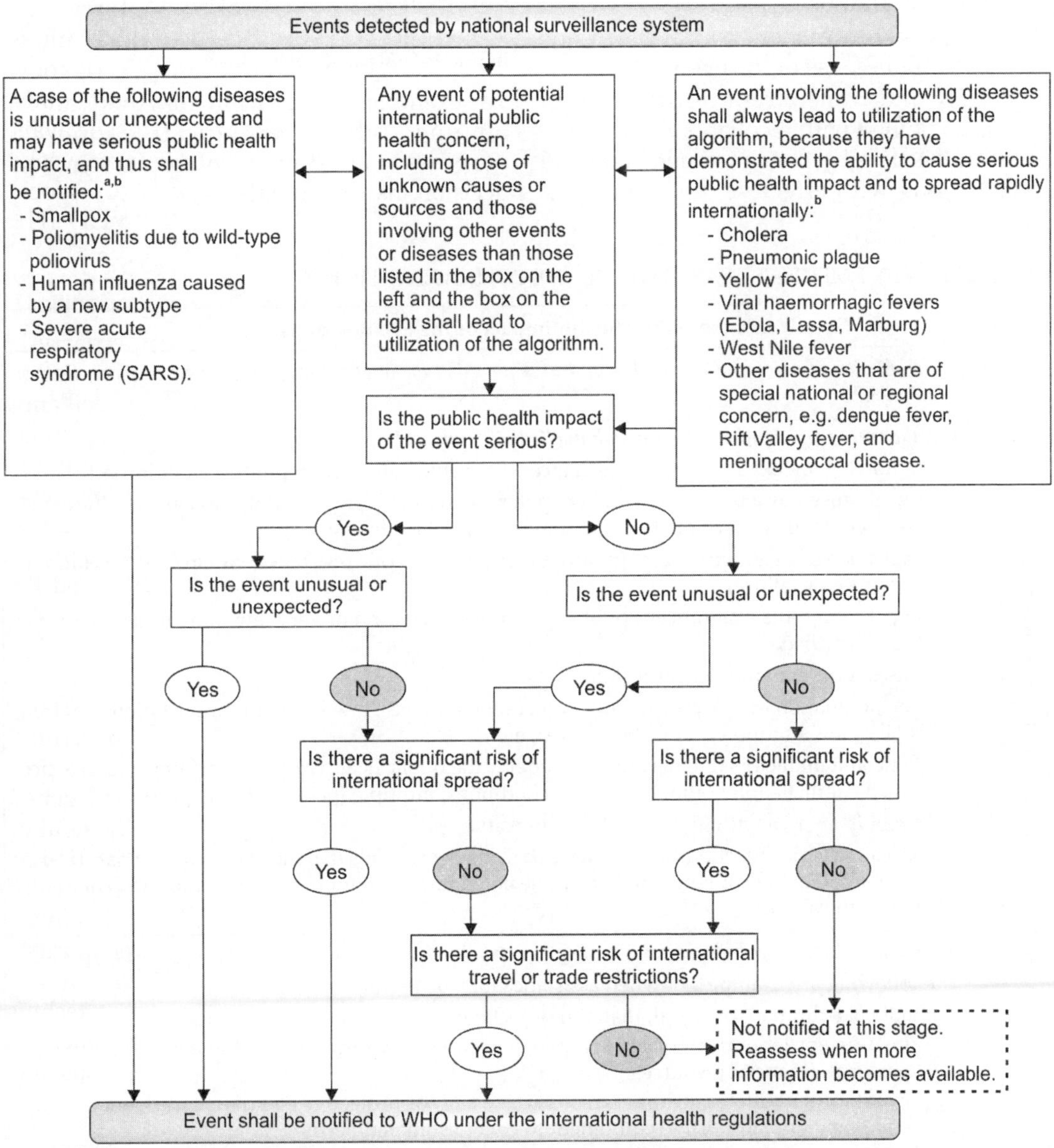

[a]As per WHO case definitions.

[b]The disease list shall be used only for the purposes of these regulations.

Fig. 18.1: Annex 2—decision instrument for the assessment and notification of events that may constitute a public health emergency of international concern

events which may constitute a Public Health Emergency of International Concern (PHEIC) based on the following criteria.

a. Seriousness of the public health impact of the event;
b. Unusual or unexpected nature of the event;
c. Potential for the event to spread internationally; and/or
d. The risk that restrictions to travel or trade may result because of the event.

Timely and transparent notification of events combined with a collaborative assessment of the risks by the concerned state and WHO, along with effective risk communication will reduce the potential for international disease spread and the likelihood of unilateral imposition of trade or travel restrictions by other countries.

EXAMPLES FOR THE APPLICATION OF THE DECISION INSTRUMENT FOR THE ASSESSMENT AND NOTIFICATION OF EVENTS THAT MAY CONSTITUTE A PUBLIC HEALTH EMERGENCY OF INTERNATIONAL CONCERN[2]

The examples appearing in this Annex are not binding and are for indicative guidance purposes to assist in the interpretation of the decision instrument criteria.

DOES THE EVENT MEET AT LEAST TWO OF THE FOLLOWING CRITERIA?

Is the public health impact of the event serious?

I. Is the public health impact of the event serious?

1. *Is the number of cases and/or number of deaths for this type of event large for the given place, time or population?*

2. *Has the event the potential to have a high public health impact?*

   The following are examples of circumstances that contribute to high public health impact.
   - ✓ Event caused by a pathogen with high potential to cause epidemic (infectiousness of the agent, high case fatality, multiple transmission routes or healthy carrier).
   - ✓ Indication of treatment failure (new or emerging antibiotic resistance, vaccine failure, antidote resistance or failure).
   - ✓ Event represents a significant public health risk even if no or very few human cases have yet been identified.
   - ✓ Cases reported among health staff.
   - ✓ The population at risk is especially vulnerable (refugees, low level of immunization, children, elderly, low immunity, undernourished, etc.).
   - ✓ Concomitant factors that may hinder or delay the public health response (natural catastrophes, armed conflicts unfavourable weather conditions, multiple foci in the state party).
   - ✓ Event in an area with high population density.
   - ✓ Spread of toxic, infectious or otherwise hazardous materials that may be occurring naturally or otherwise that has contaminated or has the potential to contaminate a population and/or a large geographical area.

3. *Is external assistance needed to detect, investigate, respond and control the current event, or prevent new cases?*

   The following are examples of when assistance may be required.
   - ✓ Inadequate human, financial, material or technical resources—in particular:
     - insufficient laboratory or epidemiological capacity to investigate the event (equipment, personal, financial resources);
     - insufficient antidotes, drugs and/or vaccine and/or protective equipment, decontamination equipment, or supportive equipment to cover estimated needs;
     - existing surveillance system is inadequate to detect new cases in a timely manner.

IS THE PUBLIC HEALTH IMPACT OF THE EVENT SERIOUS?
Answer 'yes' if you have answered 'yes' to questions 1, 2 or 3 above.

Is the event unusual or unexpected?

II. Is the event unusual or unexpected?

4. *Is the event unusual?*

   The following are examples of unusual events.

   ✓ The event is caused by an unknown agent or the source, vehicle, route of transmission is unusual or unknown.
   ✓ Evolution of cases more severe than expected (including morbidity or case-fatality) or with unusual symptoms.
   ✓ Occurrence of the event itself unusual for the area, season or population.

5. *Is the event unexpected from a public health perspective?*

   The following are examples of unexpected events.

   ✓ Event caused by a disease/agent that had already been eliminated or eradicated from the state party or not previously reported.

IS THE EVENT UNUSUAL OR UNEXPECTED?
Answer 'yes' if you have answered 'yes' to questions 4 or 5 above.

Is there a significant risk of international spread?

III. Is there a significant risk of international spread?

6. *Is there evidence of an epidemiological link to similar events in other states?*

7. *Is there any factor that should alert us to the potential for cross border movement of the agent, vehicle or host?*

   The following are examples of circumstances that may predispose to international spread.

   ✓ Where there is evidence of local spread, an index case (or other linked cases) with a history within the previous month of:
   – international travel (or time equivalent to the incubation period if the pathogen is known);
   – participation in an international gathering (pilgrimage, sports event, conference, etc.);
   – close contact with an international traveller or a highly mobile population.

   ✓ Event caused by all environmental contamination that has the potential to spread across international borders.

   ✓ Event in an area of intense international traffic with limited capacity for sanitary control or environmental detection or decontamination.

IS THERE A SIGNIFICANT RISK OF INTERNATIONAL SPREAD?
Answer 'yes' if you have answered 'yes' to questions 6 or 7 above.

Risk of international restrictions

IV. Is there a significant risk of international travel or trade restrictions?

8. *Have similar events in the past resulted in international restriction on trade and/or travel?*

9. *Is the source suspected or known to be a food product, water or any other goods that might be contaminated that has been exported/imported to/from other states?*

10. *Has the event occurred in association with an international gathering or in an area of intense international tourism?*

11. *Has the event caused requests for more information by foreign officials or international media?*

IS THERE A SIGNIFICANT RISK OF INTERNATIONAL TRADE OR TRAVEL RESTRICTIONS?
Answer 'yes' if you have answered 'yes' to questions 8, 9, 10 or 11 above.

States parties that answer 'yes' to the question whether the event meets any two of the four criteria (I–IV) above, shall notify WHO under Article 6 of the international health regulations.

THE LEGAL FRAMEWORK ESTABLISHED BY IHR

Under the WHO Constitution, all WHO member states were automatically bound by the new IHR because they did not affirmatively opt-out within a limited time period and only a very small number made reservations. According to the procedures established in the IHR (2005), reservations are evaluated by other WHO member states within a defined time period. Because one-third of the other states did not object to the reservation(s), the regulations entered into force for the states that filed them subject to the reservation(s).

THE ROLES, RESPONSIBILITIES AND OBLIGATONS OF STATES PARTIES AND WHO UNDER THE IHR[4]

The responsibility for implementing the IHR (2005) rests upon all states that are bound by the regulations and WHO. The state is responsible, including all of its sectors, ministries, levels, officials and personnel for implementing the regulations at the national level. WHO collaborates with and supports states in the implementation of the regulations.

Key Obligations for States

States parties to the IHR (2005) are required:

- to designate a national IHR focal point;
- to assess events occurring in their territory and to notify WHO of all events that may constitute a public health emergency of international concern;
- to respond to requests for verification of information regarding events that may constitute a public health emergency of international concern; to respond to public health risks which may spread internationally;
- to develop, strengthen and maintain the capacity to detect, report and respond to public health events; to provide routine facilities, services, inspections and control activities at designated international airports, ports and ground crossings to prevent the international spread of disease; to report to WHO evidence of a public health risk identified outside their territory which may cause international disease spread, manifested by exported/imported human cases, vectors carrying infection or contamination, contaminated goods;
- to respond appropriately to WHO-recommended measures;
- to collaborate with other states parties and with WHO on IHR (2005) implementation.

Key Obligations for WHO[4]

Laying down the rules for global public health security, the IHR (2005) confer on WHO new roles and responsibilities. WHO has strengthened its ability to fulfill these fresh obligations by:

- designating WHO IHR contact points at the headquarters or the regional level;
- conducting global public health surveillance and assessment of significant public health events, and disseminating public health information to states, as appropriate;
- offering technical assistance to states in the irresponse to public health risks and emergencies of international concern;
- supporting states in their efforts to assess their existing national public health structures and resources, as well as to develop and strengthen the core public health capacities for surveillance and response, and at designated points of entry;
- if required, determining whether or not a particular event notified by a state under the regulations constitutes a public health emergency of international concern, with advice from external experts;
- if a PHEIC is declared, developing and recommending the critical health measures for implementation by states parties during such an emergency (with advice from external experts);
- monitoring the implementation of IHR (2005) and updating guidelines so that they remain scientifically valid and consistent with changing requirements.

IHR—PROTECTING PEOPLE EVERY DAY

The IHR represents an agreement between 196 countries, including all WHO member states, to work together for global health security. Under the IHR, all countries must report events of international public health importance.

The IHR require that all countries can (Fig. 18.2):

- **Detect:** Make sure surveillance systems and laboratories can detect potential threats
- **Assess:** Work together with other countries to make decisions in public health emergencies
- **Report:** Report specific diseases, plus any potential international public health emergencies
- **Respond:** Respond to public health events

We share a responsibility to protect our world from outbreaks of infectious diseases and other health threats. The goal of the IHR is to stop events in their tracks before they become emergencies.

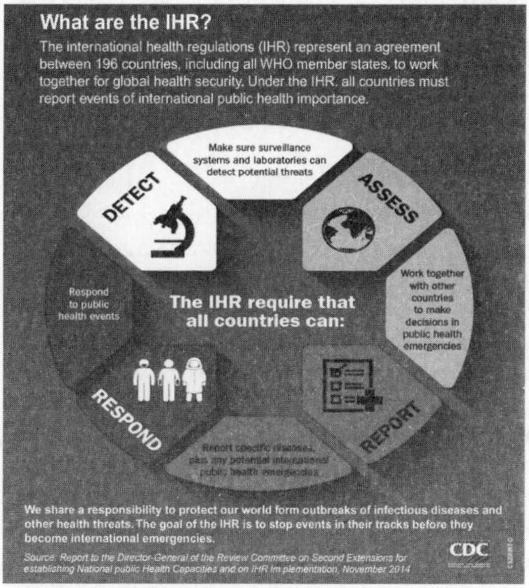

Fig. 18.2: International health regulations (IHR) protecting people every day

International health regulations (IHR) are a framework to help countries better report and respond to public health emergencies that have the potential to cross borders.

IHR TIMELINE[2,3,5]

The idea that a health threat in one part of the world can impact other parts of the world is not new. Over time, there have been a series of agreements between countries to address the potential spread of disease, beginning with the International Sanitary Convention in 1892 and continuing until today with the international health regulations. The IHR were originally written in 1969, and were revised in 2005, following the 2003 enrolled as reporting units epidemic of severe acute respiratory syndrome (SARS). After the SARS epidemic, it became clear that stronger systems were needed to detect, assess, report, and respond to public health events.

The original timeline for IHR implementation is as follows:

- May 2005: World Health Assembly approved revised IHR
- December 2006: United States accepted the revised IHR
- June 15, 2007: Initial start date for revised IHR
- June 2009: Within 2 years after IHR enters into force, member countries complete assessment of the ability of their national structures and resources to meet minimum core capacities
- 2012: Within 5 years after IHR enters into force, member countries achieve the required minimum level of core capacities, unless WHO grants an extension
- 2014: End of 2-year extensions on achieving core capacity, unless an exceptional circumstance exists and a further extension is granted by WHO
- 2016: End of final 2-year extensions (for exceptional circumstances) on achieving core capacities

When countries committed to the IHR in 2005, the first target date for achieving its goals was set for 2012. By that date, however, fewer than 20% of countries had met IHR goals. After a 2 year extension, in 2014, 64 countries reported fully achieving the IHR core capacities. Only about one-third of the countries in the world currently have the ability to assess, detect and respond to public health emergencies.

TRAVEL AND TRADE UNDER IHR[4]

International Travel and Trade

The extent of international travel in the modern world presents an extraordinary opportunity for international disease transmission. Global trade has implications in terms of potential food-borne disease or other contaminated goods. While health measures to control disease spread at borders remain one important element of the regulations, evidence shows that rapid response at the source is the most effective way to secure maximum protection against international spread of diseases.

One of the objectives of the IHR (2005) is to minimize unnecessary restrictions to travel and trade by specifying, in real-time, the appropriate public health measures for the assessed risk. WHO's neutral expert guidance in assessing and controlling public health risks is key to limiting unnecessary restrictions on trade and travel. During a public health emergency of international concern, however, application of time-limited measures affecting international travel and trade may be recommended.

Individual Travellers

The IHR (2005) aims at preventing the international spread of diseases while limiting unnecessary restrictions on the free movement of travellers. During public health emergencies of international concern or in connection with specific public health risks, measures affecting travel may be recommended to avoid the international spread of disease. Health information, basic examinations and vaccination documentation may be requested of a traveller by states. At the same time, under the IHR (2005), states are required to treat travellers with respect for their dignity, human rights and fundamental freedoms together with confidential treatment of their personal data.

States parties are required to designate international airports and ports and may designate certain ground crossings for capacity strengthening purposes under the IHR:[4] Large-scale growth of travel and trade in recent years has increased the potential and opportunities for international disease spread. Although rapid response at the source is the most effective way to prevent disease from crossing borders, routine public health measures applied to international conveyances and at airports, ports and ground crossings may further reduce the risk of spread. States parties are, therefore, required to designate the key international airports and ports to develop and strengthen the capacities provided in Annex 1 of the IHR. Additionally, where justified for public health reasons, states parties may designate ground crossings that shall develop these capacities. These designations should be made as soon as possible because the timelines established in the regulations started running on 15 June 2007.

Collaboration Under IHR[4]

Under the IHR (2005), states recognize that the regulations and other relevant agreements should be compatible. The IHR (2005) provide for cooperation between WHO and other competent inter-governmental organizations or international bodies in the implementation of the regulations. WHO, therefore, continues to foster its long-standing working relationships with a number of organizations such as the International Atomic Energy Agency, the International Air Transport Association, the International Civil Aviation Organization, the International Maritime Organization, the World Tourism Organization, Food and Agriculture Organization of the United Nations, the Office International d'Epizooties (World Organisation for Animal Health) and the

World Trade Organization. In addition to these specialized organizations, WHO works with regional economic integration organizations such as the European Union and the Mercado Común del Sur (MERCOSUR) in implementing the regulations in the countries of their respective regions.

How has the IHR (2005) affected the Model Deratting and Deratting Exemption certificates, Maritime Declaration of Health, International Certificate of Vaccination or Revaccination against Yellow Fever and the Health Part of the Aircraft eneral Declaration?[3,4]

- **Model ship sanitation/ship sanitation exemption certificate replaces the deratting/deratting exemption certificate:** Ship Sanitation/Ship Sanitation Exemption Certificates in the IHR (2005) replaced the narrower Deratting/Deratting Exemption Certificates in the IHR (1969) on 15 June 2007.
- **Model Maritime Declaration of Health:** The Maritime Declaration of Health was updated to reflect the broader scope of the IHR and currently accepted technical standards and terminology.
- **Model International Certificate of Vaccination or Prophylaxis replaces the International Certificate of Vaccination or Revaccination against Yellow Fever:** Yellow fever remains the only disease specifically designated under the IHR (2005) for which proof of vaccination or prophylaxis may be required for travellers as a condition of entry to a state. The international certificate was revised as follows—on 15 June 2007, the 'International Certificate of Vaccination or Revaccination against Yellow Fever' was replaced by the 'International Certificate of Vaccination or Prophylaxis'. Clinicians issuing the certificate should note that the main difference from the old certificate is that they have to specify in writing in the space provided that the disease for which the certificate is issued is 'yellow fever'. The current certificate no longer contains references to a designated vaccination centre and its period of validity is limited to the date indicated on the certificate for the particular vaccine or prophylaxis.

Health part of the Aircraft General Declaration: This is a document of the International Civil Aviation Organization (ICAO), a United Nations agency. The document is periodically reviewed by ICAO member states, and has historically, for practical purposes, been reproduced in the annexes of the IHR. Consequently, the revised version of this Declaration submitted by ICAO to WHO has been reproduced in the second edition of the IHR (2005), published in 2008.

SPECIFIC DISEASES UNDER THE IHR[3,4]

How do the IHR help to address the risk of an influenza pandemic in humans?

Under the IHR (2005), all cases of these four diseases must be automatically notified to WHO—smallpox, poliomyelitis due to wild-type poliovirus, SARS and cases of human influenza caused by a new subtype. Case definitions for each of these four diseases have been prepared by WHO.

What kind of yellow fever vaccines are valid under the IHR (2005) and must they be administered at a vaccination centre designated by the state or at a listed WHO-approved vaccination centre?

Under IHR (2005), each state must designate at least one yellow fever vaccination centre, but, if it so wishes, no longer has to restrict the issuance of yellow fever vaccination certificates to such an officially-designated centre. The yellow fever vaccine used must be approved by WHO. The WHO no longer maintains a list of vaccinating centres designated for the administration of yellow fever vaccine and for the issue of International Certificates of Vaccination or Revaccination against yellow fever.

INTERNATIONAL PUBLIC HEALTH HAZARDS: INDIAN LEGISLATIVE PROVISIONS

(Excerpts from WHO, SEARO—international public health hazards—Indian Legislative Provisions, 2015).[6]

The international health regulations (IHR 2005) came into force in June 2007 and India is one of the signatory member states.

The Indian Legislative Structure

India follows a quasi-federal system of governance, where there is a division of power at the federal and the state level. While the federal/central/union government governs the union of 28 states and 8 union territories, the state governments govern their respective states under the Indian Constitution (Fig. 18.3).

The Government of India constitutes three branches namely:

1. The Executive headed by the President of India and the Governor as executive head at the state level;
2 The Parliament for the central government and state legislatures which comprise the *Rajya Sabha* (the Upper House) and the *Lok Sabha* (the Lower House) at the centre (central government) and *Vidhan Sabhas* in the state (state legislatures).
3. The judiciary comprising the Supreme Court at the apex, the highcourts in the states and the district courts at the district level.

The legal system includes statutory laws as well as the common law, which administer the rights and duties of the citizens as enshrined inthe Constitution of India.

National Centre for Disease Control (NCDC), as National Focal Point[6] in India for International Health Regulations

The activities at the national level include the designation of the national IHR focal point, initially assigned to the National Institute of Communicable Diseases (NICD) under the Ministry of Health and Family Welfare. In 2009, NICD transformed into the National Centre for Disease Control (NCDC), with a larger mandate for controlling emerging and re-emerging diseases.

NCDC has the following departments.

a. Centre for AIDS and related diseases
b. Integrated disease surveillance project
c. Division of epidemiology

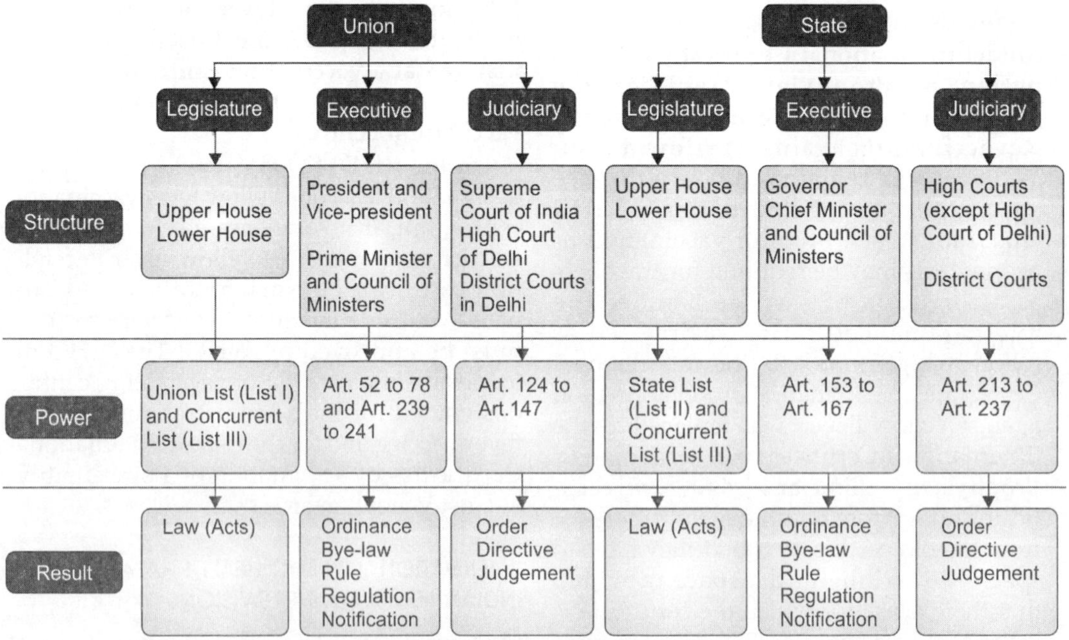

Fig. 18.3: Diagrammatic representation of the legislating powers of the Government of India, as laid down in the Constitution[6]

d. Division of biochemistry and biotechnology
e. Centre for medical entomology and vector management
f. Division of microbiology
h. Division of malaria and coordination
i. Division of parasitic diseases
j. Division of planning, budget and administration

The mandate of NCDC is also to notify public health emergencies of international concern (PHEIC) to WHO, to respond to requests for verification of information of such events, support field investigations for early diagnosis and technical guidance to the states for the timely and effective response to PHEIC.

The notification of an outbreak to WHO is based on the identification of any two of the four point criteria of determination of PHEIC:

1. Unusual or unexpected event
2. An event that seriously impacts public health
3. Event with a significant risk of international spread and
4. Event with a significant risk of international spread requiring travel and trade restrictions.

In India, there are 124 relevant laws/legislation which comprise 67Acts, the rest being rules, regulations, administrative orders, notifications, etc.[6] The Acts are administered by the concerned ministry. However, certain Acts are governed by more than one ministry. These are:

- Drugs and Cosmetics Act 1940—Ministry of Health and Family Welfare and Ministry of Chemicals and Fertilizers
- Environment (Protection) Act 1986—Ministry of Environment and Forests and Ministry of Science and Technology
- Infant Milk Substitutes, Feeding Bottles and Infant Foods (Regulation of Production, Supply and Distribution) Act, 1992—Ministry of Food Processing and Ministry of Women and Child Development
- The Destructive Insects and Pests Act, 1914—amended in 1992—Ministry of Agriculture and Ministry of Rural Development

The Laws/Legislation also comprise 36 Rules, 8 Regulations, 3 Guidelines, 3 Orders, 1 Notification, 2 International Conventions, 1 Handbook, 2 Standards and 1 Policy.

Therefore, to identify the provisions in Indian legislation that may promote IHR implementation, it becomes imperative to review the legislative bodies, the legislation and the authority designated under each of the legislations, from time to time for an effective system based on a series of SOP for IHR.

References

1. Park's Textbook of Preventive and Social Medicine, 23rd edn.
2. WHO, 2016. International health regulations (2005)—3rd edn. WHO Press, Geneva.
3. Singh Sujeet Kumar, Kumar Sudhir. International Health Regulations: A Major Paradigm Shift from 1969 to 2005; J Commun Dis 2009;41(2):113–16.
4. WHO. Frequently asked questions about the International Health Regulations (2005) https://www.who.int/ihr/about/FAQ2009.pdf
5. WHO; International Health Regulations (2005). http://www.who.int/ihr/publications/9789241596664/en/
6. World Health Organization, Regional Office for South-east Asia international public health hazards: Indian legislative provisions. 2015.

Chapter

19

Systematic Review and Meta-Analysis

Sanjay P Zodpey and Himanshu Negandhi

This chapter is an introductory chapter for readers to be acquainted with the overview and the steps involved in conducting a systematic review and a meta-analysis. Multiple publications are available in the literature that comprehensively describe the details about undertaking a systematic review and a meta-analysis. This chapter is written from the perspective of fresh post-graduates who wish to learn about the basic principles and steps involved in a systematic review and meta-analysis.

Why are Systematic Reviews Growing in Popularity?

We believe that the popularity of systematic reviews and meta-analysis is particularly driven by three principal reasons.

The modern times have witnessed an exponential growth in the publication of scientific research in the field of medicine. This growth is reflected in the form of a large body of written research, in the print and digital space. This growth in the medical research has also found wider means of access. There are increasing number of journals that are devoted to publish this work. This expansion in the scientific conduct and the publication has positive impact on the healthcare of citizens.

It is documented that against a background of such a tremendous growth, medical practitioners and researchers would have to devote a much larger block of time to keep themselves constantly updated in recent advances within their professions. An older publication authored by Mulrow in the 1994 has noted that "over 2 million articles are published annually in the biomedical literature in over 20,000 journals". These numbers would have substantially increased against the background of this rapid surge of information.

It would become humanly impossible to stay abreast of this information in the near future. Medical professionals would need access to good quality summaries in order to make correct judgements. The summaries would be expected to capture the information from a variety of sources, identify valid results, and followed by creating easily understandable summary information.

While the information overload is important factor driving the popularity of systematic reviews, conventional narrative reviews are frequently prone to reporting select literature that is driven by the author of the review. Such narrative reviews prone to reviewers preference for certain kind of results, methodology, or the journals where these results are published. In an ideal situation, we would expect that all reviews are completely free of such prejudice or bias on behalf of the author. Most often, authors would not have reviewed the entire body of evidence before arriving at a particular opinion. Systematic reviews have predefined steps towards conducting a comprehensive search. This ensures that the entire body of evidence is collected and the decision is taken in the background of complete information rather than selected bits of published information that is readily available.

The third reason for the popularity of systematic reviews and meta-analysis can be attributed to the fact that summaries also use standardized methods to identify high quality individual studies, whereby they are able to provide results that are closer to the truth. This is accomplished through systematic and transparent efforts which are pre-decided. This transparency that begins with the process of selection of the articles and continues till the creation of the final summary is an additional advantage that provides the readers and decision-makers about the comprehensiveness and the process of the creation of the summary.

Indeed, we believe that in contrast to narrative reviews, well conducted systematic reviews and meta-analysis give us reliable information that can be meaningfully used to make informed decisions in the health space. This is vitally important in every context and can help identify the most effective therapy or interventions that should be offered to those seeking health care.

What are the Steps in Conducting a Systematic Review?

The Cornell University Library lists seven steps in conducting a systematic review.[1] It begins with: Identify your research question; define inclusion and exclusion criteria; search for studies; select studies for inclusion-based on pre-defined criteria; extract data from included studies; evaluate the risk of bias of included studies, present results and assess the quality of evidence.

a. **Identify your research question:** This is a very important step that sets the stage about what is the specific research question that is expected to be answered through the systematic review. As a part of this step, it is recommended that the study team should frame a well-defined and answerable research question using the PICO format.[2]
b. **Define inclusion and exclusion criteria:** Eligibility criteria are a combination of aspects of the clinical question plus specification of the types of studies that have addressed these questions. The participants, interventions and comparisons in the clinical question usually translate directly into eligibility criteria for the review.[3]
c. **Search for studies:** This is a crucial step in the process of conducting the review. It is vitally important to note that the search for studies and evidence has to be a comprehensive search. The search is expected to identify all the possible evidence that is existent. The search strategy should make an attempt to identify these relevant sources and devise a search strategy for each of these sources separately. For example, authors will have to devise a separate search strategy for Medline, EMBASE, etc.
d. **Select studies for inclusion based on predefined criteria:** Start with a title/abstract screening to remove studies that are clearly not related to your topic using inclusion/exclusion criteria to screen the full-text of studies.[1] It is highly recommended that two independent reviewers screen all studies, resolving areas of disagreement by consensus.[1]
e. **Extract data from included studies:** A data extraction tool is designed which helps the authors to extract the relevant data from the individual papers/studies. Subsequently, this extracted data from individual studies may be entered into a spreadsheet, or a software that collects this information.
f. **Evaluate the risk of bias of included studies:** This is a recommended step which ultimately contributes towards the inclusion of valid study results in the systematic

review and meta-analysis. The Cochrane Risk of Bias tool is a highly recommended tool for undertaking this work.[4] It covers important domains such as selection bias; performance bias; detection bias; attrition bias; reporting bias; other biases.

g. **Present results and assess the quality of evidence:**[1] Clearly present your findings, including detailed methodology (such as search strategies used, selection criteria, etc.) such that your review can be easily updated in the future with new research findings. Perform a meta-analysis if the studies allow. Provide recommendations for practice and policy-making if sufficient, high quality evidence exists, or future directions for research to fill existing gaps in knowledge or to strengthen the body of evidence.

Writing a Systematic Review Protocol

The actual conduction of a systematic review is preceded by the writing of the systematic review protocol. This step ensures that the authors clearly state in advance about how they will proceed with their work without being influenced by the results of the review. The Cochrane collaboration suggests that[3] "in order to minimize the potential for bias in the review process, these judgements should be made in ways that do not depend on the findings of the studies included in the review." Published guidelines for writing the protocol are available since the publication of the PRISMA for systematic review protocols (PRISMA-P).[5,6]

PRISMA-P was published in 2015 aiming to facilitate the development and reporting of systematic review protocols. The detailed steps about the contents of the protocol are pre-specified. Journals insist authors to pre-publish their systematic review protocols in standardized formats and register it on international prospective.

Register of Systematic Reviews (PROSPERO) which is an online portal through which to register the intention to conduct a systematic review, with health-related outcomes, before it is initiated.[7] PRISMA-P is a guideline to help authors prepare protocols for planned systematic reviews and meta-analyses that provides them with a minimum set of items to be included in the protocol.[5] A protocol is intended to provide the rationale for the review and pre-planned methodological and analytic approach, prior to embarking on a review.[5]

Searching for Studies

The search for studies is a much longer phase than what is anticipated by most study teams. This stage usually lasts the longest, and entails a pains-taking effort on behalf of the study team to devise a strategy for searching for all the available evidence. This step must not be hurried through and should be devoted time. Each database has a different structure and needs special skills for its search. The search specialist should have a familiarity with the database before devising the search strategy. The recommended sources for search can be classified into: Bibliographic databases; journals and other non-bibliographic database sources; unpublished and ongoing studies. The Cochrane Collaboration suggests that "CENTRAL is considered to be the best single source of reports of trials for inclusion in Cochrane reviews. The three bibliographic databases generally considered to be the most important sources to search for studies for inclusion in Cochrane reviews are CENTRAL, MEDLINE and EMBASE. National, regional and subject-specific databases should be selected for searching according to the topic of the review." In addition to these sources, there should be an effort to also identify evidence that may be available in grey literature, masters level dissertations, unpublished studies, conference abstracts, etc. These efforts towards the search should also be well documented and are an essential step in the conduction of a good systematic review.

Selecting Studies and Data Extraction

A systematic review includes studies that meet pre-specified criteria for inclusion. Since each study may have been reported in several articles, abstracts or other reports, a comprehensive search for studies for the review may identify many reports from potentially relevant studies[3] necessitating that "Two distinct processes are therefore required to determine which studies can be included in the review;... link together multiple reports of the same study; and the other is to use the information available in the various reports to determine which studies are eligible for inclusion." In order to accomplish this step, the reviewers pains-takingly go through the searched titles and abstracts to filter those results that are relevant to the research question. The studies that meet this criteria are then subjected to a detailed read of the full-text of the article. It is recommended that this step be undertaken independently by two reviewers so as to limit the potential for reviewer biases or wrong judgements. In many developing countries where there is limited access to free full-text articles, it becomes even more challenging since the study team may have to make payments for each individual article that they have selected as a part of the process.

Assessing the Quality of Included Studies

The overall results of a systematic review and meta-analysis are considered to be superior to the results of the individual studies. This faith in the results of the systematic review and meta-analysis is created by the overall transparency and objectivity in the process of the conduct of the review. However, the overall results of a systematic review and meta-analysis are likely to be biased if the results of the participating studies are of poor quality or are not free from biases. In such a situation, the statistical pooling of the results of the studies will not correct the inherent biases within the pooled result. In such a situation, it is extremely important to consider the quality of the included studies in a systematic review. Historically, this has been one of the most crucial elements that has made systematic reviews provide valid and unbiased findings. In such a situation, study teams have to be well equipped to assess the quality of the studies that they plan to include in their analysis.

From a practical standpoint, randomized controlled trials offer the highest quality evidence among the primary study designs. This is due to their ability to also limit the effect of selection bias which is not adequately controlled in other primary research designs. Therefore, an aggregation of randomized controlled trials, particularly those randomized controlled trials which have 'good quality' is likely to give us answers closer to the truth. Various methods and scoring systems have been used in the past to assess the quality of the included studies. In the opinion of the authors, the methodology that is advocated by the Cochrane Collaboration is sound and the most appropriate approach towards assessing the quality of included studies. The Cochrane Collaboration advocates the use of the risk of bias tool, which is integrated into the Revman software and offers reviewers with the ability to undertake this assessment. The risk of bias tool[3] covers the domains that are responsible for the introduction of the most important biases into the overall pooled results. The tool encourages reviewers to carefully examine each of the searched studies (that merit inclusion) against the domains indicated in the Risk of Bias framework. The tool provides for a standard definition of 'low risk of bias', 'high risk of bias and 'unclear' for each of the domains. The studies that merit inclusion are then marked under each domain to provide an overall assessment of the presence of bias in particular domains. When the risk of bias assessment is undertaken for all the studies, reviewers have the option to graphically present this information for reading.

Undertaking a Meta-analysis

The meta-analysis is the statistical pooling of the results of the systematic review. The meta-analysis represents the step where the extracted results of the studies are mathematically combined to provide a single overall pooled effect of the intervention. An important consideration that precedes the statistical pooling is to determine whether pooling should actually be undertaken in the situation. Sometimes, the individual studies produce results that are very different from one another. This variability, referred to as heterogeneity, may be very high in some cases since the included studies may have been undertaken in different populations, using dissimilar intervention doses or using different methods during study conduct. If the heterogeneity between studies is very large (and beyond the effect of chance), the meta-analysis is not recommended.

Fixed and Random Effect Models

The Cochrane Collaboration identifies the principles that guide the conduct of a meta-analysis whereafter the estimation of the effect measure for each individual study, a weighted average of the individual studies gives us the pooled summary measure. "The combination of intervention effect estimates across studies may optionally incorporate an assumption that the studies are not all estimating the same intervention effect, but estimate intervention effects that follow a distribution across studies. This is the basis of a random-effects meta-analysis. Alternatively, if it is assumed that each study is estimating exactly the same quantity a fixed-effect meta-analysis is performed."[3] Reviewers are expected to have stated a priori in their protocol about whether they plan to conduct a fixed-effect meta-analysis or a random-effects meta-analysis with their data.

CONCLUSION

Systematic reviews and meta-analysis are sound methods that enable the health community to access high quality summary of the evidence. This enables them to make informed decisions about providing the most appropriate care to their cases and deliver effective interventions. The science of systematic reviews and meta-analysis is beyond the mere statistical pooling of the results. It is essential to understand that like all research methods, systematic reviews also need a well-defined protocol to guide the decisions. The review team must carefully undertake the steps that lead to the final results.

References

1. Ghezzi-Kopel K. LibGuides: A Guide to Conducting Systematic Reviews: Steps in a Systematic Review [Internet]. [cited 2018 Sep 27]. Available from: //guides.library.cornell.edu/c.php?g=459012&p=3142201
2. Howard C. Subject & Course Guides: Evidence Based Medicine: PICO [Internet]. [cited 2018 Sep 27]. Available from: https://researchguides.uic.edu/c.php?g=252338&p=3954402
3. Higgins JPT, Green S (editors). *Cochrane Handbook for Systematic Reviews of Interventions* Version 5.1.0 [updated March 2011]. The Cochrane Collaboration, 2011. Available from www.cochrane-handbook.org.
4. Assessing Risk of Bias in Included Studies [Internet]. [cited 2018 Sep 28]. Available from: /bias/assessing-risk-bias-included-studies.
5. PRISMA-P Group, Moher D, Shamseer L, Clarke M, Ghersi D, Liberati A, et al. Preferred reporting items for systematic review and meta-analysis protocols (PRISMA-P) 2015 statement. Systematic Reviews [Internet]. 2015 Dec. [cited 2018 Sept. 28];4(1). Available from: http://systematicreviewsjournal.biomedcentral.com/articles/10.1186/2046-4053-4-1.
6. Shamseer L, Moher D, Clarke M, Ghersi D, Liberati A, Petticrew M, et al. Preferred reporting items for systematic review and meta-analysis protocols (PRISMA-P) 2015: elaboration and explanation. BMJ. 2015 Jan 2;349 (jan02 1):g7647–g7647.
7. PROSPERO. International prospective register of systematic reviews [Internet]. [cited 2018 Sept. 27]. Available from: https://www.crd.york.ac.uk/prospero/

Chapter
20

Ethical Issues in Epidemiological Studies

Ram Chandra Goyal

INTRODUCTION

Ethics is knowing the difference between what you have a right to do and what is right to do.

—*Potter Stewart*

The first step in the evolution of ethics is a sense of solidarity with other human beings.

—*Albert Schweitzer*

As per Collins dictionary, the ethics is derived from the Greek word **ethos**, or 'behaviour'. An ethos is the set of ideas and attitudes that is associated with a particular group of people or a particular type of activity.

Merriam-Webster *described the meaning of Ethos* as 'custom' or 'character' in Greek. As originally used by Aristotle, it referred to a man's character or personality, especially in its balance between passion and caution. Today *ethos* is used to refer to the practices or values that distinguish one person, organization, or society from others (Fig. 20.1).

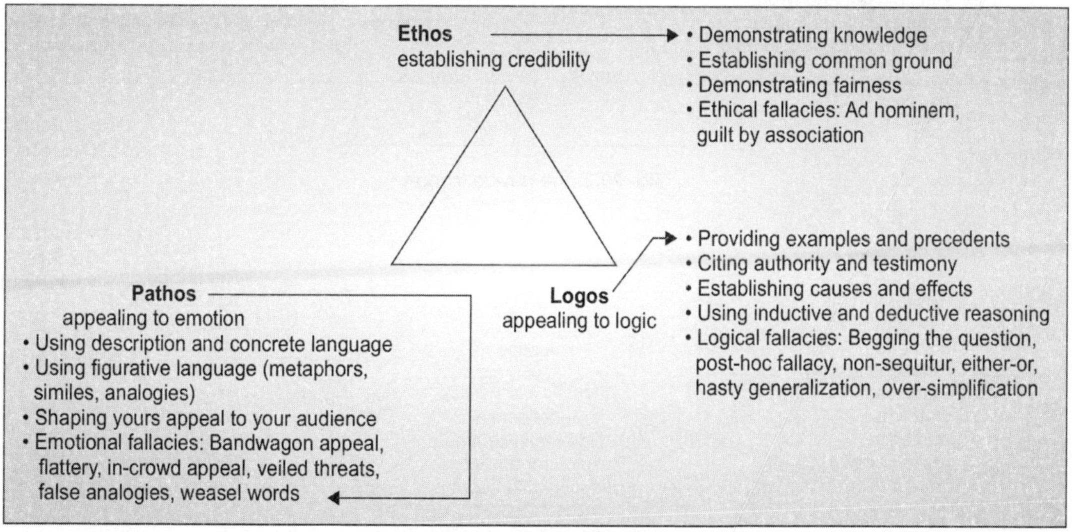
Ethos
establishing credibility
• Demonstrating knowledge
• Establishing common ground
• Demonstrating fairness
• Ethical fallacies: Ad hominem, guilt by association
Pathos
appealing to emotion
• Using description and concrete language
• Using figurative language (metaphors, similes, analogies)
• Shaping yours appeal to your audience
• Emotional fallacies: Bandwagon appeal, flattery, in-crowd appeal, veiled threats, false analogies, weasel words
Logos
appealing to logic
• Providing examples and precedents
• Citing authority and testimony
• Establishing causes and effects
• Using inductive and deductive reasoning
• Logical fallacies: Begging the question, post-hoc fallacy, non-sequitur, either-or, hasty generalization, over-simplification

Fig. 20.1: The rhetorical triangle

Ethics is an integral part of the human life, the way of living, behaving, communicating, judging, and acting and so on.

Ethics deals with right versus wrong actions where values conflict (e.g. ethical dilemmas) arises, those are systematically analyzed and finally conflicts resolved.

The trinity of research is based on **'divine triangle'** (Fig. 20.2).

The very nature of the **health ethics** is the interdisciplinary which serves the purpose of understanding the values, taking decisions and actions in healthcare, health research and health policy, to provide guidance for action when these values conflict (Fig. 20.3).

Medical ethics is concerned with ethical issues in the clinical context related to the care of specific patients.

Bioethics refers to ethical issues arising from the creation and maintenance of the health of all living things.

Health ethics has broader approach in ethical issues encountered by health professionals, health policymakers and health researchers, as well as by patients, families, and communities in a range of contexts related to health, including clinical care, health services and systems, public health, epidemiology, information technology and the use of animals in research.[1]

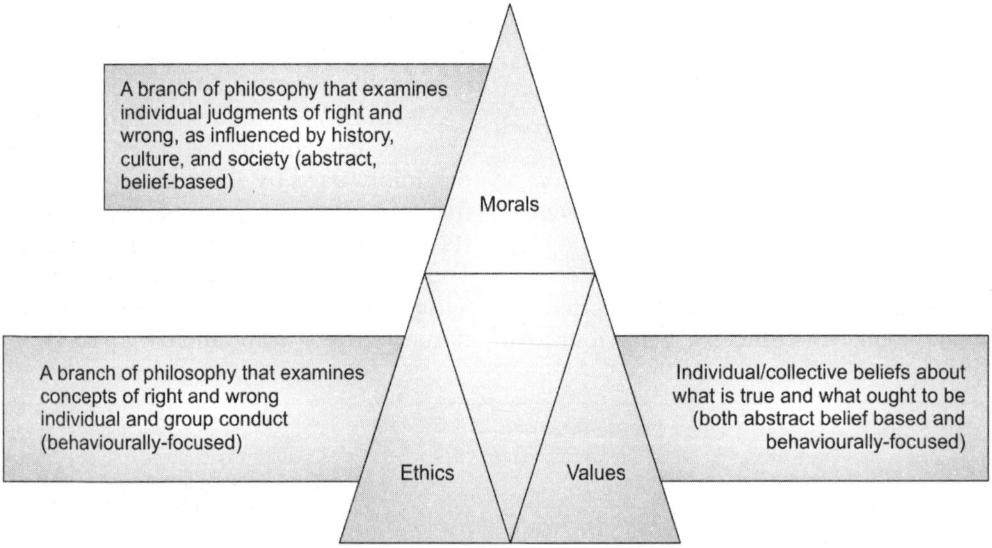

Fig. 20.2: The devine triangle

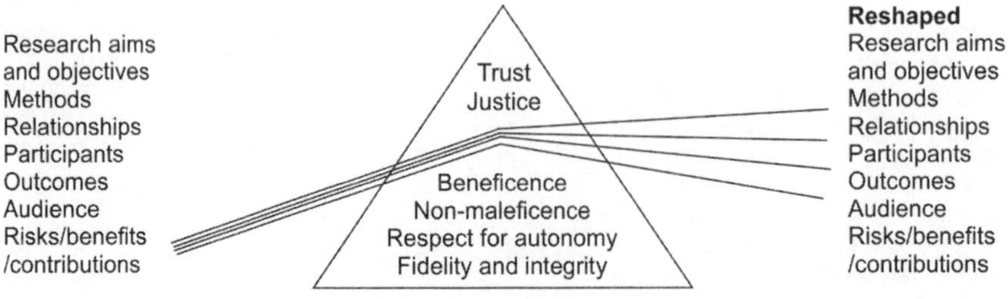

Fig. 20.3: Ethics as prism

Health Ethics and the Law

Both ethics and law are normative frameworks, i.e. they define how people/government/society/organization should behave and act. Ethics and law are often complementary and it remains a foundation for law, and often provides a justificatory basis for legal norms.

Law is the system of rules which a particular country or community recognizes as regulating the actions of its members and which it may enforce by the imposition of penalties.

OR

A law is a rule or set of rules for good behaviour which is considered right and important by the majority of people for moral, religious, or emotional reasons and a **rule** is defining correct procedure or behaviour.

Ethical, Social and Personal Values in Health

Various common values include autonomy, fairness, equity, compassion, honesty, freedom, solidarity, trust and respect. It is observed that different societies may have different values and practices. However, it is also important to note that not all personal or societal values have equivalent moral status. If conflict arises then it is worth taking time to understand and discuss divergent points of view for agreeable and appropriate actions.

Social and personal values—honesty, trust, courage, caring, fairness, respect, compassion, cooperation, positivity, enthusiasm, vitality, concern, etc.; these all forms the basis of the ethics (Fig. 20.4).

Health Ethics, Human Rights and Health Rights

Human rights are "those rights which are inherent to the human being". The adoption of the Universal Declaration of Human Rights in 1948, and led to the adoption of treaties and other sources of law "protecting individuals and groups against actions which interfere with fundamental freedoms and human dignity".

Human rights encompass what are known as civil, cultural, economic, political and social rights. Governments have an affirmative obligation to respect, protect, and fulfil human rights. The obligation to respect human rights means that government must not interfere, directly or indirectly, with individuals' enjoyment of human rights.

Rights

Justified claims made by individuals or groups upon others and based on a system of rules authorizing us to affirm or demand what is due. Possessing a right validly constrains

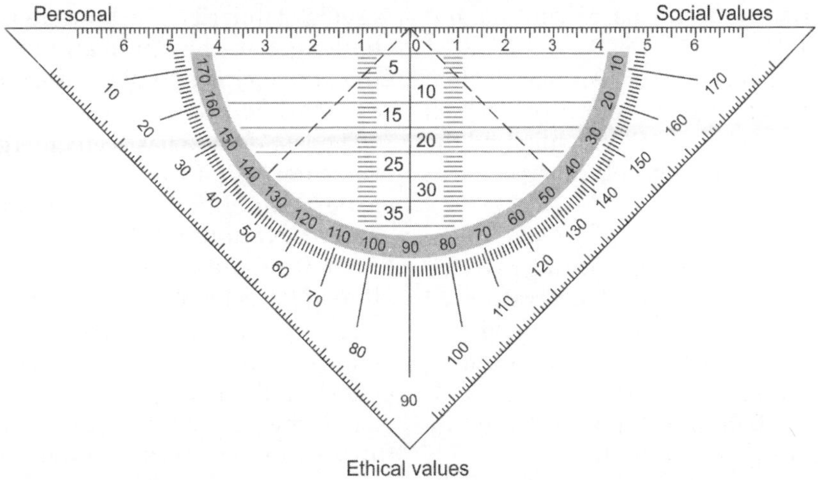

Fig. 20.4: Ethical, social and personal values in health

others from interfering with the exercise of that right. Moral rights are claims justified by moral principles and are correlated with obligations. In public health, a broadly defined set of human rights are often asserted.[2]

The Constitution incorporates provisions guaranteeing everyone's right to the highest attainable standard of physical and mental health. Article 21 of the Constitution guarantees protection of life and personal liberty to every citizen. The Supreme Court has held that the right to live with human dignity, enshrined in Article 21, derives from the directive principles of state policy and therefore includes protection of health.[3]

Right to healthcare covers a wide canvas, encompassing issues of preventive, curative, rehabilitative and palliative healthcare across rural and urban areas, infrastructure availability, health human resource availability, as also issues extending beyond health sector into the domain of poverty, equity, literacy, sanitation, nutrition, drinking water availability, etc.

Medical profession is probably the oldest one to prescribe ethical guidelines.

The code of conduct for physicians was well laid out in traditional Indian systems of medicine and do no harm was the underlying universal principle besides other principles applicable to the prevalent culture and the class systems of the society. Such guidelines were provided both in Charaksamhita and Susrutasamhita.

The Nuremberg code[4] of 1947 was the first international treatise on the ethics of research involving human beings and highlighted the essentiality of obtaining voluntary consent (Appendix I).

In 1964, the World Medical Association formulated guidelines on conducting research on humans, known as the **Declaration of Helsinki.**[5] This has undergone seven revisions with the latest version being issued in October 2013 at Fortaleza, Brazil (Appendix II).

In 1979, the **Belmont Report**[6] released by the National Commission for the Protection of Human Subjects of Biomedical and Behavioural Research in the United States of America (USA), for the first time enunciated the three basic ethical principles for research involving human subjects: Respect for persons, beneficence and justice (Appendix III).

The Department of Health and Human Services (DHHS), USA, released the Federal Policy for the Protection of Human Subjects as the 'Common Rule' in 1991 (revised in 2017). The International Conference on Harmonization (ICH) brought out the Good Clinical Practice Guidelines E6 (R1) in 1996 revised as E6 (R2) in 2016.

The National Bioethics Advisory Commission, USA (2001), the Council for International Organizations of Medical Sciences (CIOMS), Geneva (2002 revised in 2016), and the Nuffield Council of Bioethics, United Kingdom (2002) released recommendations/guidelines relevant to research in developing countries. UNESCO's Universal Declaration on Bioethics and Human Rights (2005) and other international instruments on human rights further defined the Universal Codes of Ethics to be adopted by the member countries.

The revised ICMR ethical guidelines (2017)[7] have adapted important points from these international guidelines keeping in mind the diverse socio-cultural milieu of our country (Box 20.1).

The socio-cultural ethos in India and its varying standards of healthcare pose unique challenges to the application of universal ethical principles to biomedical and health research.

The last decade has seen emerging ethical issues necessitating further revision of the earlier guidelines and preparation of the current National Ethical Guidelines for Biomedical and Health Research Involving Human Participants, 2017.

These guidelines have covered some newer areas like public health research, social and behavioural sciences research for health and responsible conduct of research, and research during humanitarian emergencies and

Box 20.1: General principles

1. **Principle of essentiality** whereby after due consideration of all alternatives in the light of existing knowledge, the use of human participants is considered to be essential for the proposed research. This should be duly vetted by an ethics committee (EC) independent of the proposed research.
2. **Principle of voluntariness** whereby respect for the right of the participant to agree or not to agree to participate in research, or to withdraw from research at any time, is paramount. The informed consent process ensures that participants' rights are safeguarded.
3. **Principle of non-exploitation** whereby research participants are equitably selected so that the benefits and burdens of the research are distributed fairly and without arbitrariness or discrimination. Sufficient safeguards to protect vulnerable groups should be ensured.
4. **Principle of social responsibility** whereby the research is planned and conducted so as to avoid creation or deepening of social and historic divisions or in any way disturb social harmony in community relationships.
5. **Principle of ensuring privacy and confidentiality** whereby to maintain privacy of the potential participant, her/his identity and records are kept confidential and access is limited to only those authorized. However, under certain circumstances (suicidal ideation, homicidal tendency, HIV positive status, when required by court of law, etc.), privacy of the information can be breached in consultation with the EC for valid scientific or legal reasons as the right to life of an individual supersedes the right to privacy of the research participant.
6. **Principle of risk minimization** whereby due care is taken by all stakeholders (including but not limited to researchers, ECs, sponsors, regulators) at all stages of the research to ensure that the risks are minimized and appropriate care and compensation is given if any harm occurs.
7. **Principle of professional competence** whereby the research is planned, conducted, evaluated and monitored throughout by persons who are competent and have the appropriate and relevant qualification, experience and/or training.
8. **Principle of maximization of benefit** whereby due care is taken to design and conduct the research in such a way as to directly or indirectly maximize the benefits to the research participants and/or to the society.
9. **Principle of institutional arrangements** whereby institutions where the research is being conducted, have policies for appropriate research governance and take the responsibility to facilitate research by providing required infrastructure, manpower, funds and training opportunities.
10. **Principle of transparency and accountability** whereby the research plan and outcomes emanating from the research are brought into the public domain through registries, reports and scientific and other publications while safeguarding the right to privacy of the participants. Stakeholders involved in research should disclose any existing conflict of interest and manage it appropriately. The research should be conducted in a fair, honest, impartial and transparent manner to guarantee accountability. Related records, data and notes should be retained for the required period for possible external scrutiny/audit.
11. **Principle of totality of responsibility** whereby all stakeholders involved in research are responsible for their actions. The professional, social and moral responsibilities compliant with ethical guidelines and related regulations are binding on all stakeholders directly or indirectly.
12. **Principle of environmental protection** whereby researchers are accountable for ensuring protection of the environment and resources at all stages of the research, in compliance with existing guidelines and regulations.

[*Source:* Dr Roli Mathur (Ed.). National Ethical Guidelines for Biomedical and Health Research Involving Human Participants. Published by Director-General, Indian Council of Medical Research, New Delhi, 2017, www.icmr.nic.in]

disasters while a few other specialized areas like informed consent process, biological materials, bio-banking and datasets and vulnerability have been expanded into separate sections.

Ethics and Epidemiology

Progress in medical care and disease prevention depends upon an understanding not only of physiological and pathological processes but also of the social, cultural, economic, and other environmental determinants of health, including the effects of the healthcare system and other social institutions. Producing that understanding requires performing research involving human subjects. Such research should be carried out only by, or strictly supervised by, suitably qualied and experienced investigators under accepted ethical guidelines.

Ethical guidelines assist both investigators and ethical review committees in acting responsibly. Investigators, with whom rests the primary duty to protect the rights and welfare of research subjects and to ensure the scientic quality of research, can benet through better design and administration of their protocols, including the processes for obtaining consent and communicating their research endings, while ethical review committees can benet through improved evaluation and oversight of studies. In their respective roles, each has a duty to see that research plans are transparent, that subjects' data and biological samples are actually used for valid studies, that study results are made publicly available, and that unnecessary administrative obstacles to research—should they occur—are effectively removed.

Because of their merely observational nature, epidemiological studies in the past were widely regarded as not raising any signicant ethical issues and were commonly carried out without approval of an ethical review committee. However, recent years have brought increased attention to the ethical conduct of research generally, greater awareness of the potential harms to research subjects including non-physical harm from disclosures of health-related information and hence increased efforts to protect privacy. All of these have implications for observational epidemiological research. Investigators and review committees need to take differences between interventional and observational studies into consideration in designing and approving observational studies. In some cases, the differences can simplify the ethical review process; in others, additional considerations are raised.

INTERNATIONAL ETHICAL GUIDELINES FOR EPIDEMIOLOGICAL STUDIES PREPARED BY THE COUNCIL FOR INTERNATIONAL ORGANIZATIONS OF MEDICAL SCIENCES (CIOMS) IN COLLABORATION WITH THE WORLD HEALTH ORGANIZATION (WHO), GENEVA, 2009[8]

GENERAL ETHICAL PRINCIPLES

There are four general ethical principles for research/studies:

1. ***Respect for individuals:*** It incorporates at least two fundamental ethical considerations, i.e.
   a. Respect for autonomy, which requires that those who are capable of deliberation about their personal choices should be treated with respect for their capacity for self-determination; and
   b. Protection of persons with impaired or diminished autonomy, which requires that those who are dependent or vulnerable be afforded security against harm abuse.
2. ***Beneficence* (do good)** is the ethical obligation to maximize possible benefits and to minimize possible harms and wrongs. This principle gives rise to norms requiring that the risks of research be reasonable in the light of the expected benefits, that the research design be sound, and that the investigators be competent both to conduct the research and to assure the well-being of the research subjects.
3. ***Non-maleficence* (do no harm)** holds a central position in the tradition of medical

ethics, and guards against avoidable harm to research subjects.

4. *Justice* requires that cases considered to be alike be treated alike, and that cases considered to be different be treated in ways that acknowledge the difference. When the principle of justice is applied to dependent or vulnerable subjects, its main concern is with the rules of *distributive justice.* The rules of distributive justice are applicable within and among communities. Studies should be designed to obtain knowledge that benefits the class of persons of which the subjects are representative—the class of persons bearing the burden should receive an appropriate benefit, and the class primarily intended to benefit should bear a fair proportion of the risks and burdens of the study.

Although these principles are well accepted, they must be seen in a broader context. Research is needed because people have the right to know about hazards to their health and to make evidence-based choices concerning treatment and prevention. From an ethical point of view, it may sometimes be preferable that no research is done, but this is not normally the case. There are many epidemiological research projects in which the ethical concerns of not doing the study far outweigh those of doing it. Research must also be of good quality. Bad research may lead to wrong decisions that may have a profound impact on people's health (Fig. 20.5).

A brief account of the international ethical guidelines for epidemiological studies prepared by the CIOMS in collaboration with the WHO, Geneva, 2009, are given in Box 20.2.

Guideline 1: *Ethical justification and scientific validity of epidemiological research involving human subjects*—finding out the new means to improve the health of individuals, groups and populations, the research can be ethically justifiable only if it respect and protect, and fair to research subjects and acceptable within the communities.

Guideline 2: *Ethical review committees (ERC)*—ERC should ensure the scientific merit and ethical acceptability of the proposed epidemiological study. The investigator must obtain their approval or clearance before undertaking the research. The ethical review committee should conduct further reviews during the course of the research, including monitoring the progress of the study.

Guideline 3: *Ethical review of externally sponsored research*—externally sponsored research refers to research undertaken in one

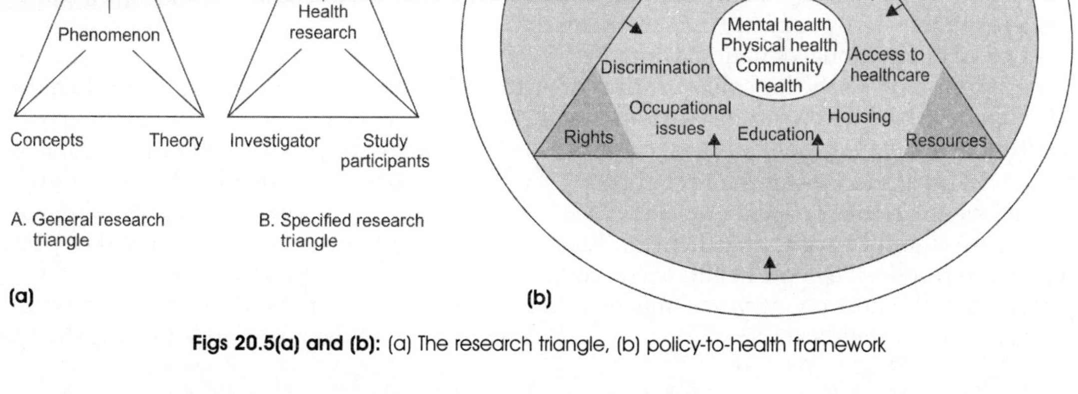

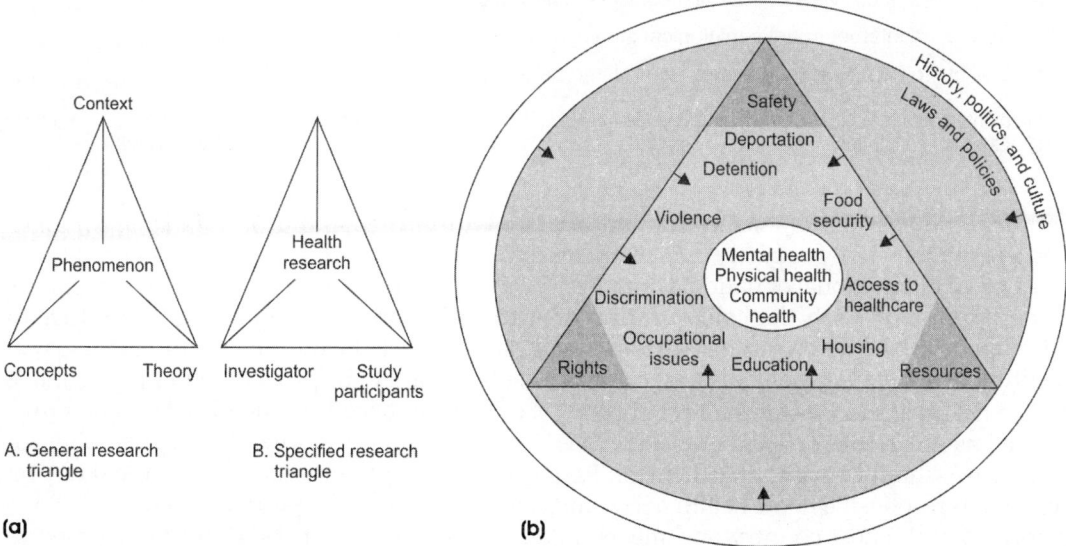

Figs 20.5(a) and (b): (a) The research triangle, (b) policy-to-health framework

Box 20.2: List of guidelines by CIOMS in collaboration with the WHO 2009

1. Ethical justification and scientific validity of epidemiological research involving human subjects
2. Ethical review committees
3. Ethical review of externally sponsored research
4. Individual informed consent
5. Obtaining informed consent: Essential information for prospective research subjects
6. Obtaining informed consent: Obligations of investigators and sponsors
7. Compensation for participation
8. Benefits, harms and risks of study participation
9. Special limitations on risk when research involves individuals who are not capable of giving informed consent
10. Research in populations and communities with limited resources
11. Choice of control in clinical trials
12. Equitable distribution of burdens and benefits in the selection of groups of subjects in research
13. Research involving vulnerable persons
14. Research involving children
15. Research involving individuals who by reason of mental or behavioural disorders are not capable of giving adequately informed consent
16. Women as research participants
17. Pregnant women as research participants
18. Safeguarding confidentiality
19. Right of injured subjects to treatment and compensation
20. Strengthening capacity for ethical and scientific review and epidemiological research
21. Ethical obligation of external sponsors to provide healthcare services
22. Disclosure and review of potential conflicts of interest
23. Use of the internet in epidemiological studies
24. Use of stored biological samples and related data

(*Source:* International Ethical Guidelines for Epidemiological Studies Prepared by the CIOMS in collaboration with the WHO, Geneva, 2009,https://cioms.ch/wp-content/uploads/2017/01/International_Ethical_Guidelines_LR.pdf.)

country (the host) but sponsored, financed, and sometimes wholly or partly carried out by an external international or national organization or company with the collaboration or agreement of the appropriate authorities, institutions and personnel of the host country.

The health authorities of the host country, as well as a national or local ethical review committee, should ensure that the proposed research is responsive to the health needs and priorities of the host country and meets the requisite ethical standards.

Guidelines 4 and 5: *Individual informed consent* (Table 20.1, Boxes 20.3 and 20.4)—respect for individuals in research entails accepting an individual's right to refuse to participate; to be informed about the research subject; and to be properly equipped to make a decision based on the best possible information. The principle of informed consent rests on the principle of autonomy and respect for those who take part in research.

Informed consent is a continuous process involving three main components—providing

Table 20.1: Essential and additional elements of an informed consent document

An informed consent form must include the following	*In addition, the following elements may also be required, depending on the type of study*
1. Statement mentioning that it is research 2. Purpose and methods of the research in simple language 3. Expected duration of the participation and frequency of contact with estimated number of participants to be enrolled, types of data collection and methods 4. Benefits to the participant, community or others that might reasonably be expected as an outcome of research 5. Any foreseeable risks, discomfort or inconvenience to the participant resulting from participation in the study 6. Extent to which confidentiality of records could be maintained, such as the limits to which the researcher would be able to safeguard confidentiality and the anticipated consequences of breach of confidentiality 7. Payment/reimbursement for participation and incidental expenses depending on the type of study 8. Free treatment and/or compensation of participants for research-related injury and/or harm 9. Freedom of the individual to participate and/or withdraw from research at any time without penalty or loss of benefits to which the participant would otherwise be entitled 10. The identity of the research team and contact persons with addresses and phone numbers (for example, PI/Co PI for queries related to the research and Chairperson/Member Secretary/ or helpline for appeal against violations of ethical principles and human rights)	1. Any alternative procedures or courses of treatment that might be as advantageous to the participant as the ones to which she/he is going to be subjected 2. If there is a possibility that the research could lead to any stigmatizing condition, e.g. HIV and genetic disorders, provision for pretest-and post-test counselling 3. Insurance coverage if any, for research-related or other adverse events 4. Foreseeable extent of information on possible current and future uses of the biological material and of the data to be generated from the research. Other specifics are as follows: a. Period of storage of the sample/data and probability of the material being used for secondary purposes b. Whether material is to be shared with others, this should be clearly mentioned c. Right to prevent use of her/his biological-sample, such as DNA, cell-line, etc. and related data at any time during or after the conduct of the research d. Risk of discovery of biologically sensitive information and provisions to safeguard confidentiality e. Post-research plan/benefit sharing, if research on biological material and/or data leads to commercialization f. Publication plan, if any, including photographs and pedigree charts

relevant information to potential participants, ensuring competence of the individual, ensuring the information is easily comprehended by the participants and assuring voluntariness of participation.

Written informed consent should be obtained when the research involves risks—the purpose should be to inform the study participants, not to protect the researcher against possible claims for compensation if something goes wrong.

Formal written consent is unnecessary if the research is carried out in settings that pose no threat to the potential participants, when it is stated that taking part is voluntary and it is obvious that no benefits are at risk of being lost if potential participants refuse to take part.

Such situations often arise in studies based on self-administered questionnaires or telephone interviews where providing the data involves giving *de facto* consent.

Box 20.3: Essential information provided to study participants while obtaining informed consent

Before requesting an individual's consent to participate in research, the investigator must provide the following information, in language or another form of communication that the individual can understand:

1. That the individual is invited to participate in research, the reasons for considering the individual suitable for the research, and that participation is voluntary;
2. That the individual is free to refuse to participate and will be free to withdraw from the research at any time without penalty or loss of benefits to which he or she would otherwise be entitled;
3. The purpose of the research, the procedures to be carried out by the investigator and the subject, and an explanation of how the research differs from routine medical care;
4. For controlled trials, an explanation of features of the research design (e.g. randomization, double-blinding), and that the subject will not be told of the assigned treatment until the study has been completed and the blind has been broken;
5. The expected duration of the individual's participation (including number and duration of visits to the research centre and the total time involved) and the possibility of early termination of the trial or of the individual's participation in it;
6. Whether money or other forms of material goods will be provided in return for the individual's participation and, if so, the kind and amount;
7. That, after the completion of the study, subjects will be informed of the findings of the research in general, and individual subjects will be informed of any finding that relates to their particular health status;
8. That subjects have the right of access to their data on demand, even if these data lack immediate clinical utility (unless the ethical review committee has approved temporary or permanent non-disclosure of data, in which case the subject should be informed of, and given, the reasons for such non-disclosure);
9. Any foreseeable risks, pain or discomfort, or inconvenience to the individual (or others) associated with participation in the research, including risks to the health or well-being of a subject's spouse or partner;
10. The direct benefits, if any, expected to result to subjects from participating in the research;
11. The expected benefits of the research to the community or to society at large, or contributions to scientific knowledge;
12. Whether, when and how any products or interventions proven by the research to be safe and effective will be made available to subjects after they have completed their participation in the research, and whether they will be expected to pay for them;
13. Any currently available alternative interventions or courses of treatment;
14. The provisions that will be made to ensure respect for the privacy of subjects and for the confidentiality of records in which subjects are identified;
15. The limits, legal or other, to the investigators' ability to safeguard confidentiality, and the possible consequences of breaches of confidentiality;
16. Policy with regard to the use of results of genetic tests and familial genetic information, and the precautions in place to prevent disclosure of the results of a subject's genetic tests to immediate family relatives or to others (e.g. insurance companies or employers) without the consent of the subject;

(Contd.)

17. The sponsors of the research, the institutional affiliation of the investigators, and the nature and sources of funding for the research;
18. The possible research uses, direct or secondary, of the subject's medical records and of biological specimens taken in the course of clinical care;
19. Whether it is planned that biological specimens collected in the research will be destroyed at its conclusion, and, if not, details about their storage (where, how, for how long, and final disposition) and possible future use, and that subjects have the right to decide about such future use, to refuse storage, and to have the material;
20. Whether commercial products may be developed from biological specimens, and whether the participant will receive monetary or other benefits from the development of such products;
21. Whether the investigator is serving only as an investigator or as both investigator and the subject's physician;
22. The extent of the investigator's responsibility to provide medical services to the participant;
23. That treatment will be provided free of charge for specified types of research-related injury or for complications associated with the research, the nature and duration of such care, the name of the organization or individual that will provide the treatment, and whether there is any uncertainty regarding funding of such treatment;
24. In what way, and by what organization, the subject or the subject's family or dependants will be compensated for disability or death resulting from such injury (or, when indicated, that there are no plans to provide such compensation);
25. Whether or not, in the country in which the prospective subject is invited to participate in research, the right to compensation is legally guaranteed;
26. That an ethical review committee has approved or cleared the research protocol.

There may also be instances where informed consent is impossible, difficult, or even unethical to obtain. There may even be circumstances where requiring specific information poses a threat to the participants and to the validity of research, e.g. in the use of already existing data.

Process for Obtaining Consent

a. ***Providing information:*** The process starts with an initial contact a prospective subject and continues throughout the course of the study. By informing the prospective subjects, by repetition and explanation, by answering their questions as they arise, and by ensuring that each individual understands each procedure, investigators elicit their informed consent and in so doing manifest respect for their dignity and autonomy. Each individual must be given as much time as is needed to reach a decision, including time for consultation with family members or others. Adequate time and resources should be set aside for informed-consent procedures. There should be adequate disclosure of information to enable the potential participant to make an informed choice.

b. ***Use of language:*** Providing the information while obtaining a consent must not be simply a ritual, the investigator/researcher must provide information whether verbal or in writing, in a manner (as per the level of understanding) and language (as far as possible in a local language), so that an individual can understand. The understanding depends on the individual's maturity, intelligence, education and belief system. It depends also on the investigator's ability and willingness to communicate with patience and sensitivity.

Box 20.4: Responsibility of researchers

1. The researcher should only use the EC approved version of the consent form, including its local language translations.
2. Adequate information necessary for informed consent should be communicated in a language and manner easily understood by prospective participants.
3. In case of differently abled participants, such as individuals with physical, neurological or mental disabilities, appropriate methods should be used to enhance the participants' understanding, e.g. Braille for the visually impaired, sign language for deaf, etc.
4. There should be no restriction on the participant's right to ask questions related to the study or to discuss with family and friends or take time before coming to a decision.
5. The researcher should not give any unjustifiable assurances or influence or intimidate a prospective participant to enroll in the study.
6. The researcher must ensure that the participant is competent and has understood all aspects of the study and that the consent is given voluntarily. Where the participant and/or the LAR are illiterate, an impartial literate person, not connected to the research, should be present throughout the consent process as witness.
7. The researcher should administer a test of understanding whenever possible for sensitive studies. If need be, the test may be repeated until the participant has really understood the contents.
8. When a participant is willing to participate but not willing to sign or give a thumb impression or cannot do so, then verbal/oral consent may be taken on approval by the EC, in the presence of an impartial witness who should sign and date the consent document. This process can be documented through audio or video recording of the participant, the PI and the impartial witness, all of whom should be seen in the frame. However, verbal/oral consent should only be taken in exceptional circumstances and for specific, justifiable reasons with the approval of the EC. It should not to be practiced routinely.
9. Re-consent or fresh informed consent of each participant must be taken under some circumstances.
10. The researcher must assure prospective participants that their decision whether or not to participate in the research will not affect their rights, the patient–clinician relationship or any other benefits to which they are entitled.
11. Reimbursement may be given for travel and incidental expenses/participation in research after approval by the EC. The researcher should ensure free treatment for research-related injury (disability, chronic life-threatening disease and congenital anomaly or birth defect) and if required, payment of compensation over and above medical management by the investigator and/institution and sponsor(s), as the case may be.
12. The researcher should ensure that the participant can continue to access routine care even in the event of withdrawal of the participant.

[*Source:* Dr. Roli Mathur (Ed.). National Ethical Guidelines for Biomedical and Health Research Involving Human Participants. Published by Director-General, Indian Council of Medical Research, New Delhi, 2017, www.icmr.nic.in]

c. ***Comprehension:*** Individuals should be able to understand what they are told and to make a reasoned choice based on that information. Too much information may be given in excessive detail, mainly to protect the researcher and the institution. The investigator should give each one full opportunity to ask questions and should answer them honestly, promptly and completely.

d. ***Documentation of consent:*** The subject may imply consent by voluntary actions, express consent orally, or sign a consent form. As a general rule, the subject should sign consent form, or, in the case of incompetence, a legal guardian or other duly authorized representative should do so. Their wording should be cleared by the ethical review committee. When consent has been obtained orally, for example, in a telephone interview, investigators are responsible for providing documentation or proof of consent. ERC can do waiver of the consent, if there no less than minimal risk to participants.

The details of renewing consent, cultural considerations, consultation with community members, community review and permission for studies, and use of medical records and biological specimens collected for other purposes may be studied from the CIMOS guidelines.[8]

Waiver of Consent Requirements in Epidemiological Studies[7,9,10]

Researchers/investigators should not begin epidemiological research involving human participants without explicit approval of ethical review committee or authorized person by legislation or competent authorities in accord with the ethical principles in these guidelines.

Categories of epidemiological research for which consent may be waived include:

- The use of personally non-identifiable materials;
- The use of personally identifiable materials with special justification;
- Studies performed within the scope of regulatory authority;
- Studies using health-related registries that are authorized under national regulations; cluster-randomized trials.

Beneficence, non-maleficence and justice may all be involved when considering whether subjects should be informed about all aspects of a study. In general, sufficient information must be given so that, when the interview or examination is completed, or when the research results are published, participants do not feel they have been misled. Information was insufficient if, at that stage, participants express regret that they took part and think they would have made a different decision had they been better informed.

Participants must also have the right to withdraw their consent at any time during the study without being obliged to give their reasons. Non-participation or withdrawal of consent should never result in disadvantage for these individuals. Informed consent should be given freely without external pressure and without unreasonable inducements. There should always be an assessment of what incentives, if any, should be offered to potential respondents for participating in the study. Although the distinction is not clear-cut, a balance between reasonable reimbursements, such as travel costs, and unreasonable remuneration must be struck. Incentives that include more than payment for actual costs are acceptable only in studies that carry no risk for the participants.

In the clinical setting, where patients may not feel free to refuse a request from their doctor to take part in a study, mechanisms to counteract undue influence must be established. These might include letting an outside person give the information or waiting until patients return to their own environment to ask for consent.

Although people have the right to say no, it should be permissible to try to contact people who do not respond to an invitation to take part.

Consent should not be required for use of information in the public domain, although countries and communities differ in their definition of what type of information about citizens is regarded as public.

Data gathered for administrative purposes do not require consent from the subjects if obtaining consent could cause undue concerns, be impractical or too expensive. This type of research requires, however, that standards of data protection are followed to reduce any possible risks of disclosure of personal data.

Research ethics committee or a similar authority could, under special conditions, give consent for children and other individuals who are temporarily or permanently unable to give informed consent by themselves. It has been suggested that research data should be made available to participants but there must be some caveats to this idea. It could present a threat to data security and would require stringent identity checks.

Do Good, Do No Harm

A central aim of epidemiological research is to improve people's opportunities for making choices that will improve their health. Individuals have the right to choose between different preventive and therapeutic actions. To do this effectively, they need to know about health hazards related to the different procedures in order to obtain optimal treatment in the healthcare system. Without research they cannot exercise these rights.

The most basic ethical principle is the moral obligation to cause no harm, whether physical or psychological, to participants in epidemiological research. Although the risk of harm to those who take part in an epidemiological investigation is usually minimal, most participants gain no personal benefit and often do not have a disease that needs treatment. In recognition of this altruism, they should be treated well and with respect.

Important findings from the research should, therefore, be made available in an understandable form. Results may reveal information on individual participants that is of importance and value for these individuals alone and such data should be made available to them. In research that does not involve risky invasive procedures; the greatest risk to individuals is a disclosure of personal data that could be misused by the media, an employee, an insurance company or someone else.

Confidentiality and Privacy

Medical confidentiality is a set of rules that limits access to information discussed between a person and their healthcare practitioners/researcher. With only a few exceptions, anything you discuss with your doctor must, by law, be kept private between the two of you and the organization they work for.

Privacy in a healthcare means that what you tell your healthcare provider, what they write down about you, any medication you take and all other personal information is kept private. You have a legal right to this privacy, and there are laws that guide health service providers in how they collect and record information about your health, how they must store it, and when and how they use and share it.

In terms of epidemiological research studies, privacy is the right of an individual to control or influence the information that can be collected and stored and by whom and to whom that information may be disclosed or shared. Confidentiality is the obligation of the researcher/research team/organization to the participant to safeguard the entrusted information. It includes the obligation to protect information from unauthorized access, use, disclosure, modification, loss or theft.

- The researcher should safeguard the confidentiality of research-related data of participants and the community.
- Potential limitations to ensure strict confidentiality must be explained to the participant.
- Any publication arising out of research should uphold the privacy of the individuals by ensuring that photographs or other information that may reveal the individual's identity are not published. A specific re-consent would be required for publication, if this was not previously obtained.
- Some information may be sensitive and should be protected to avoid stigmatization and/or discrimination (for example, HIV status; sexual orientation such as lesbian, gay, bisexual, and transgender (LGBT); genetic information; or any other sensitive information).
- While conducting research with stored biological samples or medical records/data, coding or anonymization of personal information is important and access to both samples and records should be limited.
- Data of individual participants/community may be disclosed in certain circum-

stances with the permission of the EC such as specific orders of a court of law, threat to a person's or community's life, public health risk that would supersede personal rights to privacy, serious adverse events (SAEs) that are required to be communicated to an appropriate regulatory authority, etc.[9,10]

STATEMENT OF SPECIFIC PRINCIPLES FOR EPIDEMIOLOGICAL STUDIES

(As per Indian Council for Medical Research Policy, 2009)

INTRODUCTION

Epidemiological studies are of primary importance in a large developing country like ours where the natural history, incidence, prevalence and impact on morbidity and mortality of a variety of diseases are not known. It has usually been considered that epidemiology of infectious diseases is of prime importance in our country. However, the evolving pattern of change in the society with upward economic mobility and increasing number of middle classes would mean that a significant number of life-style related diseases such as ischaemic heart disease are increasing. There is very little information about this and it would be useful to undertake long-term cohort studies in different population groups.

Epidemiological studies are generally considered in two categories. These are as below (Fig. 20.6).

Observational and Experimental

Designs of these studies are based on cross-sectional, case-control or cohort approaches. Epidemiological studies cover research, program evaluation and surveillance. Scope of ethical guidelines for epidemiological studies is concerned with epidemiological research. Ethics in epidemiological studies is multidimensional covering clinical medicine, public health and the social milieu.

Perhaps the code of ethics is much better understood for clinical research, where the interaction between a patient and a clinical researcher is of supreme importance. In epidemiological research the researcher is dealing with a group of individuals and the questions faced by an epidemiologist are more of a professional nature.

These questions would pertain to interactions with individual subjects, sources of

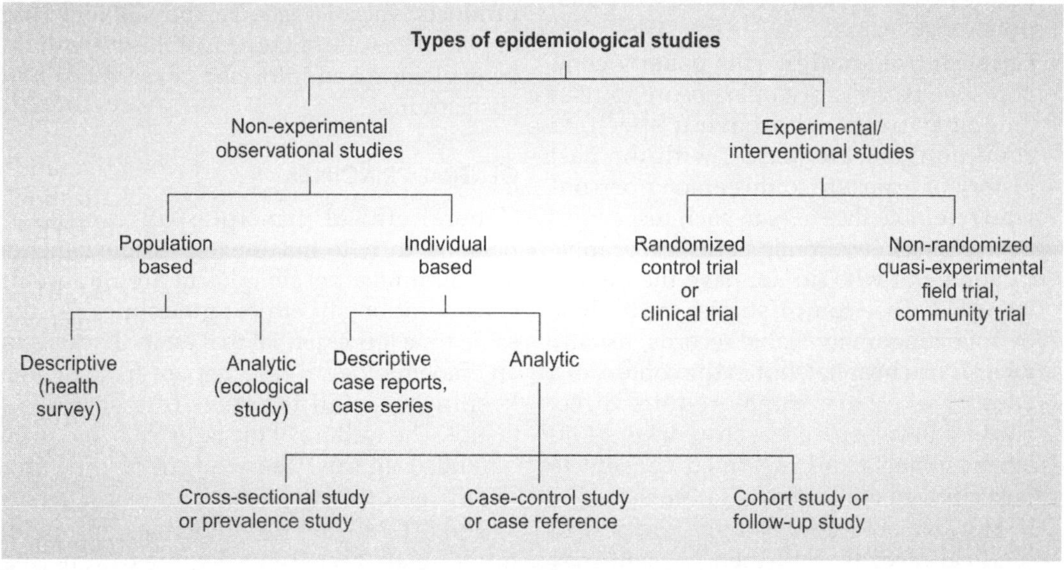

Fig. 20.6: Types of epidemiological studies

funding or employer, fellow epidemiologist and the society at large. Need for a code of ethics for epidemiologists is being recognized globally and the issues for such a code in the context of epidemiological research in India deserve attention.

Epidemiological research differs from clinical research in the context of the large number of study subjects and generally a long time frame. If some mistakes or aberrations get detected during the course of conduct of such studies, repeating the whole exercise will be expensive, time consuming and may not even be feasible. Hence utmost care needs to be taken for various aspects—technical, practical and ethical.

DEFINITIONS

Observational Epidemiology

This includes the following types.

a. **Cross-sectional studies (surveys):** This is primarily population based and involves selecting random samples of the population to be representative based on census data and then applying questionnaires to understand the prevalence of various diseases. Its aim is to assess aspects of the health of a population or to test hypotheses about possible cause of disease or suspected risk factors.

b. **Case-control studies:** This usually compares the past history of exposure to risks among patients who have a specified condition/disease (cases) with the past history of exposure to this among persons who resemble the cases in such respects as age, sex, socio-economic status, geographic location, but who do not have the disease (controls). Case-control studies can be done by following up available records, usually records in a hospital, but in the context of a country like ours, it may require direct contact between research workers and study subjects and informed consent to participation in the study is necessary.

However, if it entails only a review of medical records, informed consent may not be required and indeed may not be feasible.

c. **Cohort studies:** These are longitudinal or prospective studies of a group of individuals with differing exposure levels to suspected risk factors. They are observed over a long period usually several years. The rate of occurrence of the condition of interest is measured and compared in relation to identified risk factors. It requires a study of large number of subjects for a long time and involves asking questions, usually routine medical examination and sometimes laboratory investigations. Individuals are being followed up as the cohort and it is essential to identify precisely every individual to be studied.

Experimental Epidemiology

In experimental epidemiology the investigators alter one or more parameters under controlled conditions to study the effects of the intervention. These are usually randomized controlled trials done to test a preventive or therapeutic regimen or the efficacy of a diagnostic procedure. Although these are strictly speaking epidemiological studies they come under the purview of clinical evaluation of drugs/devices/products/vaccines, etc. The possibility of use of placebo as one of the arm of the trial should be explained and informed consent taken in such studies.

GENERAL PRINCIPLES

General ethical principles of respect for persons, duty to maximize possible benefits and minimize possible harm are important considerations in ethical guidelines. At the same time it is essential that all individuals in an epidemiological research are treated alike keeping in mind the rules of distributive justice. The welfare of the individual has to be balanced against the welfare of the community and society at large.

The CIOMS/WHO Guidelines for epidemiological research assumes that the individuals or population being studied are capable of giving informed consent understanding the implications of the study. With large segments of our population, given their level of education, the full understanding in the sense of industrialized countries may not be achievable. How the principle of 'do no harm' is ensured under such circumstances without being paternalistic is a major issue that has to be taken into consideration in ethical guidelines.

In cohort or survey techniques for incidence and prevalence of various diseases, a major issue that has to be considered is how much of intervention is justified and whether one is justified in withholding interventions. For example, if you are looking at longitudinal morbidity in a population group, should you give them health education that is well established with regard to preventive aspects, or should you leave them alone so that the natural evolution of the disease can be studied? Health education or other interventions including non-health interventions can be quite expensive. An alternate strategy that may be followed is to make curative therapy available to the population at their own request. This usually involves running a clinic, which is readily accessible to the population without any other intervention. However, it is generally considered unethical to withhold intervention or services.

SPECIFIC PRINCIPLES

1. **Informed consent:** When individuals are to be the subject of any epidemiological studies, the purpose and general objectives of the study has to be explained to them keeping in mind their level of understanding. It needs to be ensured that privacy will be maintained.

   In the context of developing countries, obtaining informed consent has been considered many times as difficult/impractical/not meeting the purpose on various grounds such as incompetence to comprehend the meaning or relevance of the consent and culturally being dependent on the decision of the head of the family or village/community head. However, there is no alternative to obtaining individual's informed consent but what should be the content of the informed consent is also a crucial issue.

   In spite of obtaining informed individual consent, it is quite likely that the subjects/patients may not be fully aware of their rights. In this context, the role of investigator is crucial and he/she should remain vigilant and conscious of his/her obligations towards the subjects/patients, all through the course of the studies.
2. In most epidemiological research it would be necessary to have the consent of the community which can be done through the Village Leaders, the Panchayat head, the tribal leaders, etc.
3. In obtaining the consent of individuals or communities it is important to keep in mind that working through peer groups or through Panchayat, etc. may mean that the individuals or community would feel reluctant to disagree and refuse to give consent because of societal pressures. This is something that has to be carefully avoided.
4. Particularly in a country like India, with the level of poverty that is prevalent it is easy to use inducements, especially financial inducements, to get individuals and communities to consent. Such inducements are not permissible. However, it is necessary to provide for adequate compensation for loss of wages and travel/other expenses incurred for participating in the study.
5. All risks involved including the risk of loss of privacy must be explained to the participants in an epidemiological study.
6. The design of the study should ensure that the benefits of the study are maximized for the individuals and communities taking part in the study. This means that at the onset itself the investigators should design the way in which the results of the study are going to be communicated and also

decide whether individuals identified at particular risk during the course of the studies would be informed. It may also be necessary in some instances to inform the concerned family members about the results. For example, as in AIDS, STD, etc. It may not always be possible to communicate study results to individuals but research findings and advise should be publicized by appropriate available means. It is also important that the beneficial results of epidemiological studies are fed into the health system and necessary training modules should be developed as part of the epidemiological project.

7. All attempts should be made to minimize harm to the individuals and society at large. Special consideration for the cultural characteristics of the communities that are being studied is essential to prevent any disturbance to cultural sensitivities because of the investigation.
8. Maintaining confidentiality of epidemiological data is absolutely essential. A particular concern is the fact that some population based data may also have implications to issues like national security and these need to be carefully evaluated at the beginning.
9. In all situations where there is likely to be conflicts of interest it must be ensured that the interest of the individuals involved in the study are protected at all cost.
10. Scientific objectivity should be maintained with honesty and impartiality, both in the design and conduct of the study and in presenting and interpreting findings. Selective withholding of data and similar practices are unethical.
11. Ethical review procedures: In all ethical committees at least one or two individuals with an understanding of the principles of epidemiological ethics should review the proposal.

THE ROLE OF ETHICS COMMITTEES

The IEA fully respects the important role of ethics committees and all research should be based on accepted ethical standards and be of high quality. Poor research may do more harm than no research at all. There must, however, be flexibility and an acknowledgement that different types of research will require different levels of ethical appraisal. One size definitely does not fit all.

Much epidemiological research requires simple observation of populations and study participants and does not involve risky or invasive procedures. Such research can be threatened by time-consuming, over-exhaustive and costly ethical appraisal that may only be necessary for research that involves invasive and/or risky procedures.

It is our contention that ethical evaluation criteria should be appropriate to the type of study under consideration. Criteria governing randomized clinical trials, which involve invasive interventions, should not be the same as those applied to simple observational studies where the sole risk to participants might be that of unwanted disclosure of personal data. It seems unreasonable to treat all protocols alike for ethical appraisal purposes, regardless of risks and benefits.

Experience has also shown that standards vary widely between difference ethical committees and large multi-centre studies must follow procedures acceptable to all relevant committees. This rigid approach can threaten the validity and conduct of a study. We would argue for procedures in this area to be streamlined, especially for research that covers several geographical regions and, is, therefore, subject to a multiplicity of ethics committees. We would further suggest that ethical approval for observational epidemiological research might be more appropriately addressed by experts in data protection and that consent to participate in research can be given in a broad sense without the need for repeated consents in studies with repeated analyses over time.

It is an unfortunate fact that there are rare instances where researchers have violated important ethical standards. This should not, however, result in unduly bureaucratic procedures that absorb unreasonable amounts of time and resources and impoverish epidemiological research as a whole.

The role of ethics committees should be to ensure that high quality epidemiological research of benefit to the public health can be carried out, after a level of scrutiny appropriate to the particular protocol involved.

A brief note on public health research and social and behavioral sciences research for health (as per New National Ethical Guidelines for Biomedical and Health Research Involving Human Participants—ICMR 2017).

PUBLIC HEALTH RESEARCH

Ethics in public health apply to both practice and research, both of which utilize epidemiology and methods of other disciplines to ensure better societal conditions for healthier lives. Therefore, public health protects both the individual and the population at large, since the benefits and risks are not limited to an individual, but influence communities, populations and the environment.

Public health practice involves data collection through surveillance, vital statistics, disease reporting and registries; investigation of outbreaks including contact tracing, use of preventive interventions and health promotion; monitoring and program evaluation; and enforcing of mandatory requirements, such as screening, treatment, immunization, notifying diseases and, sometimes, quarantine depending upon the situation.

Spatial epidemiology, including use of GIS technology, in health is an evolving area and the related ethical issues that may emerge need to be addressed as experience grows.

Principles of Public Health Research Ethics

Basic principles of the ethical issues in biomedical research including public health along with epidemiological studies should also observe all the prescribed guidelines with some justifiable variations depending on situation(s).

The situation like ethical issues of epidemiological and public health research study designs, surveillance, program monitoring data and program evaluations, demographic surveillance sites and registries, and implementation research have to be dealt with utmost care while conducting the research as perception of various health laws are varied and vivid.

Demonstration projects: These types of projects should be need based with anticipated outcome based on sound research designs keeping in mind human rights and research ethics principles. The relevant consent and decision on the exemption from review and consent waiver be taken on a case-by-case basis.

Community trials: These studies target the community as a whole and the randomization is also at community level and usually the method is useful in order to study public health interventions or disease prevention models.

In all public health research along with epidemiological studies where community as whole or part thereof are involved, informed consent issues are complex.

Generally consent is taken at two levels:

i. Local head of *Panchayati Raj* system in India/the guardian/authority of the local community and
ii. Is individual participants

There are three types of consent in such circumstances:

1. **Verbal/oral consent:** For research on sensitive topics, verbal/oral consent with a fictitious name may be suitable with appropriate approval of the EC and with proper documentation.
2. **Broad consent:** Providing an individual opt-out option, consultation may be held with only a small representative group of the population of interest.
3. **Group consent:** Cluster randomized trials (CRT), IR, and demonstration projects are examples where ECs have to decide on

the complex issues of feasibility and type of consent to be obtained from the participants.

Consent in public health research may be waived under following situations.

- Surveillance data and or administrative data with prior information to concern;
- Impracticability for obtaining consent, e.g. non-identifiable data personal, administrative data or any other material.
- Studies performed within the scope of regulatory and public health authorities
- Health-related registries data for studies that are authorized under national regulations; and
- Large geographical clusters studies.

Social and Behavioural Sciences Research for Health

The context of health research using methods from the social and behavioural sciences is often different from clinical, biomedical and public health research. Social and behavioural sciences include anthropology, sociology, psychology, philosophy, political science, economics, history, communications and education, etc. Many of these researches are mid-to-long term (Box 20.5) for knowledge production, science and society. Such research efforts will also have scholarship value besides relevance for policy and program development, providing a deeper understanding of explanatory factors.

Box 20.5: Important ethical issues in social and behaviour sciences studies

1. Non-measurable risks
2. Dynamic in nature
3. EC approval difficulty—data sharing related to incidental findings and post-research benefits
4. Ancillary care—EC approval to be given as and when required
5. Difficulty in dissemination of unacceptable practices and behaviour observed and documented, or observed.
6. Observation/practice of suicidal tendency or infanticide to reported to the concerned authorities, EC to approve.

It has now emerged as a cross-cutting area of enquiry relevant to almost every type of medical, biomedical, clinical and health research such as clinical trials, epidemiological research, program evaluations, implementation research, genetics, research on disaster and conflict contexts.

Ideally triangulation approach to be adopted for data collection in all kind of researches, however most of the time qualitative research is adopted in social and behavioural sciences.

Informed Consent in Social and Behavioural Sciences Research

- **Community consent/gatekeeper consent/ individual consent**—as discussed under heading community trials.
- **Participant consent**—As per the standard requirement under informed consent process.
- **Participant refusal**—sometime it is difficult for study participants to express refusal to participate. Researchers should be aware of cultural symbols of refusal, such as body language, silence, monosyllabic replies, or restlessness that communicate discomfort.
- **Relational autonomy:** In India, person's identity is known by socio-cultural determinants, such as caste, class, ethnicity and gender. Right to autonomy must be understood in relation to substantive equality of opportunity, sufficient social support and conditions for self-respect.
- **Waiver of informed consent:** As discussed previously under guidelines on consent (CIMOS).

Studies Using Deception (deception means fraud, fraudulence, cheating)

Deception occurs when researchers provide false or incomplete information to participants for the purpose of misleading them so as to achieve the study objectives and for larger public good. Research employing any type of deception should undergo full committee review. Types of deception are given in Box 20.6.

Box 20.6: Types of deception

Active deception: Selective withholding of the information/hypothesis of the study in the consent form along with giving incorrect information for achieving public good without influencing the outcome of the study, e.g. psychology, neuro-behavioural, behaviour intervention study.

Incomplete disclosure: If research involves incomplete disclosure but no deception.

Authorized deception: This provides the participants an opportunity to decide whether or not to participate on these terms.

Research involving any kind of deception should:

- Pose no more than minimal risk;
- Not adversely affect the welfare and safety of the participants;
- Be conducted only when the research cannot be carried out without deception;
- Have an adequate plan for debriefing the participants after completion of the study, if appropriate;
- Disseminate results of research to the participants, if applicable; and
- Be carefully reviewed by the EC.

Safety of Participants and Research Teams in the Field

If the research is conducted on sensitive or in sensitive area or personal information such as mental health, gender based violence and social exclusion and discrimination, in such a situation proper communication, adequate counselling, police protection, etc. may be required.

Similarly the **safety of the research team** is the responsibility of the institution, sponsors and local authorities. Besides providing safety, including insurance coverage, and setting up community advisory boards could be helpful to ease the situation.

CONCLUSIONS

Biomedical research including epidemiological research is based on basic principles of Research triangle, i.e. ethicality, morality and values. Epidemiological research is needed in healthcare, disease prevention and health promotion. The research should be need based and justifiable. The epidemiological research shall encompass all dimensions along with the determinants of health, therefore research only directed towards physical health will never be complete for an individual or nation. All types of research should practice national and international guideline to best. This research should be of good quality, done in a timely manner and follow recognized ethical standards.

References

1. Global Health Ethics. Key issues, WHO Press, World Health Organization, 20 Avenue Appia, 1211 Geneva 27, Switzerland) Website: http://www.who.int/ethics/en/
2. Weed DL, McKeown RE. Ethics in epidemiology and public health I. Technical terms, J Epidemiol. Community Health 2001;55:855–857.
3. Mathiharan K. Health and Law: The Fundamental Right To Health Care, Issues in Medical Ethics 2003;XI(4):123.
4. The Nuremberg Code [from Trials of War Criminals before the Nuremberg Military Tribunals under Control Council Law No. 10. Nuremberg, Oct. 1946–April 1949. Washington, DC: US GPO. 1949–1953.]
5. WMA Declaration of Helsinki–Ethical Principles for Medical Research Involving Human Subjects: https://www.wma.net/policies-post/wma-declaration-of-helsinki-ethical-principles-for-medical-research-involving-human-subjects/19th March 2018
6. Belmont report: https://www.hhs.gov/ohrp/regulations-and-policy/belmont-report/read-the-belmont-report/index.html
7. Roli Mathur (Ed.). National Ethical Guidelines for Biomedical and Health Research Involving Human Participants. Published by Director-General, Indian Council of Medical Research, New Delhi, 2017, www.icmr.nic.in
8. International Ethical Guidelines for Epidemiological Studies Prepared by the CIOMS in collaboration with the WHO, Geneva, 2009, https://cioms.ch/wp content/uploads/2017/01/International_Ethical_Guidelines_LR.pdf.
9. WHO. Ethics in epidemics, emergencies and disasters: Research, surveillance and patient care: training manual, 2015, WHO Press, WHO, 20 Avenue Appia, 1211 Geneva 27, Switzerland(http://apps.who.int/iris/bitstream/handle/10665/196326/9789241549349_eng.pdf)
10. Girish Menon R, Richard Cash, Research involving medical records review: an Indian perspective Indian Journal of Medical Ethics Vol III No 2 April-June 2006. http://ijme.in/wp-content/uploads/2016/11/1171-5.pdf

APPENDICES

Appendix I: The Nuremberg Code (Permissible Medical Experiments)

The great weight of the evidence before us is to the effect that certain types of medical experiments on human beings, when kept within reasonably well-defined bounds, conform to the ethics of the medical profession generally. The protagonists of the practice of human experimentation justify their views on the basis that such experiments yield results for the good of society that are unprocurable by other methods or means of study. All agree, however, that certain basic principles must be observed in order to satisfy moral, ethical and legal concepts:

1. The voluntary consent of the human subject is absolutely essential. This means that the person involved should have legal capacity to give consent; should be so situated as to be able to exercise free power of choice, without the intervention of any element of force, fraud, deceit, duress, over-reaching, or other ulterior form of constraint or coercion; and should have sufficient knowledge and comprehension of the elements of the subject matter involved as to enable him to make an understanding and enlightened decision. This latter element requires that before the acceptance of an affirmative decision by the experimental subject there should be made known to him the nature, duration, and purpose of the experiment; the method and means by which it is to be conducted; all inconveniences and hazards reasonably to be expected; and the effects upon his health or person which may possibly come from his participation in the experiment.

   The duty and responsibility for ascertaining the quality of the consent rests upon each individual who initiates, directs or engages in the experiment. It is a personal duty and responsibility which may not be delegated to another with impunity.
2. The experiment should be such as to yield fruitful results for the good of society, unprocurable by other methods or means of study, and not random and unnecessary in nature.
3. The experiment should be so designed and based on the results of animal experimentation and a knowledge of the natural history of the disease or other problem under study that the anticipated results will justify the performance of the experiment.
4. The experiment should be so conducted as to avoid all unnecessary physical and mental-suffering and injury.
5. No experiment should be conducted where there is a priori reason to believe that death or disabling injury will occur; except, perhaps, in those experiments where the experimental physicians also serve as subjects.
6. The degree of risk to be taken should never exceed that determined by the humanitarian importance of the problem to be solved by the experiment.
7. Proper preparations should be made and adequate facilities provided to protect the experimental subject against even remote possibilities of injury, disability, or death.
8. The experiment should be conducted only by scientifically qualified persons. The highest degree of skill and care should be required through all stages of the experiment of those who conduct or engage in the experiment.
9. During the course of the experiment the human subject should be at liberty to bring the experiment to an end if he has reached the physical or mental state where continuation of the experiment seems to him to be impossible.
10. During the course of the experiment the scientist in charge must be prepared to terminate the experiment at any stage, if he has probably cause to believe, in the exercise

of the good faith, superior skill and careful judgment required of him that a continuation of the experiment is likely to result in injury, disability, or death to the experimental subject.

Of the ten principles which have been enumerated our judicial concern, of course, is with those requirements which are purely legal in nature—or which at least are so clearly related to matters legal that they assist us in determining criminal culpability and punishment. To go beyond that point would lead us into a field that would be beyond our sphere of competence. However, the point need not be labored. We find from the evidence that in the medical experiments which have been proved, these ten principles were much more frequently honored in their breach than in their observance. Many of the concentration camp inmates who were the victims of these atrocities were citizens of countries other than the German Reich. They were non-German nationals, including Jews and 'asocial persons', both prisoners of war and civilians, who had been imprisoned and forced to submit to these tortures and barbarities without so much as assemblance of trial. In every single instance appearing in the record, subjects were used who did not consent to the experiments; indeed, as to some of the experiments, it is not even contended by the defendants that the subjects occupied the status of volunteers. In no case was the experimental subject at liberty of his own free choice to withdraw from any experiment. In many cases experiments were performed by unqualified persons; were conducted at random for no adequate scientific reason, and under revolting physical conditions. All of the experiments were conducted with unnecessary suffering and injury and very little, if any, precautions were taken to protect or safeguard the human subjects from the possibilities of injury, disability, or death. In every one of the experiments the subjects experienced extreme pain or torture, and in most of them they suffered permanent injury, mutilation, or death, either as a direct result of the experiments or because of lack of adequate follow-up care.

Obviously all of these experiments involving brutalities, tortures, disabling injury, and death were performed in complete disregard of international conventions, the laws and customs of war, the general principles of criminal law as derived from the criminal laws of all civilized nations, and Control Council Law No. 10. Manifestly human experiments under such conditions are contrary to "the principles of the law of nations as they result from the usages established among civilized peoples, from the laws of humanity, and from the dictates of public conscience."

Whether any of the defendants in the dock are guilty of these atrocities is, of course, another question. Under the Anglo-Saxon system of jurisprudence every defendant in a criminal case is presumed to be innocent of an offense charged until the prosecution, by competent, credible proof, has shown his guilt to the exclusion of every reasonable doubt. And this presumption abides with the defendant through each stage of his trial until such degree of proof has been adduced. A 'reasonable doubt' as the name implies is one conformable to reason—a doubt which a reasonable man would entertain. Stated differently, it is that state of a case which, after a full and complete comparison and consideration of all the evidence, would leave an unbiased, unprejudiced, reflective person, charged with the responsibility for decision, in the state of mind that he could not say that he felt an abiding conviction amounting to a moral certainty of the truth of the charge.

If any of the defendants are to be found guilty under counts two or three of the indictment, it must be, because the evidence has shown beyond a reasonable doubt that such defendant, without regard to nationality or the capacity in which he acted, participated as a principal in, accessory to, ordered, abetted, took a consenting part in, or was connected with plans or enterprises involving the commission of at least some of the medical experiments and other atrocities which are the subject matter of these counts. Under no other circumstances may he be convicted.

Before examining the evidence to which we must look in order to determine individual culpability, a brief statement concerning some of the official agencies of the German Government and Nazi Party which will be referred to in this judgment seems desirable.

Source: The Nuremberg Code. (from *Trials of War Criminals before the Nuremberg Military Tribunals under Control Council Law No. 10.* Nuremberg, October 1946–April 1949. Washington, DC: US GPO, 1949–1953.)

Appendix II: WMA Declaration of Helsinki (Ethical Principles for Medical Research Involving Human Subjects)

Preamble

1. The World Medical Association (WMA) has developed the Declaration of Helsinki as a statement of ethical principles for medical research involving human subjects, including research on identifiable human material and data.

   The Declaration is intended to be read as a whole and each of its constituent paragraphs should be applied with consideration of all other relevant paragraphs.
2. Consistent with the mandate of the WMA, the Declaration is addressed primarily to physicians. The WMA encourages others who are involved in medical research involving human subjects to adopt these principles.

General Principles

3. The Declaration of Geneva of the WMA binds the physician with the words, "The health of my patient will be my first consideration," and the International Code of Medical Ethics declares that, "A physician shall act in the patient's best interest when providing medical care."
4. It is the duty of the physician to promote and safeguard the health, well-being and rights of patients, including those who are involved in medical research. The physician's knowledge and conscience are dedicated to the fulfilment of this duty.
5. Medical progress is based on research that ultimately must include studies involving human subjects.
6. The primary purpose of medical research involving human subjects is to understand the causes, development and effects of diseases and improve preventive, diagnostic and therapeutic interventions (methods, procedures and treatments). Even the best proven interventions must be evaluated continually through research for their safety, effectiveness, efficiency, accessibility and quality.
7. Medical research is subject to ethical standards that promote and ensure respect for all human subjects and protect their health and rights.
8. While the primary purpose of medical research is to generate new knowledge, this goal can never take precedence over the rights and interests of individual research subjects.
9. It is the duty of physicians who are involved in medical research to protect the life, health, dignity, integrity, right to self-determination, privacy, and confidentiality of personal information of research subjects. The responsibility for the protection of research subjects must always rest with the physician or other health care professionals and never with the research subjects, even though they have given consent.
10. Physicians must consider the ethical, legal and regulatory norms and standards for research involving human subjects in their own countries as well as applicable international norms and standards. No national or international ethical, legal or regulatory requirement should reduce or eliminate any of the protections for research subjects set forth in this Declaration.
11. Medical research should be conducted in a manner that minimises possible harm to the environment.
12. Medical research involving human subjects must be conducted only by individuals with the appropriate ethics and scientific education, training and qualifications. Research on patients or healthy volunteers requires the supervision of a competent and appropriately qualified physician or other healthcare professional.
13. Groups that are under-represented in medical research should be provided appropriate access to participation in research.
14. Physicians who combine medical research with medical care should involve their patients in research only to the extent that this is justified by its potential preventive, diagnostic or therapeutic value and if the physician has good reason to believe that participation in the research study will not adversely affect the health of the patients who serve as research subjects.
15. Appropriate compensation and treatment for subjects who are harmed as a result of participating in research must be ensured.

Risks, Burdens and Benefits

16. In medical practice and in medical research, most interventions involve risks and burdens.

    Medical research involving human subjects may only be conducted if the importance of the objective outweighs the risks and burdens to the research subjects.

17. All medical research involving human subjects must be preceded by careful assessment of predictable risks and burdens to the individuals and groups involved in the research in comparison with foreseeable benefits to them and to other individuals or groups affected by the condition under investigation.

    Measures to minimise the risks must be implemented. The risks must be continuously monitored, assessed and documented by the researcher.

18. Physicians may not be involved in a research study involving human subjects unless they are confident that the risks have been adequately assessed and can be satisfactorily managed.

    When the risks are found to outweigh the potential benefits or when there is conclusive proof of definitive outcomes, physicians must assess whether to continue, modify or immediately stop the study.

Vulnerable Groups and Individuals

19. Some groups and individuals are particularly vulnerable and may have an increased likelihood of being wronged or of incurring additional harm.

    All vulnerable groups and individuals should receive specifically considered protection.

20. Medical research with a vulnerable group is only justified if the research is responsive to the health needs or priorities of this group and the research cannot be carried out in a non-vulnerable group. In addition, this group should stand to benefit from the knowledge, practices or interventions that result from the research.

Scientific Requirements and Research Protocols

21. Medical research involving human subjects must conform to generally accepted scientific principles, be based on a thorough knowledge of the scientific literature, other relevant sources of information, and adequate laboratory and, as appropriate, animal experimentation. The welfare of animals used for research must be respected.

22. The design and performance of each research study involving human subjects must be clearly described and justified in a research protocol.

    The protocol should contain a statement of the ethical considerations involved and should indicate how the principles in this Declaration have been addressed. The protocol should include information regarding funding, sponsors, institutional affiliations, potential conflicts of interest, incentives for subjects and information regarding provisions for treating and/or compensating subjects who are harmed as a consequence of participation in the research study.

    In clinical trials, the protocol must also describe appropriate arrangements for post-trial provisions.

Research Ethics Committees

23. The research protocol must be submitted for consideration, comment, guidance and approval to the concerned research ethics committee before the study begins. This committee must be transparent in its functioning, must be independent of the researcher, the sponsor and any other undue influence and must be duly qualified. It must take into consideration the laws and regulations of the country or countries in which the research is to be performed as well as applicable international norms and standards, but these must not be allowed to reduce or eliminate any of the protections for research subjects set forth in this Declaration.

    The committee must have the right to monitor ongoing studies. The researcher must provide monitoring information to the committee, especially information about any serious adverse events. No amendment to the protocol may be made without consideration and approval by the committee. After the end of the study, the researchers must submit a final report to the committee containing a summary of the study's findings and conclusions.

Privacy and Confidentiality

24. Every precaution must be taken to protect the privacy of research subjects and the confidentiality of their personal information.

Informed Consent

25. Participation by individuals capable of giving informed consent as subjects in medical research must be voluntary. Although it may be appropriate to consult family members or community leaders, no individual capable of giving informed consent may be enrolled in a research study unless he or she freely agrees.
26. In medical research involving human subjects capable of giving informed consent, each potential subject must be adequately informed of the aims, methods, sources of funding, any possible conflicts of interest, institutional affiliations of the researcher, the anticipated benefits and potential risks of the study and the discomfort it may entail, post-study provisions and any other relevant aspects of the study. The potential subject must be informed of the right to refuse to participate in the study or to withdraw consent to participate at any time without reprisal. Special attention should be given to the specific information needs of individual potential subjects as well as to the methods used to deliver the information.

    After ensuring that the potential subject has understood the information, the physician or another appropriately qualified individual must then seek the potential subject's freely-given informed consent, preferably in writing. If the consent cannot be expressed in writing, the non-written consent must be formally documented and witnessed.

    All medical research subjects should be given the option of being informed about the general outcome and results of the study.
27. When seeking informed consent for participation in a research study the physician must be particularly cautious if the potential subject is in a dependent relationship with the physician or may consent under duress. In such situations the informed consent must be sought by an appropriately qualified individual who is completely independent of this relationship.
28. For a potential research subject who is incapable of giving informed consent, the physician must seek informed consent from the legally authorised representative. These individuals must not be included in a research study that has no likelihood of benefit for them unless it is intended to promote the health of the group represented by the potential subject, the research cannot instead be performed with persons capable of providing informed consent, and the research entails only minimal risk and minimal burden.
29. When a potential research subject who is deemed incapable of giving informed consent is able to give assent to decisions about participation in research, the physician must seek that assent in addition to the consent of the legally authorised representative. The potential subject's dissent should be respected.
30. Research involving subjects who are physically or mentally incapable of giving consent, e.g. unconscious patients, may be done only if the physical or mental condition that prevents giving informed consent is a necessary characteristic of the research group. In such circumstances, the physician must seek informed consent from the legally authorised representative. If no such representative is available and if the research cannot be delayed, the study may proceed without informed consent provided that the specific reasons for involving subjects with a condition that renders them unable to give informed consent have been stated in the research protocol and the study has been approved by a research ethics committee. Consent to remain in the research must be obtained as soon as possible from the subject or a legally authorised representative.
31. The physician must fully inform the patient which aspects of their care are related to the research. The refusal of a patient to participate in a study or the patient's decision to withdraw from the study must never adversely affect the patient–physician relationship.
32. For medical research using identifiable human material or data, such as research on material or data contained in biobanks or similar repositories, physicians must seek informed consent for its collection, storage and/or reuse. There may be exceptional situations where consent would be impossible or impracticable to obtain for such research. In such situations the research may be done only after consideration and approval of a research ethics committee.

Use of Placebo

33. The benefits, risks, burdens and effectiveness of a new intervention must be tested against those of the best proven intervention(s), except in the following circumstances.
    - Where no proven intervention exists, the use of placebo, or no intervention, is acceptable; or
    - Where for compelling and scientifically sound methodological reasons the use of any intervention less effective than the best proven one, the use of placebo, or no intervention is necessary to determine the efficacy or safety of an intervention and the patients who receive any intervention less effective than the best proven one, placebo, or no intervention will not be subject to additional risks of serious or irreversible harm as a result of not receiving the best proven intervention.

    Extreme care must be taken to avoid abuse of this option.

Post-trial Provisions

34. In advance of a clinical trial, sponsors, researchers and host country governments should make provisions for post-trial access for all participants who still need an intervention identified as beneficial in the trial. This information must also be disclosed to participants during the informed consent process.

Research Registration and Publication and Dissemination of Results

35. Every research study involving human subjects must be registered in a publicly accessible database before recruitment of the first subject.
36. Researchers, authors, sponsors, editors and publishers all have ethical obligations with regard to the publication and dissemination of the results of research. Researchers have a duty to make publicly available the results of their research on human subjects and are accountable for the completeness and accuracy of their reports. All parties should adhere to accepted guidelines for ethical reporting. Negative and inconclusive as well as positive results must be published or otherwise made publicly available. Sources of funding, institutional affiliations and conflicts of interest must be declared in the publication. Reports of research not in accordance with the principles of this Declaration should not be accepted for publication.

Unproven Interventions in Clinical Practice

37. In the treatment of an individual patient, where proven interventions do not exist or other known interventions have been ineffective, the physician, after seeking expert advice, with informed consent from the patient or a legally authorised representative, may use an unproven intervention if in the physician's judgement it offers hope of saving life, re-establishing health or alleviating suffering. This intervention should subsequently be made the object of research, designed to evaluate its safety and efficacy. In all cases, new information must be recorded and, where appropriate, made publicly available.

Source: https://www.wma.net/policies-post/wma-declaration-of-helsinki-ethical-principles-for-medical-research-involving-human-subjects/19th March 2018

Appendix III: The Belmont Report (Ethical Principles and Guidelines for Research Involving Human Subjects)

Scientific research has produced substantial social benefits. It has also posed some troubling ethical questions. Public attention was drawn to these questions by reported abuses of human subjects in biomedical experiments, especially during the Second World War. During the Nuremberg War Crime Trials, the Nuremberg code was drafted as a set of standards for judging physicians and scientists who had conducted biomedical experiments on concentration camp prisoners. This code became the prototype of many later codes intended to assure that research involving human subjects would be carried out in an ethical manner.

The codes consist of rules, some general, others specific that guide the investigators or the reviewers of research in their work. Such rules often are inadequate to cover complex situations; at times they come into conflict, and they are frequently difficult to interpret or apply. Broader ethical principles will provide a basis on which specific rules may be formulated, criticized and interpreted.

Three principles, or general prescriptive judgments, that are relevant to research involving human subjects are identified in this statement. Other principles may also be relevant. These three are comprehensive, however, and are stated at a level of generalization that should assist scientists, subjects, reviewers and interested citizens to understand the ethical issues inherent in research involving human subjects. These principles cannot always be applied so as to resolve beyond dispute particular ethical problems. The objective is to provide an analytical framework that will guide the resolution of ethical problems arising from research involving human subjects.

This statement consists of a distinction between research and practice, a discussion of the three basic ethical principles, and remarks about the application of these principles.

Part A: Boundaries between Practice and Research

It is important to distinguish between biomedical and behavioural research, on the one hand, and the practice of accepted therapy on the other, in order to know what activities ought to undergo review for the protection of human subjects of research. The distinction between research and practice is blurred partly because both often occur together (as in research designed to evaluate a therapy) and partly because notable departures from standard practice are often called 'experimental' when the terms 'experimental' and 'research' are not carefully defined.

For the most part, the term 'practice' refers to interventions that are designed solely to enhance the well-being of an *individual patient or client* and that have a reasonable expectation of success. The purpose of medical or behavioural practice is to provide diagnosis, preventive treatment or therapy to particular individuals. By contrast, the term *'research'* designates an activity designed to test a hypothesis, permit conclusions to be drawn, and thereby to develop or contribute to *generalizable knowledge* (expressed, e.g. in theories, principles, and statements of relationships). Research is usually described in a formal protocol that sets forth an objective and a set of procedures designed to reach that objective.

When a clinician departs in a significant way from standard or accepted practice, the innovation does not, in and of itself, constitute research. The fact that a procedure is 'experimental,' in the sense of new, untested or different, does not automatically place it in the category of research. Radically new procedures of this description should, however, be made the object of formal research at an early stage in order to determine whether they are safe and effective. Thus, it is the responsibility of medical practice committees, e.g. to insist that a major innovation be incorporated into a formal research project.

Research and practice may be carried on together when research is designed to evaluate the safety and efficacy of a therapy. This need not cause any confusion regarding whether or not the activity requires review; the general rule is that if there is any element of research in an activity, that activity should undergo review for the protection of human subjects.

Part B: Basic Ethical Principles

The expression 'basic ethical principles' refers to those general judgments that serve as a basic justification for the many particular ethical prescriptions and evaluations of human actions. Three basic principles, among those generally accepted in our cultural tradition, are particularly relevant to the ethics of research involving human subjects—the principles of respect of persons, beneficence and justice.

1. Respect for persons: Respect for persons incorporates at least two ethical convictions—first, that individuals should be treated as autonomous agents, and second, that persons with diminished autonomy are entitled to protection. The principle of respect for persons thus divides into two separate moral requirements—the requirement to acknowledge autonomy and the requirement to protect those with diminished autonomy.

An autonomous person is an individual capable of deliberation about personal goals and of acting under the direction of such deliberation. To respect autonomy is to give weight to autonomous persons' considered opinions and choices while refraining from obstructing their actions unless they are clearly detrimental to others. To show lack of respect for an autonomous agent is to repudiate that person's considered judgments, to deny an individual the freedom to act on those considered judgments, or to withhold information necessary to make a considered judgment, when there are no compelling reasons to do so.

However, not every human being is capable of self-determination. The capacity for self-determination matures during an individual's life, and some individuals lose this capacity wholly or in part because of illness, mental disability, or circumstances that severely restrict liberty. Respect for the immature and the incapacitated may require protecting them as they mature or while they are incapacitated.

Some persons are in need of extensive protection, even to the point of excluding them from activities which may harm them; other persons require little protection beyond making sure they undertake activities freely and with awareness of possible adverse consequence. The extent of protection afforded should depend upon the risk of harm and the likelihood of benefit. The judgment that any individual lacks autonomy should be periodically reevaluated and will vary in different situations.

In most cases of research involving human subjects, respect for persons demands that subjects enter into the research voluntarily and with adequate information.

In some situations, however, application of the principle is not obvious. The involvement of prisoners as subjects of research provides an instructive example. On the one hand, it would seem that the principle of respect for persons requires that prisoners not be deprived of the opportunity to volunteer for research. On the other hand, under prison conditions they may be subtly coercedor unduly influenced to engage in research activities for which they would not otherwise volunteer. Respect for persons would then dictate that prisoners be protected. Whether to allow prisoners to 'volunteer' or to 'protect' them presents a dilemma. Respecting persons, in most hard cases, is often a matter of balancing competing claims urged by the principle of respect itself.

2. Beneficence: Persons are treated in an ethical manner not only by respecting their decisions and protecting them from harm, but also by making efforts to secure their well-being. Such treatment falls under the principle of beneficence. The term 'beneficence' is often understood to cover acts of kindness or charity that go beyond strict obligation. In this document, beneficence is understood in a stronger sense, as an obligation. Two general rules have been formulated as complementary expressions of beneficent actions in this sense—(1) do not harm and (2) maximize possible benefits and minimize possible harms.

The Hippocratic maxim 'do no harm' has long been a fundamental principle of medical ethics. Claude Bernard extended it to the realm of research, saying that one should not injure one person regardless of the benefits that might come to others. However, even avoiding harm requires learning what is harmful; and, in the process of obtaining this information, persons may be exposed to risk of harm. Further, the Hippocratic Oath requires physicians to benefit their patients "according to their best judgment." Learning what will in fact benefit may require exposing persons to risk. The problem posed by these imperatives is to decide when it is justifiable to seek certain benefits despite the risks involved, and when the benefits should be foregone because of the risks.

The obligations of beneficence affect both individual investigators and society at large, because they extend both to particular research projects and to the entire enterprise of research. In the case of particular projects, investigators and members of their institutions are obliged to give forethought to the maximization of benefits and the reduction of risk that might occur from the research investigation. In the case of scientific research in general, members of the larger society are obliged to recognize the longer term benefits and risks that may result from the improvement of knowledge and from the development of novel medical, psychotherapeutic, and social procedures.

The principle of beneficence often occupies a well-defined justifying role in many areas of research involving human subjects. An example is found in research involving children. Effective ways of treating childhood diseases and fostering healthy development are benefits that serve to justify research involving children—even when individual research subjects are not direct beneficiaries. Research also makes it possible to avoid the harm that may result from the application of previously accepted routine practices that on closer investigation turn out to be dangerous. But the role of the principle of beneficence is not always so unambiguous. A difficult ethical problem remains, e.g. about research that presents *more than minimal risk* without immediate prospect of direct benefit to the children involved. Some have argued that such research is inadmissible, while others have pointed out that this limit would rule out much research promising great benefit to *children in the future*. Here again, as with all hard cases, he different claims covered by the principle of beneficence may come into conflict and force difficult choices.

3. Justice: Who ought to receive the benefits of research and bear its burdens? This is a question of justice, in the sense of "fairness in distribution" or "what is deserved." An injustice occurs when some benefit to which a person is entitled is denied without good reason or when some burden is imposed unduly. Another way of conceiving the principle of justice is that equals ought to be treated equally. However, this statement requires explication. Who is equal and who is unequal? What considerations justify departure from equal distribution? Almost all commentators allow that distinctions based on experience, age, deprivation, competence, merit and position do sometimes constitute criteria justifying differential treatment for certain purposes. It is necessary, then, to explain in what respects people should be treated equally.

There are several widely accepted formulations of just ways to distribute burdens and benefits. Each formulation mentions some relevant property on the basis of which burdens and benefits should be distributed. These formulations are:

1. To each person an equal share
2 To each person according to individual need
3. To each person according to individual effort
4. To each person according to societal contribution
5. To each person according to merit.

Questions of justice have long been associated with social practices such as punishment, taxation and political representation. Until recently these questions have not generally been associated with scientific research. However, they are foreshadowed even in the earliest reflections on the ethics of research involving human subjects. For example, during the 19th and early 20th centuries the burdens of serving as research subjects fell largely upon poor ward patients, while the benefits of improved medical care flowed primarily to private patients. Subsequently, the exploitation of unwilling prisoners as research subjects in Nazi concentration camps was condemned as a particularly flagrant injustice. In this country, in the 1940s, the Tuskegee syphilis study used disadvantaged, rural black men to study the untreated course of a disease that is by no means confined to that population. These subjects were deprived of demonstrably effective treatment in order not to interrupt the project, long after such treatment became generally available.

Against this historical background, it can be seen how conceptions of justice are relevant to research involving human subjects. For example, the selection of research subjects needs to be scrutinized in order to determine whether some classes (e.g. welfare patients, particular racial and ethnic minorities, or persons confined to institutions) are being systematically selected simply because of their easy availability, their compromised position, or their manipulability, rather than for reasons directly related to the problem being studied. Finally, whenever research supported by public funds leads to the development of therapeutic devices and procedures, justice demands both that these not provide advantages only to those who can afford them and that such research should not unduly involve persons from groups unlikely to be among the beneficiaries of subsequent applications of the research.

Part C: Applications

Applications of the general principles to the conduct of research leads to consideration of the following requirements—informed consent, risk/benefit assessment, and the selection of subjects of research.

1. Informed consent: Respect for persons requires that subjects, to the degree that they are capable, be given the opportunity to choose what shall or shall not happen to them. This opportunity is provided when adequate standards for informed consent are satisfied.

While the importance of informed consent is unquestioned, controversy prevails over the nature and possibility of an informed consent. Nonetheless, there is widespread agreement that the consent process can be analyzed as containing three elements—information, comprehension and voluntariness.

Information—most codes of research establish specific items for disclosure intended to assure that subjects are given sufficient information. These items generally include—the research procedure, their purposes, risks and anticipated benefits, alternative procedures (where therapy is involved), and a statement offering the subject the opportunity to ask questions and to withdraw at any time from the research. Additional items have been proposed, including how subjects are selected, the person responsible for the research, etc.

However, a simple listing of items does not answer the question of what the standard should be for judging how much and what sort of information should be provided. One standard frequently invoked in medical practice, namely the information commonly provided by practitioners in the field or in the locale, is inadequate since research takes place precisely when a common understanding does not exist. Another standard, currently popular in malpractice law, requires the practitioner to reveal the information that *reasonable persons* would wish to know in order to make a decision regarding their care. This, too, seems insufficient since the research subject, being in essence a volunteer, may wish to know considerably more about risks gratuitously undertaken than do patients who deliver themselves into the hand of a clinician for needed care. It may be that a standard of 'the reasonable volunteer' should be proposed—the extent and nature of information should be such that persons, knowing that the procedure is neither necessary for their care nor perhaps fully understood, can decide whether they wish to participate in the furthering of knowledge. Even when some direct benefit to them is anticipated, the subjects should understand clearly the range of risk and the voluntary nature of participation.

A special problem of consent arises where informing subjects of some pertinent aspect of the research is likely to impair the validity of the research. In many cases, it is sufficient to indicate to subjects that they are being invited to participate in research of which some features will not be revealed until the research is concluded. In all cases of research involving incomplete disclosure, such research is justified only if it is clear that (1) incomplete disclosure is truly necessary to accomplish the goals of the research, (2) there are no undisclosed risks to subjects *that are more than minimal*, and (3) there is an adequate plan for debriefing subjects, when appropriate, and for dissemination of research results to them. Information about risks should never be withheld for the purpose of eliciting the cooperation of subjects, and truthful answers should always be given to direct questions about the research. Care should be taken to distinguish cases in which disclosure would destroy or invalidate the research from cases in which disclosure would simply inconvenience the investigator.

Comprehension—the manner and context in which information is conveyed is as important as the information itself. For example, presenting information in a disorganized and rapid fashion, allowing too little time for consideration or curtailing opportunities for questioning, all may adversely affect a subject's ability to make an informed choice.

Because the subject's ability to understand is a function of intelligence, rationality, maturity and language, it is necessary to adapt the presentation of the information to the subject's capacities. Investigators are responsible for ascertaining that the subject has comprehended the information. While there is always an obligation to ascertain that the information about risk to subjects is complete and adequately comprehended, when the risks are more serious, that obligation increases. On occasion, it may be suitable to give some oral or written tests of comprehension.

Special provision may need to be made when comprehension is severely limited—for example, by conditions of immaturity or mental disability. Each class of subjects that one might consider as incompetent (e.g. infants and young children, mentally disable patients, the terminally ill and the comatose) should be considered on its own terms. Even for these persons, however, respect requires giving them the opportunity to choose to the extent they are able, whether or not to participate in research. The objections of these subjects to involvement should be honored, *unless* the research entails providing them a therapy unavailable elsewhere. Respect for persons also requires seeking the permission of other parties in order to protect the subjects from harm. Such persons are thus respected both by acknowledging their own wishes and by the use of third parties to protect them from harm.

The third parties chosen should be those who are most likely to understand the incompetent subject's situation and to *act in that person's best interest.* The person authorized to act on behalf of the subject should be given an opportunity to observe the research as it proceeds in order to be able to withdraw the subject from the research, if such action appears in the subject's best interest.

Voluntariness—an agreement to participate in research constitutes a valid consent only if voluntarily given. This element of informed consent requires conditions free of coercion and undue influence. Coercion occurs when an overt threat of harm is intentionally presented by one person to another in order to obtain compliance. Undue influence, by contrast, occurs through an offer of an excessive, unwarranted, inappropriate or improper reward or other overture in order to obtain compliance. Also, inducements that would ordinarily be acceptable may become undue influences if the subject is especially vulnerable.

Unjustifiable pressures usually occur when persons in positions of authority or commanding influence—especially where possible sanctions are involved—urge a course of action for a subject. A continuum of such influencing factors exists, however, and it is impossible to state precisely where justifiable persuasion ends and undue influence begins. But undue influence would include actions such as manipulating a person's choice through the controlling influence of a close relative and threatening to withdraw health services to which an individual would otherwise be entitle.

2. Assessment of risks and benefits: The assessment of risks and benefits requires a careful arrayal of relevant data, including, in some cases, alternative ways of obtaining the benefits sought in the research. Thus, the assessment presents both an opportunity and a responsibility to gather systematic and comprehensive information about proposed research. *For the investigator, it is a means to examine whether the proposed research is properly designed.* For a review committee, it is a method for determining whether the *risks that will be presented to subjects are justified.* For prospective subjects, the assessment will assist the determination whether or not to participate.

The nature and scope of risks and benefits— the requirement that research be justified on the basis of a favourable risk/benefit assessment bears a close relation to the principle of beneficence, just as the moral requirement that informed consent be obtained is derived primarily from the principle of respect for persons. The term 'risk' refers to a possibility that harm may occur. However, when expressions such as 'small risk' or 'high risk' are used, they usually refer (often ambiguously) both to the chance (probability) of experiencing a harm and the severity (magnitude) of the envisioned harm.

The term 'benefit' is used in the research context to refer to something of positive value related to health or welfare. Unlike, 'risk,' 'benefit' is not a term that expresses probabilities. Risk is properly contrasted to probability of benefits, and benefits are properly contrasted with harms rather than risks of harm. Accordingly, so-called risk/benefit assessments are concerned with the probabilities and magnitudes of possible harm and anticipated benefits. Many kinds of possible harms and benefits need to be taken into account. There are, for example, risks of psychological harm, physical harm, legal harm, social harm and economic harm and the corresponding benefits. While the most likely types of harms to research subjects are those of psychological or physical pain or injury, other possible kinds should not be overlooked.

Risks and benefits of research may affect the individual subjects, the families of the individual subjects, and society at large (or special groups of subjects in society). Previous codes and Federal regulations have required that risks to subjects be outweighed by the sum of both the anticipated benefit to the subject, if any, and the anticipated benefit to society in the form of knowledge to be gained from the research. In balancing these different elements, the risks and benefits affecting the immediate research subject will normally carry special weight. On the other hand, interests other than those of the subject may on some occasions be sufficient by themselves to justify the risks involved in the research, so long as the subjects' rights have been protected. Beneficence thus requires that we protect against risk of harm to subjects and also that we be concerned about the loss of the substantial benefits that might be gained from research.

The systematic assessment of risks and benefits—it is commonly said that benefits and risks must be 'balanced' and shown to be 'in a favorable ratio.' The metaphorical character of these terms draws attention to the difficulty of making precise judgments. Only on rare occasions will quantitative techniques be available for the scrutiny of research protocols. However, the idea of systematic, non-arbitrary analysis of risks and benefits should be emulated insofar as possible.

This ideal requires those making decisions about the justifiability of research to be thorough in the accumulation and assessment of information about all aspects of the research, and to consider alternatives systematically. This procedure renders the assessment of research more rigorous and precise, while making communication between review board members and investigators less subject to misinterpretation, misinformation and conflicting judgments. Thus, there should first be a determination of the validity of the presuppositions of the research; then the nature, probability and magnitude of risk should be distinguished with as much clarity as possible. The method of ascertaining risks should be explicit, especially where there is no alternative to the use of such vague categories as small or slight risk. It should also be determined whether an investigator's estimates of the probability of harm or benefits are reasonable, as judged by known facts or other available studies.

Finally, **assessment of the justifiability of research** should reflect at least the following considerations—(i) brutal or inhumane treatment of human subjects is never morally justified. (ii) Risks should be reduced to those necessary to achieve the research objective. It should be determined whether it is in fact necessary to use human subjects at all. Risk can perhaps never be entirely eliminated, but it can often be reduced by careful attention to alternative procedures. (iii) When research involves *significant risk* of serious impairment, review committees should be extraordinarily insistent on the justification of the risk (looking usually to the likelihood of benefit to the subject—or, in some rare cases, to the manifest voluntariness of the participation). (iv) When vulnerable populations are involved in research, the appropriateness of involving them should itself be demonstrated. A number of variables go into such judgments, including the nature and degree of risk, the condition of the particular population involved, and the nature and level of the anticipated benefits. (v) Relevant risks and benefits must be *thoroughly arrayed in documents and procedures used in the informed consent process.*

3. Selection of subjects: Just as the principle of respect for persons finds expression in the requirements for consent, and the principle of beneficence in risk/benefit assessment, the principle of justice gives rise to moral requirements that there be fair procedures and outcomes in the selection of research subjects.

Justice is relevant to the selection of subjects of research at two levels—the social and the individual. *Individual justice* in the selection of subjects would require that researchers exhibit fairness: thus, they should not offer potentially beneficial research only to some patients who are in their favour or select only 'undesirable' persons for risky research. *Social justice* requires that distinction be drawn between classes of subjects that ought, and ought not, to participate in any particular kind of research, based on the ability of members of that class to bear burdens and on the appropriateness of placing further burdens on already burdened persons. Thus, it can be considered a matter of social justice that there is an order of preference in the selection of classes of subjects (e.g. adults before children) and that some classes of potential subjects (e.g. the institutionalized mentally infirm or prisoners) may be involved as research subjects, if at all, only on certain conditions.

Injustice may appear in the selection of subjects, even if individual subjects are selected fairly by investigators and treated fairly in the course of research. Thus, injustice arises from social, racial, sexual and cultural biases institutionalized in society. Thus, even if individual researchers are treating their research subjects fairly, and even if IRBs are taking care to assure that subjects are selected fairly within a particular institution, unjust social patterns may nevertheless appear in the overall distribution of the burdens and benefits of research. Although individual institutions or investigators may not be able to resolve a problem that is pervasive in their social setting, they can consider distributive justice in selecting research subjects.

Some populations, especially institutionalized ones, are already burdened in many ways by their infirmities and environments. When research is proposed that involves risks and does not include a therapeutic component, other less burdened classes of persons should be called upon first to accept these risks of research, *except* where the research is directly related to the specific conditions of the class involved. Also, even though public funds for research may often flow in the same directions as public funds for healthcare, it seems unfair that populations dependent on public healthcare constitute a pool of preferred research subjects if more advantaged populations are likely to be the recipients of the benefits.

One special instance of injustice results from the involvement of vulnerable subjects. Certain groups, such as racial minorities, the economically disadvantaged, the very sick, and the institutionalized may continually be sought as research subjects, owing to their ready availability in settings where research is conducted. Given their dependent status and their frequently compromised capacity for free consent, they should be protected against the danger of being involved in research solely for administrative convenience, or because they are easy to manipulate as a result of their illness or socio-economic condition.

- **Since 1945, various codes for the proper and responsible conduct of human experimentation in medical research have been adopted by different organizations.** The best known of these codes are the Nuremberg Code of 1947, the Helsinki Declaration of 1964 (revised in 1975), and the 1971 Guidelines (codified into Federal Regulations in 1974) issued by the US Department of Health, Education, and Welfare Codes for the conduct of social and behavioural research have also been adopted, the best known being that of the American Psychological Association, published in 1973.
- Although practice usually involves interventions designed solely to enhance the well-being of a particular individual, interventions are sometimes applied to one individual for the enhancement of the well-being of another (e.g. blood donation, skin grafts, organ transplants) or an intervention may have the dual purpose of enhancing the well-being of a particular individual, and, at the same time, providing some benefit to others (e.g. vaccination, which protects both the person who is vaccinated and society generally). The fact that some forms of practice have elements other than immediate benefit to the individual receiving an intervention, however, should not confuse the general distinction between research and practice. Even when a procedure applied in practice may benefit some other person, it remains an intervention designed to enhance the well-being of a particular individual or groups of individuals; thus, it is practice and need not be reviewed as research.
- Because the problems related to social experimentation may differ substantially from those of biomedical and behavioural research, the commission specifically declines to make any policy determination regarding such research at this time. Rather, the commission believes that the problem ought to be addressed by one of its successor bodies.

[**Note:** The above *Belmont Report* was also mandated by the 1974 *National Research Act* to be used as the foundation for the new federal OPRR (later OHRP) regulations for the use of human subjects in research, and the following OHRP federal regulations are currently in use. Note the 'exceptions'. In fact, the Secretary of DHHS has the authority to waive certain informed consent requirements, even with the opposition of the President or members of Congress. Among many other problems and concerns, note also the false scientific definitions inserted into the original OPRR regulations (admittedly done so by Richard Doerflinger of the USCCB) and preserved continuously to the present OHRP regulation updates. The two false scientific definitions are 'foetus' and 'pregnancy', both erroneously defined as 'beginning at implantation'. 'Foetus' is also defined as the 'product of *conception*' (which usually means 'fertilization', or 'sexual reproduction', fusion of sperm and oocyte). In the real world, implantation takes place about a week after the new human embryo begins to exist at the beginning of fertilization in the woman's fallopian tube, and by implantation is about a week old (consisting of about 100+ cells at the blastocyst stage of development). Therefore a woman is really already pregnant before implantation in normal sexual relations. And a 'foetus' is accurately defined as the developing human being beginning at 9 weeks post-fertilization (when the 'fetal period' begins) until birth. Also, the 'product of conception' applies only to sexually reproduced human beings; it does not apply to any asexually reproduced human beings (i.e. reproduced without the immediate use of any sperm or oocytes), e.g. all cloned or otherwise genetically engineered human beings asexually reproduced naturally *in vivo* (identical twins) or asexually reproduced artificially *in vitro* in IVF/ART research laboratories or 'infertility' clinics.

Thus, these federal regulations (1) would not consider women 'pregnant' before the already existing embryo implants into her uterus. (2) They would not cover any asexually reproduced human embryos or foetuses at any age. All asexually reproduced human embryos and foetuses would not be 'human subjects' needing protection and legally disappear. (3) They are falsely claiming that it is the *foetus* that implants into her uterus—which is absurd, since it is the 'embryo' at the blastocyst stage of development that implants into her uterus. The developing human being is not considered a 'foetus' until 9 weeks post-fertilization. (4) Therefore, these federal regulationswould not legally recognize even the sexually reproduced ('conception') developing human being during the embryonic period at all as a 'human subject of research' from fertilization until the end of the 8th week post-fertilization. Even the 'human embryo' sexually reproduced is not a 'human subject of research' needing protection and legally simply disappears. [See Irving: FERTILIZATION and IMPLANTATION of the Early Human Embryo: Accurate Scientific Resources (May 8, 2013), at: *http://www.lifeissues.net/writers/irv/irv_212accuratere sources1.html;* also, 'Individual testimony before the NIH Human Embryo Research Panel' (March 14, 1994); reprinted in *Linacre Quarterly*, 61(4):82–89 (Nov. 1994), at: *http://www.lifeissues.net/writers/irv/irv_32indi vidualtestimony.html;* PMID: 11652834 [PubMed-indexed for MEDLINE]; also, 'Invited Submission: Maryland state proposed statute for research using' decisionally incapacitated 'human subjects: The legalization of normative bioethics theory'; submitted to State of Maryland Attorney General J Joseph Curran Jr, Asst. Attorney General Jack Schwartz, in response to the *Initial Report of the Attorney General's Research Working Group* (June 30, 1998); submitted to the State of Maryland General Assembly, March 1999, at: *http://www.lifeissues.net/writers/irv/irv_70incapacitated1.html]*. The current US federal regulations for the use of human subjects in research are the following:]

V. OHRP—Federal Regulations for the Use of Human Subjects in Research (informed consent):

Appendix 4 (US Federal Guidelines): The Federal Policy and 45 CFR 46 (see page 3 of original document for beginning, page 8 read "informed consent"): *http://www.hhs.gov/ohrp/humansubjects/regbook2013. pdf.pdf*

General Requirements for Informed Consent (§46.116)

Except as provided elsewhere in this policy, no investigator may involve a human being as a subject in research covered by this policy unless the investigator has obtained the legally effective informed consent of the subject or the subject's legally authorized representative. An investigator shall seek such consent only under circumstances that provide the prospective subject or the representative sufficient opportunity to consider whether or not to participate and that minimize the possibility of coercion or undue influence. The information that is given to the subject or the representative shall be in language understandable to the subject or the representative. No informed consent, whether oral or written, may include any exculpatory language through which *the subject or the representative* is made to waive or appear to waive any of the subject's legal rights, or releases or appears to release the investigator, the sponsor, the institution or its agents from liability for negligence.

a. ***Basic elements of informed consent:*** *Except as provided in paragraph (c) or (d)* of this section, in seeking informed consent the following information shall be provided to each subject.
   1. A statement that the study involves research, an explanation of the purposes of the research and the expected duration of the subject's participation, a description of the procedures to be followed, and identification of any procedures which are experimental;
   2. A description of any reasonably foreseeable risks or discomforts to the subject;
   3. A description of any benefits to the subject or to *others* which may reasonably be expected from the research;
   4. A disclosure of appropriate alternative procedures or courses of treatment, if any, that might be advantageous to the subject;
   5. A statement describing the extent, if any, to which confidentiality of records identifying the subject will be maintained;
   6. For research involving more than minimal risk, an explanation as to whether any compensation and an explanation as to whether any medical treatments are available if injury occurs and, if so, what they consist of, or where further information may be obtained;
   7. An explanation of whom to contact for answers to pertinent questions about the research and research subjects' rights, and whom to contact in the event of a research-related injury to the subject; and
   8. A statement that participation is voluntary, refusal to participate will involve no penalty or loss of benefits to which the subject is otherwise entitled, and the subject may discontinue participation at any time without penalty or loss of benefits to which the subject is otherwise entitled.
b. ***Additional elements of informed consent:*** When appropriate, one or more of the following elements of information shall also be provided to each subject:
   1. A statement that the particular treatment or procedure may involve risks to the subject (or to the *embryo* or *foetus*, if the subject is or may become pregnant) which are currently unforeseeable;

2. Anticipated circumstances under which the subject's participation may be terminated by the investigator without regard to the subject's consent;
3. Any additional costs to the subject that may result from participation in the research;
4. The consequences of a subject's decision to withdraw from the research and procedures for orderly termination of participation by the subject;
5. A statement that significant new findings developed during the course of the research which may relate to the subject's willingness to continue participation will be provided to the subject; and
6. The approximate number of subjects involved in the study.

c. An *IRB may approve a consent procedure which does not include, or which alters, some or all of the elements of informed consent set forth above, or waive the requirement* to obtain informed consent provided the IRB finds and documents that:
   1. The research or demonstration project is to be conducted by or subject to the approval of state or local government officials and is designed to study, evaluate, or otherwise examine—(i) public benefit or service programs; (ii) procedures for obtaining benefits or services under those programs; (iii) possible changes in or alternatives to those programs or procedures; or (iv) possible changes in methods or levels of payment for benefits or services under those programs; and
   2. *The research could not practicably be carried out without the waiver or alteration.*

d. An IRB may approve a consent procedure which does not include, or which alters, some or all of the elements of informed consent set forth in this section, or waive the requirements to obtain informed consent provided the IRB finds and documents that:
   1. The research involves no more than minimal risk to the subjects;
   2. The waiver or alteration will not adversely affect the rights and welfare of the subjects;
   3. *The research could not practicably be carried out without the waiver or alteration*; and
   4. Whenever appropriate, the subjects will be provided with additional pertinent information after participation.

e. The informed consent requirements in this policy are not intended to pre-empt any applicable federal, state, or local laws which require additional information to be disclosed in order for informed consent to be legally effective.

f. Nothing in this policy is intended to limit the authority of a physician to provide emergency medical care, to the extent the physician is permitted to do so under applicable federal, state, or local law. (Approved by the Office of Management and Budget under Control Number 0990-0260.) (56 FR 28012, 28022, June 18, 1991, as amended at 70 FR 36328, June 23, 2005).

Documentation of Informed Consent (§46.117)

a. *Except as provided in paragraph (c)* of this section, informed consent shall be documented by the use of a written consent form approved by the IRB and signed by the subject or the subject's legally authorized representative. A copy shall be given to the person signing the form.

b. *Except as provided in paragraph (c)* of this section, the consent form may be either of the following.
   1. A written consent document that embodies the elements of informed consent required by §46.116. This form may be read to the subject or the subject's legally authorized representative, but in any event, the investigator shall give either the subject or the representative adequate opportunity to read it before it is signed; or
   2. A short form written consent document stating that the elements of informed consent required by §46.116 have been presented orally to the subject or the subject's legally authorized representative. When this method is used, there shall be a witness to the oral presentation. Also, the IRB shall approve a written summary of what is to be said to the subject or the representative. Only the short form itself is to be signed by the subject or the representative. However, the witness shall sign both the short form and a copy of the summary, and the person actually obtaining consent shall sign a copy of the summary. A copy of the summary shall be given to the subject or the representative, in addition to a copy of the short form.

c. An IRB may waive the requirement for the investigator to obtain a signed consent form for some or all subjects if it finds either:
   1. That the only record linking the subject and the research would be the consent document and the principal risk would be potential harm resulting from a breach of confidentiality. Each subject will be asked whether the subject wants documentation linking the subject with the research, and the subject's wishes will govern; or
   2. That the research presents no more than minimal risk of harm to subjects and involves no procedures for which written consent is normally required outside of the research context. In cases in which the documentation requirement is waived, the IRB may require the investigator to provide subjects with a written statement regarding the research.

(Approved by the Office of Management and Budget under Control Number 0990-0260.) (56 FR 28012, 28022, June 18, 1991, as amended at 70 FR 36328, June 23, 2005)

*(**Note** again that both 'foetus' and 'pregnancy' are extremely misdefined in the next section as 'beginning at implantation'. — DNI)*

Subpart

Additional Protections for Pregnant Women, Human Foetuses and Neonates Involved in Research Source: 66 FR 56778, Nov. 13, 2001, unless otherwise noted.

a. *Foetus* means the product of conception from *implantation until delivery*.
b. Neonate means a newborn.
c. Non-viable neonate means a neonate after delivery that, although living, is not viable.
d. *Pregnancy* encompasses the period of time *from implantation until delivery*. A woman shall be assumed to be pregnant if she exhibits any of the pertinent presumptive signs of pregnancy, such as missed menses, until the results of a pregnancy test are negative or until delivery.

Index